Foundations of Nursing

An Integrated Approach

Foundations of Nursing
An Integrated Approach

Edited by Cliff Evans and Emma Tippins

McGraw-Hill
Higher Education

London Boston Burr Ridge, IL Dubuque, IA Madison, WI New York San Francisco St. Louis
Bangkok Bogotá Caracas Kuala Lumpur Lisbon Madrid Mexico City Milan Montreal New Delhi
Santiago Seoul Singapore Sydney Taipei Toronto

Foundations of Nursing: An Integrated Approach
Cliff Evans and Emma Tippins

ISBN-13 978–0-33–522525–5 (pb) 978–0-33–522524–8 (hb)
ISBN-10 0–33–522525-X (pb) 0–33–522524–1 (hb)

**McGraw-Hill
Higher Education**

STAMPS	✓
TRIGGER	✓
CLASS	✓
SPINE	✓

Published by McGraw-Hill Education
Shoppenhangers Road
Maidenhead
Berkshire
SL6 2QL
Telephone: 44 (0) 1628 502 500
Fax: 44 (0) 1628 770 224
Website: www.mcgraw-hill.co.uk

British Library Cataloguing in Publication Data
A catalogue record for this book is available from the British Library

Library of Congress Cataloguing in Publication Data
The Library of Congress data for this book has been applied for from the Library of Congress

Commissioning Editor: Rachel Crookes
Development Editor: Karen Harlow
Product Manager: Bryony Skelton
Senior Production Editor: James Bishop
Text design by HL Studios
Cover design by Pointing Design
Printed and bound in Great Britain by Bell and Bain Ltd., Glasgow

ISBN-13 978–0-33–522525–5 (pb) 978–0-33–522524–8 (hb)
ISBN-10 0–33–522525-X (pb) 0–33–522524–1 (hb)

Brief Contents

Detailed Contents

Guided tour

Chapter 3 Learning Objectives

- Gain knowledge and insight into the anatomy and physiology of the respiratory system
- Gain insight into several common conditions affecting these systems
- Apply theory to practice by understanding the physical manifestation of these illnesses in patients
- Gain understanding of commonly used medications to either prevent or treat respiratory conditions
- Learn essential practical skills that can be easily applied within clinical practice
- Learn to apply a solid structured approach to the patient assessment process
- Construct solid evidence of professional development for your growing portfolio

Learning Objectives

Each chapter opens with a set of learning objectives, summarising what knowledge, skills or understanding you should acquire from each chapter.

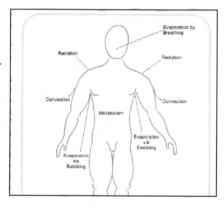

Figures and Tables

Each chapter provides a number of figures, illustrations and tables to help you to visualise the concepts and procedures explained.

speech, language comprehension, writing and analytical thought. The right dominates in perception, generalised thought, non-verbal and spatial perception; the more creative and insightful side. The dominance of activity between left and right sides is known as **cerebral dominance**.

The sensory and motor areas are located within the cerebral cortex, spanning the left and the right hemispheres, the motor area in the **precentral gyrus** and the sensory area in the **postcentral gyrus** (Figure 5.6). The sensory area's function is to perceive sensation and the motor area's function is to control movement. The fibres controlling sensation and movement cross over, or **decussate**, from left to right, thus, perception of sensation and control of movement occurs on the opposite side of the body; is contralateral. The whole body can be spatially represented in the sensory and motor cortex

Key Terms

These are highlighted throughout the chapter in bold and definitions are provided in a glossary of terms at the end of the book.

Applying Theory to Practice: Exercise 2.1

Before commencing this chapter:

- Identify which organs or glands you already know that are involved in maintaining homeostasis
- Compose a list of diseases that you already know that affect the body's ability to maintain homeostatic function in relation to temperature, blood pressure, water balance, glucose control and acid base
- Add this list to your developing portfolio and on completion of this chapter expand your portfolio with the new disorders you have gained knowledge on and elaborate on how these

Applying Theory to Practice boxes

These boxes aim to show how a particular concept or idea works in practice to make you act on the theory you are learning.

Anatomy & Physiology in Action: **A+P**
Exercise 3.8

Compare the breathing of different individuals;
there are many influencing or contributing factors to
why an individual breathes in a certain way.
■ Compare the rhythm and depth of breathing of
 a very obese patient with someone with a petite
 build
Remember what is considered normal for one
person can be very abnormal for another.
■ What is sleep apnoea?
■ Which group of individuals are at particular risk
 of experiencing this?

Anatomy and Physiology in Action boxes

These demonstrate how the anatomy and physiology learned in the chapters relates to nursing practice.

Scenarios

Brief scenarios are included in each chapter to place concepts in a real-life context and to set the scene for further analysis.

Scenario 3.2

Chronic Obstructive Pulmonary Disease

Joan Middleton is a 63-year-old woman who is
brought into the emergency department at 02.00
after experiencing shortness of breath and a
purulent cough for three days. She is unable to
complete a sentence; she appears alert although
very anxious. Her respiratory rate is shallow, rapid
and irregular at 38 breaths per minute. She appears
to be nearing exhaustion, demonstrated by the
heavy use of the accessory muscle of respiration,
her neck veins are protruding and she adopts the
tripod position (sitting, leaning forward with arms
on thighs). Mrs Middleton has evidence of

Developing and Delivering
Expert Care: Exercise 6.7

Obtaining a Mid-Stream Urine Sample (MSU)

A urinalysis provides a quick and simple overview
of the urine. If a potential infection is identified a
further specimen should be ascertained. This
sample requires a mid-stream sample of the urine
so that contaminates like bacteria that colonise
around the end of the urethra are not included. The
sample will be sent to a microbiology laboratory so
that the bacteria can be grown and identified. The
specimen is sent for micro-culture and sensitivity
(MC&S, which means the identification of the
bacteria (micro-culture) and what the specific
bacterium is sensitive to, i.e. which antibiotic will

Delivering and Developing Expert Care boxes

These boxes indicate how and where you could develop and improve your knowledge and practice to become a better nurse.

Questioning Clinical Practice boxes

These boxes encourage critical thinking by inviting you to think in more detail about procedures and how they could be improved.

Questioning Clinical Practice:
Exercise 4.16

There are several important phrases used within
clinical practice to describe both the act of
resuscitation and the legal terminology surrounding
care.

Using the correct terminology is paramount as
misunderstandings can lead to distress and
confusion in an area commonly described as one of
the most sensitive that clinicians, patients and family
members may have to face.

■ Find out the clinical meaning of the terms
 below and locate a copy of the DNAR policy
 your trust employs
■ What is the difference between a patient

Chapter 6 Summary Quiz

1. The renal system is composed of:

A. Two kidneys, two ureters, and a bladder
B. Two kidneys, a common ureter, a bladder and the ure
C. Two kidneys, two ureters, a bladder and the urethra
D. Two kidneys, two ureters, two bladders and a urethra

2. Each nephron contains an extremely intricate pathway
renal function. These include:

A. The collecting duct, the distal convoluted tubule, the
Boatman's capsule and glomerulus
B. The distal convoluted tubule, the loop of Henle, the P
glomerulus
C. The distal convoluted tubule, the loop of Henle, the I

Summary Quizzes

The text includes brief summary quizzes at the end of chapters to enable you to test the knowledge you have gained from that chapter. Answers are found at the end of the book.

Technology to enhance learning and teaching

Online Learning Centre (OLC)

After completing each chapter, log on to the supporting Online Learning Centre website. Take advantage of the study tools offered to reinforce the material you have read in the text, and to develop your knowledge in a fun and effective way.

Resources include:
Testbank of Multiple Choice Questions
PowerPoints
Video interviews with Cliff Evans and a Patient Relations Manager

Visit www.openup.co.uk/foundationsofnursing today

Preface

Identifying a new philosophy

Welcome to a book designed specifically for nursing students. The focus of this book is to assist developing nurses to gain the essential knowledge and practical understanding necessary to excel as a newly qualified nurse. The initial knowledge and skill base required on qualification by a modern nurse can appear unachievable; when commencing your chosen course the university structure will be divided into many subsets or faculties, each one will consider itself the pinnacle of your development and show little regard for the workload and deadlines you will experience from the combination of them all.

I, Cliff Evans, have written and taught both pre- and post-registration nursing courses as an adult-branch lecturer specialising in both emergency care and acute cardiology. Emma Tippins has been employed predominately as a senior sister and practice educator within emergency care; this includes facilitating both advanced life support and advanced trauma courses. More recently Emma has developed the role of the modern matron within emergency care. Our combined theoretical and practice experience has enabled us to write this book with an underpinning philosophy centring on assisting student nurses to be fit for practice or fit for purpose by the end of their initial academic study and clinical placements.

When placed within clinical practice, many students can be bewildered by what may appear the total disparity between what is taught within the classroom and what is delivered in clinical practice. This theory/practice divide is not a new phenomenon and has had serious implications for students over many years. The Nursing and Midwifery Council (NMC 2005), Duffy (2003), and many providers of healthcare (healthcare trusts), have recognised this and as a direct result have had to introduce post-registration educational programmes for newly qualified nurses enabling them to develop the skills and knowledge to be fit for purpose. This can have a negative effect on the newly qualified nurse, who understandably may feel aggrieved after having spent three years in full-time education and having amassed considerable debt to be told they are unfit to practise safely.

Why are there inconsistencies between the Nursing and Midwifery Council's requirements, pre-registration courses and the skills and knowledge necessary to deliver quality care?

Although it may initially appear that a person or an organisation must be held accountable for this inconsistency, this may not be the case. Over recent years the role, knowledge base, and clinical skills required by nurses have expanded at an incredible rate. It is almost unbelievable to imagine that in 1969, the year in which I was born, it was common practice for only doctors to record blood pressures. Today nurses have taken on many tasks traditionally undertaken by other disciplines such as medical physicians and made them their own by developing research- and evidence-based initiatives surrounding these actions. Traditionally, doctors learnt following the see one, do one, teach one basis. Within the nursing profession you will find almost a contrary approach, with a study day, a competency document and a period of supervised practice mandatory for many 'advanced' or 'extended' tasks. Although this may appear unfair, this culture of education and underpinning rationales has had a dramatic effect on care delivery and the confidence and respect that nurses receive. To fully understand the development of nursing as a profession it is necessary to look back into the not so distant past and visualise how nursing education has developed and how it will continue to do so. On completion of this book I hope you will realise that nursing education was and remains mainly experiential, and that to become a dynamic and proactive practitioner your education will continue until you retire; this is termed lifelong learning and is at the centre of good clinical practice.

The team of contributors to this book all currently practise or deliver educational programmes. This inspiring mix of educators and healthcare providers has come together to produce a book that combines the best of both worlds by applying theory to clinical practice and, through the use of scenarios, demonstrating not only the physical

skills associated with nursing, but also the considerable knowledge base a modern nurse requires.

Using the Book

This book is split into three distinct parts. Part 1 is an introduction to nursing which includes a reflective account of the many changes one nurse has experienced over her 40-year career.

Part 2 provides a 'systems'-based approach to understanding modern healthcare. By understanding the basic functioning of a physiological system of the body, a nurse can easily anticipate and recognise the associated clinical signs and symptoms when a particular system begins to fail. This foundation of anatomical and physiological knowledge is essential to practising nurses. The clinical application of this knowledge, in association with a structured assessment process, can result in both increasingly effective care and reduced morbidity and mortality rates (Evans & Tippins 2007). This section has been designed with particular components to assist the student with fundamental elements of their educational programme. These learning activities consist of individual exercises with common themes designed to facilitate this process. Activities include:

- Applying theory to practice
- Developing and delivering expert care
- Anatomy and physiology in action
- Questioning clinical practice.

Many of these activities have identified outcomes designed to facilitate the early development of a comprehensive personal and professional portfolio. The student can reflect on and visualise previous levels of understanding and practice and clearly demonstrate evidence of their progression from novice to expert (Benner 2001). Each chapter presents common patient scenarios clearly demonstrating how the student can apply a solid knowledge base to their clinical practice, thereby improving the care patients receive. This approach will aid the student in acquiring a holistic view of the needs of individuals and provide the clinical skills, theoretical knowledge base, and critical analysis techniques required to pass their chosen academic programme and become a competent and knowledgeable practitioner.

The importance of a research and evidence base to rationalise modern healthcare will be emphasised to familiarise students at an early stage of their training in a questioning approach to the care they deliver and to introduce students to 'best practice' initiatives geared to improving and standardising patient outcomes. These include government-driven initiatives such as the national service frameworks that currently underpin many areas of healthcare delivery, structuring local healthcare delivery strategies, through to internationally agreed guidelines delivered via the World Health Organization.

Part 3 details the separate but intrinsically linked branches of nursing. All nurses need to gain insight into all specialties, as they will encounter varying patients throughout their careers with a multitude of needs; in order to provide a quality of care, individuals must be seen as a whole (holism).

Part 3 is also designed to assist student nurses in gaining some of the associated skills required by nurses that are not always part of a university's curriculum (although this may be changing in the near future). These skills focus on a detailed understanding of medications and their administration, and the ability to provide effective first aid both within and outside the hospital setting.

Online resources designed to develop the facilitator–student relationship are also presented. This is achieved by the provision of a PowerPoint presentation for each chapter which can be used by lecturers within the academic setting or by the students for quick reference. A selection of other materials is also available to aid the learning process.

All chapters begin with identified learning outcomes; the student can then identify their own abilities and areas for development by completing the end of chapter quiz, the answers to which can be found at the back of the book. Each chapter shares common themes: these include in-depth patient scenarios detailing how complex patient management can be, activity boxes highlighting best practice initiatives, and the integration of anatomy and physiology and theory into clinical practice. The activity boxes are also designed to encourage students to question their practice, rationales, and the evidence base of care delivery. This enquiry-based approach treats students as adults and encourages individuals to seek further understanding for themselves. This requires discipline: by completing the exercises in this book at their own pace, individual students will gain the essential professional skills associated with lifelong learning and remain fit for practice.

Acknowledgements

Our thanks go to the following reviewers for their comments at various stages in the text's development:

Tonks Fawcett, University of Edinburgh
Dawn Freshwater, University of Leeds
Ray Higginson, University of Glamorgan
Helen Iggulden, University of Salford
Mary Law, University of Bradford
Paul Lowe, Middlesex University
Paul Mills, University Campus Suffolk
Sean Roe, Queen's University Belfast
Jenny Temple, University of Plymouth
Anne Waugh, Napier University

Contributors

Cliff Evans BSc RN

Cliff Evans is the Emergency Care Matron at Heatherwood & Wexham Park Hospitals. This role includes clinical, managerial and innovative components. Cliff has had a broad career encompassing mental health, acute medicine and cardiology, and is a qualified medical practitioner/specialist and Emergency Care/Acute Cardiology Lecturer. Cliff has had several publications including 'The Foundations of Emergency Care' (Open University Press/McGraw-Hill Education 2007) and has undertaken a consultancy role for the DoH.

Emma Tippins MSc RN

Emma Tippins has worked as an Emergency Care Sister, Practice Development Educator and recently as a Modern Matron within Emergency Care. Emma is also both an Advanced Life Support and Advanced Trauma Nursing Course instructor. Emma is an established writer with several publications including 'The Foundations of Emergency Care' (Open University Press/McGraw-Hill Education 2007). Emma's current role encompasses raising a 6-month-old baby boy!

Lucy Tebbit Dip RN

Lucy Tebbit is part of the Practice Development team at Heatherwood & Wexham Park Hospitals. Lucy is a registered Emergency Nurse Practitioner and has an extensive history within Emergency Care. Lucy leads on several in-house educational modules and is a pioneer of introducing evidence-based practice into the clinical setting. Lucy also has a keen interest in the local community and is Chair of Governors at a local Children's school.

Dimple Charters Grad Dip Sc. A33 RN

Dimple Charters is a Senior Sister and Team Leader at Heatherwood & Wexham Park Hospitals. Dimple has a keen interest in minor injuries and illness and teaches on several in-house educational programmes. Dimple is a registered Emergency Nurse Practitioner and leads on both Asthma and Cardiac best practice initiatives.

Susie Scott BA (Hons) ENB 100 ENB 998 RN

Susie Scott (formerly Clear) is a Clinical Practice Educator within Critical Care at Imperial College Healthcare NHS Trust in London, where she has been in post since 2004. Susie's career in critical care nursing has spanned over 11 years and as well as working in London, she has worked in Oxford and Sydney, Australia. Susie is currently studying for an MSC in advanced practice, education, at Kings College, London. Susie has a passion and enthusiasm for Intensive and Critical Care nursing, as well as in facilitating other nurses to learn and develop.

Andrew Frazer MSc RN

Andrew Frazer is an Emergency Nurse Consultant at Newham University Hospital NHS Trust in East London. He carries a clinical caseload of Emergency patients and has research and educational components to his role. He is an honorary Lecturer at City University, and an Advanced Life Support and Advanced Trauma Nursing Course instructor. In addition Andrew is an independent Nurse Prescriber and an established Author.

Paul Newcombe, BA (Hons), PG Cert (HE), RN

Paul Newcombe is Senior Lecturer at Kingston University and St George's, University of London. He is Critical Care Pathway leader and module leader for Continuing Professional Development (CPD) courses in Acute and Emergency Care. He is also responsible for teaching across pre-registration nursing and other CPD courses. Previous publications include a chapter entitled Acute Surgical Emergencies in 'The Foundations of Emergency Care' (Open University Press/ McGraw-Hill Education 2007).

Nick Wrycraft MSc BA (Hons), RMN

Nick Wrycraft is a Senior Lecturer at Anglia Ruskin University. Nick's current roles include Module Tutor for Module one of the Common Foundation Programme for pre-registration nursing, and admissions Tutor for Mental Health nursing. Nick has a keen interest in Mental Health nursing education and practice and the role of reflection, clinical supervision and other support mechanisms in developing capable practitioners. Other areas of interest include qualitative research methods, service design and development and new and generic roles including the Associate Practitioner.

Alex McClimens, PhD

Alex McClimens, wannabe writer and aspiring literary giant, is senior research fellow with Sheffield Hallam University where he divides his time between writing research proposals, teaching and drinking coffee.

Clare Culpin MSc RN

Clare is an established pioneer within practice development, Clare's passion centers on working in partnership with patients and developing the team and organizational culture to support this. Clare has a keen interest in leadership and has led many leadership development programmes for nurses and midwives. Clare's current role of Assistant Director of Nursing includes practice and professional development, encompassing both pre and post registration nursing.

Karen Chivers BSc (Hons) ENB 199,998,934 RN

Karen Chivers is employment at Heatherwood & Wexham Park Hospitals as a Clinical Practice Development Nurse. Karen is an Advanced Trauma Nursing Course instructor and a registered Emergency Nurse Practitioner. Karen's role includes formally and informally educating nursing students, nursing colleagues and other members of the multidisciplinary team. Karen leads on innovating clinical practice and delivers in-house programmes designed to empower and develop senior nurses.

Andrea Blay RGN, ENB 100, MSc

Andrea is currently working as Consultant Nurse specialising in Critical Care at Chelsea & Westminster NHS Foundation Trust. Andrea has an extensive history within critical care and leads a Critical Care Outreach Service.

Part 1
The role of the nurse

1 The role of the nurse
Cliff Evans and Emma Tippins

The role of the nurse

Cliff Evans and Emma Tippins

Chapter 1 Learning Objectives

- Gain insight into how the historical role of the nurse has led to the creation of the modern reflective practitioner
- Understand the importance of questioning care practices and applying theory to decision making and clinical practice
- Provide qualitative care through gaining insight and understanding into the importance of 'rationales' to underpin practice
- Understand the role of the Nursing and Midwifery Council (NMC) and gain insight into principal publications
- Gain insight into the principles of research, thereby gaining skills associated with the true professions and lifelong learning
- Understand the rationale of having a reflective practice portfolio and begin constructing this essential tool to professional development
- Gain insight into modern educational techniques and the core nursing curriculums
- Gain insight into how politics affect healthcare delivery
- Gain understanding of the nursing career ladder

This introductory chapter includes a reflective account of nursing education and practice written by Penny Russell, a friend and colleague, who during her 40-year nursing career has lived through and partaken in many of the changes that have resulted in the modern nurse. Penny discusses how many external and internal influences have heralded dramatic transformation in both nursing education and the very act of nursing, thereby revolutionising modern healthcare delivery. This section provides the reader with insight into why a theory/practice divide exists and how, throughout recent times, many have tried to bridge this divide. Throughout the following chapters our contributors, all of whom are specialists in their fields,

will introduce the reader to many methods of applying a theoretical underpinning to clinical practice, thereby delivering evidence-based clinical care.

This chapter identifies many aspects relevant to the everyday practice of the nurse including:

- The Nursing and Midwifery Council (NMC) and the Nursing Register
- Portfolio development and maintaining clinical knowledge and competence
- Educational techniques
- Clinical decision making
- The nursing process
- Government legislation and health policies (a modern approach to healthcare delivery)
- The importance of ethical decision making
- The introduction of research and an evidence base to nursing practice
- Nursing career potentials.

The Nursing and Midwifery Council and the Nursing Register

The Nursing and Midwifery Council (NMC) was established in April 2002, taking over from the United Kingdom Central Council and the four national boards (UKCC). The NMC published its new rules on registration in August 2004 entitled *Code of Professional Conduct: Standards for Conduct, Performance and Ethics* (NMC 2004a). This document identifies the basis of nursing practice thereby forming a crucial component of your professional development. The NMC is the UK regulator for nurses and midwives. Once you have fulfilled the learning outcomes of your chosen university course, you will need to be registered with the NMC before you can practise as a nurse. The NMC's key responsibilities are to protect the public by establishing standards of performance, nursing education and conduct (NMC 2004a). During training, student nurses also have standards of practice that they must abide by NMC (2005a): although they are not

cont. on page 10

The role of the nurse

Penny Russell, former Head of Nursing (Adult Branch) at Thames Valley University

This piece follows a personal reflective journey, through entry to nursing, the experiences of training in the 1960s, changes in clinical practice and nursing responsibilities, and nurse education. The influences of the changing health needs and expectations of society and how these have influenced and driven political and legal changes will be briefly explored, particularly where they have affected the role of the nurse.

Why do you want to become a nurse?

This question has been asked of every new nursing recruit since schools of nursing began in the United Kingdom in the middle of the 19th century. Individual answers would be slightly different but most would contain the wish to care for the sick and their families. I had never been a patient or visited a hospital before I entered nurse training. What I knew about the nurse's role was gleaned from watching *Emergency Ward 10* on television or reading Monica Dickens's book *Two Left Feet*. However, I had insight into illness and the needs of the chronically sick from my early years, particularly from visiting my grandparents. My grandfather was responsible for forming a great deal of my early values and feelings about life. He was a retired general practitioner who won the Military Cross for his medical services in the Great War. I never knew him without crutches and I often looked at his gnarled and deviated hand joints and wondered how they had got like that. I knew my grandmother had to help him wash and dress and that he took soluble aspirin for pain. He was a gentle and knowledgeable man who spent endless hours with his granddaughter explaining about cultures and peoples as we placed stamps in my stamp album. These experiences formed my early values and beliefs about peoples, places and, essentially, about sickness and health. Rheumatoid arthritis is indeed a cruel disease. Unfortunately, my grandmother and mother were similarly affected. My father died at the age of 46 from a heart attack. It was through these experiences that I was able to discuss how suffering, early death and bereavement had affected my family and myself at my interview, which contributed to my entry into nurse training.

Nurse training, 1966–1969

Twenty-five young women and I commenced nurse training at a London teaching hospital in March 1966. The preliminary training school was in the leafy suburbs of west London and was really very like my boarding school with a clearly defined timetable for classes and meals. Theory was largely anatomy, physiology and some public health. Psychology with some sociology was discreetly applied in the practical classes. We were only allowed out of the school grounds until 10.30pm at night. Afterwards we had to ring the doorbell, have our name taken and be reported to the Senior Tutor (or Matron) and given a suitable lecture on lateness and how such trends had to change and not transfer into our ward experiences. The practical sessions were challenging since a great deal of understanding was required to follow procedures accurately. A visual demonstration was followed by repeated practice: bandaging with hip spicas, reverse spirals, simple spirals, etc. Some of the learning was also experiential such as nursing observations, bed baths and feeding of each other. We all regarded these classes as 'real nursing' and seemed to absorb the theory that went with it, particularly as we were told 'lives depended on accuracy'. Our visits to the hospital were by coach once a week where we were introduced to 'real' patients. The ward sisters always seemed formidable with starched hats, cuffs, aprons and numerous badges. Several senior staff would prove to be quite eccentric with certain foibles that we needed to be aware of. However, the ward sister was mistress of all she surveyed; I can well remember new junior doctors and the ward orderly being put straight on several points with the consequence that patients, staff and the ward environment were all respected and kept in proper order. Students were set to work under close supervision and we busied ourselves with applying only what we had learnt, i.e. moving patients using the Australian lift (now banned), bed baths and

→

←

patient observations. We learnt about the ward routine, religiously cleaning bedpans and sluices, also, essentially, the giving out of meals, on the instructions from the ward sister. We also helped patients to eat and drink. These were exciting times and we could not wait to get on the wards at the end of our three months in the training school. We felt confident, secure and supported.

Being a first-year student nurse was intermixed with trial and error, learning while doing, and a great deal of watching, listening and learning. There was also a subculture of trying to keep on the right side of sister and the senior staff nurses. Each placement was a new adventure. However, all nursing care followed the medical diagnosis and an unwritten protocol of patient care management. The ward sister managed nursing care with tasks being allocated according to experience via a workbook. Each student learnt from a more senior student, the 'sitting next to Nellie' method, and developed their skills and knowledge through the clinical placements with a stern test of each using a buff-coloured nursing schedule book which recorded observing, practising and proficiency of prescribed procedures and skills over the three-year training period. However, much unrecorded learning was gleaned from the context and the lived personal experience of being a young person endeavouring to care for sick and dying people in a regimented and 'professional' environment. There was little discussion on the traumatic issues that either patients or nurses had faced on a shift except informally with peers in the nurses home. Peers supported, comforted and saw to it that emotion gave way to common sense and a sense of perspective. In many cases fellow trainee nurses became lifelong friends through their shared experiences. A continuum of personal and professional growth was fostered throughout each year of the course through an advancement of knowledge of the disease processes, and the nursing response to symptoms, ever-increasing complexity of skills and increasing responsibility for patient care. There was security in this system as everyone knew their place and all students knew what they were supposed to be doing, although often patient care was seen as a set of tasks and applied to anatomical parts rather than as a whole person. Graduation to staff nurse was a natural process with the end of the third year spent on night duty in charge of the ward with a night sister on call. Teaching junior students, assigning and monitoring nursing care, reporting to the medical staff and ordering of medicines and essential equipment were expectations of a third year student to ensure that they were fit for purpose on completion of their course. Most of us were confident and had carefully chosen our first staff nurse post when our letter came through from the General Nursing Council.

Thus it was that nurse training in an apprenticeship model largely achieved its aim of producing a staff nurse who would carry on the old traditions and practise the skills using the medical diagnosis as the guide. The art and science of nursing itself was limited until challenges to the accepted nursing protocols began to ask serious questions of certain nursing practices.

Questioning clinical practice

Early nursing studies followed the quantitative research model almost exclusively favoured by the medical profession, based on large data gathering exercises; it took a further decade for the art of nursing to be acknowledged through the lived experience of the patient. The early qualitative research approach based on in-depth questioning, observation studies and empirical knowledge remained an area of scepticism outside nursing; within the profession they were well used to develop nursing care and patient well-being. The 'doctor's handmaiden' role of the nurse changed with greater professional confidence, almost alongside the introduction of more men into nursing and the changes to the role of women in society. Thus, postmodernism was to affect nursing with many challenges and moves for change through the 1970s.

→

←

Changes in nursing care management

The introduction of the Nursing Process and Care Planning made attempts to consider patients as a whole rather than parts in the biological, psychological and social dimensions. This was later confused by the introduction of nursing models where new aspects of 'the person' could be viewed in different ways and a nursing response generated therefrom. Initially, the United Kingdom adopted the 'Activities of Daily Living' as a model and assessment tool (Roper et al. 1980). For those trying to assess the patient and plan care using the nursing process, adopting different formats to assess an individual patient's needs was sometimes confusing. It was often felt that 'the cart had come before the horse' since it would have been more fitting for the nursing model to be adopted first, with its specific assessment tools rather than the nursing process format.

Fundamentally, all nursing models assess patient need in a multidimensional fashion and the nursing response is generated from that assessment. Nursing care management moved from a series of tasks performed by selected individuals to being team orientated. The team was an eclectic mix of staff nurses, enrolled nurses, students and auxiliary nurses. Teams were secure and discharged their responsibilities for a group of patients in a corporate and responsible fashion. Although, it must be said, that sometimes the staff mix or staff numbers did not match the patient care requirements. Various tools were used to ensure that proactive staffing was achieved but none of these proved to be accurate enough for every situation. Thus, the anticipation of nursing needs was planned by those on the previous shift. Specific patient allocation in accident and emergency and intensive care units was, and still is, the patient care management pattern. However, individualised patient care was soon to become part of nursing care philosophy. This was followed by a flirtation with 'primary nursing'. This process required knowledgeable and experienced nursing practitioners to assess, plan and oversee care, and evaluate outcomes in a systematic and scientific fashion. Nurses needed time and education to be able to take on patient management from admission to discharge. However, the adoption of primary nursing care into busy surgical and medical wards was problematic since it was expensive and required a considerable number of top grade nurses. Visitors to the wards became confused as to who was in charge as the ward sister role became absorbed into that of ward coordinator.

The patient's named nurse (derived from the Patient's Charter which was abolished in 2000 – http://www.pfc.org.uk/node/633) was not 'on duty' 24 hours a day, although they were responsible for patient care for that time. Patient care became fragmented with the nursing handover not including all patients. The true success of primary nursing was seen in care of the elderly units where staffing was constant and access to outside agencies easy. But it was an exciting time to be a senior staff nurse with so many different ways to look at patient care, and with the sphere of responsibility for patient care increasing to allow for specialisation and the emergence of the specialist nurse role.

In the early 1990s the idea of having a more controlled and predictable patient care pathway was introduced through 'patient-focused' care and the arrival of patient care protocols. At this time my career moved into education and I was an educational manager in a school of nursing surrounded by a hospital introducing this type of patient management. The training of staff became crucial to its implementation, as the protocols were to be central to patient care, and I was involved in some of the staff assessments. It was expected that all the staff within a unit or ward, be they healthcare assistants, staff nurses or physiotherapists, would be able to address the patient's needs. This caused considerable debate and disharmony among professional groups, as they each had their own body of knowledge and professional boundaries. Some protocols proved successful and beneficial to patient care, particularly for patients such as those coming into hospital in sickle-cell crisis. The success of this particular philosophy was that it was generated by those working at the coalface and not from outside the unit. Patient focus as a form of patient care management, although inspirational, did not survive to be embraced

→

across nursing. However, the idea of multi-professional patient protocols to guide staff and patients along the recovery pathway was adopted with great success in many areas. Today we see the emphasis in the management of patient care being that of 'the patient's journey'. The need for nurses to assume some of the junior doctors' role is not new but is legitimised through the reduction of junior doctor hours and the developing expertise of specialist nurses. In specialist units nurses' and junior doctors' roles have often merged for the good of the patient. Nurses have acquired knowledge and skills at the bedside with the expert tuition from lecturer practitioners and hospital consultants. To some extent the ward nurse has been left behind, possibly because of poor vision by educationalists and managers alike. Many find the interesting parts of their role being taken over by the nurse specialist, such as the diabetic nurse, the tissue viability and wound specialist nurse, or the cardiac rehabilitation nurse.

Contemporary teaching and learning

Being a clinical teacher was one of the roles that I enjoyed most. Teaching at the bedside and involving the patients and their relatives in the discussion and management of care was immensely satisfying. Not being responsible for the management of the ward provided essential time to demonstrate how procedures should be done. Afternoon tutorials during the patients' rest hour ensured that students applied and demonstrated their knowledge. They also allowed individual patient care to be critically discussed and for students to ask questions. Unfortunately, in the 1980s a clinical teacher was considered to be neither a tutor nor a clinician and, therefore, no career structure was developed and the role, like so many others created for a need at the time, fell away. It was supplanted by the lecturer practitioner, which added university support and development to the role while allowing knowledge and skills to be imparted at the bedside. This was particularly successful in units and distinct areas of clinical practice. Again, many lecturer practitioners enjoy their roles for the same reasons as the clinical teacher but they are an expensive resource and universities are short of money as are the National Health Service Trusts, making them an easy target in times of crisis.

Nursing and higher education

It is sometimes difficult to distinguish what has influenced nursing care and nurses most over the past 40 years. The training and education debate has almost gone full circle from the apprenticeship and learning on the job, through the introduction of the Project 2000 curriculum in 1989, following the Judge Report (1983). In this curriculum other academic disciplines were taught in their pure form and then applied to nursing, particularly sociology, law and ethics, physiology and psychology. At times, being a teacher of adult nursing was a juggling act to provide the essentials of nursing while applying the other disciplines. Patient Scenarios became the only way of bringing parts together to see the patient as whole through a multidimensional lens.

The Diploma of Nursing curriculum set out to mould nurses into 'knowledgeable and questioning doers' not just 'doers'. Thus, students were encouraged to enquire and develop their own knowledge base in the practice setting. This would have worked well had the existing workforce been prepared to diploma level, and indeed for the enquiring student. Many hours have since been spent by teachers, on their clinical visits, smoothing over areas of difficulty and situations where the assertive, enquiring student had asked the wrong question at the wrong time. Clinical staff have rightly felt threatened by the challenge to their knowledge and experience, especially as many had not had a basic training which reached diploma level. Post-basic education was slow to address the academic needs of the already qualified nurse other than by advancement of clinical skills.

There is no doubt that the closure of schools of nursing on the hospital sites in the mid-1990s had a profound effect on nursing students, teachers and indeed the way nursing education was perceived. Many hospital staff

→

←

were glad that 'the school' was no longer omnipresent, since the demands on them with the close monitoring of the learning environment was, and still is, somewhat of a threat. Nurse teachers had to apply for the new university posts. Several schools of nursing had to merge and, therefore, downsize with inevitably job losses resulted. University life brought with it many changes of boundaries. Teachers were now lecturers, sharing large offices with colleagues they hardly knew, and had their workload redesigned into modules or units of learning. Joining a large establishment and feeling part of higher education depended on interactions with other lecturers in the university. Our faculty, as with many health science or nursing faculties, was run and kept largely separate, which meant that it took time for us to feel as though we belonged. Many lecturers of nursing found it hard to treat students differently and as independent learners, since we had always fostered learning and nurturing individuals through their difficulties. This simply was not possible in terms of the numbers of students and lecturer time. The political agenda and therefore university strategy to recruit as many students as possible meant that the student population changed markedly to include many nationalities, some fleeing oppressive regimes in Europe and Africa and others with complex family situations. Mastery of the English language and numeric skills soon became a huge problem in terms of examination success and patient safety. Although the education of nursing students was now within higher educational institutes, it could appear to the established nursing workforce that the abilities of the modern student nurse (other than to question) in basic skills such as written English and mathematics were diminishing. On qualification, nurses were now unable to perform many of the traditional basic nursing tasks, had a poor understanding of the human body and were seen to be fit only for essay writing and not the delivery of care.

A nurse that is both fit for purpose/practice and demonstrates a higher level of thinking

Fitness for practice and purpose is clearly the political agenda at the present time (NMC 2005a) but teaching and learning at the bedside are not necessarily consistent. This is due to the lack of clinical staff and sometimes the student's inability to observe and communicate effectively their learning needs to their mentor. Mentors have many students and they are not necessarily on duty at the same time. Mentors are also usually staff nurses; although they may be able to perform at an expected level, they may not be able to convey the theoretical components of many illnesses or situations to others, complicating the learning process. No matter what the fashion in nurse teaching, be it 'chalk and talk', lectures followed by seminars, experiential learning, enquiry- or problem-based learning, or structured reflection, the successful student manages their own time and learning agenda, making sure appropriate assessment takes place at the due time. They also then develop their own professional and personal schemata of what is optimum care and best practice. Learning to be a responsible professional should be a fundamental goal.

In the early years of my nursing training, patients were subservient, compliant and totally trusted their doctors and nurses to act in their best interests. Society regarded nursing as a respectable career, and indeed nursing in return tried to fulfil the criteria of a profession with its own body of knowledge and an active register of practitioners. It also had inculcated professional standards, which were monitored by the General Nursing Council. As a staff nurse on a busy 33-bed surgical ward, the nature of surgery was significant because often it was the only option in the treatment of tumours or gastrointestinal conditions. Coupled with the effects of anaesthesia, big procedures with large wounds and drains, patients spent considerable time in hospital.

The nurse's role in aiding recovery was specific, particularly in respect of observations, pain relief, wound care, fluid replacement, early mobility and acute reporting. Patients routinely could expect help from nurses with their personal hygiene, mouth care and toileting. Discharge planning was undertaken when the medical staff decided that a level of recovery had been sustained for the patient to manage at home. The hospital bed demand was not

→

the issue that it is today and nurses were reassured that patients had reached their optimum recovery before discharge. They were also able to discuss fully with district nurses what ongoing care might be required. The introduction of non-invasive surgical procedures, advances in medicine, anaesthetics and wound closure and care have altered surgical nursing fundamentally. Today, most surgical procedures can be performed as a day case, the stay in hospital being minimal.

Discharge is planned simultaneously with admission and protocols are adhered to, ensuring patients move along the recovery pathway in a uniform and predicted fashion. General practitioner surgeries and 'walk-in clinics' now also perform surgical procedures, which means that the role of the surgical nurse is now extremely focused and the relationship with the patient is often transient and fleeting. Nursing care has needed to change to reflect the health needs of society. These have changed significantly with the speed and demands of everyday life. The concept of the family has moved from the traditional two parents with two children to now involve a broad spectrum of participants with partners, significant others, the community, and various agencies playing active parts to support parents and children. Patients are now often well informed and know that they are empowered to make choices. Successive governments have promoted patient empowerment and choice, which has meant that nurses have to be skilled at giving patients information and putting forward alternatives, ensuring that the patient's experience is one that they agree with and partake in. Many patients find this hard, preferring others to make choices for them: 'You're the nurse/doctor, you tell me what the best option is.'

The introduction of National Service Frameworks/National Strategies

The National Service Frameworks generated by the Department of Health have helped address the needs of various patient groups, including the elderly, the diabetic patient group, the cardiac patient, the mental health patient and those with cancer or chronic illness. The targets have proved invaluable in setting and monitoring a uniform agenda to prevent, treat and manage particular illnesses. Nurses were somewhat surprised to have a review of essential nursing care with dignity and privacy, record taking and nutrition being some of the central issues to be brought into focus with the Department of Health's *Essence of Care* (DH 2001, revised 2003). *The Essence of Care* was designed to support the measures to improve quality and contribute to the introduction of clinical governance at local level. The benchmarking process outlined in *The Essence of Care* assists practitioners to take a structured approach to sharing and comparing practice, enabling them to identify the best practice and to develop action plans to remedy poor practice. Hospitals systematically reviewed their procedures, setting up task groups and setting appropriate standards as a result of this exercise. Many nurses trained in times past were aghast at how poor essential care had become since it was so much part of our conditioning in the apprenticeship model. Nursing education and training have, to me, never lost the continuum explored in Patricia Benner's book *From Novice to Expert* (Benner 2001). It illustrates the acquisition of knowledge and skills through exemplars which demonstrate that there is no substitute for experience in nursing, but in my view this must be supported by the willingness of the individual nurse to learn through academic enquiry, and above all, from observation and critical reflection on and in action. The application of acquired knowledge and skills to each individual patient situation makes nursing the unique art and science that it is.

Conclusion

Being part of the nursing care environment working alongside patients, relatives and colleagues remains a privilege and has been central to my career as both a nurse and a teacher. Caring first about family, then patients, colleagues and students has never been far from my mind in all that I have endeavoured to do because it has given me such pleasure and enormous satisfaction. No other career could have given me more.

Penny Russell, 2007

not professionally accountable, students can be called to account by their university or by the law for the consequences of their actions or omissions. Nurses need to re-register with the NMC each year; absurdly the cost of this process is not met by the public, which the NMC serves to protect, but by nurses themselves. Over recent years the now annual cost has far exceeded inflation and is an area of much contention. The nurses' part of the register has marks to identify the branch of nursing practice in which the nurse has achieved the standards of proficiency.

The NMC and pre-registration

The NMC state that pre-registration nursing programmes should be designed to prepare students to apply knowledge, understanding and skills to provide the nursing care that patients require in a safe and effective manner, thereby assuming the responsibility and accountability necessary for the protection of the public. This is achieved by setting standards; these standards are considered the minimum expected level to enable the registrant to be competent to deliver safe and effective practice (NMC 2004a). The basic principles underpinning educational programmes are that:

- Evidence should inform practice through the integration of relevant knowledge
- Students should be actively involved in nursing care delivery under supervision
- Research should underpin practice
- The importance of lifelong learning and professional development is recognised.

The NMC monitors and approves the detailed programmes that demonstrate how the standards of education enable the NMC standards of proficiency to be achieved within the context of practice in each of the four branches or specialties of nursing. This quality assurance monitoring process is undertaken each year. The pre-registration nursing education programmes have to ensure that their individual programmes adhere to these guidelines, as their status is mandatory in accordance with statutory legislation.

Course design and the branches

All nursing students study together in the first year in a 'common foundation programme' (CFP). Many universities have made this not only a collaboration of nursing specialities but also multidisciplinary by including future doctors, physiotherapists and occupational therapists. On the completion of the first year, students must be seen to have met pre-designated outcomes or essential skill clusters (ESC) to enable progression into their chosen specialty or branch. The second set of outcomes or ESC are identified as the prerequisite level of knowledge to clinically practise. These are achieved in several ways during the educational programme and will include constructing a portfolio of professional development and practice (see next section). In addition, several clinical competencies must be achieved while on practice placements, making the educational programme 50% theoretical and 50% clinically based. These include ESC based on medication delivery, aspects of care and communication. The four branches of nursing are:

- **Adult nursing**: caring for those 18 and above, this includes various clinical settings and levels of patient dependency. Philosophically, care should be in partnership with the patient, be patient centred, and should acknowledge the individuality of patients. Nurses require skills to address the physical, psychological and social needs of patients; in addition, spiritual or religious requirements should be both respected and catered for when planning care. The nurse is seen as a pivotal member of the multidisciplinary team and supports patients through care pathways by working closely with other professions to maximise opportunities for recovery, and future avoidance of ill health through programmes of health education and promotion.
- **Mental health nursing**: centres on the provision of care for those experiencing mental distress through the application of therapeutic relationships directed at providing support and understanding for those afflicted. Mental health nurses work as part of a multi-agency/disciplinary team that seeks to involve service users and their carers in all aspects of their care and treatment.
- **Learning disabilities nursing**: aims to influence behaviours and lifestyles of a vulnerable client group to enable optimum health. This includes positive promotion of the cause and actively supporting the inclusion of those afflicted within society as equal and deserving citizens. The use of expert communication skills will engage the user group and establish

individual care packages. Learning disability nurses will work in various settings establishing support for clients and their families.

- **Children's nursing**: centres on the development of family-centred care and the belief that children should be cared for by people they know and, whenever possible, within their home environment. The empowerment of children and their families is a key element to promoting and providing safe, effective and informed care. Children's nurses play a fundamental role in the collaboration of key professionals to contribute to child protection. A central philosophy is respecting and promoting the rights of the child.

The NMC has published several pertinent documents that the student will be required to familiarise him- or herself with:

- *Code of Professional Conduct: Standards for Conduct, Performance and Ethics* (NMC 2004a)
- *Guidelines for the Administration of Medicines* (NMC 2004b)
- *Guidelines for Records and Record Keeping* (NMC 2004c)
- *An NMC Guide for Students of Nursing and Midwifery* (NMC 2006).

The identification of new learning opportunities and taking the onus to develop one's own knowledge and skill base are essential components of both modern adult education and nursing practice.

The NMC and mentorship

Your chosen course will be composed of 50% theory and 50% clinical practice. It is therefore imperative that the clinical provider, whether a healthcare trust, privately run concern or a primary care trust (PCT), provide you with a 'coach' or supervisor within that particular area. In 1993, the then statutory body for nursing (the UKCC) recommended the introduction of a formally recognised local support system for newly qualified nurses. This heralded the formal introduction of the preceptor, an experienced practitioner who would assist student nurses or newly qualified nurses in the transitional period between novice and capable practitioner.

Today an experienced nurse will be designated your mentor; the word mentor derives from Greek. In Greek mythology, Mentor was a famous figure whose name is proverbial for a faithful and wise adviser. Mentor was a man of integrity, an excellent friend to his friends, he did not deal in lies, and he could speak out if necessary. Mentor was a firm believer in acquiring knowledge from positive reflection, and was therefore in an ideal position to speak freely and unhindered about the actions of others. Mentor was a firm believer in addressing injustices, one of which was that he believed that to be aware of injustice and not act was also a crime. This could be directly applied to clinical practice today in that if a practitioner witnesses poor practice or abuse and does not act on it, they become part of the act itself (NMC 2004a).

The modern role of the mentor can be defined as a professional relationship that is dependent on joint, dynamic, sharing characteristics. The choice of mentor should be determined by the mentee as the mentoring philosophy is based on common ground (Morton-Cooper 2000). The initiation of this relationship is based on individuals who are brought together by common characteristics, abilities or recognition of shared values. Therefore the mentee will need to work for a period of time before they can identify their personal mentor. Although this process of identification is suited to the circumstance of the newly qualified nurse, it does not suit the requirements of students on short placements where a supervisor is identified for them. This individual was previously referred to as a clinical preceptor although in some areas the terminology will still exist.

The key to developing the mentor–student relationship

Respect is the key to both building a strong professional relationship and gaining the most from your placements. Some of your mentors will be keen to teach and facilitate your needs; others will see you as an unnecessary addition to their workload and may be unhelpful to your development. It is a mandatory requirement of the Code of Conduct (NMC 2004a) that all qualified nurses facilitate students; do not, therefore, tolerate individuals who demonstrate no interest in your learning outcomes for that placement, as this will be detrimental to your current needs and future learning. Give and take is the key to success; be seen as part of the team, seek every opportunity to show that you are both a hard worker and an inquisitive student. Use psychology and the understanding of others.

Your mentor will have a set of priorities to complete each shift; be seen to assist them with their workload and they will then be free to assist you in yours. The early implementation of action plans based on the clinical outcomes identified within your clinical placement or proficiency booklet is essential, as identifying them late within the placement can come back to haunt you. Action plans and fixed deadlines agreed by you and the mentor are easy to refer back to if either party is unreliable and they provide a solid structure for your placement.

Link lecturers can play a pivotal role in both the development of a unit's philosophy towards students and education and the student's acceptance in a particular placement. On commencement of a placement, identify the link lecturer's details, which should be on display on the education board, identify which days they are in clinical practice, and meet them early within the placement. They will be your first point of contact if you encounter any problems; they are also the first point of contact for the nurses if they encounter difficulties with you. Before commencing a placement, call to ascertain when you are off duty, make yourself known, and if possible identify your intended mentor. Be aware of both your presentation and your time keeping. Gain knowledge of the specialty of the placement by conducting a quick internet search and identify common medications used within that area; this will show you are not just another run of the mill student but a dynamic thinker. Nurses will treasure your keen interest and this will be rewarded by their placing a greater level of trust in you, so you will be entrusted to undertake roles and acts such as administering medications while others are undertaking more mundane tasks. Although this may appear unfair, remember that your mentor's actions and their delegation of tasks to you will be a direct result of how you present your current understanding. By demonstrating little understanding of that particular specialty or the needs of the patients, the student's abilities are limited and the mentor will identify this as they are professionally responsible for the delegation of tasks undertaken by you and will be held accountable if things go wrong.

The NMC and public protection

The NMC has a wide range of powers designed to protect the public. These include the ability to remove a registrant by the evoking of a 'striking off order'; they can impose a 'suspension order', or a 'conditions of practice order'; in addition, a caution of between one and five years can be imposed (NMC 2005b). Students and qualified nurses are allowed to view NMC disciplinary hearings held in London. By viewing this process one can gain insight into how things can go very wrong and the nurse can be held accountable for their practice and actions and failure to act.

The *NMC Advice for Delegation to Non-regulated Healthcare Staff* sets out ten principles for nurses and midwives to follow when delegating to non-regulated healthcare staff. The full set of principles can be viewed at http://www.nmc-uk.org/aArticle.aspx?ArticleID=2582.

Portfolio development and maintaining clinical knowledge and competence

Nurses and other healthcare professionals work in an area of constant change as a direct result of increasing technological and scientific advances, expanding roles and society's demands, in combination with political strategies. The ability and dedication to meeting these challenges by updating one's knowledge and skills base are therefore crucial to providing evidence-based care. The construction of a portfolio demonstrating the individual's professional knowledge and competence to cope with these demands is an essential part of professional development and an easy access point for regulation. Professional development is linked to the registration process through post-registration education practice (PREP) standards. These identify lifelong learning and the nurse's developing professional practice built upon the basic requirements for entry to the register. On qualification all newly registered nurses will have a comprehensive portfolio demonstrating their experience and evidence of competence in basic nursing skills, as this will be a requirement of their pre-registration course. This developing portfolio will be beneficial for career planning, assist in promoting you for career options and highlighting transferable skills. In addition, the portfolio will serve as direct evidence of locally agreed achievements for your future individual performance reviews.

The portfolio contains both personal and professional components. The personal portfolio is a private document and includes individual records of the development of the nurse's skills, knowledge, attitudes, understanding and achievements. It may also include structured written reflective accounts of individual case studies and critical

reviews of practice (critical implies an open-minded, reflective appraisal that takes account of different experiences, perspectives and assumptions). The professional profile is seen as a public document, which may involve a combination of the above structured with the consideration that this document is open to scrutiny. It may include accounts of professional experience and direct observations of practice development. It can include evaluations of new working practices and critical incident reviews. Reflective pieces should focus on various topics and be seen to demonstrate positive aspects of practice as well as incidents that could be worth re-evaluation.

Recognising the limitations of one's knowledge or skills base is an essential element of professional development and self-recognition (NMC 2004d). The NMC refer to PREP as an essential component to providing best care for your future patients. The ability of an individual practitioner to reflect on both their clinical encounters and on new learning is a central component in applying theory to practice and improving one's practice.

Reflection in action

Learning and applying reflection to your daily practice will be a major component of your pre-registration course. Initially this key skill enables the individual to re-evaluate an encounter, their actions and the outcome of a situation, interaction or event. To actively reflect on your clinical practice creates the possibility of making sense of the past and present with the focus being the identification of an informed future; this 'higher level' of thinking is at the centre of professional development and an essential component of postgraduate higher educational courses. Smith (1995) identifies that by reviewing past events the individual can enhance good standards through the avoidance of actions that led to inferior outcomes in the past. Schön (1995) refers to reflection in action as the responses that skilful practitioners bring to their practice. This reflection consists of strategies of action, understanding of phenomena, and ways of framing the situations encountered in day-to-day experience.

This 'reflection-in-action' may take the form of problem solving, theory building, or re-appreciation of the situation (Schön 1995). Reflecting on practice therefore involves passing judgement on your own actions and reaching an understanding of your experiences, and then learning from them. It is an active process that should result in real outcomes in terms of changing your understanding of a situation and increasing your knowledge. It also involves developing action plans for future practice. In short, professional reflection involves the critical analysis of clinical practice (Johns & Freshwater 1998). In order to fulfil their professional development requirements, it is mandatory for all registered nurses to maintain a personal and professional portfolio. Within this personal and professional portfolio it is essential to provide demonstrable evidence of some structured and written reflective work (NMC 2004a).

Although this is a professional obligation, there are also many positive aspects to professional reflection, an example being that practitioners can gain insight into their own actions and beliefs in order to be able to build on existing strengths and take appropriate future action. Action should be the focal point, as analysis of past and present practice should be the driving force behind improved future practice. Reflection can be made easy and fluent by applying a structured approach to critical analysis (in this context the word critical refers to the ability to critique, not the seriousness of the situation). There are many models or structural frameworks the practitioner can use; your chosen university will discuss this with you. Taylor (2006) discusses these in detail; the reader is therefore directed to this source as a point of reference. Within the context of their chosen course the student will be asked to reflect on the application of new theory within their clinical practice. The aim of this is to make the student think of how important the application of evidenced-based information is to their expanding knowledge base, and to provide a rationale to their clinical practice. In addition, evidence of this learning opportunity will form the foundation for their developing portfolio. Having knowledge does not necessarily demonstrate understanding, as many practitioners have a solid knowledge base, but fail to apply this within the clinical arena, hence the importance of professional structured reflection (Evans & Tippins 2007).

Educational techniques – methods of learning

The enquiry-based approach

In recent years there have been several different approaches employed to educate student nurses. In the early 1990s, Burnard (1992) identified three types of knowledge:

- **Propositional**: relating to academic and scientific theory. Permits students to understand basic concepts, the 'what is' and 'why'
- **Practical**: relating to the acquisition of practical skills and the application of technology. Permits students to demonstrate 'how to'.
- **Experiential**: relating to the application of propositional and practical knowledge, which through time and experience allows the addition of reasoning which permits flexible application and considered practice.

Today these three basic principles are utilised in the delivery of enquiry-based learning (EBL). This approach to education refers to styles of learning motivated by a process of enquiry, where the learner is introduced pragmatically to a potentially complex problem or clinical case scenario. The learning ethos throughout this book centres on the enquiry-based approach to learning that provides the reader with certain cues or triggers which, through further reading and clinical experience, enable further exploration in order both to develop relevant knowledge and to gain the ability to research independently or in small groups. The EBL approach is composed of several supportive networks for the student; these can include workshops, chaired or facilitated presentations and simulations of real-life professional problems to stimulate students' learning. The facilitator's, or tutor's, role is purely to facilitate learning and provide guidance. Key sessions incorporate structures and forms of support to help students carry out enquiries. This can take several forms including analysis, problem solving and research. This approach enables students of nursing to obtain the ability to seek new knowledge, understanding and skills for themselves (an essential part of lifelong learning).

Clinical decision making

Nurses make multiple decisions rapidly in highly complex environments in order to deliver expert individualised care. A patient's condition can change rapidly and, therefore, demands intelligent and decisive decision making from nurses in short time frames. Despite this there remains minimal research on the clinical decision-making skills of nurses, and consequently much of the content and structure of nurses' decision making remains unclear (Fonteyn & Ritter 2000).

Clinical decision making can be defined as the process nurses use to gather patient information, evaluate that information and make a judgement that results in the provision of patient care (White et al. 1992). This process involves collecting information through the use of both scientific and intuitive assessment skills. This information is then interpreted by utilising knowledge and past experiences (Cioffi 2000, Tippins 2005).

There are many theories on how to teach these essential and dynamic skills; however, learning or the acquisition of new knowledge does not necessarily guarantee the clinical application of expert practice or critical thinking (Tippett 2004). Many theories on teaching and learning the art of critical thinking and expert clinical decision making are found; behaviourist, cognitive, and humanistic are the three commonly recognised (Sheehy & McCarthy 1998). The behaviourist theory relates to reactionary learning whereby the learning occurs when an unmet need causes the learner to embrace the learning process; unfortunately the inclination to learn is often stimulated by the learner feeling inadequate due to uncertainty and a lack of confidence. The cognitive theory relates to the interaction between the learner and their immediate environment, i.e. learning through experience and professional stimulation. The humanistic theory relates to adult-based learning where the focus is clearly on the learner ascertaining new knowledge through the process of self-discovery. A teacher who understands the present organised subject matter which is relevant to the learner's need will, therefore, encourage learning. The expert practitioner perceives the situation as a whole, uses past concrete situations as paradigms and moves to the accurate solution of the problem without wasteful consideration of a large number of irrelevant options.

The nursing process

The nursing process is a tool used by nurses to assist with decision making and to predict and evaluate the results of nursing actions (Reeves & Paul 2002). The deliberate intellectual activity of the nursing process guides the professional practice of nursing by providing care in a systematic manner. The nursing process has developed in recent years to incorporate five or six phases or stages (Lindberg et al. 1994, Oermann 1996, Wilkinson 2001, Reeves & Paul 2002).

Movement between these phases is unusually linear; there is free movement among the phases during clinical practice. Once an assessment begins, the nurse should begin to formulate some diagnoses and eliminate others.

Applying Theory to Practice: Box 1.1

Several key skills have been identified that facilitate the process of learning and empower the learner to independently further their own knowledge and understanding.

These key learning skills include:

- Information technology – literature searching skills, data retrieval, email, use of online resources and websites

- Communication – history taking and establishing a rapport, presentation of patient assessments and multidisciplinary team involvement

- Application of number – assessment of patient's clinical status using numerical data such as pain scoring, biochemistry results and the interpretation of individual's vital sign data

- Working with others – developing the ability to work within a small group, as part of a multidisciplinary team and to build short-term but mutually beneficial relationships with preceptors/mentors

- Improving own learning and performance – students need to reflect on new learning and evaluate their own performance within this area and simultaneously the amount of effort they used to achieve this

- Problem solving – developing the key skill of critical analysis and effective/decisive decision making.

The Nursing Process

1. Assessment – collection of subjective and objective clinical data to provide a rationale for care

2. Nursing/working diagnosis – analysis of physical presentation confirmed by scientific fact (data collection results)

3. Planning/outcome identification – plan of care and realistic goals discussed with patient

4. Implementation – performing interventions, reassess plan following each intervention to determine initial response

5. Evaluation – have expected outcomes been achieved? Determine patients level of clinical need and regularity of subsequent assessment

As more information is gathered, through physical and technological findings, the practitioner should begin to narrow the possibilities. The worst possible diagnosis should be paramount in the practitioner's hypotheses, as this must be addressed and eradicated before moving on. By using a systematic approach, patient problems can be identified and acted upon in the most effective way to ensure the best possible outcome for the patient. Examples of a systematic approach are those adopted by the Resuscitation Council (2006) on the Advanced Life Support (ALS) course with the ABC mnemonic: airway, breathing and circulation; and ABCDE: airway, breathing, circulation, disability and environment, taught on the Acute Life Threatening Events: Recognition and Treatment (ALERT) course, and by the American College of Surgeons (2005) in the Advanced Trauma Life Support (ATLS) course.

An obvious nursing diagnosis, such as difficulty in breathing with acute exacerbation of asthma, may be developed while data collection is still ongoing. In this situation implementation of life-saving actions (such as administration of oxygen therapy and bronchodilators) in which the desired outcome is obvious, may have begun before the assessment, diagnosis, outcome identification, and planning phases can be verbalised. Throughout the phases, reassessment can lead to immediate changes in any of the previous phases. Reassessment and the further collection and analysis of data are a continuous, ongoing dynamic process and should not be confused with evaluation, which measures outcomes. Reassessment may lead to a change in the working diagnosis, which in turn could lead to a change in outcome identification, planning, implementation and evaluation as the process continues. Although this process may appear complex, the novice can quickly begin to structure their patient assessment leading to early identification, action and evaluation.

Legislation and health policies

There have been massive improvements in health and life expectancy in recent years. A child born in Britain today on average will live nine years longer than one born when the NHS was first established in 1948 (Council for Science and Technology 2006). The current UK government have identified healthcare as an essential area of development, with healthcare being a focal point of their manifesto. In 2000, they published *The NHS Plan*, a White Paper identifying a 10-year plan for healthcare reform and development (DH 2000). *The NHS Plan* is available in a digestible format (executive summary) from the Department of Health's (DH) website dh.gov.uk. The government have also introduced several think tanks designed to introduce best practice and national standards based on the evaluation of both research and cost effectiveness; these include NICE (National Institute for Health and Clinical Excellence, formerly National Institute for Clinical Excellence). *The NHS Plan* identified:

- A lack of national standards
- Old-fashioned demarcations between staff and barriers between services
- A lack of clear incentives to improve performance
- The current approach to patient care delivery actually disempowered patients.

Of particular importance to nurses was the development of their role; this included the statement that in all areas of healthcare nurses would have the opportunity to extend their roles and that by 2004 over half of practising nurses would be able to supply medicines (under Patient Group Directions, Chapter 14).

The Government have recently established three core principles relating to public health:

- Informed choice
- Personalisation
- Working together (DH 2004).

The central focus is designed to assist individuals in making choices about their lifestyle that have a positive impact on their health. Providing healthcare within the community and assisting individuals in maintaining their independence are also contributory elements.

Do current government-driven health policies have an evidence base?

The improvement of the health of the entire population while simultaneously combating health inequalities should be central to any health philosophy. This requires well-informed and evidence-based policies, produced in combination with user groups and the professional organisations representing practitioners. In many areas where health policy has been dictated, it has demonstrated little clinical credibility by being unaudited and subsequently unevaluated. The setting of unrealistic goals has led to the development of unrealistic public expectations (DH 2001). The government's lack of clarity on many health topics and the failure of different government departments to act in unison have led to the Council for Science and Technology (2006) stating that both mechanisms for training government policy makers in the wider determinants of health and the use of evidence to assess them are needed.

In the modern era with evidence underpinning ever-increasing areas of healthcare it is unacceptable to think political parties can introduce both laws and local policies built upon obtaining short-term public accolade or demonstrating unfounded personal beliefs rather than introducing policies built upon a solid evidence base. This is reinforced by the Council for Science and Technology (2006) who state that the evidence base of government departments, not least the Department of Health, is at best patchy, at worst non-existent. Lord Darzi in his recently published interim review states that change should only be initiated when there is a clear and strong clinical basis for doing so. This may herald a new approach for ministers when examined in combination with the findings of the Council for Science and Technology (DH 2007).

The introduction of research and an evidence base to nursing practice

For many years healthcare delivery has been dependent on the particular skill base and subjective beliefs of individual practitioners (DH 2000). The modern approach to healthcare centres on each practitioner being able to work in unison with the patient to deliver a plan of care that envisages the patient as the central focus, and also involves an evidence base and cost effectiveness.

The argument surrounding the clinical application of

theoretical knowledge has continued throughout nursing and healthcare education. *The NHS Plan* (DH 2000) identified the NHS as deficient in national evidence-based standards and, therefore, much of the practice was subject to individual interpretation. This initiated the current protocol-driven approach to care which aims to provide practitioners, and subsequently patients, with evidence-based objective treatment regimens, in contrast to individual subjective preferences. A prime example is demonstrated by the advanced life support algorithms, which have revolutionised multidisciplinary care delivery.

Changing practice within the vast institution of healthcare is a monumental task and to this end clinical governance was established. The clinical governance initiative is put into clinical practice by the National Institute for Health and Clinical Excellence (NICE). NICE, in conjunction with several specialist professional institutions, have released numerous national guidelines on specific patient presentations or illnesses. These are also supplemented by the DH's National Service Frameworks (NSF), which set clinical standards in relation to specific disorders, and specialist organisations such as the British Thoracic Society, which promote 'best practice'. These initiatives have combined to produce a constantly progressive clinical arena in which novice practitioners and students can easily become lost.

There is, therefore, a clear need to implement a tool or structure to the diagnostic process directly aimed at facilitating practitioners with the ability to base their clinical findings on objective rather than subjective data. This facilitation centres on two components: firstly, a solid understanding of the signs and symptoms associated with physical illness, and secondly, the application of critical thinking to practice. The first component is demonstrated throughout this book by experienced practitioners who discuss their own experiences in the form of patient scenarios which highlight both common clinical encounters and the frameworks and protocols they use to prioritise and manage patients quickly, appropriately and effectively. In addition, the clinicians discuss the associated anatomy and physiology, providing the reader with several key words or triggers. This enquiry-based learning approach promotes lifelong learning by encouraging the reader to seek key texts listed at the end of each chapter, thereby gaining further knowledge and understanding of the topics.

The importance of ethics in clinical decision making

'The ethics incorporated into good nursing practice are more important than knowledge of the law; practising ethically saves the effort of trying to know all the laws' (Hall 1996). Making decisions that are ethically sound can be extremely taxing for inexperienced nurses who seek to provide the best care for their patients. There are several tools a nurse can use to structure and re-evaluate their decisions (Tingle & Cribb 2007). Beauchamp and Childress (1994) provide a set of five basic principles to guide practitioners.

Non-maleficence
The first principle, non-maleficence, means to do no harm; this is directly linked to the nurse's duty to protect the patient's safety. Born out of the Hippocratic oath, this principle dictates that practitioners allow no harm to their patients.

Beneficence
The second principle, beneficence, is at the heart of everyday nursing practice. Beauchamp and Childress (1994) identify that beneficence requires taking action by 'helping or preventing harm, removing harm and promoting good'. A crucial component of beneficence centres on paternalism, which can be categorised as 'weak' or 'strong'. Weak paternalism implies protecting the patient when the patient is vulnerable and unable to make decisions. Strong paternalism involves interactions intended to benefit a person despite the fact that the person's risky choices and actions are informed, voluntary and autonomous (Beauchamp & Childress 1994).

Autonomy
The third ethical principle, autonomy, means that an individual has a right to self-determination, that is, to make decisions and choices about their health or life without interference from others.

Justice
The fourth ethical principle, justice, indicates giving each person, or group, what they are due. Justice is measured in terms of fairness and equality. In nursing, justice frequently focuses on impartial access to care and on the fair distribution of scarce resources. The postcode lottery and failure of clinical governance in many areas of care

throughout the United Kingdom in recent times have made a mockery of 'just' decisions.

Privacy and confidentiality

The fifth ethical principle relates to privacy and confidentiality. Privacy is a fundamental right of each individual and, as such, it cannot be taken away from that person unless they choose to share it. Confidentiality, on the other hand, means that information shared with other persons regarding the patient will be used only for the purposes intended. A patient's sharing of private information imposes a duty of confidentiality on healthcare providers. That duty means providers will share information only on a need-to-know basis (NMC 2004a).

Nursing: career potentials

Nursing in the 21st century offers the student a diverse and rewarding career, second to none. Once qualified, and a consolidatory period of practice established, the nurse is ready to begin planning their future. Many specialist areas of practice will have a prerequisite that nurses have six months relevant experience prior to commencing with them. This is usually due to higher than normal patient dependency or the technical demands of the specialty. Teaching and educating others plays a major component of the nursing role; many nurses, therefore, undertake a coaching or mentoring course early in their career. There are many teaching pathways within nursing, with practice development or lecturing being two prime examples. These two roles offer the nurse great reward as they influence the knowledge and skills base of other practitioners and indirectly affect the care patients receive. The reintroduction of the matron role was seen by many as a paper exercise but this high-profile role does offer a focal point for professionals and patients. In addition, junior nurses have an easily identifiable role model and clear pathway of progression from staff nurse to senior staff nurse/junior sister/charge nurse to senior sister/charge nurse. Many areas also have a senior nurse supervising an area of practice and a matron overseeing several clinical areas. The roles of the nurse specialist, and the areas encompassed, have proliferated over recent years; most clinical areas will now have experienced nurses working at an advanced level. The grades of these specialists vary, with the role of the consultant nurse seen as the pinnacle position (DH 2000).

This chapter has discussed many key issues surrounding modern nursing including professional regulations, the importance of lifelong learning and maintaining an evidence-based approach established through the construction of a portfolio directly demonstrating professional development including clinical and ethical decision-making skills. Throughout the following chapters the reader can work at his or her own pace to gain extensive insight into the essential knowledge base required to deliver what can be called 'basic nursing care'. Undertaking the learning activity boxes and completing the end of chapter quizzes can assist in the development of this essential knowledge and skills base. As the reader progresses through their chosen educational programme, they will soon realise there is nothing basic about 'basic nursing care'. The ability to care for others in moments of their life when they have been affected by trauma, illness or psychological stress can provide the nurse with great satisfaction and self-fulfilment. Patients and their relatives are frequently vulnerable and require the demonstration of both professionalism and humanity from their nurse. The combination of these skills, which include information sharing and empathy, demonstrates a clinically knowledgeable nurse and a caring individual.

Work through the chapters at your own pace and return to the topics as you encounter them on your clinical placements, this will increase your understanding of clinical conditions and the potential care needs of the individual. Each chapter highlights methods of assessing and treating patients in an individual and dignified manner; in addition, each chapter provides several pertinent sources of further reading, including links to educational websites that convey best practice or relevant educational materials. I hope you enjoy this book and gain as much pleasure from it as we did writing it.

Further reading

Benner, P. (2001) *From Novice to Expert: Excellence and Power in Clinical Practice.* Commemorative Edition. Prentice Hall: USA.

Boud, D., Keogh, R. & Walker, D. (1985) *Reflection: Turning Experience into Learning.* Kogan Page: London.

Department of Health (2000) *The NHS Plan: A Plan for Investment, a Plan for Reform.* Department of Health: London.

Department of Health (2003) *The Essence of Care: Patient-focused Benchmarks for Clinical Governance.* Department of Health: London. http://www.dh.gov.uk/en/Publicationsandstatistics/Publications/PublicationsPolicyAndGuidance/DH_4005475

Nursing and Midwifery Council (NMC) (2006) *An NMC Guide for Students of Nursing and Midwifery.* NMC: London. http://www.nmc-uk.org/

Taylor, B. (2005) *Reflective Practice: A Guide for Nurses and Midwives.* Open University Press: Maidenhead.

References

American College of Surgeons Committee on Trauma (2005) *Advanced Trauma Life Support for Doctors: Student Course Manual*, 7th edn. American College of Surgeons: Chicago.

Beauchamp, T.L. & Childress, J.F. (1994) *Principles of Biomedical Ethics*, 4th edn. Oxford University Press: New York.

Benner, P. (2001) *From Novice to Expert: Excellence and Power in Clinical Practice.* Commemorative Edition. Prentice Hall: New Jersey.

Burnard, P. (1992) Learning nursing knowledge. In: Robinson, K. & Vaughan, B. (eds) *Knowledge for Nursing Practice.* Butterworth Heinemann: Oxford.

Cioffi, J. (2000) Recognition of patients who require emergency assistance: A descriptive study. *Heart and Lung* 29(4): 262–8.

Council for Science and Technology (2006) *Health Impacts – A Strategy across Government.* Council for Science and Technology: London.

Department of Health (2000) *The NHS Plan: A Plan for Investment, a Plan for Reform.* Department of Health: London.

Department of Health (2001) *Reforming Emergency Care.* Department of Health: London.

Department of Health (2003) *The Essence of Care: Patient-focused Benchmarks for Clinical Governance.* Department of Health: London. http://www.dh.gov.uk/en/Publicationsandstatistics/Publications/PublicationsPolicyAndGuidance/DH_4005475

Department of Health (2004) *Choosing Health – Making Healthy Choices Easier.* Department of Health: London.

Department of Health (2007) *Our NHS. Our Future.* NHS Next Stage Review Interim Report: Summary. Department of Health: London.

Evans, C. & Tippins, E. (2007) *The Foundations of Emergency Care.* Open University Press: Maidenhead.

Fonteyn, M. & Ritter, B. (2000) Clinical reasoning in nursing. In: Higgs, J. & Jones, M. (eds) *Clinical Reasoning in the Health Professions.* Butterworth Heinemann: Oxford, pp. 107–16.

Hall, J. (1996) *Nursing Ethics and Law.* Saunders: Philadelphia.

Johns, C. & Freshwater, D. (1998) *Transforming Nursing Through Reflective Practice.* Blackwell: Oxford.

Lindberg, J.B., Hunter, M.L. & Kruszewski, A.Z. (1994) *Introduction to Nursing: Concepts, Issues and Opportunities*, 2nd edn. Lippincott: Philadelphia.

Morton-Cooper, A. & Palmer, A. (2000) *Mentoring Preceptorship and Clinical Supervision: A Guide to Professional Support Roles in Clinical Practice*, 2nd edn. Blackwell Science: Oxford.

Nursing and Midwifery Council (NMC) (2004a) *Code of Professional Conduct: Standards for Conduct, Performance and Ethics.* NMC: London.

Nursing and Midwifery Council (NMC) (2004b) *Guidelines for the Administration of Medicines.* NMC: London.

Nursing and Midwifery Council (NMC) (2004c) *Guidelines for Records and Record Keeping.* NMC: London.

Nursing and Midwifery Council (NMC) (2004d) *The PREP Handbook.* NMC: London.

Nursing and Midwifery Council (NMC) (2005a) *Consultation on Proposals Arising from a Review of Fitness for Practice at the Point of Registration.* NMC: London. http://www.nmc-uk.org/aFrameDisplay.aspx?DocumentID=920 (accessed 28/09/07).

Nursing and Midwifery Council (NMC) (2005b) *Fitness to Practise Annual Report 2004–2005.* NMC: London. http://www.nmc-uk.org/aFrameDisplay.aspx?DocumentID=1102

Nursing and Midwifery Council (NMC) (2006) *An NMC Guide for Students of Nursing and Midwifery.* NMC: London.

Oermann, M.H. (1996) *Professional Nursing Practice: A Conceptual Approach*, 2nd edn. Lippincott: Philadelphia

Parada, C. (1993) *Genealogical Guide to Greek Mythology* (Studies in Mediterranean Archaeology, Vol 107). Coronet Books: New Jersey.

Reeves, J.S. & Paul, C. (2002) Nursing theory in clinical practice. In: George, J.B. (ed.) *Nursing Theories: The Base for Professional Nursing Practice.* Prentice Hall: New Jersey, pp. 21–41.

Resuscitation Council (UK) (2006) *Advanced Life Support Course Provider Manual*, 5th edn. RSUK: London.

Roper, N., Logan, W. & Tierney, A. (1980) *Elements of Nursing.* Churchill Livingstone: London.

Schön, D.A. (1995) *The Reflective Practitioner: How Professionals Think in Action.* Arena: Aldershot.

Sheehy, C. & McCarthy, M. (1998) *Advanced Practice Nursing Emphasizing Common Roles.* Davis Co: Philadelphia.

Smith, C. (1995) Evaluating nursing care; reflection in practice. *Professional Nurse* 10(11): 723–4.

Tingle, J. & Cribb, A. (2007) *Nursing Law and Ethics*, 3rd edn. Blackwell Publishing: Oxford.

Tippett, J. (2004) Nurses' acquisition and retention of knowledge after trauma training. *Accident and Emergency Nursing* 12: 39–46.

Tippins, E. (2005) How emergency department nurses identify and respond to critical illness. *Emergency Nurse* 13(3): 24–33.

White, J., Nativo, D.G., Kobert, S.N. et al. (1992) Content and process in clinical decision making by nurse practitioners. *Image* 24:153–8.

Wilkinson, J.M. (2001) *Nursing Process: A Critical Thinking Approach*, 3rd edn. Prentice-Hall: New Jersey.

Part 2
Body systems

Homeostasis

Andrea Blay

2

Chapter 2 Learning Objectives

- To gain knowledge and insight into the physiology related to the systems involved in maintaining homeostasis
- To gain insight into conditions related to dysfunction of these systems
- To apply theory to practice by understanding the clinical presentation when homeostatic failure occurs in patients
- To gain insight into pharmacological preparations to either prevent or treat relevant conditions
- To follow a structured approach to patient assessment thereby identifying homeostatic failure at a treatable stage
- To demonstrate evidence of professional development within your portfolio in relation to understanding homeostasis and homeostatic mechanisms
- To continue to develop the ability to question and critique the evidence base and effectiveness of plans of care for patients with a variety of problems affecting homeostatic problems

Introduction

Homeostasis refers to the state of functional equilibrium within the body's internal environment, namely the cells, tissues, organs and fluids (Clancy & McVicar 2002).

Maintenance of homeostasis depends primarily on providing an internal environment suitable for normal cellular function. Certain stimuli can result in alterations to the internal physical environment referred to as stressors, all of which have the ability to affect cellular function pathologically. Insults range from compromise to a specific cellular function, through to multi-organ failure and death. As a result, the internal environment is constantly changing or adapting; this is a direct result of physical, psychological and environmental stressors.

This chapter will define homeostasis and the homeostatic mechanisms essential to the normal functioning of healthy cells, which preserve the fundamental processes necessary to maintain cell, tissue and organ function i.e. life. One such example is the regulation of carbon dioxide, an acid and waste product of cellular metabolism which, if it accumulates, can lead to respiratory depression, hypoventilation or a low respiratory rate (<10 breaths/minute). Healthy lungs excrete carbon dioxide in water, which we exhale. Any diseases that affect the lung tissue or reduce the diffusion of gases across the alveolar–capillary membrane may affect the ability of the lungs to excrete carbon dioxide (Chapter 3).

The human body has many homeostatic mechanisms: thermal, chemical, neural and hormonal, which govern a multitude of cellular processes. Some processes are more familiar to us and more common than others, such as the production of insulin, the regulation of food intake, water and electrolyte balance, the hypothalamic control of body temperature, the maintenance of cardiac output, oxygen and carbon dioxide levels, and the balance between acidity and alkalinity as a consequence of metabolism. Others are less known but are of no less importance, such as calcium homeostasis for the remodelling and repair of bones (Chapter 8). A myriad of hormones released by the thyroid gland control growth, the sleep–wake cycle, and the body's response to stress and illness to maintain health.

Throughout the 24-hour cycle the body continuously adjusts all of these mechanisms, and many others, to maintain equilibrium and optimum cell function. During illness or excessive or prolonged exposure to stressors, the ability of the body to self-regulate and maintain an optimum internal environment by manipulating these finely tuned mechanisms is exceeded and cells and organs dysfunction; this can manifest as acute or chronic disease.

There are many different symptoms and clinical presentations associated with homeostatic failure; in fact most of the clinical conditions presented by patients are as a result of a failure on some level. This chapter will

demonstrate how homeostatic failure is related to specific diseases, such as diabetes; case examples will illustrate the complexity of such clinical presentations and relevant investigations, and the clinical care required will be reviewed. The challenge for nurses is to be able to link the symptoms to the altered pathophysiology of the many diseases associated with homeostasis, and to understand the role of the nurse in supporting patients with a variety of clinical problems as a result of homeostatic failure. Questions should focus on understanding which assessments and investigations the patient may undergo. Which observations should be performed in the acute stages of homeostatic failure? How should treatment and management plans be constructed and evaluated? What information is required by the patient from healthcare professionals to adjust life styles such as those with newly diagnosed diabetes or renal failure?

Applying Theory to Practice: Exercise 2.1

Before commencing this chapter:

- Identify which organs or glands you already know that are involved in maintaining homeostasis

- Compose a list of diseases that you already know that affect the body's ability to maintain homeostatic function in relation to temperature, blood pressure, water balance, glucose control and acid base

- Add this list to your developing portfolio and on completion of this chapter expand your portfolio with the new disorders you have gained knowledge of and elaborate on how these disorders affect physiological function and how to recognise homeostatic failure

- This might include the patient's history, clinical presentation and tests such as blood analysis

Homeostatic feedback mechanisms: a matter of balance

As a nurse you need to understand how the different hormones and chemicals are 'switched' on and off, or how they are regulated up or down in response to a stimulus. These mechanisms operate on feedback systems that either result in a positive or negative response. For a system to operate, there must be detectors and effectors, which are ultimately coordinated by nerve centres, most often the hypothalamus in the brain. A feedback mechanism is one in which a positive effect is seen, with the release of chemicals or hormones which target specific cells or organs to achieve the desired effect.

Detectors are mostly nerve receptors that detect changes and monitor the variable that needs to be controlled. An example of a detector would be baroreceptors or stretch receptors that detect changes in blood volume by the amount of 'stretch' or volume of blood in the carotid sinus and arch of the aorta. When the circulating blood volume falls, as in haemorrhage, the baroreceptors send impulses back to the brain, or coordinating centre. In turn, via the autonomic nervous system, several mechanisms are stimulated, all aimed at increasing and redirecting the circulating volume and restoring blood pressure (Figure 2.1).

An effector is a gland, organ or muscle that will bring about or 'effect' the change (Figure 2.1). The release of catecholamines, such as noradrenaline and adrenaline, from sympathetic nerve endings causes an increase in heart rate in an attempt to raise cardiac output. When we review the mechanisms of hypotension, there are many effectors that come into play to try to raise the blood pressure; these will be discussed later in the chapter.

A negative feedback system is designed to respond in the opposite direction of the deviation so that the deviation is reduced in potency or shut off, causing the opposite effect to occur i.e. a drop in blood pressure. The deviation feeds back to the cardiovascular system, in this case via the brain, to reverse or alter the direction of the deviation or reduce its potency, in other words, to halt the hypotension. Equilibrium is achieved as the blood pressure is restored to normal, achieving homeostasis.

A positive feedback system responds in the same direction as the initial stimulus, enhancing the potency of and amplifying the stimulus rather than controlling, reducing or shutting off the deviation. An example would be the activation of the clotting cascade in response to haemorrhage. The up-regulation and production of clotting factors are amplified to control bleeding and achieve haemostasis.

Failures in homeostatic mechanisms can lead to life-threatening clinical emergencies such as severe hypotension, hypo- or hyperglycaemia, haemorrhage, and acid-base imbalances, which can cause patients to

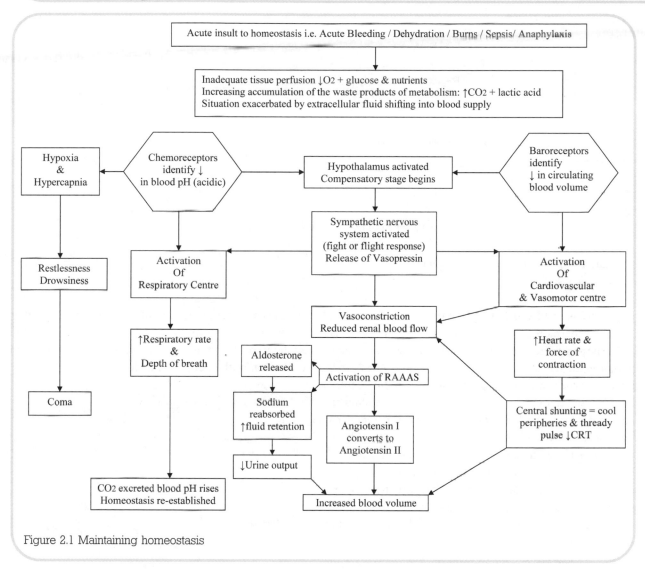

Figure 2.1 Maintaining homeostasis

develop renal failure and ultimately cardiac arrest or death. Extreme homeostatic failure can lead to the development of multi-organ dysfunction syndrome (MODS) necessitating admission to intensive care units.

The hypothalamus

One of the most important homeostatic regions of the body is the hypothalamus, situated below the thalamus on top of the brain stem and comprising the base of the third ventricle. It is the nerve control centre for many autonomic responses, which include respiratory rate and depth, heart rate and force of contraction, blood pressure and gut motility. Metabolic control includes body temperature regulation, water balance and thirst control,

hunger and fullness mechanisms, which are linked to glucose and insulin levels, and regulation of the sleep–wake cycle or 'biological clock'. Emotional responses such as fear, rage and pleasure are also under hypothalamic control as the hypothalamus sits within the limbic centre, an area responsible for emotional responses, which are relayed via the autonomic nerve pathways of the hypothalamus (Figure 2.2).

The hypothalamus exerts its effects through two main mechanisms: the release of hormones and activation of nervous pathways to achieve the desired effect. The hypothalamus is in close contact with other important centres, the pituitary gland and the mammillary bodies or nuclei that are involved in the sense of smell (olfactory pathways).

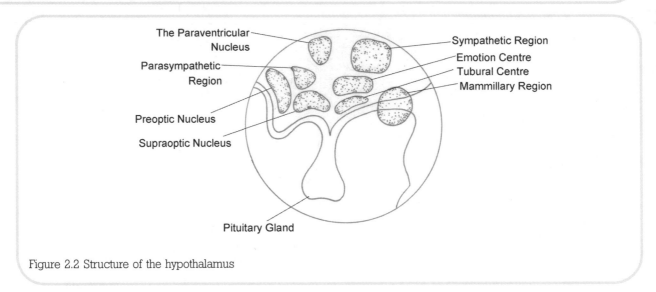

Figure 2.2 Structure of the hypothalamus

Regulation and control of temperature

The main thermoregulation centre in the hypothalamus is the preoptic region (Figure 2.2), which regulates temperature via the autonomic nervous system (ANS). This area comprises of a heat-loss and heat-promoting centre or the thermoregulatory centre. Humans maintain a constant core temperature about 37ºC which is independent of the surrounding environment. We are capable of living in extreme climates with the external temperature ranging from −52ºC to +49ºC (Hinchliffe et al. 1999).

The core temperature is shared between the organs within the skull, thoracic and abdominal cavities; these deep-seated organs have the highest temperature. The shell or periphery is the heat loss surface; the organs and deeper vessels are separated from the skin by a layer of fatty tissue, which acts as an insulating layer during cold weather. The skin has the lowest temperature and this can range from 27ºC on the toes to 34ºC on the forehead (Hinchliffe et al. 1999). A temperature gradient therefore exists between the core and the periphery. Sometimes patients who have severe infections can have a high core temperature of >39ºC but peripherally they can be cold demonstrating peripheral shutdown, often a sign of severe sepsis and circulatory collapse. Exercising skeletal muscles can generate 30–40 times more heat compared to the rest of the body (Marieb 1998). Heat or cold is detected by peripheral receptors (afferents) located in the skin and central thermoreceptors that detect blood temperature are located in the core.

The hypothalamus responds to input via autonomic efferent pathways. The nature of the stimulus will determine the character of the physiological response; whether to gain heat by shivering and vasoconstriction of the periphery or to promote heat loss by sweating and vasodilation of the periphery. (Figure 2.3).

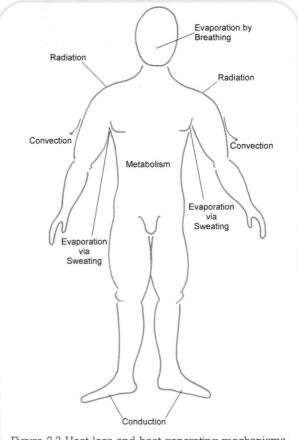

Figure 2.3 Heat loss and heat-generating mechanisms

Anatomy and Physiology in Action: Box 2.1

Maintaining Homeostatic Balance of Heat Loss and Heat Gain		
Radiation: heat is lost as infrared waves from the body to the air. A dense object like the body will transfer heat to the environment. Energy flow is always from warmer to cooler air/ objects (Marieb 1998).	Conduction or convection: the transfer of heat between objects in contact with each other. It involves molecule-to-molecule contact. Thermal energy moves through a medium such as fluid. Convection is the transfer of heat to the air, causing warm air to expand and rise. The cooler air becomes denser and falls: the warmed air is continually replaced by cool air. This mechanism enhances the exchange of heat from the body surface to air – as the cooler air absorbs heat by conduction. That is how a summer breeze on a hot day cools the skin.	Evaporation: the conversion of water from a liquid into a gas or water vapour. Water molecules absorb heat from the environment – called the heat of vaporisation. The kinetic energy or temperature of the liquid will determine how much energy is generated and hence water vapour produced. An example is demonstrated by huskies in the Antarctic – as the huskies exhale, heat is lost as water vapour and because the surrounding air temperature is −28°C the water vapour is visible.
	Conduction and convection account for 15–20% of heat loss (Marieb 1998). Think about this statement – what might that mean for patients? Patients who experience fever are often fanned: this is called forced convection – fanning enhances the heat loss process. Patients should not be directly fanned as this can cause shivering and generate heat to inadvertently raise the temperature. Try the experiment on yourself or a colleague. Keep the fan on one part of the body for 10 minutes or more and see the effects.	Insensible water loss. Water vapour is lost via respiration, the mucosa of the mouth and skin. A patient with a chest infection on oxygen with a respiratory rate of 40 breaths/minute can lose water vapour due to the high respiratory rate and pulmonary secretions. This is exacerbated by the drying effects of oxygen and enhances the feeling of dehydration. During vigorous exercise the body can perspire and evaporate up to 2L of water just through sweat. In normal resting conditions and in environmental temperatures of 31°C–32°C the sweat glands produce 0.5L sweat/day. Sweat output increases up to 12L of body water/day depending on the external temperature and degree of humidity.

Heat-generating mechanisms

The peripheral receptors send impulses when the blood is cooler than the hypothalamic set point to the posterior heat-promoting centre.

Applying Theory to Practice: Exercise 2.2

- How does the body generate heat in response to cold external temperatures or following immersion in cold water or an infusion of cold fluids during a blood transfusion or prolonged resuscitation?

Administering cold intravenous fluids can quickly cause hypothermia in an already compromised patient.

- How can this be prevented?

Under the control of the sympathetic nervous system, vasoconstriction of the periphery is activated, diverting blood flow away from the skin surface to deeper tissues and vessels by closing precapillary sphincters and reducing blood flow to the skin. Patients who are very cold may have white, marble-like skin which may be cyanosed; this is caused by the trapping of blood in the periphery with loss of oxygen from the blood to the tissues, hence the blue tinge of the skin (Hinchliffe et al. 1999). The hairs or pili on our skin play a part in trapping heat; each hair follicle is attached to erector muscles which help to lift the hair follicle – the trapped heat acts as an insulting layer. This makes our hairs stand on end and also gives us goose pimples or bumps.

Another effective way of raising the core body temperature is shivering. Any muscle activity will increase the body temperature; shivering is activated by the hypothalamus when the shell temperature falls below 35°C. Shivering is much more effective as a mechanism at higher temperatures as the muscles become weak and uncoordinated at lower temperatures. In the elderly, shivering is much reduced due to an ineffective response to sympathetic activity. The elderly can lose heat over a period of time and therefore may not take effective measures to raise the body temperature.

Thyroxine (T_4) is an important hormone secreted by the thyroid gland that stimulates metabolically active cells

Applying Theory to Practice: Exercise 2.3

Review the warming devices in your clinical areas that are available to warm patients and fluids

- Which mechanisms of heat production are employed?
- Which is the most effective?

to consume oxygen; this is called the calorigenic effect (Ganong 1995) and is effective in raising the basal metabolic rate (BMR). Chemicals such as adrenaline and noradrenaline also raise the body temperature by increasing the BMR and heat is gained. Another provider of heat is the powerhouse of the body, the liver. Through its enzymatic functions and processes it provides a constant source of heat.

Anatomy and Physiology in Action: Exercise 2.4

Thyroxine is an important hormone released by the thyroid gland. Identify the anatomical position of the thyroid gland and make a list of the functions of the different hormones released by the gland.

Removal of the thyroid is called a thyroidectomy

- For what reasons can this occur?

Heat loss mechanisms

During warmer weather the increased air temperature causes vasodilation of dermal blood vessels bringing the vessels close to the skin surface so that heat can be lost via conduction, radiation and convection. In addition, stimulation of the sweat glands via sympathetic fibres helps to cool the body by the process of evaporation. This negative feedback system is finely tuned to maintain the hypothalamic set point; during warmer weather the heat promoting centre is inhibited and the heat loss centre is activated.

Anatomy and Physiology in Action: Exercise 2.5

- Using Figure 2.1 apply the feedback pathway to the regulation of temperature. Draw the pathway and insert the mechanisms that are related to the homeostatic control of temperature.
- What and where would the receptors and effectors be located?
- What effectors are found within the skin that result in sweating and shivering?
- Make a list of the factors that affect heat gain and heat loss.

Developing and Delivering Expert Care: Box 2.2

Normal Body Temperature

The body can only function within a narrow temperature range between 35.6°–37.8°C despite changes in air temperature.

Body temperature fluctuates about 1 degree in 24 hrs. It is lowest in the early morning and highest in the early evening.

Temperature helps maintain optimal enzymatic function for effective cell metabolism.

Increases in the temperature will increase enzymatic activity or catalysis – therefore each rise of 1°C results in a 10% increase in chemical reactions (Marieb 1998).

Temperatures above 41°C can cause convulsions. The upper limit for life is 43°C although there are case reports of patients surviving beyond this upper limit. At this temperature proteins begin to denature and cell function is destroyed.

Hypothermia is a core temperature below 35°C. Heat-generating mechanisms are activated such as shivering and erector pili muscles.

At 34°C intense shivering occurs, there is difficulty in the movement of digits, changes in skin colour – cyanosis and some confusion or behavioural changes may occur.

At 30°C–32°C shivering progressively ceases. There is increased sleepiness, bradycardia or slowed heartbeat, shallow respirations and moderate confusion.

At 28°C the patient may appear dead. If uncorrected, coma, cardiac arrest from severe rhythm disturbances or respiratory arrest and death will occur when the body temperature approaches 21°C.

Pathology of fever

Fever is also known as pyrexia or controlled hyperthermia. It is derived from the Latin word *febris* or febrile. Fever occurs when the body temporarily fails to maintain the temperature within normal limits. The set-point is elevated by 1–2° C and is a symptom of many medical conditions. White blood cells and macrophages release endogenous (internal) pyrogens (fire starters) or cytokines into the bloodstream. These chemicals act directly on the thermostat in the hypothalamus causing the release of prostaglandins and elevating or re-setting the set-point. Fever also increases the basal metabolic rate; it inhibits the growth of bacteria thus assisting the body's defence mechanisms to fight invading pathogens, eating is inhibited (anorexia) and proteins are denatured which can result in irreversible brain damage.

Figure 2.4 Mercury thermometer

Developing and Delivering Expert Care: Exercise 2.6

Classification of Fever

Pyrexia (fever) can be classed as

- Low-grade: 38–39°C (100.4–102.2°F)
- Moderate: 39–40°C (102.2–104°F)
- High-grade: >40°C (>104°F)
- Hyperpyrexia: >42°C (>107.6°F) (a medical emergency)

During clinical placements identify patients who have changes in temperature.

- Can you identify the causes?
- What treatments are required to manage patients with hypothermia and hyperpyrexia?

Applying Theory to Practice: Exercise 2.7

Causes of Fever

Under the following three headings identify some of the micro-organisms, diseases or therapies that might cause a fever:

- Infections: ..
- Inflammation: ..
- Allergic reactions: ..

Cancer and chemotherapy treatments can also induce a fever due to tumour necrosis. Brain injuries can cause fever that is unresponsive to cooling measures and anti-pyretics. Why might that be?

Review the location of the hypothalamus.

Immunological diseases like lupus erythematosus, sarcoidosis and inflammatory bowel diseases can also cause fever.

The destruction of tissues which can occur in **haemolysis**, surgery, myocardial infarction, crush syndrome, **rhabdomyolysis** and cerebral hemorrhage may induce fever.

- In clinical practice see if you can identify patients who have experienced some of the diseases or treatments mentioned.

Drugs can also cause a 'drug fever' either as a direct consequence of the drug or as an adverse reaction to the drug (e.g. antibiotics). Discontinuation of some drugs like heroin can induce a fever.

The homeostatic control of blood pressure

Before discussing the compensatory mechanisms deployed to control blood pressure we need to review some commonly used definitions. Blood pressure is defined as the force or pressure exerted on blood vessel walls by the circulating volume of blood in a closed system. Blood pressure is a hydrostatic pressure as the blood is confined within a closed system; confined liquids exert a pressure against the walls of the container and therefore any changes in flow, viscosity, resistance and structure will influence the pressure. See Chapter 4 for a more in-depth review of the cardiac cycle.

Applying Theory to Practice: Exercise 2.8

Thermometers

The first thermometers were used nearly 300 years ago based on the principles of a liquid (mercury) expanding in a sealed glass bulb (Figure 2.4). The temperature is recorded along a scale on the thermometer. There are two temperature scales in use today, Fahrenheit and Celsius. In the UK, Celsius is commonly used.

Mercury thermometers were used to take the temperature orally: from the axilla, mouth and rectum. There was also a low-grade thermometer, which had a blue-coloured bulb for easy identification. Today there are many alternatives to thermometry.

- Identify which thermometers are used within your practice areas.
- How are they cleaned? Does this affect their reliability?
- Why do they use this system? Are they research based?

Developing and Delivering Expert Care: Exercise 2.9

Recording the Temperature

Normal Temperature Readings:

Rectal temperature 0.5°C higher than the oral temperature

Otic temperature or tympanic (ear) is at, or higher than 38°C (100.4°F)

Oral temperature is at, or higher than 36.5°C–37.5°C (99.5°F)

Axillary temperature is at, or higher than 37.2°C (99°F)

- Identify in your clinical area which methods are utilised to measure the temperature (chemical, digital, tympanic or temporal).
- How is temperature monitored during surgery?
- Identify what alternatives may be used to monitor unconscious patients who cannot shiver or change their body temperature due to anaesthesia.

The 'gold standard' of temperature measurement is either the pulmonary artery catheter (PAC) or any device that can measure the blood temperature directly. The problem with these devices is that they are highly invasive and are only available in high dependency and intensive care settings.

Pulse pressure

The pulse pressure is the difference between the maximal systolic pressure and minimal diastolic pressure (Klabunde 2005). The pulse pressure is affected by the stroke volume and the elasticity of the arteries. If the 'normal' blood pressure in healthy adults is 120/80mmHg, then the 'normal' pulse pressure is roughly 40mmHg. Increases in heart rate and contractility can widen the pulse pressure as can head injuries associated with raised intracranial pressure. A narrowed pulse pressure is seen in hypovolaemia, septic shock, in patients on glycerine trinitrate (GTN) infusions (a potent vasodilator), or during major haemorrhage when the systolic pressure falls due to reduced arterial stretch; the diastolic pressure may drop slightly but often remains fairly constant. If you refer to the case study of Mark Bradbury on p. 32, his blood pressure has dropped to 85/45mmHg, he has a narrowed pulse pressure of 30mmHg. The clinical significance of severe blood loss resulting in a reduced or narrowed pulse pressure is that oxygen delivery to the tissues and subsequently the cell is compromised, resulting in cellular dysfunction.

Scenario 2.1

Major Haemorrhage

Mr Mark Bradbury, a 35-year-old Caucasian man is admitted to the emergency department following a road traffic accident. He sustained an open fractured right femur, ruptured spleen and a fractured pelvis, resulting in internal bleeding, and lacerations to his face and hands.

On examination he is pale, cold and clammy

His vital signs are:

Airway – Clear

Breathing – Respiratory rate 36, SpO2 95% on 12L/minute O_2 via non-rebreathe system

Circulation – Pulse 120, weak, regular. Blood pressure 85/45mmHg. Capillary refill time >4 seconds. Blood glucose 4.8mmols/L.

Disability – Patient responds only to voice on the AVPU scale = V. Pupils – Pupils equal and reactive to light (PEARL)

Exposure – Open/compound fracture right leg. Distended abdomen, tender with evidence of guarding in left upper quadrant. Lacerations to face and hands Temperature 35.6°C.

Past medical history (PMH): Nil of note

Social – Smokes 30/day. Alcohol: 20 units/week. Lives alone.

Mean arterial pressure (MAP)

Another important pressure recording is the mean or average arterial blood pressure (MAP). It is often recorded in brackets beside the blood pressure reading on monitors. The MAP reflects the perfusing pressure needed to maintain arterial blood flow and hence oxygen delivery to tissues and organs during each cardiac cycle. A MAP of 60mmHg is necessary to supply the coronary and cerebral arteries and the kidneys, which are more sensitive to pressure changes than other organs. The normal mean arterial pressure range is 70–110mmHg. At normal resting heart rates it can be calculated simply as the following equation in Anatomy and Physiology in Action: Box 2.3.

helpful in assessing how the organs are being perfused guiding clinical judgement and interventions.

In Scenario 2.1 Mr Bradbury's current cardiovascular status is reduced; this is identified through the reduced capillary refill time and the MAP, which is calculated at 56mmHg. In a young and fit person this MAP is relatively normal and is well tolerated, but even the young and fit can experience renal compromise if the insult is sustained or the MAP is reduced even further over a number of hours causing renal impairment and failure of other organs.

Anatomy and Physiology in Action: Box 2.3

MAP = systolic + (diastolic x 2)/3

Normal diastolic filling time is twice as long as the systolic time and is therefore measured twice. In patients who are unstable, this is a less accurate method but trends are

Developing and Delivering Expert Care: Exercise 2.10

Calculate the pulse pressure and MAP from the following blood pressure recordings

120/80 mmHg =
90/50 mmHg =
160/90 mmHg =
70/40 mmHg =

Anatomy and Physiology in Action: Box 2.4

Mean Arterial Pressure (MAP) – Why is this so important?

Essentially there is no 'normal blood pressure' for many patients with cardiovascular disease. Healthcare professionals can get caught out if a 'normal' blood pressure is recorded which might not be 'normal' for that patient. Another way of defining 'normal' blood pressure is whatever pressure is required to maintain organ function. As we age, that will certainly rise as arteries lose their elasticity and resistance increases. If the BP drops more than 30mmHg below 'normal' or premorbid blood pressure, it should be considered as hypotension for that patient.

For example, if the BP is 180/90 –

MAP = 180 + (90 x 2) = 360/3 = 120mmHg

If the BP drops to 120/80 this would not be recognised as significant by healthcare professionals as it lies within the 'normal' range. Attempts to restore the BP are not undertaken and this can result in organ failure.

MAP = 120 + (80 x 2) = 280/3 = 89mmHg

As you can see, there is a difference of about 30mmHg between the two MAPs; for some patients this may be the difference between maintaining the fine balance between adequate blood flow to the tissues and ischaemia and MODS.

Many patients can maintain perfusion even if the blood pressure is lower than normal; the important determining factor is whether the patient can maintain sufficient cardiac output and oxygen delivery to the vital organs over a period of time. Cardiac output is very difficult to measure outside of critical care areas. A much cheaper and simpler method is urine output. The kidneys are a very good indicator of adequate perfusion; you can measure the volume hourly, observe the colour and concentration, analyse the blood urea and electrolytes in relation to the history, clinical information and diagnosis.

Renal blood flow

Why are the kidneys so sensitive to blood pressure changes? Despite their innate ability to auto-regulate blood flow over a wide and variable blood pressure range (80–180mmHg), during periods of hypotension they cannot maintain this state for too long without ischaemia occurring. It's because they receive approximately 20–25% of the cardiac output per minute, which they are dependent upon. Normal cardiac output is roughly 5L/minute or 5000ml/minute. Renal blood flow is approximately 400ml/min/100g at rest. The kidneys require a high blood flow, as the primary function of the kidney is to filter blood and produce urine. Most of the filtration of the blood occurs in the cortex region of the kidney.

The hydrostatic pressure within the glomerular capillaries is much higher than in normal capillaries; this is important in maintaining the glomerular filtration rate within the Bowman's capsule. The kidney is richly innervated by sympathetic noradrenergic nerve fibres, which maintain the glomerular filtration rate (GFR) by altering the diameter of the afferent arterioles if arterial pressure falls. The afferent arteriole dilates to maintain blood flow and pressure within the glomerular capillary. Prostaglandin E_2 (PGE_2) is synthesised in the renal medulla cells and is a potent vasodilator. The kidney is able to maintain function and GFR by a combination of autoregulatory mechanisms across a wide range of pressures from 80–180mmHg and renal vasodilation.

In acutely unwell patients the urine output should be calculated using the following formula: 0.5ml/kg/hr.

It is essential that an accurate weight assessment is made to guide the amount of urine expected per hour.

Calculate the following:

Weight is 80kg. How much urine should the patient pass/hour?

80 x 0.5 = ml/hr

Ageing, arterial wall changes and other factors can affect the MAP, especially in the elderly; this makes it more difficult for blood to flow through the arteries due to changes in the luminal wall of the artery. As the pressure is increased along the length of the arteriole, the MAP will also increase; over time a higher MAP is required to maintain arterial circulation to the organs. A sustained fall in MAP as a result of hypovolaemia, dehydration, sepsis or myocardial injury can lead to ischaemia resulting in organ failure.

Before discussing the homeostatic control of blood pressure it is important to include a brief overview of oxygen supply and demand. Outside of intensive care units it is difficult to monitor whether the oxygen supply to the tissues is adequate or not. When patients experience an inadequate oxygen supply to metabolically active cells an oxygen debt is accrued, which, if not corrected, can lead to chest pain and myocardial infarction, rhythm disturbances, confusion, gut ischaemia, organ failure and many other clinical manifestations associated with hypoxia and lactic acidosis. It is important as nurses that we appreciate and understand our role when recording observations, particularly the respiration rate and oxygen saturations which may be the first clinical warning signs that there is a problem; we need to act on these early warning signs by communicating this in a timely fashion to medical colleagues and to ensure that appropriate interventions are commenced to correct the problem and to restore homeostasis as quickly as possible.

Oxygen delivery

The primary function of the cardiovascular system is to maintain adequate blood supply, nutrients and oxygen essential for aerobic respiration and to remove the waste products of cellular functions. The delivery of oxygen to tissues is dependent on availability in the atmosphere, diffusion of the gas across the alveolar–capillary membrane, haemoglobin-carrying capacity and finally the diffusion of oxygen down its concentration gradient across the cell membrane to be utilised by the mitochondria for energy or adenosine tri-phosphate (ATP) production.

Oxygen delivery can be represented by the equation outlined in Exercise Anatomy and Physiology in Action: Box 2.5.

The amount of oxygen delivered to the tissues in a healthy adult is about 1000ml/minute or 550ml/min/m². Normal oxygen consumption (VO_2) is 250ml/minute or 140ml/min/m² (Hinds & Watson 1996).

Anatomy and Physiology in Action: Exercise 2.11

$DO_2 = Q \ (Hb \ x \ 1.34 \ x \ SaO_2)$

DO2 = delivery of oxygen, Q = cardiac output

- Why is this important to maintain particularly in patients with homeostatic failure?
- What simple blood test is performed to analyse oxygen content in the blood?

Controlling and maintaining acid base balance

Let us now look at the acid base balance of fluids which is essentially the regulation of hydrogen (H^+) ion concentration of extracellular fluid (ECF). All cells are very sensitive to changes in H^+ ion concentration. You may have heard of the pH scale which is used to denote the H^+ ion concentration in solution or alternatively the number of moles per litre of molarity. The scale ranges from 0–14. It is logarithmic, that is, each change of one pH unit equals a tenfold increase in H^+ concentration: this is an important point to remember that can have profound clinical implications. The pH of a solution is defined as the negative logarithm of the hydrogen ion concentration [H^+] in moles/litre or $-\log$ [H^+] (Marieb 1998).

Anatomy and Physiology in Action: Box 2.5

The normal or optimal pH range for arterial blood = 7.4

Venous and interstitial fluid pH = 7.35
Intracellular fluid pH = 7.0
Arterial blood gases actually measure the true plasma pH. Any reading below 7.40 is acidosis and above 7.40 is alkalosis.

Normal Arterial Blood Gas Values:
pH = 7.35–7.45
$PaCO_2$ = 4.5–6.0 kPa (kilopascals is the unit of measurement)
PaO_2 = 10.6–13.3 kPa
HCO_3 = 22–26mmols
Base excess or deficit (BE) = –2 to +2

Carbon dioxide production, transport and excretion

A by-product of respiration is carbon dioxide (CO_2) produced in large amounts by cellular processes; it is an important influence on the pH of the blood. We produce approximately 15,000 to 20,000 mmol of CO_2 each day or 200ml/minute (Marieb 1998). The body is constantly balancing the pH of the blood and ECF to maintain equilibrium.

CO_2 is transported by three mechanisms; 60% is converted into bicarbonate (HCO_3^-) ions formed by the reaction of CO_2 and H_2O at tissue level, this forms a weak acidic solution – carbonic acid (H_2CO_3). CO_2 is transported in solution in the blood, as carbonic acid rapidly dissociates into bicarbonate (HCO_3^-) and H^+ ions in the presence of an enzyme carbonic anhydrase found mainly in red blood cells. As the blood passes across the alveolar capillary membrane, CO_2 diffuses from the capillary into the alveolar sac and is excreted by the lungs.

The body is very sensitive to minute changes in pH, CO_2 and O_2 levels. Excretion of CO_2 via the respiratory system is regulated by peripheral chemoreceptors found in the carotid bodies and aortic arch and central receptors in the medulla which are sensitive to the pH of the cerebrospinal fluid (CSF). CO_2 diffuses easily across the blood–brain barrier whereas H^+ and HCO_3^- do not. The response is mediated by the medulla, increasing impulses to the phrenic nerve which innervates the diaphragm and the intercostal nerves which innervate the intercostal muscles to increase the rate and depth of respirations within 1–3 minutes to rebalance CO_2 concentration.

Carbonate–bicarbonate buffering system

The kidneys are the main regulators of acid base along with proteins, blood (Hb) and acids which act as buffers to control sudden changes in pH. When the pH rises, H^+ ions (act as acids) are released to mop up the excess base. When the pH drops (acidosis) H^+ ions bind to raise pH back to normal. This results in shifting the blood pH within normal limits as H^+ is removed or added to blood. Why is the H^+ ion concentration so important? Essentially cells can become denatured and destroyed within a few hours if the pH is <6.8 or >8.0 even for a few hours. The kidneys may take a few hours or even days to alter the pH. What might happen to the delicate balance between acid and base if the patient has renal failure?

The phosphate buffer system is present in low concentrations in the ECF. The buffering systems include sodium salts of dihydrogen phosphate ($H_2PO_4^-$) and monohydrogen phosphate (HPO_4^{2-}) which are effective intracellular fluid buffers when phosphate levels are high. Some 75 per cent of all buffering occurs within the cells and plasma proteins. Amino acids are also involved in buffering; groups of atoms carboxyl (-COOH) dissociate and release H^+ ions as the pH rises, amino acids act as bases and accept protons (H^+) to reduce the acidity of

solutions. The kidneys have a number of functions maintaining acid-base homeostasis. They excrete other acids generated by cellular metabolism e.g. phosphoric, uric and lactic acid and ketone bodies. They regenerate new bicarbonate ions and replenish the stores as HCO_3^- is excreted from the lungs.

Developing and Delivering Expert Practice: Exercise 2.12

There are four main blood gas derangements:

- Respiratory acidosis
- Respiratory alkalosis
- Metabolic acidosis
- Metabolic alkalosis

Can you identify the causes of each of the above acid base disturbances and also determine whether the pH will be acidic or alkaline, and whether the CO_2 and HCO_3^- will be elevated or lowered? Interpreting blood gases is complicated and takes time, in your clinical areas collect some examples and see if you can work them out. Get a colleague to check your answers.

In summary

Acid base balance is a dynamic and constantly changing process. It is dependent on functioning lungs and kidneys, adequate haemoglobin and steady homeostatic states. When patients experience an insult such as Mark Bradbury has, this fine balance is disrupted and compensatory mechanisms are activated. If the insult is overwhelming despite the activation of the above mechanisms, decompensation will occur which may result in respiratory and/or cardiac arrest if uncorrected.

Control of insulin and glucose release

The pancreas is both an endocrine (consists of ductless glands that empty hormones directly into the bloodstream) and exocrine gland, releasing pancreatic juice into the small intestine for digestive purposes. Millions of pancreatic islets – the Islets of Langerhans – produce pancreatic hormones from the following cells:

- Alpha cells – Involved in glucagon synthesis
- Beta cells – Insulin production

- Delta cells – Growth hormone inhibiting factor (GHIF) somatostatin.

We are going to focus on the endocrine function of the pancreas; the release of insulin in response to raised blood glucose levels.

What is insulin?

Insulin is comprised of a 51 chain of amino acid synthesised by the beta cells. It is synthesised as a polypeptide chain proinsulin. Insulin has a very short half-life of 5 minutes. Eighty per cent of insulin is degraded by the liver and kidneys. Raised blood levels of glucose stimulate the release of insulin. The activation of insulin causes glucose to enter target cells. Insulin triggers enzyme activity which catalyses the oxidation of glucose for ATP production, enhances glycogenesis and converts glucose to fat (lipogenesis). Insulin stimulates amino acid uptake, protein synthesis and fat storage.

Developing and Delivering Expert Care: Box 2.7

Physiological effects of insulin
- Lowers blood sugar levels – (accelerates glycogenesis)
- Increases the membrane transport of glucose into cells
- Influences protein and fat metabolism

Insulin inhibits
- Glycogen breakdown to glucose (glycogenolysis)
- Amino acid and fatty acid conversion to glucose (gluconeogenesis)

Hyperglycaemia – defined as beta cells secreting insulin in response to
- Catecholamines (epinephrine)
- Growth hormone
- Glucagon
- Thyroxine

Gluconeogenesis 'new glucose'

Gluconeogenesis is the synthesis of glucose from lactic acid and non-carbohydrate molecules e.g. fatty acids, glycerol and amino acids. The release of glucose by liver cells into the blood causes the blood glucose level to rise.

The rise in blood glucose inhibits glucagon release and stimulates the secretion of insulin. Glucagon is released by alpha cells in response to a fall in blood glucose levels and is another example of a negative feedback system. Secretion is inhibited by GHIF (somatostatin). Glucose enters cells by facilitated diffusion. Normal venous glucose levels are 3.6–6.1mmol/L.

Figure 2.5 summarises the example of a negative feedback system. Patients who are experiencing high levels of stress may have a stress-induced hyperglycaemia

Developing and Delivering Expert Care: Box 2.8

Different Types of Shock

Hypovolaemic shock may result from a number of reasons, from haemorrhage as in the clinical case or from other factors as listed below:

- Exogenous – burns, trauma, sepsis
- Endogenous – interstitial loss or third space fluid shifts
- Increased capillary leakage

The main clinical characteristics are a reduction in circulating volume, reduced venous return, reduced stroke volume and cardiac output and ultimately blood pressure. The only simple bedside measurement available is blood pressure. However, as we will discover later on when we review the compensatory mechanisms for maintaining blood pressure, hypotension is often a late sign and can be misleading, as the body may have experienced a significant loss of circulating volume before the blood pressure changes.

Cardiogenic shock is defined as a systolic arterial pressure <90mmHg, and in a patient with known hypertension a fall of more than 30mmHg from their premorbid reading. Other features include reduced renal perfusion, urine output <20ml/hour, cold and peripherally vasoconstricted, changes to mental state – i.e. new onset confusion and signs of myocardial failure such as raised jugular venous pressure, pulmonary oedema and basal crepitations.

Causes:

- Acute myocardial infarction
- Cardiomyopathy
- Myocardial dysfunction post cardiac surgery
- Mitral and aortic regurgitation

Obstructive shock is defined as a fall in cardiac output due to mechanical obstruction to the circulation or by restriction of ventricular filling and ejection

- Cardiac tamponade – is the accumulation of fluid or blood in the pericardial sac. It acts like a tourniquet around the heart or myocardium reducing the force and contractility of the ventricular contraction and so less blood is ejected/beat.
- Pulmonary embolism – can completely occlude the pulmonary capillary circulation causing catastrophic circulatory collapse.

In both scenarios severe and refractory hypotension is the main clinical feature associated with distended neck veins, cyanosis, tachycardia, severe respiratory distress (in PE) and if untreated both situations can lead to cardio-respiratory arrest and death.

Distributive shock – is essentially related to the maldistribution of blood flow caused by severe and prolonged vasodilation and changes in vascular resistance as a result of anaphylactic reaction to antibiotics, blood transfusions or allergies. Other factors such as sepsis or spinal cord injury where there is a loss of vascular tone and capacitance.

Figure 2.5 Negative feedback system: blood glucose and control

as a result of sepsis, catecholamines, glucagons, cortisol and growth hormone; this is due to excessive glucose release.

Defining shock/haemodynamic collapse

Patients may experience circulatory collapse for a variety of reasons: this is commonly known as shock. Physiological shock can be defined as an inadequate circulatory volume to facilitate the oxygenation and nutritional needs of the body's cells; this internal insult is intensified by the insufficient removal of the waste products of cellular metabolism (leading to metabolic acidosis). Initially this can result in compensatory homeostatic responses, which aim to counteract the internally identified deficit or surplus of waste products. If homeostasis is not restored, the internal environment will become increasingly hypoxic and acidotic. This acidotic environment is not compatible with cellular function, initially resulting in cellular injury. Depending on the insult this process can be instantaneous or have a gradual accumulative effect escalating from cell to tissue damage, and progressing into multiorgan failure.

In clinical practice all serious illnesses have the potential to result in reduced cellular perfusion producing physiological shock.

Now that you have gained insight into the different types of shock, the chapter will progress into discussing the protective and compensatory mechanisms the body can deploy to avert the problems associated with shock such as tissue necrosis and the initial patient assessment process will be discussed, providing the reader with a

Developing and Delivering Expert Care: Box 2.9

Stages of Shock

There are essentially four stages of shock:

- **Initial stage**: tissues are poorly perfused; there is a decreased cardiac output (CO), increased anaerobic metabolism and lactic acid formation
- **Compensatory stage**: is still reversible. Low CO activates sympathetic nervous system and compensatory mechanisms are deployed to improve tissue perfusion
- **Progressive stage**: compensatory mechanisms are inadequate and failing. There is profound vasoconstriction, with severe metabolic acidosis, CNS and myocardial depression
- **Irreversible or refractory stage**: cellular necrosis and multiple organ failure are evident and non-retractable.

As healthcare professionals it is important that we can recognise the different signs and stages of shock to prevent and anticipate further problems, to communicate effectively to other professional groups and to proactively intervene with appropriate and life-saving treatments.

structured approach to patient care that can be applied throughout their developing career.

Blood pressure

Blood pressure is normally regulated by several complex and inter-related neural, chemical and hormonal mechanisms. It is an example of a negative feedback system.

In cardiogenic shock the problem is not hypovolaemia-induced hypotension but the lack of response by the heart muscle to the stimulatory effects of adrenaline and nor-adrenaline. Compensatory mechanisms are activated but are ineffective. The same is seen in septic shock when the peripheral vasculature cannot vasoconstrict the arteries in response to sympathetic stimulation, compensation is ineffective resulting in a high cardiac output, tachycardia, hypotension and vasodilation or reduced systemic vascular resistance (SVR).

Hypovolaemia-induced hypotension

Changes in blood pressure are detected by baroreceptors found in the arch of the aorta, carotid sinus and all large arteries of the neck and thorax. The first part of the reflex to be activated is the baroreceptors or 'stretch' receptors, which are sensitive to changes in the stretch or pressure exerted by fluctuations in the volume of blood. When blood pressure falls, the receptors detect a change in the amount of 'stretch', there is an increased rate of impulses firing via afferent pathways back to the vasomotor or cardio-acceleratory centre within the medulla oblongata. Cardiac output, as discussed in Chapter 4, is the heart rate multiplied by the stroke volume, stroke volume being the amount of blood ejected per ventricle per beat. The stroke volume falls during haemorrhage as does the cardiac output, what is seen clinically is a fall in systolic blood pressure, and a narrowing of the pulse pressure. To compensate for the reduction in stroke volume, the heart rate is increased to distribute less blood faster around the body to the major organs to maintain oxygen delivery, perfusion and ultimately organ function.

How is the heart rate increased?

The heart rate is usually under the autonomic control of the parasympathetic or vagal nerve fibres (see Chapter 4 for more detail). The medulla receives information from baroreceptors and chemoreceptors via afferent nerve pathways on the volume and pressure status within the cardiovascular system. During times of emotional or physical stress and illness the sympathetic nervous system, via efferent vagal fibres, induces the 'fight or flight response' by releasing noradrenaline from nerve fibres which bind to beta one (β_1) adrenoreceptors within the heart muscle to increase the force of contraction (inotropy) and the heart rate (chronotropy). The adrenal medulla synthesises adrenaline and noradrenaline, which circulate in the blood stream. Adrenaline binds to β_1 adrenoreceptors also increasing heart rate and contractility. At higher concentrations of adrenaline it binds to alpha (α_1) adrenoreceptors causing peripheral smooth muscle vasoconstriction. As the rate of impulses from the SA node is increased, the conductivity of the impulse through the AV node also has to increase. In other words the gate (AV node) is opened to let more impulses pass through so that the ventricles can contract faster to raise the cardiac output.

Noradrenaline also exerts a vasoconstricting effect on the vasculature by binding to α_1 adrenoreceptors within the tunica media (middle arterial wall lumen) to bring about vasoconstriction of the vascular smooth muscle and increased systemic vascular resistance. Vasoconstriction shunts blood away from the peripheral circulation and the gut to the core organs; the clinical signs exhibited are cold, shutdown peripheries with an increased capillary refill time, as demonstrated by the clinical case in Scenario 2.1. The redirection of blood flow away from the mesenteric circulation of the gut is very difficult to measure and quantify, but the patient may exhibit signs such as nausea and vomiting.

Developing and Delivering Expert Practice: Exercise 2.13

In the elderly due to SA node disease and conduction problems, this may not be evident.

- Why might this be a problem if a patient is bleeding and the heart rate did not increase?

Patients on beta blockers will not be able to increase their heart rate as a natural response, why not?

What effects does beta blockade have on sympathetic stimulation?

Refer to the *British National Formulary* (BNF) for your answer.

Overall, the cardiovascular effects of noradrenaline on the blood pressure are increased blood pressure, MAP and pulse pressure. The collective term for noradrenaline and adrenaline is catecholamine; high catecholamine levels in the blood also stimulate the release of renin which is an important polypeptide released in low perfusion states by the kidney as part of the compensatory mechanisms for blood pressure control. While the body is attempting to maximise and increase available circulating blood volume, it also attempts to reduce urine output and water loss by stimulating other hormones such as aldosterone and anti-diuretic hormone to conserve water.

Renin-angiotensin-aldosterone mechanisms

In response to a significant drop in renal artery pressure below 80mmHg, such as in Scenario 2.1, the low blood pressure and MAP would stimulate the kidney's own tubuloglomerular feedback mechanism which is coordinated by the macula densa cells of the juxtamedullary apparatus (JMA). The reduced stretch on the juxtaglomerular cells is similar to the effects of baroreceptors. Other mechanisms such as increased β_1 adrenoreceptor stimulation brought about by sympathetic activity from the renal nerve triggered by shock and the kidney detect haemorrhage. The vasodilation of the afferent arteriole is also another indicator that something is wrong with blood flow. When the GFR, arterial blood pressure and circulating volume fall, as in our case scenario due to haemorrhage, there is a decrease in the delivery of sodium and chloride ions to the distal convoluted tubule which is detected by the macula densa cells. Remember they control and initiate the kidney's own feedback mechanism. A fall in the plasma concentrations of sodium and potassium ions also stimulates the secretion of renin. The combination of all these mechanisms causes renin to be released from the juxtaglomerular cells. Renin has a direct action on and causes afferent arteriole constriction.

Renin's main purpose is to bring about the release of the enzyme angiotensinogen from the liver, which undergoes a catalytic change to form angiotensin I. It circulates throughout the blood; certain endothelial membranes, particularly within the lining of the lung, produce an enzyme called the angiotensin-converting enzyme (ACE). When the angiotensin comes into contact with the enzyme, it converts angiotensin I to angiotensin II, a powerful vasoconstrictor. Further peripheral vasoconstriction occurs by increasing the systemic vascular resistance and raising the blood pressure. Angiotensin II also causes vasoconstriction of the efferent arterioles increasing the glomerular capillary pressure in the Bowman's capsule to maintain GFR. The glomerular filtration rate is the amount of filtrate produced per minute by the kidneys. Normal GFR is 120–125ml/minute or about 7.5L/hour. Ninety-nine per cent of filtrate is normally reabsorbed; normal urine production per day is 1–1.5L. The reason why maintaining the GFR is so crucial is that the GFR is directly proportional to the net filtration pressure, this means that even small changes in the hydrostatic pressure of the glomerular capillary or the large surface area available for filtration will affect the rate at which solutes are removed from the filtrate and the reabsorption of water and other substances. Filtration can cease completely with relatively small changes in blood pressure. It is also important to remember that the kidneys have a high demand for oxygen and are very sensitive to changes in oxygen delivery which can result in pre-renal failure, ischaemia or acute tubular necrosis (ATN).

Angiotensin II also acts on the adrenal cortex to release aldosterone, a mineralocorticoid. The function of aldosterone is to increase the reabsorption of sodium and water in the distal convoluted tubules in the kidney in response to low blood pressure and low circulating blood volume. As a result of this, the urine becomes dark and concentrated as water is removed.

Anti-diuretic hormone

Angiotensin II also stimulates the release of anti-diuretic hormone (ADH), or vasopressin, from the posterior pituitary. Anti-diuretic hormone inhibits or affects the production of urine. The hormone is released when water needs to be conserved. ADH exerts its effect on the lining of the distal convoluted tubule (DCT) and collecting ducts by increasing water permeability. Water moves out of the DCT and collecting ducts by osmosis and is reabsorbed by the peritubular capillaries and transported into the circulation to raise the circulating volume. The removal of water also causes sodium to move across and so both water and sodium are reabsorbed. ADH is also triggered by pain and emotional stress, hypoxia, severe exercise and surgery. In the absence of ADH, dilute urine is formed, this is called diabetes insipidus. Excessive ingestion of alcohol inhibits ADH production causing the loss of large volumes of urine, intense thirst and a dry mouth.

ADH is also released by the hypothalamus in response to signals from osmoreceptors located in the

Developing and Delivering Expert Practice: Box 2.9

Diabetes insipidus is a syndrome of ADH deficiency. It is characterised by the production of large amounts of dilute urine leading to dehydration and unrelieved thirst. It can be caused by damage to the hypothalamus or the posterior pituitary gland as a result of raised intracranial pressure from head injuries.

hypothalamus, which constantly detect the concentration of solutes in the blood. When the solute concentration is increased, the osmoreceptors send impulses to the hypothalamus to secrete ADH. The thirst mechanism is also stimulated so that more water is consumed to balance the concentration of the solutes.

Structured initial assessment

One of the principal skills required by all nurses is the ability to carry out a timely, but comprehensive, patient assessment. The focal point is to ascertain the individual care needs of the patient and prioritise subsequent treatment. To function effectively the practitioner requires excellent communication skills, and a thorough understanding of how pathology and trauma can affect the internal environment and its equilibrium leading to the clinically recognised state of physiological shock.

The initial assessment

There are numerous assessment models, or mnemonics, currently adapted to suit the needs of acutely ill patients and clinical practice. The Resuscitation Council in the United Kingdom (RCUK 2006) recommends the universal adoption of the ABCDE structure (Box 2.10), where each category addresses a separate, but intrinsically linked body component.

Vital signs

Vital signs directly demonstrate the current physiological state of the patient, yet research has clearly demonstrated the inability of healthcare professionals to correctly interpret or act on recorded data. The most common mistake nurses make is to underestimate the seriousness of the clinical data they have recorded; this is of particular

importance in relation to the blood pressure due to an over-reliance on this one component. Many clinicians fail to recognise the subtle signs of deterioration associated with shock until there is a dramatic decrease in the blood pressure. The respiratory system is the first to demonstrate compensation therefore the application of the ABC approach will identify deficits early in the assessment process (the reader is referred to Evans & Tippins 2007 for

Developing and Delivering Expert Practice: Box 2.10

ABCDE Mnemonic

A = Airway and cervical spine immobilisation (Chapter 15)

When assessing a patient's potential to maintain their own airway, think about why they have been admitted or why they need assessment. This will provide vital clues as to what you might expect. For example, if the patient has been involved in an accident, they may have sustained a head injury thereby rendering them unconscious, they may have trauma to their mouth and bleeding. The mechanism of injury provides vital clues!

B = Breathing and ventilation (Chapter 3)
Refer to Chapter 3 which describes the full process

C = Circulation and haemorrhage control (Chapter 4)
A circulatory assessment should always focus on initially looking at the patient for signs of life and perfusion (Chapter 15). Always feel their pulse to ascertain the Rate, Rhythm and Depth.

D = Disability and neurological assessment (Chapter 5)
Chapter 5 provides in-depth detail on a neurological assessment. In the short term the AVPU tool can be applied.

E = Exposure and environment
No assessment is complete without recording the patient's temperature (an indicator of the internal environment); depending on the type of presentation, the nurse may need to see the front and back of the patient to look for signs of injury – remember dignity and respect, in addition, a chaperone may be required.

in-depth patient assessment techniques and scenario-based demonstrations).

Possible misleading data

Many factors can affect the reliability of vital signs data and clinicians need to take this into consideration when interpreting data. These include any other internal mechanisms that initiate the fight or flight response. These mechanisms mimic the instigation of the compensatory phase of shock, i.e. pain, fear, anxiety and stimulants. In contrast, several commonly prescribed medications can inhibit the compensatory response, these include beta blockers.

Developing and Delivering Expert Practice: Box 2.11

Level of Consciousness
A = Alert
V = Responds to a Verbal Stimulus
P = Responds to a Painful Stimulus
U = Unresponsive

Capillary refill time (CRT)

The recording of a CRT in addition to a radial pulse is an excellent indicator of peripheral perfusion. The patient's nail bed or the pulp of the finger is compressed for five seconds with sufficient pressure to cause blanching. Once pressure is released the nail bed should be engorged with blood and return to normal.

- In adults a CRT of two seconds or less will indicate good peripheral perfusion
- A prolonged CRT should be interpreted in conjunction with other circulatory parameters, such as pulse rate, blood pressure, and conscious level (RCUK 2006).

This figure can be prolonged in the elderly, in a cold environment, and in the presence of poor ambient lighting or circulation-based anomalies such as Raynaud's phenomenon.

Postural blood pressure

Under normal conditions autonomic reflexes stabilise an individual's blood pressure from the lying to sitting/standing positions. This can be seen as the initiation of quick response mediators that result in peripheral vasoconstriction and shunting of blood into the main circulation. When there is an established loss of circulating volume in the peripheries, this mechanism fails and a fall in blood pressure results, the recording of a postural blood pressure, therefore, is an excellent eliminative tool to the practitioner suspecting a patient to be in the early stages of shock.

Example of a patient experiencing reduced circulating volume:

- Lying B/P 105/70, H/R 90
- Sitting B/P 85/58, H/R 115

A positive result is achieved if the patient's blood pressure demonstrates a systolic drop of >20mmHg from lying to standing, or >15mmHg from lying to sitting, although the differential may be slightly less, this is offset by dangling the patient's legs over the trolley and the reduction in risk potential. Rises in heart rate exceeding 20 beats per minute (bpm), or a diastolic drop exceeding 10mmHg are also positive indicators.

If circumstances allow, lay the patient supine for five minutes, record a blood pressure and heart rate, then assist them to sit up, allow 1–3 minutes then record vital signs with the patient's legs dangling over the side of the trolley. Be aware of the possibility that your patient may become acutely unwell and document any changes to the initial assessment findings.

Defining the cause of shock

Defining the cause of shock will determine the focus of treatment, as the causative agent will need to be dealt with to combat the pathophysiological processes taking place. Shock is a progressive state and, therefore, early identification facilitates early intervention, which improves the patient's prognosis. A dramatic example is demonstrated in the management of meningitis. If left untreated until obvious signs like a haemorrhagic rash are evident, the long-term prognosis is poor.

Conclusion

Maintaining homeostasis is a dynamic process affecting all organs and cells of the body. It comprises complex, inter-related and interdependent systems that respond to the internal and external environment. As nurses, our role is to understand the complexities of the chemical, neural and hormonal interplay and how this can manifest as a single disease or as a result of multiple pathologies. Clinical treatments may range from simply correcting hypoxaemia or fluid deficits to the instigation of multi-organ support systems. Our role is to recognise, administer and constantly evaluate prescribed treatment until the fine balance of homeostasis is achieved.

The combined efforts of vasoconstriction of the smooth muscles, the redirection of blood flow, raising of the heart rate, and the complex interplay between the kidneys, adrenal glands and the hypothalamus, all assist in raising blood pressure and maintaining vital oxygen and nutrient supply in potential times of crisis. By applying the structured assessment process discussed, the nurse can identify varying degrees of illness at an early stage and initiate a plan of care based on a working diagnosis which is open to change as the assessment process broadens to encompass specialists and various members of the multidisciplinary team. Complete the following quiz to see direct evidence of your professional development and identify areas in need of further development.

Chapter 2 Summary Quiz

1. What is homeostasis?

A. The brain's ability to speed things up
B. The state of functional equilibrium within the body's internal environment
C. The state of gases within the body
D. The equilibrium of the venous and arterial blood supplies

2. Catecholamines describe hormones such as:

A. Noradrenaline and adrenaline
B. Glucose and oxygen
C. Blood and lymph
D. Vasopressin and methohaemoglobin

3. Normal body temperature ranges between:

A. 31.6°C–36.8°C
B. 35.6°C–37.8°C
C. 36.6°C–39.8°C
D. 35.6°C–36.9°C

4. Which of the following can result in a fever?

A. Infections
B. Inflammation
C. Allergic reactions
D. All of the above

5. A MAP of above what pressure is needed to supply the coronary and cerebral arteries and the kidneys?

A. 90mmHg

B. 10mmHg

C. 60mmHg

D. 120mmHg

6. Body fluids function optimally within a narrow range, at an arterial blood pH ranging between

A. 7.0 and 7.9

B. 0 and 14

C. 7.45 and 7.55

D. 7.35 and 7.45

7. Physiological shock can be defined as:

A. An inadequate circulatory volume to facilitate the oxygenation and nutritional needs of the body's cells

B. Not enough blood to produce urine

C. An inadequate circulatory volume to facilitate the process of haemofiltration

D. A severe fright causing stress

8. If a patient was demonstrating compensatory physiological shock, which of the following blood pressures would be expected?

A. 120/80

B. 50/30

C. 70/60

D. 84/59

9. How long should an area of skin be pressed on to identify the capillary refill time?

A. 1 minute

B. 10 seconds

C. 20 seconds

D. 5 seconds

10. What is an easy to remember tool for both respiratory and cardiovascular assessment?

A. Rate, rhythm and depth

B. Rate, listen and feel

C. Look listen and cross

D. Feel, count and write

Further reading

Cannon, W. (1932) *The Wisdom of the Body*. W.W. Norton: New York. (/http://en.wikipedia.org/wiki/Walter_Bradford_Cannon)

Evans, C. & Tippins, E. (2007) *Foundations of Emergency Care*. Open University Press: Maidenhead.

Klabunde, R.E. (2005) *Cardiovascular Physiology Concepts*. Lippincott Williams & Wilkins: Philadelphia.

Ramrakha, P. & Moore, K. (2003) *Oxford Handbook of Acute Medicine*. Oxford University Press: New York.

Saladin, K. (2007) *Anatomy and Physiology: The Unity of Form and Function*, 4th edn. McGraw-Hill Higher Education: New York.

http://www.resus.org.uk/siteindx.htm

References

Clancy, J. & McVicar, A.J. (2002) *Physiology and Anatomy: A Homeostatic Approach*, 2nd edn. Arnold: London.

Evans, C. & Tippins, E. (2007) *Foundations of Emergency Care*. Open University Press: Maidenhead.

Ganong, W.F. (1995) *Review of Medical Physiology*, 17th edn. Prentice Hall: London.

Hinchliffe, S.M., Montague, S.E. & Watson, R. (1999) *Physiology for Nursing Practice*. Baillière Tindall: London.

Hinds, C.J. & Watson, D. (1996) *Intensive Care: A Concise Textbook*, 2nd edn. WB Saunders: London.

Klabunde, R.E. (2005) *Cardiovascular Physiology Concepts*. Lippincott Williams & Wilkins: Philadelphia.

Marieb, E.N. (1998) *Human Anatomy and Physiology*, 4th edn. Benjamin-Cummings Publishing: California.

3

The respiratory system

Cliff Evans and Emma Tippins

Part 3 Learning Objectives

- Gain knowledge and insight into the anatomy and physiology of the respiratory system
- Gain insight into several common conditions affecting these systems
- Apply theory to practice by understanding the physical manifestation of these illnesses in patients
- Gain understanding of commonly used medications to either prevent or treat respiratory conditions
- Learn essential practical skills that can be easily applied within clinical practice
- Learn to apply a solid structured approach to the patient assessment process
- Construct solid evidence of professional development for your growing portfolio
- Continue developing the ability to question and critique the evidence base and effectiveness of plans of care

Introduction

In the UK, respiratory diseases are responsible for more emergency hospital admissions than diseases of any other origin (LHO 2007). Many respiratory conditions are easy to assess and treat and despite a continual reduction in mortality rates over recent years in England and Wales, respiratory disease and infections still caused 11% of deaths among those aged 15–74 in 2000 (ONS 2007). Many problems can lead to respiratory distress, ranging from obstruction of the upper airway through to infection, emotional distress, hyperventilation and hypersensitivity reactions such as asthma. One of the most prevalent diseases affecting the respiratory system is chronic obstructive pulmonary disease (COPD): this disease alone affects around 900,000 individuals within the UK and accounts for in excess of 30,000 deaths per year, making it the fastest growing cause of death in the UK (British Lung Foundation 2005, GOLD 2006).

This chapter will initially guide the reader through both the form and function of the respiratory system; this will be aided by several exercises that the reader can undertake to consolidate new learning and provide evidence of professional development. The chapter progresses into discussing several disease processes that impact on respiratory function resulting in both acute hospital and primary care presentations and a chronically reduced ability to function. Many of the chronic conditions identified within the Government's National Service Framework (NSF) for long-term conditions and the NSF for older people have a respiratory component (DH 2001, 2005). The use of clinical scenarios will provide the reader with insight into how acute respiratory conditions are initially assessed and managed, and how their long-term management and treatment can be a complex multidimensional undertaking.

Form

The form of the respiratory system centres on several vital organs and their components, which work in unison with a range of muscles to produce the act of respiration. Figure 3.1 identifies the vital components that aid the passage of oxygen in and out of the body.

The initial structures of the respiratory system are the mouth, or oropharynx, and the nose. Although the nose, which is lined with special types of tissue cells and hair to filter and moisten air, is the primary route for the conveyance of air, the mouth can also relay air into the upper airway passages leading to the lungs.

Applying Theory to Practice: Exercise 3.1

- Why is it necessary to have two air entry points?
- If an individual breathes predominantly through the mouth rather than the nose, what might the long-term consequences be?

From Figure 3.1 identify where the two air entry points converge.

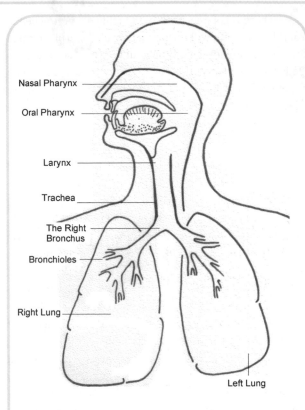

Nasal Pharynx

Oral Pharynx

Larynx

Trachea

The Right
Bronchus

Bronchioles

Right Lung

Left Lung

Figure 3.1 The main components of the respiratory system

The pharynx, larynx, trachea, bronchi and bronchioles

These structures are considered together as they form a continuous link between the air entry points and the beginning of the lungs. The 12.5cm passageway that forms the pharynx leads from the back of the mouth and nose, dividing into the oesophagus at the rear of the throat, and the larynx at the front. At the rear of the pharynx, at the base of the nose, sit small collections of **lymphoid** tissue known as the adenoids; in conjunction with similar structures called the palatine tonsils at the junction of the mouth and throat, they combine to filter invading bacteria.

Applying Theory to Practice: Exercise 3.2

Bacterial and viral infections of the airways are extremely common (BTS 2004), complete the following exercise before continuing:

- Make a list of at least three common infections that affect the upper airways
- What would be the clinical signs that someone was experiencing one of these infections?
- Do these infections need treating with drugs, if so, which ones?

The nose

The nose consists of two nasal bones and cartilage. The inside of the nostrils is lined with a **ciliated** mucous membrane (Figure 3.2). The nostrils are divided by the nasal septum composed of cartilage. This means the nose is soft on the outside and bony on the inside. The nostrils link with the paranasal sinuses, hollow air-filled spaces also lined with cilia.

The hyoid bone, which provides stability for the tongue and the epiglottis, is positioned at the top of the larynx. The epiglottis is the small movable flap that covers the airway to prevent the inhalation of particles of food and water into the airway. Some individuals can lose the

Cila
Hair-Like Projections

Ciliated
Columnar Cells

Figure 3.2 Ciliated tissues. Note that ciliated tissue opposes the flow of air resulting in foreign particles or bacteria/debris being swept away from the lower airways and lungs

Figure 3.3a The upper airway tracts

Labels: Nasal Pharynx, Oral Pharynx, Tongue, Epiglottis, Larynx, Oesophagus

males where it is larger than in the female. The trachea is around 10cm long with incomplete hyaline cartilage rings running its outside length; involuntary muscle and connective tissues form the back or posterior aspect. The trachea is lined with a rich supply of mucus-secreting goblet cells.

The airway so far has consisted of a single pathway (excluding the mouth); the bronchi are where the single passageway splits in two, one leading to the right lung and one leading to the left. The bronchi are similar in composition to the trachea, consisting of hyaline cartilage, involuntary muscle and connective tissues. The inside of the bronchi are still lined with ciliated **epithelium**. The bronchioles should be envisaged as the last segment of a continuous passageway from the nose and mouth to the lungs. These increasingly fine tubes are composed of elastic, fibrous and muscular tissue.

The lungs

The lungs lie either side of the heart; the left lung consists of two lobes (superior and inferior), the right lung has an additional lobe (the middle lobe). Lung tissue is the combination of bronchioles, blood vessels, elastic and connective tissue, nerves and alveoli. A double-layered membrane, called the pleura, individually surrounds the lungs.

ability to manage this involuntary function, which can potentially result in aspiration pneumonia.

The larynx, commonly referred to as the voice box, begins at the back of the mouth leading down the neck towards the trachea; both the larynx and trachea are composed of rings of cartilage attached by membranes and ligaments. The thyroid cartilage surrounding the larynx forms the Adam's apple, which is often visible in

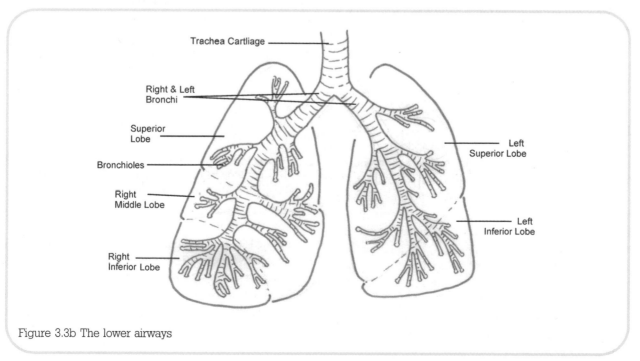

Figure 3.3b The lower airways

Labels: Trachea Cartliage, Right & Left Bronchi, Superior Lobe, Bronchioles, Right Middle Lobe, Right Inferior Lobe, Left Superior Lobe, Left Inferior Lobe

Anatomy and Physiology in Action: Exercise 3.3

Common disease processes can affect the amount of fibrous and elastic tissue as well the muscularity of the bronchioles:

- Identify one disease process that results in hypertrophy of the involuntary muscles within the bronchioles
- What are the physical consequences of a hypertrophic muscular layer within the bronchiole?

The pleurae

The two layers of the serous membrane that form the pleurae surround the lungs. The inner layer, or visceral layer, covers the surface and the outer layer, the parietal layer, adheres to the chest wall and to the diaphragm below. Between the two layers there exists a potential space containing serous fluid.

The acinus

The alveoli, of which there are an estimated 300 million within the lungs, are the point where air stops travelling and the action of respiration begins. The acinus is composed of the terminal portions of the bronchioles, which at this point are extremely fine, or one cell thick, and the alveolar ducts, which in turn open into two or three alveolar sacs, progress into several alveoli.

The muscles of respiration

Muscles that enable the act of respiration are as essential as the organs or structures that enable the passage of air to the alveoli. These muscles are so vital that if they begin to fail, the body has several reserve muscles that can also aid respiration; these are called the accessory muscles. Visualising the accessory muscles in a patient is a clear clinical indicator of respiratory distress, and individuals with chronic respiratory disease may have overdeveloped accessory muscles due to their continual use. The main muscle of respiration is the diaphragm, a large muscular sheet that separates the chest cavity from the abdominal contents. Lying beneath the lungs, the diaphragm resembles a dome and stretches across the base of the chest, attached at various points to bone for stabilisation. The sternocleidomastoid and intercostal muscles all assist in respiration.

Function

The act of respiration is a constant process that does not require conscious effort as it is driven by both voluntary and involuntary control mechanisms. In combination with the muscles of respiration, air is drawn in by active contraction of the thorax; during inhalation the diaphragm contracts downward and away from the lungs, creating more space in the chest cavity. This lowers the air pressure in the chest cavity relative to the pressure outside the body, subsequently air moves into the lungs. The diaphragm works in combination with the muscles of the neck which attach to the upper part of the sternum and clavicles; the sternocleidomastoid muscle, and the muscles between the ribs; the internal and external intercostal muscles; these increase the diameter of the chest wall, decreasing the pressure in the chest. The intercostal muscles then contract and minimise the size of the chest wall during forced exhalation.

The respiratory system is typically divided into two descriptive components: the acts of conduction and respiration; that is, a percentage of the respiratory system is dedicated to aiding the conduction of oxygen into the lungs; this function must also include warming of the air to achieve a level of heat conducive to homeostasis, the facilitation of diffusion, and the filtering of particles such as dust and contaminants. Once the air reaches the alveoli, the process of respiration can take place. The act of respiration can also be divided into two succinct parts:

- **External respiration** centres on the exchange of gases through diffusion between the alveoli and the bloodstream. A network of small blood capillaries surrounds the alveolar wall. The alveoli provide a large surface area for gaseous exchange, estimated at 70 to 80 square metres if stretched out (Shire et al. 2004). Venous or deoxygenated blood arrives at the lungs, via the right side of the heart and the pulmonary arteries, containing high levels of carbon dioxide (CO_2) and low levels of oxygen (O_2). The CO_2 diffuses into the alveoli until the point of equal pressure or equilibrium is realised. Simultaneously O_2 diffuses from the alveoli into the blood. This newly oxygenated blood is returned to the left side of the heart via the pulmonary veins. Once it reaches the heart, it is pumped to the systemic circulation to facilitate the process of internal respiration and the oxygenation of all cells. Blood flow through the capillaries is slow due to their relative

Form	Structure	Function
Nose	Composed of cartilage Lined with a ciliated mucous membrane The nasal cavity connects to the paranasal sinuses also lined with a mucous membrane	Sensual organ – smell Warms, moistens air Cilia – filter dust and foreign particles including bacteria Mucus secretion is part of the defensive inflammatory system which prevents particles entering the lungs
Pharynx	Around 12.5cm in length Composed of muscular and fibrous tissue Contains the lymphoid pharyngeal tonsils (adenoids)	Continues the process of warming, filtering and moistening air Lymphoid tissue filters and eradicates bacteria
Larynx	Tube-like structure Commonly referred to as the voice box Consisting of cartilage rings Contains the thyroid cartilage	Maintains voice production Continues the process of warming, filtering and moistening inspired air
Trachea	Continuation of the larynx Around 10cm in length Terminates to divide into the two bronchi Consists of hyaline cartilage (anteriorly) and involuntary muscle (posteriorly)	Continues the process of warming, filtering and moistening inspired air Secretes mucus from goblet cells
Bronchi	Connection points of trachea to lungs Consist of hyaline cartilage and involuntary muscle	Passageway for inspired air into the lungs
Bronchioles	Composed of muscular fibrous and elastic tissue Continually narrow until they meet the alveoli	Passageway for inspired air into the lungs
Alveoli	Composed of squamous epithelial cells Entwined with blood capillaries	Point of gaseous exchange Carbon dioxide is expelled back through the respiratory system and deoxygenated blood is circulated through the alveoli where it obtains oxygen through the process of diffusion
Lungs	The two lungs are divided into lobes, the right having superior, middle and inferior lobes, the left having just superior and inferior Lung tissue is composed of the alveoli, blood vessels, elastic connective tissue	The lungs facilitate the act of breathing In combination with the muscles of respiration the lungs inspire and expel air
Pleura	Serous membrane covering each lung Composed of an inner visceral layer and an outer parietal layer These layers are separated by a potential space lubricated with serous fluid	Prevents friction during the two layers as the lungs expand and contract. Provides structural points for the lungs

Table 3.1 Form and Function of the Respiratory System

Reproduced from Evans & Tippins (2007).

size; this allows the required time for diffusion to occur (refer to Table 3.3 for percentages of O_2 and CO_2).

- **Internal respiration** describes the process whereby gases diffuse between the blood capillaries and the cells of the body. The percentage of oxygen arriving at the tissue cells is constant with the concentration at the alveoli. This means the oxygen-rich blood creates a concentration gradient between the blood and the tissue cells, which, through the act of metabolism, are rich in CO_2 and low in O_2. O_2 diffuses from the bloodstream into the cells; simultaneously CO_2 diffuses into the extracellular fluid and into the venous capillaries and blood stream. Table 3.1 provides a quick review of both the form and functional components of the respiratory system.

Transportation of oxygen and carbon dioxide within the blood

Oxygen transport

Most of the O_2 is transported in combination with haemoglobin (Chapter 4) to form oxyhaemoglobin. When the body is active, the tissues produce excessive CO_2 and heat, oxygen is released from its bound state with the haemoglobin. This intrinsic prioritisation process allows cells with the greatest need to receive O_2 first.

Carbon dioxide transport

This waste product of metabolism is mainly carried as bicarbonate ions in the plasma (70%). In addition, around 7% is carried in a dissolved state within the blood plasma and the remaining 23% loosely combined with haemoglobin as carbaminohaemoglobin (Waugh & Grant 2007).

Central control of respiration

The act of respiration is predominantly under involuntary control, otherwise when asleep an individual would lose the governing stimulus to breath. The rate and depth of inspiration are under the control of the respiratory centre situated within the medulla oblongata within the brain stem.

Chemoreceptors

Chemoreceptors monitor blood gas tensions and respond to **hypercapnia**, **hypoxia** and **acidosis**; there are two main types of chemoreceptors:

Figure 3.4a The alveoli

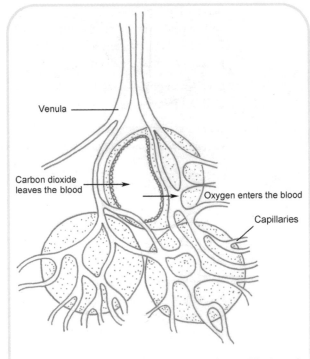

Figure 3.4b Close-up of the alveoli and the diffusion of oxygen and carbon dioxide

- Central chemoreceptors: it is estimated that 80% of the drive for ventilation is a result of stimulation of the central chemoreceptors (McGowan et al. 2003). These receptors, as the name implies, are located centrally although anatomically separate from the medullary

Anatomy and Physiology in Action: Box 3.1

There are many internal mechanisms within the human body that result in an equalisation of pressures or substances. Listed below are several basic principles that, once understood, would aid future learning.

- **Diffusion** occurs when a high concentration of a gas comes into contact with a weak concentration of the same gas (Figure 3.4). Molecules from the strong concentration will move across to the weaker area to create a balance or equilibrium; this process can only occur when the membrane lining of the lungs is moist as oxygen and carbon dioxide can only undergo the process of gaseous exchange in water-like material.
- Within the alveoli O_2 is under more pressure than the deoxygenated venous blood, therefore O_2 from the high pressure gradient moves or diffuses into the low pressure gradient until an equal balance is achieved.
- Within the venous blood the CO_2 is under higher pressure than the CO_2 level within the alveoli and therefore diffuses through the capillaries into the alveoli.
- At a cellular level the oxygenation/waste removal process continually repeats dependent on the current requirements of the body.

Anatomy and Physiology in Action: Exercise 3.4

There are several other types of receptors aiding and contributing to effective ventilation. Complete the following exercise to gain further insight into the essence of respiratory function:

Identify what effect the following limited list of receptors have on ventilation/respiration; the first is completed for you:

- **Pain receptors** have an effect on respiration by initially causing apnoea which is closely followed by hyperventilation
- **Irritant receptors**
- **Stretch receptors**
- **Arterial baroreceptors**

Once you have completed the exercise, think about how you would identify the cause of hyperventilation in an acute clinical presentation.

respiratory centre. They react to hydrogen ion levels whereby an increase results in a rise in the respiratory rate, and a decrease in hydrogen ions results in a lowering of the respiratory rate.

- Peripheral chemoreceptors: these receptors are located around the aortic arch and the carotid sinus. When stimulated, these receptors evoke both a respiratory and cardiovascular effect. They are directly affected by the blood pH, have a quick initial or compensatory effect, but have a limited systemic effect estimated at less than 10% of that of the central receptors (McGowan et al. 2003).

Now you have gained insight into both the form and functioning of the respiratory system, the chapter will broaden to discuss how the entry of air into the system can be hindered, thereby compromising oxygen delivery and the elimination of carbon dioxide. Common disease processes will then be discussed with the use of real-life clinical patient presentations to demonstrate the physical manifestations of illnesses affecting respiratory function.

Airway assessment and intervention (management)

Without an adequate constant and 'clean' supply of oxygen an individual will soon demonstrate the clinical signs of hypoxia. If a patient has an obstructed airway or fails to maintain airway patency, oxygen will not reach the lungs, leading to asphyxia. Prevention of hypoxaemia requires a protected, unobstructed flow of air into the lungs. Within the lungs it is also essential that a constant supply of blood reaches the alveoli. This balance between circulating oxygen levels and the presence of sufficient blood is referred to as the perfusion–ventilation ratio.

For a patient demonstrating an inability to maintain their own airway, prompt assessment, control of the airway, and provision of ventilation are essential. Airway compromise may be sudden and complete, insidious and partial, or progressive and/or recurrent (American College of Surgeons 2004). A compromise to air entry or flow can

Applying Theory to Practice: Exercise 3.5

Many disease processes can affect the perfusion–ventilation ratio resulting in minimal to profound hypoxaemia and cardiac arrest. Complete the following exercise to understand how common medical problems can impact on the respiratory system:

Identify at least three physiological problems that will affect the perfusion–ventilation ratio; the first is identified for you.

- If an individual has a reduced oxygen, carrying capacity within the blood due to a form of anaemia they will not be able to efficiently circulate the oxygen resulting in hypoxaemia. Interestingly their oxygen saturation level may read 100% because the red blood cells they have are fully saturated.

Once you have identified a further two abnormalities, add these to your portfolio.

occur at any level between the nose/mouth down to the bronchi. The site of obstruction varies dependent on the cause; in the unconscious patient the most common cause of airway obstruction is by the posterior displacement of the tongue at the level of the pharynx (RCUK 2006). Vomit, blood and foreign bodies commonly obstruct airflow at the site of the soft palate and epiglottis, resulting in aspiration of particles into the lungs. Obstruction can also occur at the larynx, resulting from the inflammation associated with burns and anaphylaxis. Obstruction below the larynx is also possible, but less common, and can be caused by excessive bronchial secretions, mucosal oedema, bronchospasm, pulmonary oedema, or the aspiration of gastric contents into the lungs.

Airway assessment

Assessment of the patient for signs of airway obstruction is also briefly covered in Chapter 15, as the ability to undertake a quick assessment and implement a manoeuvre can prove vital for a patient experiencing airway obstruction. The initial assessment can be achieved by applying the look, listen, and feel approach:

- **Look** for chest and abdominal movements.

- **Listen** and **feel** for airflow at the mouth and nose.

To assess effectively, put the side of your face, and ear, above the patient's nose and mouth, with your eyes facing the patient's feet for up to 10 seconds; this allows for rapid assessment of all three descriptors in one action.

Airway obstruction in an alert and conscious patient can be identified through their actions, such as grasping at their throat, clinical indicators such as central cyanosis, or obvious indicators such as the presence of vomit and blood within the oropharynx. There are also many localised noises that are synonymous with airway obstruction, which may alert the nurse when the patient is unable to communicate their compromise. These include stridor, wheeze, gurgling, snoring or crowing (Table 3.2).

Sign	Cause
Inspiratory stridor	Obstruction at laryngeal level or above
Expiratory wheeze	Obstruction of the lower airways, which can collapse and obstruct during expiration
Gurgling	Presence of liquid or semi-solid foreign material in the upper airways
Snoring	Partial occlusion of the pharynx by the tongue or palate
Crowing or stridor	Laryngeal spasm or obstruction

Table 3.2 Recognition of Airway Obstruction

Although most individuals breathe in a similar fashion, many patients present with chronically abnormal and inefficient breathing techniques.

Airway management

The administration of oxygen is pointless to a patient with an obstructed airway, as the oxygen will not enter the lower airways, irrespective of the delivered concentration.

If you identify possible airway obstruction immediate action must be taken. There are three basic manoeuvres that can be used to relieve upper airway obstruction:

head tilt, **chin lift** and **jaw thrust**. These simple repositional methods of expanding the airway are frequently successful when the cause of the obstruction is a loss of muscle tone within the pharynx; however, as with all interventions, it is crucial that following any manoeuvre the patient's ability to ventilate is reassessed by reapplying the look, listen and feel approach as described earlier.

The quick availability of suction is an absolute necessity for any patient with an actual or clear potential for airway obstruction. Suction can be used via a Yankaver tube if any visible debris is identified in the mouth. Suction should only be used in the areas of the oral cavity that can be visualised: pushing a suction catheter down an individual's throat can stimulate a conscious patient's gag reflex, and cause vomiting, further exacerbating the problem.

Basic airway adjuncts

There are several easily applied airway adjuncts readily available in most clinical areas. The two most common are the oropharyngeal and nasopharyngeal airways. These types of airway adjunct are designed to correct soft palate obstruction and backward tongue displacement.

The oropharyngeal **Guedel** airway is inserted into the mouth behind the tongue. The Guedel airway must be sized before insertion; this can be achieved by holding the flange of the airway level with the patient's incisors and the other end of the airway at the angle of the patient's jaw. See Figure 3.5.

There are two techniques for insertion, the first is to insert the airway into the oral cavity in the 'upside down' position as far as the junction between the hard and soft palate, and then rotate it through 180 degrees. The other method is to use a tongue blade to depress the tongue and then insert the airway posteriorly. The advantage of the first method is that it minimises the chance of displacing the tongue backwards and downwards, thereby exacerbating the situation (RCUK 2006). The oropharyngeal airway must not be used in a conscious patient as this can result in gagging, vomiting and aspiration. Correct and effective placement is indicated by an improvement in the patient's breathing ability and/or the

Anatomy and Physiology in Action: Exercise 3.6

Compare the breathing of different individuals; there are many influencing or contributing factors to why an individual breathes in a certain way.

- Compare the rhythm and depth of breathing of a very obese patient with someone with a petite build

Remember what is considered normal for one person can be very abnormal for another.

- What is sleep apnoea?
- Which group of individuals are at particular risk of experiencing this?

Questioning Clinical Practice: Exercise 3.7

Oxygen Therapy

There are many inconsistencies within clinical practice regarding the administration of supplementary oxygen therapy. In acutely unwell patients, regardless of any underlying aetiology such as COPD, the Resuscitation Council (UK) advocate delivering high flow oxygen at a rate of between 12–15L/min preferably via a mask attached to a reservoir bag.

- While on clinical placements identify if oxygen therapy needs to be prescribed by a practitioner with prescribing rights or if it can be administered via a patient group direction

This will prepare you for future discussions on this contentious topic.

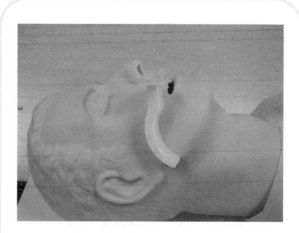

Figure 3.5 Measuring an oropharyngeal airway

eradication of the signs of obstruction identified in Table 3.2. Following any intervention always reassess and evaluate its effectiveness, in this case by applying the look, listen, feel approach as before. If an improvement is noted, supplementary oxygen should then be delivered via a facemask with reservoir bag.

The nasopharyngeal airway can be used in conscious patients, as it is not associated with initiating the gag reflex or vomiting. The RCUK (2006) recommends sizes 6–7mm as suitable for use in adults. Prior to inserting the nasopharyngeal airway the right nostril should be observed for obvious potential obstruction such as nasal polyps, blood or septal deviation; if any of these are present, the left nostril can be used. In some designs a safety pin should be inserted into the flanged end, prior to insertion, to prevent the adjunct disappearing into the airway. A water-soluble lubricant should be used to reduce localised trauma; insert the airway bevel end first,

vertically along the floor of the nose, twisting gently as this is done. Once the airway is in place and the flange is sitting at the opening of the nostril, reassessment of the airway and breathing should occur with the look, listen and feel approach with supplementary oxygen applied as before. Insertion of the nasopharyngeal airway can cause damage to the mucosal lining of the nasal airway and will result in minor bleeding in 30% of patients (RCUK 2006). Extreme caution should be used when considering the use of the nasopharyngeal airway in patients with obvious facial fractures or suspected basal skull fractures, as passage of the airway through a fracture of the skull base and into the cranial vault is possible, although extremely rare.

If at any stage the patency of the airway cannot be maintained the patient will need urgent referral to an anaesthetist for assessment and possible intubation.

Before discussing the administration of supplementary oxygen it is worth reviewing your current understanding of how much oxygen and carbon dioxide we inspire and expire with each breath.

Gas	Inspired air (%)	Expired air (%)
Oxygen	21	16
Carbon dioxide	0.04	4

Oxygen delivery devices are produced in two formats: fixed flow and non-fixed flow

Type of mask	Percentage of oxygen delivered
Fixed flow devices	
Venturi adaptors (24–60%)	These devices deliver fixed flow oxygen dependent on which adaptor is used; concentrations range between 24–60%
Non-fixed flow devices	**Estimated percentage**
Nebulising mask Ambu bag Nasal cannula Standard oxygen mask (Hudson) Oxygen mask with reservoir bag	60% at 6–10 L/min 85% at 12–15 L/min 24% at 2 L/min (higher rates not recommended) 60% at 6–10L/min 85% at 10–15L/min

Table 3.3 Oxygen Delivery Devices

Scenario 3.1

Asthma

Gary Gibbs is a 24-year-old Caucasian man who attends the local walk-in centre near where he works as a labourer, suffering from shortness of breath, which he states commenced 20 minutes before while he was shovelling broken bricks on a building site. Mr Gibbs can complete a sentence without running short of breath.

His respiratory rate is shallow, rapid and regular at 28 breaths per minute. He has an audible wheeze on expiration and does not appear to be overusing the accessory muscles of respiration. There are no signs of central or peripheral cyanosis. His pulse oximetry reading is 94% on air. He is asked if he knows his normal peak expiratory flow rate (PEFR), which is documented as 550. A current PEFR is recorded as 200. His radial pulse is strong, regular and recorded as 129 bpm, CRT is within two seconds. The initial blood pressure is recorded as 132/87.

Mr Gibbs appears anxious, sweaty and clammy. He is orientated to time and place, with an AVPU score of A. His temperature is recorded as 36.5.

Relevant medical history includes eczema and asthma for which he takes a salbutamol inhaler as required.

Assessment and analysis of patient presentation

Mr Gibbs presents with several early warning signs of respiratory compromise that, if left untreated, may lead to respiratory failure. His respiratory rate of 28, PEFR of 200 (33–50% of his normal), in conjunction with a pulse rate above 110, demonstrates compensatory shock and is classified as an acute severe presentation.

The British Thoracic Society's clarification of the severity of asthma is an excellent predictor of the severity of presenting symptoms, and also provides the assessor with a quick reference to the appropriate treatment regimen (Figure 3.6).

In this scenario there are four indicators of severe compromise: the respiratory and pulse rates, the low oxygen saturation level and the reduced PEFR. He is also sweaty and clammy in appearance. Mr Gibbs has an atopic history, meaning he has a predisposition to various hypersensitivity reactions such as asthma, eczema and rhinitis. There is also a high correlation between atopic individuals and anaphylactic reactions to common antibiotics, namely penicillins and cephalosporins.

From the presenting history and primary data gathered. Mr Gibbs appears to be experiencing an asthma attack related to his exposure to allergens from the brick dust which he would have inhaled while at work. Mr Gibbs requires emergency treatment and should be transferred to an appropriate emergency centre. If available, treatment should commence at the walk-in centre: this will include the quick administration of high flow oxygen, combined with nursing the patient in a sitting position, allowing full lung expansion. Mr Gibbs has had a PEFR recorded: this test records the maximum flow of air that can be expelled in one single expiration, it provides a convenient indicator of the amount of bronchial

Recording Peak Expiratory Flow Rates Box 3.2

Many patients with a history of asthma will undertake regular peak flow recordings at home and will know their expected score; note this but be aware of their technique.

There are several meters on the market and patients are usually advised to keep their meter and to bring it with them if they attend hospital to reduce cross-infection rates. A disposable tube should be placed on the mouthpiece, the meter reset to zero and held by the patient horizontally. The patient should be standing and directed to take a deep breath in before placing the meter in their mouth. Their lips should be applied to the mouthpiece and the air expelled in one hard, fast breath. If the breath is continual and not short and sharp it may induce coughing. This test should be repeated three times and the highest score recorded. If possible, record their PEFR before and after any nebulised interventions; this will provide quantifiable data to the effectiveness of the treatment.

constriction, although readings can be affected by a poor user technique. Box 3.2 describes how to take a PEFR reading. Patients with an established history of asthma may know their usual or best PEFR; this will provide a baseline for evaluation of their current presentation. Current PEFR recordings will be expressed as a percentage of the patient's previous best. If this information is unavailable, the PEFR should be documented as a percentage of their predicted rate; this can be achieved by using the graph predictor in Figure 3.7. The continual monitoring of the patient's respiratory rate and oxygen saturation by pulse oximetry will determine the effectiveness of the supplementary oxygen therapy; an arterial blood gas is indicated if the SpO_2 falls below 92%.

Asthma – the facts

Asthma can be defined as a chronic condition with acute exacerbations resulting in a hypersensitivity reaction. Asthma is the result of a combination of complex interactions which culminate in the hypersecretion of mucus, constriction of smooth muscle within the bronchioles, and localised inflammation resulting in compromise of the affected individual's ability to breathe. The Global Initiative for Asthma (GINA 2004) estimate that 300 million people, of all ages and races, experience asthma. The annual incidence is increasing in all age groups. GINA estimate that asthma accounts for one in 250 deaths worldwide, many of which are preventable. Suboptimal long-term medical care and delay in seeking help are the main contributing factors. Industrialised countries top the list of worldwide prevalence with the USA experiencing a prevalence rate of 11% and England and Wales 15%, accounting for an estimated 4.7 million individuals, including 590,000 teenagers (Gina 2004, NICE 2006). The UK demonstrates the worst prevalence rate in Europe in comparison to Sweden's 6%; however, the UK has a mortality rate of around 3% which is extremely low in comparison to China's 36%. There are many theories related to the causes of asthma (Currie et al. 2005) although no one factor appears solely responsible.

Pathophysiology

The pathophysiology or **pathogenesis** of asthma can be seen as a multidimensional phenomenon in which a series of internal reactions combine or accumulate to produce increasing inflammation and hyper-responsiveness of the airways. This cascade effect results in varying levels

of bronchoconstriction via smooth muscle contraction, mucus production and increased vascular permeability. Over repeated attacks the individual is exposed to the hypertrophy of several of the local tissues involved in this process, resulting in a cycle of deterioration and the potential for increasingly severe clinical symptoms (Figure 3.8).

Anatomy and Physiology in Action: Box 3.3

Pathology of Asthma
- Thickened basement membrane
- Hypertrophic goblet cells
- Hypertrophic smooth muscle
- Dilated local blood supply
- Increased eosinophils/immune/inflammatory response cells
- Increased mucus secretion resulting in mucus plugging

Theories related to the development of asthma

Environmental
The aetiology of asthma has for decades been considered to have a strong environmental link. This theory has been strengthened by studies concentrated on population migrations from areas of low prevalence to areas with an established high prevalence rate, whereby the migrating populace develop the same prevalence rate of asthma as the indigenous population (Bourke 2003).

Hand hygiene
This theory relates to the modern trend of creating of an artificially clean environment whereby children fail to develop immunologic responses to specific antigens, allergens and pathogens early in life. This failure to develop response mechanisms to common environmental factors results in an exaggerated or hypersensitive reaction later in life.

Genetic
It has been theorised that one of the components that contribute to both the development of asthma and the severity of the hypersensitivity response is genetic. The rationale is that the genes for most of the cytokines

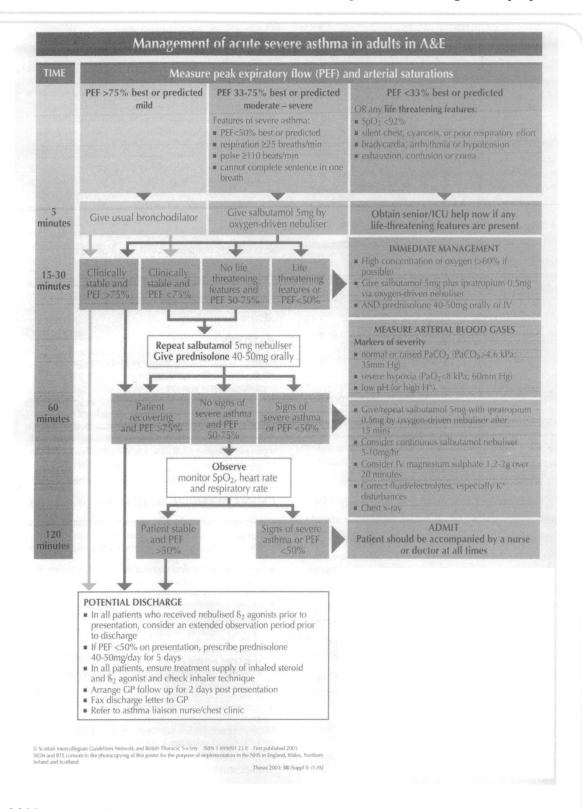

Figure 3.6 Management of acute severe asthma in adults in A&E. Source: British Thoracic Society and Scottish Intercollegiate Guidelines Network (2005)

Peak expiratory flow in normal adults

PEF L/min

Men

Women

Standard deviation men 48 litres/min
Standard deviation women 42 litres/min

In men, values of PEF up to 100 litres/min
less than predicted, and in women up to 85 litres/min
less than predicted, are within normal limits

Age in years

Nunn AJ, Gregg I. New regression equations for predicting peak expiratory flow in adults. BMJ 1989; 298: 1068-70

Figure 3.7 Predicted PEFR indicator. Source: British Thoracic Society and Scottish Intercollegiate Guidelines Network (2005)

involved in the development of asthma are found on chromosome 5, for which asthmatics have a predisposition (Lumb 2003). In addition, human lymphocyte antigens, which are involved in sensitisation of lymphocytes to specific antigens, play a major part in allowing immunological self-recognition and are inherited (Chapter 10).

Signs and symptoms

The indicative, and to an extent diagnostic, signs or symptoms of asthma are an expiratory wheeze, sometimes combined with wheezing on inspiration, shortness of breath, chest tightness and coughing.

When a patient presents in an alert and orientated condition, the assessment can begin by observing the patient's respiratory rate, depth, and the amount of effort they use to achieve effective respiration/ventilation. The

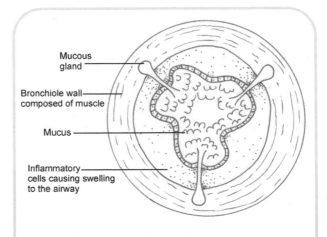

Mucous gland

Bronchiole wall—
composed of muscle

Mucus

Inflammatory—
cells causing swelling
to the airway

Figure 3.8 Bronchial hypertrophy and excessive mucus production

Applying Theory to Practice: Exercise 3.8

There are numerous outdoor and indoor environmental instigators implicated in the development of an acute attack of asthma, identify at least three from each category. The first is identified for you:

Indoor

1. **Dust mites** are commonly implicated in the development of asthma; there is now an entire industry providing bedding materials that are dust mite-free.

2.

3.

Outdoor

1. Nitrogen dioxide: the principal source of nitrogen dioxide and other oxides is motor vehicle emissions.

2.

3.

respiratory effort centres on the use of the shoulder girdle to assist breathing. Patients frequently present resting forward, with their arms outstretched in order to brace the shoulder girdle and enable the use of the accessory muscles of respiration, the sternocleidomastoid and trapezius muscles being the most evident. The ability of the patient to talk is a prime indicator of serious illness: if the patient cannot complete a sentence without stopping to draw breath, they are in a potentially life-threatening situation. In combination with the patient's level of consciousness their ability to complete a sentence is an extreme symptom. Chronic symptoms of asthma are variable, intermittent, can be worse at night, and can be provoked by certain catalysts, that is, allergens. These allergens include:

- Dust mites
- Pollen
- Chemical allergens such as paint fumes
- Exercise and cold weather.

In addition, psychological components have been extensively implicated in both provoking and exacerbating an acute asthma attack (BTS and SIGN 2005).

Psychosocial aspects

Physiological findings initially comprise the majority of the assessment process in a patient experiencing an acute asthma attack but there are other influencing and instigating factors. The BTS Guidelines (2005) state that in the assessment of asthma the assessor should note if the patient presents with one or more psychosocial factors such as a psychiatric illness (including depression), or drug and alcohol use, as these patients have a significantly increased mortality rate, making their identification paramount (BTS and SIGN 2005).

Analysis and treatment options

There is no universal approach to the prevention and management of asthma, with the UK and USA classifying the severity of asthma in different ways (Cates 2001). The UK philosophy focuses on prevention with the stepwise approach (BTS and SIGN 2005). This approach centres on increasing the use of medications titrated to the frequency and severity of symptoms and exacerbations, beginning with the use of inhaled short-acting beta 2 agonists for mild intermittent episodes, through to the daily use of oral and inhaled steroids. Recent pharmacological advances have led to the development of preventative medications that prevent, or antagonise, a major physiological instigator of asthma; these are the leukotriene antagonists.

The treatment of acute exacerbations, such as in the case of Mr Gibbs, should follow the BTS Guidelines (2005). These presentations frequently resolve with the administration of high flow oxygen and nebulised beta 2 agonists, which should be delivered within five minutes of the patient assessment; if the symptoms resolve and the PEFR returns to above 75% of the patient's predicted score, the patient can be discharged. If the patient's clinical condition slightly improves, but the PEFR remains below 75% of his best, a repeat beta 2 agonist should be administered and the patient commenced on oral steroid therapy; by strictly adhering to the guidelines, this reassessment will take place within 30 minutes and can be re-evaluated within the hour. If at any point the patient's clinical condition deteriorates, more intensive therapy should begin. This section of the algorithm includes the administration of ipratropium, an **anticholinergic** bronchodilator, recording and measuring arterial blood gases, possible administration of magnesium, and intubation if medication does not improve the patient's condition.

Scenario 3.2

Chronic Obstructive Pulmonary Disease (COPD)

Joan Middleton is a 63-year-old woman who is brought into the emergency department at 02.00 after experiencing shortness of breath and a purulent cough for three days. She is unable to complete a sentence; she appears alert although very anxious. Her respiratory rate is shallow, rapid and irregular at 38 breaths per minute. She appears to be nearing exhaustion, demonstrated by the heavy use of the accessory muscle of respiration, her neck veins are protruding and she adopts the tripod position (sitting, leaning forward with arms on thighs). Mrs Middleton has evidence of peripheral cyanosis. Her radial pulse is strong, regular and recorded as 118 bpm, CRT exceeds two seconds. Her initial blood pressure is recorded as 168/98. Mrs Middleton appears pale, sweaty and clammy. She is orientated to time and place, with an AVPU score of A. Mrs Middleton is a chronic smoker of around 30 cigarettes a day and has been an inpatient on several occasions with similar presentations related to what she describes as a chronic breathing problem. She commonly produces purulent green sputum.

Assessment and analysis of patient presentation

Mrs Middleton's presentation indicates a potentially life-threatening condition. This is demonstrated by her inability to complete a sentence, an ominous sign of impending respiratory failure. The dramatic rise in the patient's respiratory rate confirms the initial clinical findings. Her pulse and blood pressure are also raised and her CRT reduced. Her past medical history includes a chronic history of smoking and similar presentations, diagnosed as a chronic breathing problem or chronic obstructive pulmonary disease (COPD). If a patient presents with established damage to their lung function, it is essential to ascertain the current functioning ability of their heart as the two systems interlink to such an extent that it is very likely the lung compromise will also affect, at the very least, the functioning of the right side of the heart (Chapter 4).

Chronic obstructive pulmonary disease – the facts

Chronic obstructive pulmonary disease (COPD) can be defined as a chronic and debilitating disease continuum in which localised irritation of the bronchioles and lungs results in increasing airflow obstruction which is usually progressive (NCCCC 2004). COPD encompasses several lung conditions with varying causes (Table 3.4), although smoking is by far the most significant factor in its development (NICE 2004).

It is estimated that 900,000 individuals are diagnosed with COPD in the UK alone and it accounts for around 30,000 deaths each year (NICE 2004). In the USA there are an estimated 32 million affected individuals, with COPD being the fourth leading cause of death (Kleinschmidt 2005). Worldwide, COPD is the sixth leading cause of death.

Pathophysiology

COPD is a collective term for three separate disease processes: chronic bronchitis, emphysema and, to a smaller extent, chronic asthma. COPD is predominately caused by smoking, with each individual experiencing a unique mixture of these three instigators (NCCCC 2004). The two major components are identified in Table 3.4.

Symptoms are insidious and usually begin to appear in the mid-thirties proliferating with increasing age. The early warning signs or symptoms are the excessive production of phlegm and a chronic or persistent cough generally lasting in excess of three months. The diagnosis of COPD should be considered in all patients over 35 who have a chronic history of smoking, and who present with external breathlessness, a chronic cough and regular sputum production (NICE 2004). The formal diagnosis of COPD is confirmed by spirometry. Spirometry plays a pivotal role in the identification and modern management of COPD.

Due to the underpinning disease process, patients with COPD are susceptible to many illnesses that can result in a rapid deterioration of their already chronically compromised lung function. The NICE have produced specific guidelines for the treatment and management of this group of individuals (NICE 2004) (Figure 3.9).

Treatment plan

As with all serious presentations, high-flow oxygen should be administered, regardless of whether the patient may have a history of COPD. The application of high-flow

Chronic bronchitis	Emphysema
Chronic bronchial (inflammation bronchitis) leads to continuous stimulation of the immune system resulting in excessive production of mucus and hyperplasia of mucus-producing glands resulting in the obstructive component of chronic bronchitis. The internal response is to increase the cardiac output and decrease ventilation, thereby producing a ventilation–perfusion mismatch leading to hypoxaemia, hypercapnia and a mixture of respiratory and metabolic acidosis. Heart failure is a common pre-existing factor as the chronic respiratory failure causes pulmonary hypertension, and right heart enlargement (cor pulmonale). These patients have traditionally been described as 'blue bloaters' due to the clinical manifestation or picture that these internal disease processes create.	Emphysema is defined as a destruction of the distal airways. The alveoli and capillary beds that entwine them are gradually destroyed leading to the inability to oxygenate blood. There are several forms, each affecting either the distal bronchiole or different regions of the alveoli. The internal environment compensates by increasing ventilation and lowering the cardiac output, resulting in hypoxia. Due to the excessive respiratory function individuals experience chronic weight loss and muscle wasting. Traditionally described as 'pink puffers'.

Clinical presentation

Chronic bronchitis	Emphysema
Patients may be obese Frequent cough and phlegm expectoration are typical Use of the accessory muscles of respiration is common The breath sounds are often normal but upon auscultation there may be inspiratory and expiratory crackles, rhonchi (coarse gurgling) and wheezes Patients may have signs of right heart failure (i.e. cor pulmonale), such as peripheral oedema and cyanosis Similar overall appearance to heart failure	Patients may be very thin with a barrel-shaped chest (hyper-inflated) They typically have little or no cough or expectorations Breathing may be assisted by pursed lips and use of accessory respiratory muscles; they may adopt the tripod sitting position The chest may be hyper-resonant, and wheezing may be heard Overall appearance is more like classic COPD exacerbation

Table 3.4 The Main Instigators of COPD

supplementary oxygen is essential until proven otherwise (RCUK 2006) (Table 3.4). The patient should be helped to sit upright to reduce the work of breathing; this may involve the use of several pillows on conventional beds. The effectiveness of treatments should be closely monitored and evaluated; this will involve continually monitoring the patient's oxygen saturation level via a pulse oximeter, counting their respiratory rate and assessing their level of consciousness.

Medication

The initial management of exacerbations of COPD centre on the use of nebulised bronchodilators, and antibiotics if the patient is producing purulent sputum. When tachypnoea is a prominent feature, steroids are added to the therapy; these are continued for one to two weeks and decreased gradually to prevent an acute adrenal insufficiency crisis.

Maintenance of the patient's oxygen saturation above 90% is essential; this will be achieved by supplementing oxygen and dilating the bronchioles. In addition, steroids will begin to reduce the inflammation, and anti-cholinergic

Managing exacerbations of COPD

Exacerbations of COPD can be associated with increased:

- dyspnoea
- sputum purulence
- sputum volume

Initial management
- Increase frequency of bronchodilator use – consider giving via a nebuliser
- Oral antibiotics if purulent sputum
- Prednisolone 30 mg daily for 7–14 days – for all patients with significant increase in breathlessness, and all patients admitted to hospital, unless contraindicated

Hospital ← **Decide where to manage** (see table below right) → Home

Investigations
- Chest X-ray
- Arterial blood gases (record inspired oxygen concentration)
- ECG
- Full blood count and urea and electrolytes
- Theophylline level if patient on theophylline at admission
- Sputum microscopy and culture if purulent

Investigations
- Sputum culture not normally recommended
- Pulse oximetry if severe exacerbation

Further management
- Arrange appropriate review
- Establish on optimal therapy
- Arrange multidisciplinary assessment if necessary

Further management
- Give oxygen to keep SaO$_2$ above 90%
- Assess need for non-invasive ventilation:
 - consider respiratory stimulant if NIV not available
 - assess need for intubation
- Consider intravenous theophyllines if poor response to nebulised bronchodilators

Consider hospital-at-home or assisted-discharge scheme

Before discharge
- Establish on optimal therapy
- Arrange multidisciplinary assessment if necessary

Factors to consider when deciding where to manage patient		
Factor	Favours treatment in hospital	Favours treatment at home
Able to cope at home	No	Yes
Breathlessness	Severe	Mild
General condition	Poor/deteriorating	Good
Level of activity	Poor/confined to bed	Good
Cyanosis	Yes	No
Worsening peripheral oedema	Yes	No
Level of consciousness	Impaired	Normal
Already receiving LTOT	Yes	No
Social circumstances	Living alone/not coping	Good
Acute confusion	Yes	No
Rapid rate of onset	Yes	No
Significant comorbidity (particularly cardiac disease and insulin-dependent diabetes)	Yes	No
SaO$_2$ < 90%	Yes	No
Changes on the chest radiograph	Present	No
Arterial pH level	< 7.35	≥ 7.35
Arterial PaO$_2$	< 7 kPa	≥ 7 kPa

Figure 3.9 Managing exacerbations of COPD. Source: NICE (2004)

bronchodilators will reduce mucus secretion. If the patient fails to respond, there will be a need for more aggressive therapy such as non-invasive ventilation therapy or intubation; this will require expert advice and a senior anaesthetist should be sought. In the meantime a respiratory stimulant may be prescribed if the patient's level of consciousness begins to decrease. All patients presenting with sporadic bouts of coughing and purulent sputum production should be risk-assessed for tuberculosis, as this infection could be spread to other users of the emergency department or to healthcare professionals.

Non-invasive ventilation

Non-invasive ventilation (NIV) is a key component of treating severe presentations of COPD. This precise method of oxygen delivery is used to correct hypoventilation and reduce the workload of the accessory respiratory muscles; this is achieved by forcing open distal areas of lung space via a tightly fitted face mask (sometimes a nasal device may also be used) connected to either a continuous positive pressure airway (CPAP) or bi-level ventilation (BIPAP). The use of CPAP has been shown to be an effective frontline treatment (Vanpee et al. 2002). NIV assists in both the inspiratory and expiratory phases of breathing.

By providing additional assistance during the inspiratory phase of respiration alveolar ventilation is increased, thereby decreasing carbon dioxide accumulation and providing increased oxygen availability. This will also result in the patient having to work less (very beneficial when the accessory muscles are beginning to tire).

The provision of an expiratory positive airway pressure results in the alveoli being forced open at the end of expiration increasing the functional capacity of the lungs

The major drawback of this therapy is that many patients find it hard to tolerate due to the claustrophobic effect the mask can have, and as a result of the increased pressures the device delivers. Newer machines incorporate a pressure sensor to enable the machine to alter the CPAP pressure on a breath-by-breath basis, thereby making it more tolerable. If these NIV therapies fail to improve the patient's condition, the patient may need intubation (Poponick et al. 1999).

Psychosocial aspects

Smoking cessation is crucial to halting the progressive physiological lung deterioration associated with COPD; it

Oxygen Therapy Myths and Reality: Box 3.4

- Adequate oxygen should be given to relieve all cases of hypoxia

In COPD aim to maintain SpO_2 >90–93%

It is widely believed that supplementing too much oxygen can cause significant respiratory depression: multiple studies dispute this as administering high-flow oxygen causes PO_2 and PCO_2 to rise, but not in proportion to the very minor changes in respiratory drive (Kleinschmidt 2005).

Increased circulating PCO_2 can occasionally precipitate a decrease in the patient's level of consciousness; a subsequent reduction in supplementary oxygen only leads to profound hypoxia,

Patients exhibiting clinical deterioration should either receive a trial of non-invasive ventilation or be intubated.

Developing and Delivering Expert Care: Box 3.5

Orthopnoea

Patients presenting with severe respiratory compromise in the early hours of the morning are a common presentation to acute services. When a patient has a known cardiac history the obvious cause is that they have slipped down into a flatter sleeping position during the night, causing pulmonary oedema; this inability to breathe while lying flat is termed orthopnoea. Orthopnoea is most commonly associated with heart failure, but is also seen in asthma and chronic bronchitic conditions.

is therefore fundamental to the management plan of all patients experiencing COPD, regardless of their age (NICE 2004). Nurses are placed in a variety of clinical settings providing the unique opportunity to interact with patients, and the public at large, in many formats other than through a formal consultation. This provides many occasions when health promotion and education can be utilised and a clear, concise message conveyed to the listener.

Applying Theory to Practice: Exercise 3.9

Work through the following questions to develop skills in relation to educational programmes:

- How could you encourage a patient or friend to stop smoking?
- Would your programme include trying to scare them by using statistics on mortality rates and the development of cancer?
- Do you think scare tactics work?
- Now think about government initiatives such as printing 'SMOKING KILLS' on the outside wrapper of every packet sold.
- On reflection, do these initiatives work or do participants become 'conditioned' to them?

Shared decision making

Educational programmes designed to help individuals to cease smoking cannot be forced on participants, there must be an initial desire on the behalf of the patient to want to stop smoking. This may be due to many reasons or to a combination of recent events such as ill health, external pressure from family members, or due to the deteriorating health of someone they know. Government-funded organisations such as NICE (2006) and Prodigy (2007) have published several documents providing plans of care to assist practitioners in delivering effective plans of care to smokers. Primary care programmes include referral of the individual to a NHS Stop Smoking Clinic. Prodigy identify several tips on aiding an individual to stop:

- Set a date to quit, and stop smoking completely from that day
- Get rid of cigarettes, ashtrays and lighters
- Anticipate problems such as social gatherings, withdrawal symptoms, cravings, and an increase in appetite
- If possible, give up with someone else for mutual support
- Nicotine substitutes are available in several forms such as gums and transdermal patches. It is estimated that by using a nicotine substitute the success rate for quitting smoking doubles (Prodigy 2007)

Remember that encouraging a person to continue when they have stopped smoking can be extremely beneficial:

- Congratulate the person on his or her success
- Reinforce the importance of permanent cessation

Developing and Delivering Expert Care: Exercise 3.10

Smoking Cessation

Once an addiction is established, whether physical or psychological, it can be extremely difficult to stop. Therefore the best policy is prevention. Recent legislation has been directed at stopping the promotion and use of tobacco and stopping exposure to secondary cigarette smoke.

- Do you feel this is a contradiction when cigarettes are legally available throughout the retail industry?

There are several help-lines that can provide in-depth information to both healthcare professionals and individuals wanting to cease smoking:

- gosmokefree.co.uk
- smokefreeengland.co.uk
- www.givingupsmoking.co.uk

Questioning Clinical Practice: Exercise 3.11

Professional Issues Debate

Many areas of healthcare involve controversial decisions or debates; these debates can become personal when they interfere or challenge the belief systems of participants. To hold an effective debate the process must therefore be structured and overseen by a chairperson or adjudicator; identify someone who has good 'crowd control' skills! For best effect your class should be split into two groups; if this isn't possible, the same exercise can be reproduced using a few of your classroom colleagues. Group A will argue for and Group B against.

- Can nurses who smoke engage in constructive relationships with patients wishing to 'kick the habit'?

Points for consideration:

A nurse informs a patient and their family that quitting smoking is paramount to the patient's long-term survival. On their next visit the family see the nurse having a quick 'fag' break outside the ward.

- Do you think the nurse would maintain her professional creditability or is this a conflict of interests?

Scenario 3.3

Pneumonia

Robert Bassett, an 81-year-old Caucasian man, has been an inpatient for several weeks. He has been awaiting a community care bed following a stroke that has left him unable to cope independently with the activities of everyday living. His family are insistent that the care home is of the highest quality as they have read newspaper articles that have revealed how bad care standards can be in some homes.

You are allocated to care for Mr Bassett today. As you begin talking to him you notice that he appears vague, short of breath and lethargic. He has had a cough for the past two days and is expectorating green phlegm. You record his vital signs: airway patent – patient talking, respiratory rate 21, shallow and irregular with sporadic episodes of coughing. Mr Bassett's pulse is 72, strong and regular, capillary refill within two seconds and his blood pressure is recorded as 154/93. His **tympanic** temperature is 35.

You are worried that he is suffering from a chest infection. High-flow oxygen is commenced and you ask a senior nurse to auscultate his chest. The senior nurse identifies that Mr Bassett has consolidation at the base of his right lung, orders a chest X-ray and asks you to collect a sputum sample as soon as possible for microculture and sensitivity. He prescribes broad-spectrum intravenous antibiotics under a local patient group direction, attaches Mr Bassett to an intravenous infusion to hydrate him, and takes blood samples including cultures before administering the antibiotics. The senior nurse also writes an urgent referral request for physiotherapy assistance to remove some of the deep secretions within the base of Mr Bassett's lung. He assists Mr Bassett to sit upright by placing several pillows behind him.

Assessment and analysis of patient presentation

Mr Bassett is demonstrating the early signs of a severe chest infection and lobular pneumonia. The recent history of increasing shortness of breath and lethargy can indi-cate ominous signs of respiratory failure. Knowledgeable clinicians will also recognise that elderly patients are less likely than younger individuals to exhibit a temperature in response to severe infection, and that Mr Bassett may be

becoming septic (BTS 2006). The working diagnosis for Mr Bassett is hospital-acquired pneumonia (HAP), a serious consequence for all patients experiencing a prolonged stay in hospital. Mr Bassett has been prescribed the required treatments including intravenous fluids and blood tests, which need to include:

- Full blood count
- Urea and electrolytes
- Liver function test
- C reactive protein.

Blood has also been taken for microculture and sensitivity (MC&S) before broad-spectrum antibiotics are administered, as this would compromise the sensitivity of the blood result.

Pneumonia – the facts

Pneumonia can be defined as an acute inflammation of the lower respiratory tract most commonly due to bacterial and viral infection. Lobes of the lung become consolidated, resulting in an impairment of gaseous exchange (Figure 3.10). The British Thoracic Society Guidelines on the management of pneumonia include evidence of radiographic shadowing (BTS 2004).

Consolidation in the Right Inferior Lobe

Figure 3.10 Right inferior lobe pneumonia

Classification of pneumonia

Pneumonia is classified into two distinct subgroups; the reason for this is that the two groups, despite having many common features, are treated very differently:

- **Community-acquired pneumonia.** Pneumonia that is contracted outside the hospital setting often following a viral respiratory infection; it affects nearly four million adults each year. Community-acquired pneumonia is caused by a small range of bacteria, namely *Streptococcus pneumoniae* (BTS 2004). Patients within the community are treated empirically: microbial investigations are not routinely requested and sputum should only be examined if the patient fails to respond to oral antibiotics.
- **Hospital-acquired pneumonia.** Pneumonia that is contracted within the hospital environment is known as nosocomial pneumonia. Hospitalised patients are particularly vulnerable to pneumonia, a complication of bed rest and a leading secondary infection. The main pathogens responsible for disease within the hospital environment are frequently resistant to standard antibiotics; they also prove to be increasingly virulent and associated morbidity and mortality are high. Hospital-acquired pneumonia is the leading cause of death in hospitalised patients. These infections require specific antibiotic therapy depending on the identified cause, making pathogen identification essential.

The mortality rate from pneumonia is estimated at around 10% and is the fifth leading cause of death in the UK with elderly patients experiencing the most serious effects (BTS 2004). Pneumonia is the sixth leading cause of death in the USA and the leading cause of death from infection; it is also the leading hospital-acquired infection and cause of death (Pellerano 2005).

The BTS Guidelines identify a 5-point scoring system based on individual clinical features these are summarised in Box 3.6.

Pathophysiology

Pneumonia can result from a variety of different causes:

- **Viruses** which invade cells in order to reproduce. Viruses reach the lungs when airborne droplets are inhaled through the mouth and nose (many them highly contagious). Once in the lungs, the virus

The CURB-65 Scoring System: Box 3.6

(Score 1 point for each feature present)

- Confusion
- Urea >7 mmol/L
- Respiratory rate >30/min
- Blood pressure: Systolic (<90mmHg) Diastolic (<60mmHg)
- Age >65 years

A CURB-65 score of 0 is associated with a mortality rate of 1.2%.

This figure rises to 18.2% for a score of 4 (BTS 2004).

0–1	Assess suitability for home treatment
2	Consider hospital treatment
3	Or more, manage as severe pneumonia
4–5	Assess need for ITU admission

invades the alveoli, and this can result in cell destruction. The immune system responds to the viral infection by proliferating the white blood cells. This immune or inflammatory response results in fluid leaking into the alveoli. The combination of cell destruction and fluid-filled and inflamed alveoli compromises the transportation of oxygen into the bloodstream, resulting in the clinical signs of shortness of breath, pain on inspiration and excessive mucus production. Viral infections make the body more susceptible to bacterial infections; for this reason, bacterial pneumonia often complicates viral pneumonia.

- **Bacteria** enter the lungs through inhaled airborne droplets; additionally they can also reach the lungs through the bloodstream from an infection in another part of the body. Once inside the alveoli, the immune response is triggered, and this leads to the release of several different types of cell (Chapter 10), and neutrophils engulf and kill the offending organisms. The combination of immune reactions leads to clinical signs such as fever, chills and fatigue. Again oxygenation can become compromised due to inflammatory processes associated with the immune response. In severe infections bacteria can migrate from the lung into the bloodstream causing sepsis and septic shock. Bacteria can also travel to the pleural cavity causing a complication called an empyema.

Fungi and parasites can also cause pneumonia; in addition, pneumonia may also occur from chemical or physical injury to the lungs. This can include aspirational pneumonia, a common complication of a stroke or compromise to the patency of the protective mechanisms of the airway, with altered level of consciousness, neuromuscular disease or seizures. Inhalation of infectious particles is probably the most important pathogenic mechanism in the development of community-acquired pneumonia. Various pathogens can colonise the lungs and cause disease, for example, tuberculosis. The clinical signs and features associated with acute pneumonia are insidious and develop over days to weeks.

In hospital-acquired pneumonia, invasive tubes or investigations compromise the anatomical defences and result in bacteria bypassing the defence network and directly compromising the tracheobronchial tree via colonisation, leading to a massive inflammatory reaction and an increase in mucus production. This escalating reaction results in bacteria entering the bloodstream causing involvement of the systemic circulation and the affected individual will demonstrate septicaemia. Hospital-acquired pneumonia is therefore far more virulent and destructive.

Treatment

Treatment focuses on administering appropriate antibiotics to terminate the colonisation of bacteria, sustaining optimum oxygenation through simultaneously supplementing oxygen and maintaining the patient's systolic blood pressure above 100mmHg. Providing **humidified oxygen** early in the treatment plan will reduce the incidence of damage to the airways and mucus membranes associated with high-flow oxygen administration. The early intervention of specialist care – ITU and physiotherapy to assist the movement of lung consolidation – will benefit the prognosis. Keeping the patient well hydrated and nourished has also been shown to benefit patient outcomes.

Professional issues

This preventable illness is one of the serious consequences of prolonged bed rest. Complete Exercise 3.12 to gain insight into these life-threatening complications and good nursing practice.

The Department of Health recognise that elderly patients are at increased risk of iatrogenic illness and inequality in healthcare provision. Statistics show that

Developing and Delivering Expert Care: Exercise 3.12

Complications of Bed Rest/Immobility

All healthcare workers need to be aware that all hospitalised patients are at varying degrees of risk from reduced mobility.

While on clinical placements you will see that many patients are prescribed medications to prophylactically prevent some of the possible complications of bed rest. Listed below are some extremely common pathologies associated with prolonged immobility. See if you can think of ways of preventing their development:

- Pneumonia
- Deep vein thrombosis/pulmonary embolism
- Pressure-related sores
- Thrombophlebitis
- Urine infections
- Constipation
- Malnutrition

The development of most of these pathologies are often associated with poor levels of nursing care, negligence on behalf of the carers and a failure in the nurse's duty of care (NMC 2004).

Questioning Clinical Practice: Exercise 3.13

Risk Assessment Tools

There are many risk assessment tools intended to provide a safeguard against poor hospital practices by identifying those at increased risk. Complete the following exercise to extend your developing knowledge:

- What risk assessment tools are used within the clinical areas you have practised in?
- Are tools such as the **Waterlow score** completed on a regular basis?
- What is a VIP score? How often should it be evaluated?

The following websites will provide additional information:

http://www.rcn.org.uk/publications/pdf/002179.pdf

nice.org.uk/download.aspx?o=57690

http://www.worcestershirehealth.nhs.uk/Intranet1_Library/foi_internet/foi_files/class_9/

Clinical_Policies/130405IV%20medication%20policy%202005.pdf

those over 65 occupy around two-thirds of hospital beds, their lengths of stay can be three times as long as younger patients, 80% of delayed transfers affect older patients, and figures based on London's '60 worst trolley waits' indicated that half of these patients were over 65 (DH 2005). As a nurse you need to be aware of this inequality and actively represent the best interests of those placed within your care by anticipating these complications.

Conclusion

Respiratory medicine covers an enormous catalogue of disease states and potential clinical presentations. Many of these are chronic and will lead to several patient presentations, for example, **cystic fibrosis** and COPD. Nurses do not need to specialise in respiratory medicine or one of its derivatives to encounter respiratory disease as these can be encountered in virtually all primary, secondary and tertiary environments. It is essential, therefore, that all nurses have a solid foundation of knowledge of respiratory care, particularly in assessing and maintaining a patent airway. Complete the summary quiz to reinforce your developing knowledge.

Chapter 3 Summary Quiz

1. What are the vital organs and components of the respiratory system?

A. Lungs, ciliated tissue, bronchioles
B. Lungs, epithelial tissue, alveoli
C. Lungs, villi, bronchioles
D. Lungs, adipose tissue, trachea

2. How much oxygen is in the air we breathe?

A. 19%
B. 21%
C. 60%
D. 100%

3. A patient stops breathing, which oxygen device is now essential?

A. 24% Venturi device
B. A Hudson mask
C. An Ambu bag
D. An oxygen mask with a reservoir bag

4. The muscles of respiration include:

A. The diaphragm, intercostal muscles, the hamstrings
B. Sternocleidomastoid muscles, quadriceps, triceps
C. The diaphragm, intercostal muscles, sternocleidomastoid muscles
D. Intercostal muscles, latissimus dorsi, gluteus medius

5. Non-invasive ventilation (NIV) is a key component to treating severe presentations of COPD because:

A. This precise method of oxygen delivery is used to correct hypoventilation and reduce the workload of the accessory respiratory muscles
B. This precise method of oxygen delivery means the patient will always receive 24% oxygen
C. This air delivery device will mean the patient only receives room air
D. It is the only way to deliver nebulisers to COPD patients

6. Orthopnoea can be defined as:

A. The inability to breathe due to coughing
B. The inability to breathe while lying flat
C. Shortness of breath on exertion
D. The inability to complete a sentence

7. The lungs are composed of:

A. Three lobes on the left and two on the right
B. Two lobes on the right and two on the left
C. Three lobes on the right and two on the left
D. Three lobes on both sides

8. External respiration centres on:

A. The exchange of gases through diffusion between the alveoli and the blood stream

B. The exchange of gases through diffusion between the trachea and the bronchioles

C. The passage of air into the larynx

D. The osmotic reaction within the alveoli circulation

9. Internal respiration describes the process whereby:

A. A person breathes in

B. Gases diffuse between the blood capillaries and the lymphatic circulation

C. Blood renews its supply of iron

D. Gases diffuse between the blood capillaries and the cells of the body

10. Which of the following are complications associated with prolonged bed rest/immobility?

A. Deep vein thrombosis, pulmonary embolism, euphoria

B. Constipation, pressure-related sores, pneumonia

C. Malnutrition, pressure-related sores, diarrhoea

D. Pressure-related sores, cystic fibrosis, deep vein thrombosis

Further reading

Currie, G.P., Devereux, G.S., Lee, D.K.C. & Ayres, J.G. (2005) Recent developments in asthma management. *British Medical Journal* 330: 585–9.

Damiani, M. & Dixon, J. (2002) *Managing the Pressure*. King's Fund: London.

Department of Health (2007) *England Becomes Smokefree 1 July 2007*. DH: London.

Jarvis, H. (2006) Exploring the evidence base of the use of non-invasive ventilation. *British Journal of Nursing* 15(14): 756–9.

Kleinschmidt, P. (2005) Chronic obstructive pulmonary disease and emphysema. *Emedicine* http://www.emedicine.com/emerg/topic99.htm (accessed 12 May 2006).

Lumb, A.B. (2003) *Nunn's Applied Respiratory Physiology*, 5th edn. Butterworth Heinemann: Oxford.

Shire, D., Butler, J. & Lewis, R. (2004) *Hole's Human Anatomy and Physiology*, 10th edn. McGraw-Hill: New York.

http://www.brit-thoracic.org.uk

http://www.dh.gov.uk/en/Policyandguidance/Healthandsocialcaretopics/DH_4138532

References

American College of Surgeons (2004) *Advance Trauma Life Support for Doctors*, 7th edn. American College of Surgeons: Chicago.

Bourke, S.J. (2003) *Lecture Notes on Respiratory Medicine* (Lecture Notes Series), 6th edn. Blackwell Publishing: Oxford.

British Lung Foundation (2005) British Lung Foundation launches new COPD guidance for GPs. http://www.lunguk.org/news.asp. (accessed July 2007).

British Thoracic Society (2004) *BTS Guidelines for the Management of Community Acquired Pneumonia in Adults*. 2004 Update. BTS: London.

British Thoracic Society (2006) *The Burden of Lung Disease: A Statistics Report from the BTS*. 2nd edn. BTS: London

British Thoracic Society and Scottish Intercollegiate Guidelines Network (2005) *British Guidelines on the Management of Asthma: A National Clinical Guideline*. Revised edition. BTS & SIGN. London.

Cates, C. (2001) Extracts from 'Clinical Evidence': chronic asthma. *British Medical Journal* 323: 976–9.

Currie, G.P., Devereux, G.S., Lee, D.K.C. & Ayres, J.G. (2005) Recent developments in asthma management. *British Medical Journal* 330: 585–9.

Department of Health (2001) *National Service Framework for Older People*. DH: London.

Department of Health (2005) *National Service Framework for Long Term Conditions*. DH: London.

Evans, C. & Tippins, E. (2007) *The Foundations of Emergency Care*. Open University Press: Maidenhead.

Global Initiative for Asthma (GINA) (2004) *Global Strategy for*

Asthma Management and Prevention: NIH Publication No 02–3659. GINA: Hamilton, Ontario.

Global Initiative for Chronic Obstructive Lung Disease (GOLD) (2006) *Global Strategy for the Diagnosis, Management and Prevention of Chronic Obstructive Pulmonary Disease*. http:www.goldcopd.com (accessed July 2007).

Kleinschmidt, P. (2005) Chronic obstructive pulmonary disease and emphysema. *Emedicine* http://www.emedicine.com/emerg/topic99.htm (accessed 12 May 2006).

London Health Observatory (LHO) (2007) *Disease Groups – Respiratory Disease*. http://www.lho.org.uk/HIL/Disease_Groups/RespiratoryDisease.asp (accessed July 2007).

Lumb, A.B. (2003) *Nunn's Applied Respiratory Physiology*, 5th edn. Butterworth Heinemann: Oxford.

McGowan, J., Jefferies, A. & Turley, A. (2003) *Respiratory System*. Crash Course Series, 2nd edn. Mosby: Edinburgh.

National Collaborating Centre for Chronic Conditions (2004) *Chronic Obstructive Pulmonary Disease: National Clinical Guideline on Management of Chronic Obstructive Pulmonary Disease in Adults in Primary and Secondary Care*. NICE Guideline 12. *Thorax* 59: 1–232.

National Institute for Clinical Excellence (NICE) (2004) *NICE Guideline to Improve Care of Patients with Chronic Obstructive Pulmonary Disease*. NICE: London.

National Institute for Clinical Excellence (NICE) (2006) *Brief Interventions and Referral for Smoking Cessation in Primary Care and other Settings: Public Health Intervention Guidance No. 1*. NICE: London.

Office for National Statistics (ONS) (2007) Mortality: by gender and major cause, 1911–2000. *Social Trends* http://www.statistics.gov.uk/StatBase/ssdataset.asp?vlnk=5224&Pos=4&ColRank=2&Rank=272 (accessed July 2007).

Pellerano, M.E. (2005) Fast facts: respiratory tract infection, *Chest* 127: 693–84.

Poponick, J., Renston, J.P., Bennett, R.P. & Emerman, C.L. (1999) Use of a ventilatory support system (BIPAP) for acute respiratory failure in the emergency department, *Chest* 116; 166–71.

Prodigy (2007) Guidelines Smoking Cessation http://www.cks.library.nhs.uk/smoking_cessation/view_whole_guidance (accessed July 2007]

Resuscitation Council UK (2006) *Advanced Life Support*, 5th edn. RC (UK): London.

Shire, D., Butler. J. & Lewis, R. (2004) *Hole's Human Anatomy and Physiology*, 10th edn. McGraw-Hill: New York.

Vanpee, D., Khawand, C.E.L., Rousseau, L., et al. (2002) Effects of nasal pressure support on ventilation and inspiratory work in normocapnic and hypercapnic patients with stable COPD, *Chest* 122: 75–83.

Waugh, A, & Grant, A. (2007) *Ross & Wilson's Anatomy and Physiology in Health and Illness*, 10th edn. Churchill Livingstone: London.

Blood and the cardiovascular system

Cliff Evans

<div style="float:right">4</div>

Chapter 4 Learning Objectives

- Gain knowledge and insight into the anatomy and physiology related to these systems
- Gain insight into several predominant conditions related to these systems
- Apply theory to practice by understanding the physical manifestation of these illnesses in patients
- Gain insight into several commonly used medications to either prevent or treat relevant conditions
- Learn essential anatomical landmarks which can be applied in clinical practice
- Gain a solid structured approach to patient assessment
- Construct solid evidence of professional development for your growing portfolio
- Continue developing the ability to question and critique the evidence base and effectiveness of plans of care

Introduction

Disease of the cardiovascular system, or the essential fluids it carries, affects a vast percentage of the population at some time during their life (DH 2006). The physical signs are varied with many symptoms not clinically manifesting until irreversible damage has taken place.

This chapter focuses on two fundamentally important components to life: the heart and the fluid it circulates to provide nourishment, oxygenation and the removal of waste products throughout the body. For the system to be effective a transportation medium is necessary; this is the blood, which travels through a highly complex network of vessels. The lymphatic system, which complements the cardiovascular system, is also briefly discussed as the systems work in unison to maintain the internal state of homeostasis (Chapter 10 highlights the lymphatic system). Diseases related to the cardiovascular system, or

one of its components, are so common that all nurses at some time during their career will deal with the consequences within their daily practice.

This chapter commences with an overview of basic cardiovascular function, identifying the main anatomy and physiological functions of this system. Common diseases that affect the ability of the system to function will be explored, illustrating how an individual's ability to perform the basic functions of life can be compromised; ultimately these diseases can result in the individual's lifespan being shortened.

Applying Theory to Practice: Exercise 4.1

Before reading on:
- Compose a list of diseases you already know that affect the heart, vessels or blood
- Add this list to your developing portfolio. On completion of this chapter expand your portfolio with the new disorders you have gained knowledge of and elaborate on how these disorders affect physiological function. This might include blood tests, electrocardiograms (ECG) and the patient's physical presentation.

Cardiovascular function

Optimum function requires several key components working in unison; despite this, the system itself can continue in the face of severe insult and the failure of many of its components.

The heart

The heart is the pump that ejects deoxygenated blood to the lungs for oxygenation, and simultaneously oxygenated blood to the systemic circulation for essential cellular function and waste removal. The heart weighs around 300g and is positioned in the thoracic cavity in the

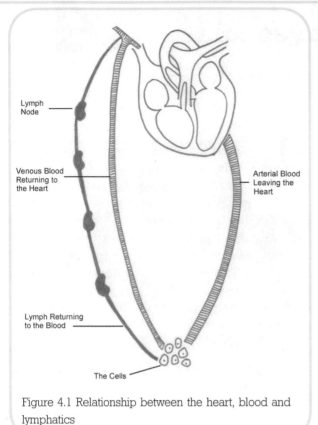

Figure 4.1 Relationship between the heart, blood and lymphatics

Lymph Node

Venous Blood Returning to the Heart

Arterial Blood Leaving the Heart

Lymph Returning to the Blood

The Cells

mediastinum, resting between the right and left lungs. The heart tilts towards the left where its main musculature sits

just above the diaphragm. It is extremely muscular and compact, disproportionately powerful for an organ roughly the size of an adult fist – a necessity for its principal action of pumping a lifetime's supply of blood.

Form

The heart has three main layers:

● **The pericardium** – composed of two sacs surrounding the heart.

 The outer layer consists of strong fibrous inelastic tissue preventing over-distension. The inner layer consists of a double-layered serous membrane (secreting fluid which prevents friction as the heart pumps). The outer layer is called the parietal pericardium and the inner layer the visceral pericardium/epicardium which runs continuously with the parietal layer. These membranes are separated by a potential space in a similar fashion to the pleural space (Chapter 3).

● **The myocardium** – this specialised muscle is only found in the heart. It is mainly under involuntary control.

 Cardiac muscle resembles skeletal muscle although each cell has a nucleus and one or more branches. Cardiac muscle appears as a sheet of muscle rather than a large number of individual cells; this is important to its function, as when an electrical

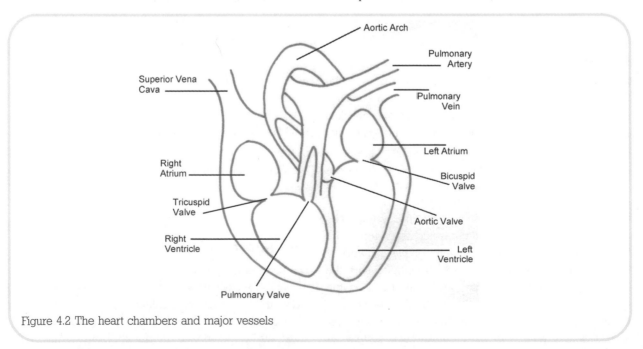

Aortic Arch

Pulmonary Artery

Superior Vena Cava

Pulmonary Vein

Left Atrium

Right Atrium

Bicuspid Valve

Tricuspid Valve

Aortic Valve

Right Ventricle

Left Ventricle

Pulmonary Valve

Figure 4.2 The heart chambers and major vessels

impulse initiates muscle contraction, the entire muscle sheet contracts simultaneously causing a huge force of contraction that can be increased or decreased depending on the body's needs.

- **The endocardium** – the inner layer of the myocardium, this layer is thin and covered with epithelial tissue in a similar way to the transport vessels, thereby preventing the adhesion of blood; this is essential otherwise the heart would be continuously firing off clotted blood into the circulation.

Figure 4.2 identifies the four hollow chambers of the heart:

- The atria (left and right)
- The ventricles (left and right).

The interatrial septum divides the two upper chambers, or atria; this partition continues downwards separating the ventricles where it becomes the interventricular septum. Each atrium is separated from the ventricles by an atrioventricular valve (the tricuspid on the right and bicuspid on the left) and horizontally between thin bands of non-conducting fibrous tissue, only allowing electrical conduction to follow one pre-designated route through to the ventricles. In comparison to the ventricles the atria are small receiving chambers for blood returning to the heart. The ventricles are large with a disproportionate amount of muscle on the left due to its increased workload. The top of the heart sits in the middle of the chest. The apex, which is mainly composed of the left ventricle, sits around the level of the left nipple.

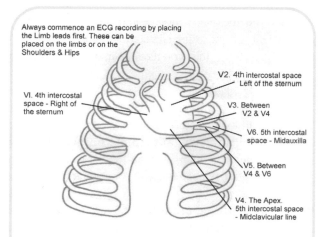

Figure 4.3 The chest and ribs with the anatomical landmarks identified for ECG recording

Anatomy and Physiology in Action: Exercise 4.2

Identification of the apex:
Located at the 5th intercostal space in the midclavicular line, left of the sternum.
Easily located by counting down the ribs from the collarbone otherwise known as the clavicle.

The clavicle counts as rib one because the first rib lies underneath it making it inaccessible. Once you have counted down and located the fifth rib, the fifth intercostal space will be between that rib and the sixth rib (Figure 4.3).
This landmark is important for the recording of electrocardiograms (ECG) and listening to heart sounds.

Practise finding and feeling this area. If you have a willing companion, ask them to undertake some aerobic exercise then locate the area again. When the heart contracts with increased power to meet the intensified cellular demands associated with physical exercise, the heart can be easily felt pounding against the chest wall.

Anatomy and Physiology in Action: Box 4.1

You can listen to the heart at the apex with a stethoscope; this process is referred to as **auscultation**.

The sounds to identify are those of particular actions within the cardiac cycle. This usually begins with:

- S1 – signifying the closure of the interventricular valves (sounds like lub)
- S2 – signifying the closure of the aortic and pulmonary valves (sounds like dub)

The first heart sound can be identified by concurrently feeling the carotid pulse and listening for the simultaneous closure of the interventricular valves (Figure 4.4 identifies the anatomical landmarks for auscultation).

There are several other heart sounds that you can learn once you have mastered the first two (Cox 2004).

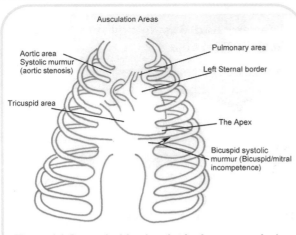

Ausculation Areas

Aortic area
Systolic murmur
(aortic stenosis)

Pulmonary area

Left Sternal border

Tricuspid area

The Apex

Bicuspid systolic
murmur (Bicuspid/mitral
incompetence)

Figure 4.4 Anatomical landmarks for heart auscultation

The muscular ventricles form the main pumping component of the heart; each ventricle communicates with a large vessel via a semilunar valve to forward the blood flow. The pulmonary valve on the right leads to the pulmonary artery and ultimately the lungs. The aortic valve on the left leads to the aorta and the systemic circulation. At the base of the aorta there are two small openings, one to the left, one to the right; these are the coronary arteries, which branch off into smaller vessels encompassing the heart and supplying the heart muscle with a dedicated blood supply.

Applying Theory to Practice: Exercise 4.3

Disease of these arteries is referred to as coronary artery disease.

- Do you know which patient groups are particularly susceptible to this illness?
- List some ways of preventing this disease process

The DH's *National Service Framework for Coronary Heart Disease* is a good place to find further information (DH 2000).

Function

The cardiac cycle
The heart has electrophysiological, mechanical and neurological properties that combine and coordinate to pro-

duce effective myocardial contraction and pumping of the blood.

Mechanical
Each complete heartbeat, or cardiac cycle, consists of two phases in response to electrical stimulation.

The pumping phase of the atria is referred to as atrial systole and the pumping phase of the ventricles as ventricular systole.

Systole is triggered by depolarisation of cardiac muscle cells, which involves a transient change in sodium and potassium ion concentration inside and outside the cells (Chapter 2). Both the superior and inferior vena cava transport deoxygenated blood into the right atrium (venous return); simultaneously the pulmonary veins return oxygenated blood from the lungs to the left atrium. The blood travels into the respective atria then continues down into the ventricles through the open atrioventricular valves. The semilunar valves are closed. The atria are stimulated by a wave of electrical conduction from the sinoatrial node to force any remaining blood down into the filling ventricles. Once an adequate pressure is exerted by the ventricles, the atrioventricular valves close and the blood in the ventricles is simultaneously ejected through the semilunar valves towards the lungs from the right ventricle and the systemic circulation via the left ventricle.

The relaxation or filling phase of the atria takes place during the ventricular systole and the ventricular filling or relaxation phase takes place during atrial systole.

Immediately after depolarisation is completed, the process reverses itself, resulting in repolarisation and a return to the resting state, this relaxation phase is referred to as diastole.

These are the mechanics behind the cycle, which is also reliant on nervous stimulation and an electrical current to drive the conduction and depolarisation processes.

Neurologic (involuntary control over the heart)
Various neurologic factors regulate heart function; the most predominant is the **autonomic nervous system** (ANS). The heart is innervated via the cardiac centres in the brain by both sympathetic and parasympathetic fibres:

- The **sympathetic branch** of the ANS stimulates the heart via cardiac or accelerator nerve fibres and the release of **norepinephrine/epinephrine**. This results in both an increase to the heart rate and force of

Anatomy and Physiology in Action: Box 4.2

Summary of the Cardiac Cycle

The cardiac cycle reflects the flow of blood through the heart during one heartbeat:

- Depolarisation = discharging
- Repolarisation = recharging
- Systole = the contraction phase
- Diastole = the relaxation phase (filling) phase

The atria contract and force blood down into the ventricles; in contrast, the ventricles need to exert a pumping force to reach their targets.

The contraction of the atria can result in 20–30% more blood entering the ventricles; in disease states such as atrial fibrillation where the atria fail to adequately contract, the individual can lose this amount of their cardiac output resulting in haemodynamic collapse.

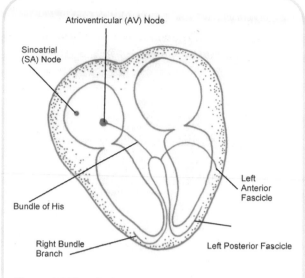

Figure 4.5 Electrical conduction within the heart

contraction (**positive inotropic effect**). This can have a profound effect with rates reaching in excess of 200 beats per minute (bpm). Sympathetic fibres also innervate the coronary arteries causing dilation and allowing increased amounts of oxygen and nutrients through.

- The **parasympathetic branch** of the ANS releases **acetylcholine** which blocks accelerator nerve fibres and causes an ionic change within the cells resulting in a slowing of the heart rate.

The levels of noradrenaline and acetylcholine are dependent on the requirements of the body at that particular moment, i.e. they either increase or decrease to maintain homeostasis. The principal force is the inhibitory effect of the parasympathetic nervous system, which slows the resting heart rate to between 60–80bpm. If the parasympathetic fibres were to totally dominate this tug of war, the heart rate might fall to a rate of between 20–30bpm. The term **vagal tone** is used to describe this slowing effect as the nerve stimulus originates in the vagus nerve. If the sympathetic nerve fibres dominate, the rate would exceed 100bpm (clearly demonstrated in exercise).

Electrophysiological (the conduction system)

The cardiac conduction system controls the route and pace, or timing, of electrical stimulation through the heart muscle. The four chambers are coordinated to work in concordance. Under normal conditions the electrical stimulation proceeds in the following sequence:

- **The sinoatrial (SA) node**: this collection of modified muscle cells (myocytes) found in the right atrium locally control or initiate each heartbeat and the rate at which the heart pumps. The SA node is commonly referred to as the heart's natural pacemaker. Under normal circumstances (at rest) the SA node will have an intrinsic rate of between 60 and 100 bpm. This intrinsic rate can be affected by exercise or intensified cellular demands: when asleep the rate will decrease. In individuals who are extremely fit the rate will be slower than normally expected due to an increase in the efficiency of the heart.
- **The atrioventricular (AV) node**: situated near the tricuspid valve acts as a bridge or gateway between the atria and ventricles. Under normal conditions this is the only entry route into the ventricles, as all other tissue between the atria and ventricles is fibrous and non-conducting.
- **The bundle of His**: this pathway, clearly identified in Figure 4.5, runs along the interventricular septum; it divides into two branches or fascicles on the left

(anterior and posterior) and one fascicle on the right travelling toward the apex of the heart.

- **The fascicles of the bundle of His/Purkinje fibres** become nerve-like processes that encompass the ventricular myocardium and form an elaborate network particularly on the disproportionately large left ventricle.

Although the SA node is the natural pacemaker of the heart, you will encounter many patients where this is not the case. Scenario 4.2 highlights a common clinical presentation where the conduction system becomes blocked.

Anatomy and Physiology in Action: Box 4.3

The Cardiac Conducting System

Under normal physiology the SA node is the heart's pacemaker, an electrical impulse instigates myocardial contraction.

The SA node determines the pace because it initiates a faster intrinsic rate of fire than any other area of the conduction system or the heart muscle; this rate ranges between 60–100bpm; the rate is affected by the body's needs via the autonomic nervous system.

If there is a failure of the SA node to conduct an impulse to the AV node, the AV node will itself instigate an impulse and become the pacemaker with an intrinsic rate of between 40–60bpm. If this back-up mechanism also fails, impulses can be generated further down the conduction system including in the bundle of His and Purkinje fibres where rates vary between 15–40bpm, but are notoriously unreliable, i.e. complete failure of the heart as a pump may ensue.

The electrical activity within the heart can be monitored via electrodes placed on the chest. Various views of the heart can be obtained depending on where the electrodes, otherwise known as leads, are positioned.

The two main formats used in clinical practice are a three-lead ECG where the viewer has three different views to choose from, and the **12-lead ECG** which uses 10 actual positions, but through combining some of these

Applying Theory to Practice: Exercise 4.4

What would the physiological consequences be for the patient if the heart fails? This may develop gradually.

Answer the following questions and add the answers to your portfolio.

- How would you expect the patient to look?
- Apart from the slow pulse rate, what effect would you expect on the other vital signs?

reveals 12 actual views of heart activity. Figure 4.3 identifies the positioning of these leads with which the nurse will need to become familiar. To begin to appreciate the ECG, the nurse needs to understand the correlation between heart function and the ECG waveforms (Table 4.1).

Heart Function	ECG Waveform
Atrial systole/depolarisationAtrial systole to commencement of ventricular activityVentricular systole/depolarisationEndpoint of ventricular systole pre-repolarisationVentricular diastole/repolarisationLength between ventricular activity de/repolarisationPossible interventricular septal repolarisation	P wavePR intervalQRS complexST segmentT waveQT intervalU wave

Table 4.1 The Correlation between Electrophysiology and ECG Waveforms

When continuously monitoring a patient on a cardiac monitor it is customary to select lead 2, which views the heart from the bottom up; therefore the electrical activity should be travelling toward this lead (think of sitting directly in the middle at the front of a cinema). When viewing the heart's electrical activity in this lead the

80

electrics should be positive because under normal conditions the conduction will be coming directly toward lead II.

Cardiac output

The cardiac output can be defined as the amount of blood ejected from the heart by each ventricle in each minute (summarised in Box 4.4).

The cardiac output varies depending on the requirements of the body. Both the stroke volume and heart rate can be increased or decreased; these can work independently or they can combine, again depending on the current requirements.

The effects of ageing

Chronic wear and tear affects the heart's ability to function in several ways. **Arteriosclerosis** is a degenerative process affecting the arteries whereby the walls of the vessel calcify and harden, resulting in a loss of elasticity, causing increased blood pressure and increased resistance and workload for the heart. As discussed, the main layer of the heart is composed of thick muscle; this muscle continually works harder to overcome the increased resistance of the arteries resulting in the insidious development of many illnesses:

Figure 4.6 ECG revealing a sinus rhythm

Anatomy and Physiology in Action: Box 4.5

The Cardiac Reserve

The Frank–Starling law of the heart identifies that the crucial factor determining stroke volume is the degree of stretch on the myocardium just before it ejects. The greater the stretch of the myocardium, the greater the force of contraction.

During strenuous exercise the stroke volume can double; in contrast if an individual is losing blood or fluid resulting in less blood returning to the heart, the stroke volume and contraction are decreased.

- The ventricles, particularly the left, can enlarge and become **hypertrophic**, resulting in less space within the chambers; as the muscle grows larger it becomes sluggish.
- Due to **calcification** and degeneration the valves within the heart lose the ability to close properly, resulting in blood being forced in the wrong direction (regurgitation).
- The electrics begin to degenerate, leading to conditions such as **atrial fibrillation** and **heart block**.
- **Atheromatous deposits** adhere to the inner artery lining causing an increase in blood pressure and the potential for varying degrees of thrombus/clot forma-

Scenario 4.1 Part I

Acute Myocardial Infarction

James Collins, a 56-year-old Caucasian man, is admitted to the emergency department after suffering severe chest pain and shortness of breath for the past 25 minutes.

On arrival, he appears grey and clammy. He has vomited in the ambulance.

On arrival, his vital signs are:

Airway – clear, patient is talking, AVPU = A
Breathing – respiratory rate 24
Circulation – pulse 102, regular
Blood pressure – 149/94
PMH: **Hypertension**. Mr Collins smokes and is grossly obese.

tion with the potential of artery occlusion and starvation of the myocardium.

- **Aneurisms** within the vessels can develop, leading to weakness in the vessel wall and splitting of the vessel; common vessels include the aorta. A dissecting or leaking aneurysm is a life-threatening emergency (Evans & Tippins 2007).

Assessment and analysis of patient presentation

Mr Collins has presented with the typical clinical signs and symptoms of heart disease and more specifically acute coronary syndromes (ACS). He has vomited in the ambulance, a common cardiac-related symptom. He has several risk factors for the development of cardiovascular disease and his physical appearance suggests the possibility of a heart attack or acute myocardial infarction (AMI).

The structured initial assessment has identified several alterations to the patient's physical state before any vital signs are recorded. This approach is essential to identifying serious illness at an early stage. Clinical data reveal tachypnoea, borderline tachycardia and hypertension.

Developing and Delivering Expert Care: Box 4.6

Clinical Signs Associated with ACS/AMI

- Chest pain – commonly central and radiating into the neck, arms or jaw
- Sweaty, clammy or ashen grey appearance
- Nausea or vomiting
- Chest pain can be masked by diabetic neuropathy
- Sudden collapse of unknown cause
- Shortness of breath/dyspnoea
- Crushing sensation to central chest
- The early identification of these signs can prove life-saving.

Heart disease – the facts

Cardiovascular disease (CVD) is the collective name given to diseases affecting the heart and circulatory system. Cardiovascular disease was responsible for in excess of 216,000 deaths in the UK in 2004 with coronary heart disease (CHD) claiming the lives of 137,000 individuals. Cardiovascular disease is the leading cause of premature

death, with more than one in three people dying from it (BHF 2006).

CVD can be split into two main types:

- Diseases affecting the heart and its circulation (coronary heart disease)
- Diseases affecting the circulation of blood to the brain (cerebral vascular accidents/stroke).

The blood distribution or supply to any area of the body can be disrupted; commonly affected areas include:

- The peripheral blood supply (arms and legs); this peripheral vascular disease is commonly precipitated by smoking
- The gut/intestines; the mesenteric artery supplies this region and can become blocked either locally by thrombus formation or by a blood clot travelling from elsewhere within the arterial system
- The deep veins of the lower and upper legs; clots can form in these areas and then travel throughout the venous system until they encounter a vessel of small diameter and become lodged; this area is commonly within the lungs resulting in a pulmonary embolism.

Pathophysiology

CHD and CVD relate to pathophysiological changes that take place within the circulatory system. In the case of CHD this process takes place within the coronary arteries directly affecting the delivery of blood to the heart. There are two closely related disease processes leading to CHD:

- **Arteriosclerosis** occurs as part of the ageing process in which arterial walls gradually become thickened, ridged and inelastic due to the deposition of fibrous tissue. The end effect of thickened and inelastic vessels is an increase in blood pressure and an inability to alter lumen size. This renders the vessel at an increased risk of rupture or occlusion, a prime example is demonstrated by aortic stenosis.
- **Atherosclerosis** is the term used to describe the deposition of lipid and cholesterol-rich atheromatous plaques within the arterial walls. Over time the inner lumen becomes increasingly clogged, resulting in a reduced **distal** blood flow. These atheromatous plaques have a serious risk of dislodgement, leading to thrombus formation and the complete occlusion of blood to an area of the heart.

Developing and Delivering Expert Care: Box 4.7

The Three Stages of Acute Myocardial Infarction Development

- Ischaemic – tissue damage caused by a lack of oxygen. Early administration of O_2 therapy can salvage the potential damage
- Injury – greater degree of damage, but still salvageable with the early instigation of treatment
- Infarction – necrotic/dead tissue, depending on timescale, damage can be limited

The early administration of oxygen saves lives!

Several theories exist as to why atheromatous plaques form or adhere to arterial walls. One theory centres on fat being the ultimate source of potential energy; it is stored throughout the body for times of need, but because of modern methods of farming and food production, with various foods being available all year round, and with increased wealth and access to food, this historically traditional period of starvation is never realised, resulting in the excessive accumulation of fatty deposits within the arteries (and elsewhere). It is accepted that if a surplus amount of fat is consumed within the diet and not utilised through energy requirements (exercise), then it is deposited not only in visible subcutaneous areas, but also within the walls of the arteries. This disease process does not occur overnight, in fact it can take decades before the

Applying Theory to Practice: Box 4.8

Risk Factors Associated with CHD

- Previous myocardial infarction
- Diabetes mellitus
- Obesity
- Genetic pre-disposition (Afro-Caribbean/Asian origination)
- Smoking
- Stimulant use (cocaine)
- Family history of CHD/CVD
- Sedentary lifestyle
- Hypertension
- Hypercholesterolaemia/lipidaemia

accumulation of atherosclerosis within the arteries actually leads to the patient experiencing chest pain due to ischaemia (cessation of blood flow). Recent studies have identified fatty deposits within the arteries as early as the teenage years (DH 2000). There are several prime predisposing factors for the development of coronary heart and vascular disease although obesity, a high fat diet, smoking, and a sedentary lifestyle, virtually guarantee its development.

The acute coronary syndromes

Figure 4.7 provides an overview of the acute coronary syndromes (ACS), an umbrella term used to describe the varying degrees of acute ischaemia that can result from this insidious disease process, disrupting blood flow to the heart, thereby compromising myocardial function.

The acute coronary syndromes reflect a disease continuum comprising three distinct but interchangeable stages of disease progression. Figure 4.7 identifies the potential outcomes when fat deposits within the coronary arteries dislodge.

The immediate treatment options depend on the extent of damage to the heart. If the episode fails to demonstrate changes on an ECG, and the patient's blood results fail to

show a rise in the cardiac enzymes that are released into the bloodstream when the myocardium is damaged, the episode is referred to as unstable angina. The next stage, as identified in Figure 4.7, is non S-T elevated myocardial infarction (NSTEMI). The difference between NSTEMI and unstable angina centres on a specific blood result: if levels of **troponin** are raised in the blood, a myocardial infarction is indicated and the patient will require further treatment such as angioplasty. If the blood results reveal a raised troponin level and there is evidence of ECG changes associated with acute myocardial infarction (namely S-T segment elevation), then this is an S-T elevated myocardial infarction (STEMI).

Acute myocardial infarction – the facts

Thirty-three per cent of men and 25% of women who suffer an AMI die instantaneously. Post-myocardial infarction 50% of patients will go on to die within 30 days of the event (MINAP 2004). These alarming statistics are only the tip of the iceberg, as all of those that survive will still develop varying degrees of long-term heart failure.

In March 2000 the Department of Health published the *National Service Framework for Coronary Heart Disease*. Since its introduction the National Service Framework

Figure 4.7 Acute coronary syndromes
(Adapted from Evans & Tippins 2007)

Applying Theory to Practice: Box 4.9

Summary of Pharmaceutical Treatments

- **Anticoagulants**: unfractionalised (UFH) and low molecular weight heparin (LMWH): true anticoagulants prolonging clotting time, reducing further clotting, enabling thrombus to disperse.
- **Anti-platelet agents**: aspirin and clopidogrel used together to reduce platelet aggregation in response to internal arterial damage (NICE 2004). Glycoprotein IIb/IIIa inhibitors are also used prior to percutaneous coronary interventions (PCI) and in the treatment of NSTEMI; their use is currently under review by NICE.
- **Thrombolytics**: directly decompose the thrombus. Time-dependent reduction in morbidity and mortality rates.
- **Morphine/diamorphine**: reduce pain, anxiety and pre-load thereby removing potential strain on the heart
- **Anti-emetics**: reduce nausea and vomiting thereby preventing further strain on the heart
- **Glyceryl trinitrate** (GTN): short-acting nitrate (vasodilators), which dilate coronary arteries, reduce myocardial oxygen demand and reduce both pre- and afterload
- **Percutaneous coronary interventions**: direct dilation of the affected artery and use of stents to maintain artery patency
- **Beta blockers**: reduce heart rate and lower blood pressure, prevention of further coronary events
- **Statins**: reduce cholesterol levels in the blood and possibility of further events

(NSF) has directly affected the care this group of patients receive. Specific guidelines dictate strict timescales within which patients must be seen and treated. The traditional treatment for AMI centres on delivering an intravenous drug to decompose the thrombus, referred to as a thrombolytic. In many hospitals a newer therapy involving directly accessing the occluded vessel and either removing or squashing the thrombus, or inserting a stent has proven to be increasingly effective (ESC 2005). These

forms of treatment are called percutaneous coronary interventions or **angioplasty**.

In 2003, 75% of patients eligible for thrombolysis were treated within 20 minutes of arrival, more than double for the same period in 2000 (MINAP 2004).

The early treatment of AMI prevents and reduces the amount of death the myocardium experiences, thereby limiting the future development of heart failure (ESC 2005). The Resuscitation Council (UK) advocate the use of the acronym MONA as a quick and easy aide-mémoire for the effective initial treatment of cardiac chest pain.

Psychosocial aspects

Many patients have stated that the initial feelings they experience during an AMI centre on impending doom and a real feeling that they are going to die. Nurses throughout their career will encounter patients experiencing varying levels of anxiety and fear. It is paramount to listen to the patient's fears and communicate in a way they will understand; the minimal use of medical terminology is essential. By beginning to construct a good rapport with patients at an early stage of their presentation a relationship based on

Developing and Delivering Expert Care: Box 4.10

Excellent tools for curtailing AMI, are:

- Morphine
- Oxygen
- Nitrates
- Anti-platelet agents

Questioning Clinical Practice: Exercise 4.6

When Patients Benefit from Immediate PCI

In your clinical placements you will find many treatments on offer for particular diseases: however, this does not mean they are necessarily the most effective.

- Identify a treatment in your current placement, and research alternatives.
- NICE and NSFs provide national standards but what about international 'best practice'?

mutual respect can begin, this relationship will benefit both as the nurse will ascertain in-depth knowledge about the patient's needs and the patient will feel increasingly secure in the knowledge that the nurse is both interested in their case and is showing that they actually care about what the person is experiencing. Do not underestimate the profound effect this relationship-building phase can have on the entire patient journey!

Individuals respond very differently when faced with a potential serious illness: some will become hysterical, others will deny. It is the nurse's responsibility as the patient's main advocate to explain both the disease process (keep this brief and concise) and the immediate treatment options. Patients will frequently ask what treatment you would like to have in the same circumstance. This can be a particularly difficult question for the nurse to answer due to some serious ethical considerations that currently plague the National Health Service. Available treatments can be limited to certain regions; others may only be available privately, leaving the nurse in a compromising position in their ability to convey honest information.

Mr Collins's treatment will depend on which hospital he attends. Some will assess his needs and transfer him to another hospital where he could immediately undergo angioplasty; others may have angioplasty facilities; less-equipped areas will treat him with thrombolysis despite knowing this is not entirely in his best interest. Modern healthcare is littered with such clinical complexities and as the first line of contact for patients it is the nurse who will face most of the questions.

Professional issues

In emergency presentations the immediate priority is to assess and treat the patient's presenting problem, pain and vomiting caused by AMI in this case. Lifestyle choices are responsible for many of today's healthcare presentations. The worst culprits are smoking (Chapter 3) and obesity (DH 2006). The lifestyle choices of Mr Collins are literally killing him; his heart disease could have been completely preventable if he had adopted a healthier lifestyle. What influence can the healthcare professional have on individual choice? Does the government in a political democracy have the right to impinge on the social behaviours/habits of the public?

Recent healthcare initiates are directed at providing patients with an informed choice; if patients do not follow the guidance of the case managers (normally medical

Scenario 4.1 Part II

Acute Myocardial Infarction (4 days post-presentation)

Mr Collins has received treatment for his acute presentation and is making a good recovery. He is now on the cardiac care ward, mobile and feeling well.

Family members who have brought him his favourite meal of steak and ale pie with chips are visiting. As his nurse walks past, Mr Collins is pouring salt onto his chips and talking with his family members.

The nurse knows that Mr Collins needs to rest and recuperate, but by continuing to eat a high fat diet with added salt he is putting himself at direct risk of a repeat episode of AMI.

The nurse begins discussing the issue with both the patient and his family. Mr Collins becomes upset and leaves the ward for some fresh air. On return the nurse can smell he has been smoking.

Questioning Clinical Practice: Exercise 4.7

What do you consider to be the role of nurses in promoting health?
- If nurses actively encourage healthier lifestyles, does this mean they need to abide by the same standards they are advocating?
- Do you smoke? Are you overweight? Do you binge drink alcohol or take recreational drugs? Does this compromise on your credibility as a nurse?

consultants/nurse specialists), they may limit their future choices. This is clearly demonstrated by local policies whereby a consultant cardiologist may refuse to undertake a second angioplasty on Mr Collins if he continues to smoke. This raises many ethical concerns for both the healthcare professional and the patient.

Analysis

Healthcare professionals are in an ideal position to provide essential information to patients for their long-term well-being. This health education or health promotion is vital, particularly for those with limited understanding of their conditions or limited resources (Rutter & Quine 2002). According to Rutter & Quine (2002), changing health behaviour is a complex process involving several stages:

- The patient needs to want the desired change to their lifestyle
- They must acknowledge the link between the identified high-risk behaviour and their predicament
- They need to visualise a clear pathway leading to the outcome whereby they have an action plan of avoidance and distraction when tempted to recommence the behaviour
- This includes identifying potential obstacles, resources and opportunities that will either assist or hinder their attempted change

Gollwitzer (1999) discusses how the construction of implementation intentions can further goal attainment. This can be a complex part of the patient's secondary phase of care, as confronting patients with news they would rather not hear can often be ignored or greeted with anger and denial.

In the case of Mr Collins, we know the disease process that brought him to hospital is related to the accumulation of fat within his coronary blood vessels; this could have killed him. By continuing to smoke, consuming a high-fat and calorie-rich diet, Mr Collins will be at increased risk of experiencing another heart attack or a cerebral vascular accident (stroke).

In the acute phase these matters are not usually addressed for two reasons: first, there may not be adequate time as medical and nursing staff are prioritising care; second, during this period of stress and anticipation, potentially blaming the patient for the illness would be viewed as unkind and inconsiderate. In addition, it is highly unlikely that Mr Collins would be in a fit mental state to comprehend such information. Regardless, the issue must be confronted during his time in hospital and should be a priority in his care plan during the secondary phase of his stay in hospital. Some hospitals will employ specialists (usually nurses) to address these issues and follow up patients either in the community or as outpatients.

All nurses have a moral and ethical obligation to confront actions by patients that may lead to direct harm; therefore, in this scenario the nurse should discuss the matter with both Mr Collins and his family, as these are the people he will be living with. If his current behaviour continues, they may well be living without him. Nurses must be professional and conscious of portraying themselves in a patronising manner. The point should be made that by encouraging Mr Collins to continue eating high-fat foods, his family are aiding the disease process that has led to his heart attack and that next time he may not be so lucky.

The family may view this presentation as a warning sign and take the matter seriously. It is important to educate patients about their illnesses and how they can prevent further exacerbations; this provides them with ownership of their fate. This patient empowerment is central to the modern philosophy of the Department of Health (2005). The DH has three main principles on promoting health in the NHS identified in *Shaping the Future of Public Health* (2005) which contributes to the delivery of the *Choosing Health* White Paper (DH 2004):

- Help people to make and maintain informed health choices
- Empower and mobilise local communities for health
- Develop health programmes and services, especially to reduce inequalities in health

By consulting with the patient and forming a mutually realistic plan of action, patient compliance can be improved; this process must include the patient understanding the plan and being satisfied with the affective aspects. These will include the support of his family, and counselling or belonging to a group with a common goal. Ogden (2004) centres the plan of care on information sharing and personalised information: when making statements about the benefits or risks of a particular action, it should be directly related to the patient's case so they can directly visualise the potential impact. Many patients will take the warning seriously and adopt healthier lifestyles, others will deny the cause and blame the condition on other less intrusive parts of their personality such as modern living and stress. It is important not to push the patient too far on these issues otherwise they may shun the health services completely and fail to seek help in the future.

The obesity epidemic and cardiovascular disease

Obesity and the associated long-term increase to both morbidity and mortality have led to this condition being the number one public health issue in the developing world. The clinical consequences primarily include heart disease and type 2 diabetes.

Obesity – the facts

The Department of Health have constructed a National Service Framework focusing on reducing clinical obesity, a phenomenon which is escalating at a prolific rate. In 2003, within the UK, 22% of men and 23% of women were clinically obese (DH 2006).

Questioning Clinical Practice: Exercise 4.8

You will need to ascertain which tools or systems are used to identify clinical and morbid obesity.
- Are these systems foolproof?
- Will certain user groups be given false information by the test components?

Scenario 4.2

Complete Heart Block

Ronald Mwete, a 72-year-old man of African origin, has been hospitalised for four days since collapsing at home where he lives with his wife.

Mr Mwete was found to have complete heart block; subsequently a pacemaker was inserted.

You are caring for him today and start your duties by undertaking a quick assessment of his current needs and by recording his vital signs.

On arrival his vital signs are recorded as:

Airway – clear, patient is talking, AVPU = A
Breathing – respiratory rate 16
Circulation – pulse 70, regular
Blood pressure – 149/94
Temperature – 37.9
PMH: hypertension and hypercholesteraemia

Assessment and analysis of patient presentation

Mr Mwete appears to be in a stable condition following the insertion of a mechanical pacemaker. His vital signs demonstrate that the pacemaker is functioning with an intrinsic rate set at 70. Mr Mwete has been found to have a slightly raised temperature; this could be due to an underlying infection. A source of infection should be sought. This will include observation of the pacemaker insertion sight and any indwelling invasive lines such as venous cannulae.

Applying Theory to Practice: Exercise 4.9

Venous cannulae and urinary catheters are common sites for infection (NICE 2003, NAO 2000). This is because they by-pass the body's natural defences and allow bacteria to proliferate and enter sterile sites. They should only be in place for as short a period as possible; this depends on the make and material type of the device.

- What is the life expectancy of the makes used within your clinical area?
- What cardinal signs are associated with infection?
- Identify which tests are regularly requested within your clinical placement areas and the laboratories they are sent to and for what kind of analysis.
- What is a VIP score?

Psychosocial aspects

There are two pertinent points for consideration in the care of Mr Mwete.

- First, it has been identified that many patients are frightened at the prospect of being hospitalised, sometimes due to adverse publicity, or to the real threat of developing a hospital-acquired infection (Washer & Joffe 2006). Healthcare professionals should rationally discuss patient fears about catching resistant bacteria while in hospital. Nurses must remain professional when questioned, with patient education the onus; simultaneously the nurse must be aware that hospital-acquired infections do pose a real and significant threat to both patient morbidity and

mortality rates, with currently one in ten hospitalised patients affected (NICE 2003).

● Second, Mr Mwete must learn to come to terms with the device planted within his body. Most pacemakers will only be slightly noticeable to those unaware of their presence; despite this, the patient will initially be constantly aware of its presence.

Nurses are in an ideal position to discuss the psychosocial aspects of patient care, particularly when the patient is susceptible to the information. This is not necessarily within the initial period when the medical team may have conveyed relevant although technical data. Patients often take time to absorb information and frequently require the same explanation several times (Hollinworth & Hawkins 2002). Patients will commonly require reassurance about the potential alteration to body image, alterations to lifestyle and technical information.

The plan of care

Mr Mwete's plan of care will be based on the activities of living described by Roper et al. (2000: Chapter 1). Using a model provides the nurse with prompts to deliver a holistic approach to his care. Case management will include assisting Mr Mwete to return to his own home as soon and as safely as possible. This will be a multidisciplinary effort with several members of the team providing expert opinions on his potential needs via assessment processes. The initial plan of care centres on ensuring the pacemaker is providing an adequate level of stimulus to meet his physiological demands. This is demonstrated via vital sign analysis.

Mr Mwete was found to have a localised skin infection at the site of his pacemaker insertion. The area became red, inflamed and a purulent discharge was noted when the dressing was changed. A swab was taken of the discharge and sent to the microbiology laboratory for microculture and sensitivity examination (MC&S). Antibiotics were commenced and, depending on the results of the laboratory tests, the antibiotics might be replaced by a specific drug that would eradicate the infection. Mr Mwete was discharged home once his temperature had resolved. He was still taking oral antibiotics and was told to see his GP if the site became inflamed or if he felt unwell. An outpatient appointment was made to assess the effectiveness of his pacemaker.

Pacemakers – the facts

Pacemakers are common although most people are not aware of the crucial role they play in assisting an individual to lead a normal lifestyle. A permanent artificial pacemaker is a small, battery-operated device inserted below the skin on the patient's chest. There are a variety of different types of pacemakers available depending on the initial compromise. These include:

● Single-wire pacemakers, which sit inside one of the heart's chambers
● Two-chamber pacemakers are generally used when the individual requires additional support: one of those wires goes in the atrium; the other wire goes in the ventricle
● Three-lead pacemakers are used when the muscle of the heart fails to be powerful enough to maintain an adequate cardiac output.

The pulse generators can be set to a fixed-rate (asynchronous) or demand (synchronous) mode.

Although pacemakers are generally inserted when a patient has such a slow heart rate that they might collapse without warning due to insufficient blood flow to their brain (symptomatic bradycardia), they are also inserted for heart rates that can become dangerously fast (tachyarrhythmias). These devices can initiate an electrical charge designed to restart the heart in its normal sequence thereby curtailing the abnormal and potentially life-threatening rhythm (arrhythmia). These devices are referred to as indwelling defibrillators.

Applying Theory to Practice: Exercise 4.10

While on clinical placement identify how long the battery lasts in the types of pacemakers used in your area.

● How does one change the batteries?

Pathophysiology

The conduction sequence and its relationship to heart function are commonly affected by disease. These disease processes are synonymous with ageing and degeneration of areas of the conduction sequence, although several other predisposing factors have been identified

Figure 4.8 Bradycardia algorithm. Source: Resuscitation Council UK (2006). Reproduced with permission.

(Ariyarajah et al. 2005, Levine & Brown 2006). These disease processes manifest in several different ways depending on the origin of the anomaly and the current health status of the individual. There are two distinct types of arrhythmia: those that increase the heart rate (tachyarrhythmias) and those that slow the heart rate (bradyarrhythmias).

Bradyarrhythmias

There are several independent factors that can result in an excessively slow heart rate and for physically fit individuals (particularly runners) a very slow heart rate can be normal. Therefore, when assessing a patient's heart rate, take into consideration other relevant factors such as levels of fitness, medications such as beta blockers that will slow the heart rate, and hypothermia that may also have a pronounced effect. There is, therefore, a distinct need to separate the term bradycardia (purely meaning

slow heart rate) into symptomatic or non-symptomatic bradycardia. Common causes of symptomatic bradycardia include:

- Drug toxicity – commonly digoxin and beta blockers
- Vagal over-stimulation
- Blocks within the electrical conduction pathway (referred to as heart block)
- Myocardial infarction.

The Resuscitation Council (UK) have identified an algorithm that identifies best practice when confronted by a patient demonstrating bradycardia (Figure 4.8).

Heart block – the facts

There are varying classifications of heart block referred to as degrees, with some simply being variants of normal and producing no physical effects. Others will result in profound effects including haemodynamic collapse and cardiac arrest. Heart block has a variety of causes. It can be a consequence of a congenital defect or **cardiomyopathy**, although it is commonly associated with myocardial infarction (Ghuran et al. 2003).

Tachyarrhythmias

Tachyarrhythmias encompass several pertinent abnormal cardiac rhythms. It does not include sinus tachycardia, as this is not an abnormal rhythm and therefore not an arrhythmia. The most prevalent tachyarrhythmia is atrial fibrillation, the most famous or infamous is ventricular tachycardia:

Atrial fibrillation (AF) is associated with an increased risk of embolus-related stroke due to clot formation within the atria, heart failure due to a reduced cardiac output and premature death (Bilal Iqbal et al. 2005). AF affects approximately 4% of over 65-year-olds in the USA; this figure increases to 15% by age 75 (Ezekowitz 1999). Majeed et al. (2001) suggest there are approximately 650,000 individuals diagnosed with AF in England and Wales. This is probably an underestimate as many people live with undiagnosed AF until a symptom manifests.

Stewart et al. (2004) state that the prevalence of AF is increasing and that 1% of the UK population experience AF; this increases to 10% in the elderly. Most patients with AF require long-term pharmacological treatment, often including anticoagulants, which require monitoring. The prevalence of AF-related hospitalisations has increased

**Questioning Clinical Practice:
Exercise 4.11**

- How might a symptom of AF manifest?
- Which is the most common illness directly associated with AF?

**Applying Theory to Practice:
Box 4.11**

Causes of Atrial Fibrillation

- Coronary heart disease
- Alcohol
- Hyperthyroidism
- Cardiomyopathy
- Infection (sepsis)
- AF can be **idiopathic**

Atrial fibrillation can be easily felt at the patient's radial pulse. The pulse will feel irregular and possibly thready if the individual has a significantly reduced cardiac output. This vital datum will not be identified if you rely solely on machines to record vital signs.

threefold over recent years (Stewart et al. 2004). Patients experiencing AF commonly present in one of three ways;

- Lethargic and weak; this is due to the reduction in cardiac output that the patient can experience
- In a collapsed state due to a combination of established heart disease and the impact of a reduced cardiac output
- Following a stroke or a cerebral event: due to insufficient contraction of the atria, blood stagnates resulting in clot formation; these clots are eventually fired around the circulation commonly resulting in a **stroke**.

Figure 4.9 demonstrates a **narrow complex tachyarrhythmia** with an irregular ventricular response. When a tachyarrhythmia is identified, there are two main points that need to be clarified:

- Does the patient exhibit signs of circulation? If not, the advanced life support algorithm should be commenced.

Figure 4.9 Atrial fibrillation (Evans & Tippins 2007)

■ Is the patient haemodynamically compromised or incapacitated?

AF is a complex presentation to treat and its management is dependent on potential risk factors. NICE are currently reviewing AF guidelines published in 2007. The emergency management phase is covered within the Resuscitation Council (UK) tachycardia algorithm (Figure 4.10).

In chronic AF the prospect of cardioversion being successful is greatly reduced and drugs may be prescribed to reduce the ventricular response. Depending on the risk factors the patient may be prescribed long-term anticoagulant therapy.

Cardiac arrest

Ventricular tachycardia (VT) implies that the ventricles, which form the major pumping force of the heart, are beating at an exaggerated rate exceeding 120–150bpm. Strictly speaking, only a limited number of beats originating from within the ventricles constitute ventricular tachycardia, but in reality the rhythm is continuous, with the individual commonly experiencing a sense of impending doom, or collapsing due to a reduction of their cardiac output, whereby the ventricles are pumping so fast that they do not have enough time to fill with sufficient blood.

Ventricular tachycardia, also known as **broad complex tachycardia**, can continue even after the individual

has suffered such a haemodynamic insult that they lose their cardiac output and pulse. This is referred to as pulseless ventricular tachycardia; one of the four cardiac arrest rhythms.

Developing and Delivering Expert Care: Exercise 4.12

All healthcare staff need to be able to identify critical illness and deliver basic life support (DH 2001).

■ You will need to develop expert skills within this area. The RC (UK) have a website with extensive information and easy to follow algorithms on serious emergencies such as choking and anaphylaxis through to cardiac arrest.
■ Visit their site and download the algorithms guiding current practice.
■ Practise drawing the electrical rhythms associated with cardiac arrest; add these to your portfolio.
■ www.Resus.org.uk

Cardiac arrest synopsis

Cardiac arrest can be defined as the sudden cessation of cardiac function, resulting in the loss of effective circulation and therefore incompatible with life. The Resuscitation Council (UK) have published guidelines on advanced life support (RCUK 2006). These guidelines

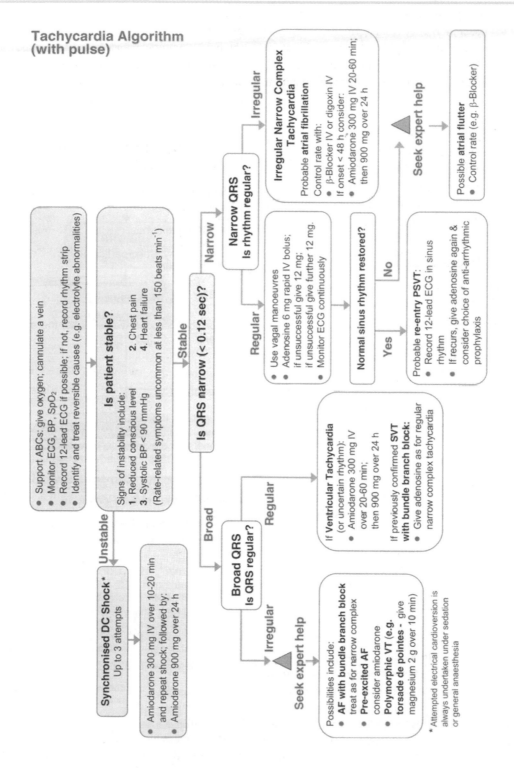

Figure 4.10 Tachycardia algorithm (with pulse). Source: Resuscitation Council UK (2006). Reproduced with permission.

provide healthcare practitioners with a structured approach to the emergency management of patients experiencing cardiac arrest (Figure 4.11). Most cardiac arrests within the hospital environment are predictable events, with many early warning signs and symptoms (RCUK 2006).

The ALS guidelines are initially based on the chain of survival outlined in Table 4.2.

Chapter 2 identified many of the early warning signs synonymous with physical deterioration and cardiac arrest; the following section describes the arrest rhythms and the associated ECG changes. The reader is referred to the RC (UK) guidelines for in-depth guidance.

Advanced life support

The treatment of cardiac arrest centres on achieving cerebral and vital organ perfusion until definitive treatment such as defibrillation can be delivered or an instigating cause identified and treated. Life support becomes 'advanced' once a defibrillator/cardiac monitor is available.

Shockable rhythms (defibrillation)

This requires a cardiac monitor to identify an underlying rhythm. If the rhythm is **pulseless ventricular tachycardia** (PVT) or **ventricular fibrillation** (VF), the application of an electrical current or **defibrillation** of the heart muscle may result in the chaotic rhythm and fibrillating muscle mass becoming organised again, with the patient regaining a cardiac output/pulse. VF and PVT are commonly associated with AMI and have the lowest mortality rate when early treatment is initiated. Therefore if the cause of the cardiac arrest is due to electrical faults such as ventricular fibrillation, defibrillation is the key to management (Figure 4.11).

Non-shockable rhythms

Two other rhythms are associated with the arrested patient. The first is **asystole**, which means without output, i.e. an absence of electromechanical activity throughout the heart. This, therefore, cannot be defibrillated and the management centres on basic life support. It is traditionally referred to as a 'flat line' and hence there is a need to check lead attachments are correct. This arrhythmia has the highest mortality rate. Causes include vagal over-stimulation. The second is **pulseless electrical activity** (PEA). PEA can be defined as an organised electrical rhythm without a cardiac output/pulse, i.e. the patient is pulseless despite a potentially normal electrical rhythm. Common causes include hypovolaemia and hypoxia. In PEA the cause must be identified and addressed in order to restore a spontaneous circulation. Exercise 4.13 lists the reversible causes of cardiac arrest.

Applying Theory to Practice: Exercise 4.13

**Reversible Causes of Cardiac Arrest
4 Hs and 4 Ts**

- **H**ypovolaemia
- **H**ypothermia
- **H**ypoxia
- **H**ypo/hyperkalaemia (electrolyte imbalances)
- **T**ension pneumothorax
- **T**amponade – cardiac
- **T**hromboembolic
- **T**oxins

Memorise this list and add it to your portfolio. By structuring your clinical decision making around these causes you may save lives!

Questioning Clinical Practice: Exercise 4.14

There are several important phrases used within clinical practice to describe both the act of resuscitation and the legal terminology surrounding care.

Using the correct terminology is paramount as misunderstandings can lead to distress and confusion in an area commonly described as one of the most sensitive that clinicians, patients and family members may have to face.

- Find out the clinical meaning of the terms and locate a copy of the DNAR policy your trust employs
- What is the difference between a patient receiving active treatment and a patient not being resuscitated in the event of a cardiac arrest?

Figure 4.11 Adult advanced life support algorithm. Source: Resuscitation Council UK (2006). Reproduced with permission.

Action	Rationale
Early recognition of associated signs and call for help	Prevention is better than cure
Early **cardiopulmonary resuscitation** (CPR)	Cerebral oxygenation while buying time
Early defibrillation	To restart organised electrical activity and cardiac output
Post-resuscitation care	To maintain adequate circulation
	To prevent further arrests
	To restore quality of life

Table 4.2 The Chain of Survival

A. Asystole

B. Ventricula fibrillation

C. Ventricula Tachycardia into Ventricula fibrillation

D. Sinus Rhyth but no cardiac output

Figure 4.11 The four electrical rhythms synonymous with cardiac arrest

Professional issues
Cardiac arrest and Do Not Attempt Resuscitation Orders (DNAR)

Television programmes can portray an unrealistic view of cardiac arrest and the act of resuscitation: most patients survive after receiving defibrillation in response to the flat line seen on a cardiac monitor. As you will have already read, asystole is a non-shockable rhythm. In reality, even within an acute hospital environment fewer than 20% of patients who experience a cardiac arrest survive (RCUK 2006).

Every patient should be resuscitated following a diagnosis of cardiac arrest unless a patient has explicitly refused cardiopulmonary resuscitation (CPR), an example being the patient has a valid advanced directive/living will, or if their individual circumstances limit the potential benefits of CPR: this could include the patient being in the terminal stage of an illness, or having a chronic condition whereby the burdens of CPR outweigh the benefits.

Nurses need to be able to distinguish between the act of actively treating a patient, withdrawing active treatment and not resuscitating in the event of cardiac arrest. Patients and those close to them may misinterpret DNAR as a withdrawal of care. A DNAR order, which must be written by a consultant or the most senior doctor present, only relates to the act of administering CPR (it is assumed that senior nurses will also soon be decision makers). Many patients are admitted to hospital with complex

needs; in younger patients these may be congenital defects. In the ageing population these may be due to a lifetime's wear and tear.

When a serious diagnosis is confirmed and cannot be cured, the patient's care management may change from cure to symptom control. Care is never withdrawn but the focus changes dependent on the individual's needs. In nursing terms this has been classically described as allowing the patient to die with both dignity and comfort. Pain control, symptom relief and psychological care become the central care focus. Withdrawing treatment centres on stopping treatments or investigations aimed purely at gaining a diagnosis or prolonging the quantity, rather than quality, of life. The patient's needs are still addressed and their plan of care may include surgery or radiotherapy for symptom control.

The Department of Health have issued guidelines on this sensitive issue. These include removing subjectivity from the decision-making process and involving the patient and those close to them as much as possible (BMA 2001). A DNAR decision should be considered when patients:

- Have previously stated they do not want to be resuscitated in the event of cardiac arrest
- Are unlikely to survive the cardiac arrest.

All UK hospitals should have an agreed DNAR policy, based on national guidelines (NHS Executive 2000). Healthcare workers need to attend regular mandatory updates on both the delivery of basic life support and on the clinical application of DNAR orders.

Analysis

DNAR orders can cause great distress to both patients and their families or loved ones. This can be exacerbated if they have not been involved or informed about the decision. It is considered best practice to involve the individual, next of kin or family in decisions affecting them, although legally the ultimate decision is a medical one (RCUK 2006).

The blood

The blood can be viewed as a fluid and mobile connective tissue. This tissue is composed of two prime components – cells and **plasma**.

Form

The components of blood are bathed and transported in the plasma. Plasma constitutes 55% of the blood volume. It is a thick and straw-coloured fluid; its main component is water (90–92%), the remaining volume being the transportation enzymes and the plasma proteins:

- Albumin
- Fibrinogen
- Prothrombin
- Globin.

Plasma transports several essential components to where they are required within the body, these include:

- Oxygen and carbon dioxide, dissolved within the plasma
- Hormones and enzymes – these chemical messengers and catalysts assist in the maintenance of homeostasis by influencing organs to return a state of internal equilibrium
- Antibodies and antitoxins – complex proteins programmed to attack specific antigens
- Waste – urea, carbon dioxide and lactic acid are transported to the liver to be broken down and to the kidneys for excretion
- Mineral salts or electrolytes – maintain nerve conduction and acid/water balance
- Nutrients – amino acids, essential fatty acids, glucose and vitamins are distributed to the cells for energy, cellular reproduction and repair.

The blood cells are composed of three distinct types of cell (Table 4.3).

Function

- Transports oxygen, hormones, enzymes and nutrients throughout the body
- Removes waste products from every region of the body and transports them to the organs of excretion
- Contains clotting factors, white blood cells and antibodies

Anaemia – the facts

Anaemia is a collective term used to describe the end result of many disease processes in which the blood cannot carry enough oxygen, either resulting from a decrease in the number of RBCs or because each RBC is unable to carry sufficient oxygen due to the depletion of

Erythrocytes (red blood cells/RBC)	**Leucocytes** (white blood cells/WBC)	**Thrombocytes** (platelets)
Biconcave cells that do not contain a nucleus Produced in the red bone marrow, containing haemoglobin which absorbs oxygen, providing blood with its distinctive red colour On average, circulate for 120 days when they are broken down by the spleen and iron recycled by the liver	Split into two groups: Granulocytes and non-granular leucocytes Irregularly shaped cells, largest of the blood cells Active role in preventing infection and repairing damage Can proliferate dramatically through mitosis when confronted by infection	Small, easily damaged cells with no nucleus The instigators to blood clotting Produced within the red bone marrow

Table 4.3 The Blood Cells

Pernicious anaemia	**Iron deficiency anaemia**	**Aplastic anaemia**
An insidious process in which a vital component for the absorption of vitamin B_{12} is lost This failure in the production of intrinsic factor in the stomach is associated with a reduction in hydrochloric acid production The end result is the circulation of large cells within the blood circulation that do not contain haemoglobin and cannot, therefore, carry oxygen The cause has been associated with an autoimmune response in the gastric mucosa Treatment centres on replacing vitamin B_{12} via slow-releasing intramuscular injections (cyanocobalamin)	A deficiency of dietary iron, the main component of haemoglobin, leads to the world's leading nutritional deficiency and the most common cause of anaemia (Clancy & McVicar 2002) A common cause is heavy periods (menorrhagia); 1% of women become anaemic at some time in their life due to this (Ramrakha & Moore 2004) Diseases related to a slow loss of blood e.g. peptic ulcers (often associated with the long-term use of NSAIDs) Some bowel conditions, e.g. coeliac disease or chronic diarrhoea, cause poor absorption of iron Low dietary iron can lead to anaemia, although there are many sources of iron, including meat, green vegetables, milk, flour and eggs Worldwide, hookworm infestation is the leading cause due to the worms feeding inside the intestines (Easton 1999); although mostly prevalent in tropical countries hookworm infestation can be seen in those who have recently been to tropical areas.	A failure in the production process of red blood cells in the bone marrow. Has been linked to certain classes of drugs i.e. sulphonamides, chloramphenicol, and the effects of radiation. Over a period of time the bone marrow becomes atrophied and ineffective Treatment ranges from discontinuing the identified cause to administering blood transfusions for the anaemia All the common forms of anaemia result in similar signs and symptoms

Table 4.4 Common Classifications of Anaemia

essential components, such as haemoglobin. The most prevalent forms of anaemia are summarised in Table 4.4.

Anaemia is associated with several common signs and symptoms:

- Breathlessness, increasing with activity
- Tiredness or lethargy
- Dizziness, particularly on standing
- Rapid pulse and palpitations (irregular heartbeats)
- Pallor (dependent on severity)
- Red, inflamed tongue
- Reduced CRT
- Jaundice.

Applying Theory to Practice: Exercise 4.15

- List what changes to a patient's lifestyle you would expect from this chronic or insidious disease process. Think about the symptoms previously discussed.
- Read the scenario 4.3 and compare your findings.

Scenario 4.3

Sickle Cell Disease

Chantal Ferguson, a 24-year-old woman, has been referred to the acute medical unit after experiencing increasing abdominal pain over the past two days. She has taken dihydrocodeine, which is prescribed by her GP for periodic acute attacks of sickle cell pain.

During the initial assessment Chantal appears pale, clammy and is crying with pain. Her respiratory rate is 29, regular and bilaterally shallow. There are no signs of central or peripheral cyanosis. Her radial pulse is weak, regular and recorded as 115 bpm; this is in conjunction with a CRT of three seconds. Her blood pressure is recorded as 148/79.

Miss Ferguson appears frightened. She adopts the fetal position and guards her abdomen, which is soft to touch. She is alert and orientated to time and place. Her pupils are equal and reactive to light. Temperature is 38.1.

She is allergic to penicillin, has lactose intolerance and a PMH of sickle cell anaemia.

Assessment and analysis of patient presentation

Miss Ferguson appears to be demonstrating the early stages of compensatory shock, identified by the rapid rise in her respiratory rate. Her radial pulse is weak and her CRT reduced. Her pale, sweaty appearance may be due to pain, or a severe ischaemic event making this presentation serious. A patient exhibiting severe pain is always a cause for concern due to the underpinning pathophysiology associated with pain development. Although sickle cell anaemia is a chronic disease process, the effects can result in acute exacerbations. She is at risk of vaso-occlusive, haematological and infectious processes, which can be extremely painful, leading to organ failure and ultimately an early death.

Applying Theory to Practice: Exercise 4.16

What would your initial plan of care involve for Chantal Ferguson?

- Identify her needs and prioritise your care delivery.
- Many healthcare trusts have a local policy on best practice – identify the one in your area.

As with all potentially critically ill patients, high-flow oxygen (12–15L/min) should be commenced via a reservoir bag and mask. Intravenous access will need to be established as sickle cell presentations commonly involve dehydration, with the associated decrease in peripheral circulation precipitating the red blood cells to sludge. The administration of analgesia should be a priority and all progressive units will have a set protocol to follow. Her pain will need to be assessed, analgesia administered and its effect evaluated.

Developing & Delivering Expert Care: Box 4.12

When administering intravenous **opiates** the drug should be given slowly to ascertain the desired effect and reduce the possibility of respiratory depression. This is called the titration of drugs, and is an essential component in the delivery of quality care.

Administering appropriate pain relief is an essential part of nursing practice. This assessment should be based on the World Health Organization's step approach to analgesics (WHO 1996). There are many pain assessment scales available, and it is recommended that acute areas use a minimalist approach to the assessment process due to the clinical symptoms, demonstrated in Table 4.5 (Evans & Tippins 2007).

Pain score	Appropriate analgesia
0 = No pain	None indicated
1 = Mild pain	Non-opioid analgesia
2 = Moderate pain	Weak opioid combinations
3 = Severe pain	Stronger opioid combination
4 = Very severe pain	Opioids titrated to pain

Table 4.5 Categorical Rating Scale for Acute Pain

Many studies have identified that analgesia administration to patients in pain is inadequate, mainly due to the subjective opinions of practitioners (Davies & McVicar 2000, Nurmikko et al. 1999). The categorical rating scale directly links theory to practice through the correlation between the identified pain score and the choice of analgesia. As with the assessment of all patients in pain, objective findings, such as those associated with the sympathetic response, should be included in your assessment. There are many theories related to how patients interpret pain, and how their interpretation can be based on childhood experiences and learnt behaviour through to cultural beliefs and ethnicity (Edwards et al. 2001).

Sickle cell disease – definition and prevalence

Sickle cell disease is a genetically inherited disorder. Sufferers inherit two variant haemoglobin genes, one from each parent. It mainly affects individuals of Afro-Caribbean heritage, although similar genetic pathologies exist within Mediterranean countries and the Middle East. The high incidence of the sickle cell gene in these regions of the world is due to the sickle cell's ability to make RBCs resistant to the malaria parasite (Clancy & McVicar 2002). Thirty years ago the life expectancy of a sufferer was around 14 years; today with modern treatments it exceeds

Questioning Clinical Practice: Exercise 4.17

Explore your own experiences of pain.
- List some of the alternatives to drugs for pain relief.
- While on clinical placement identify local methods of pain relief.
- What tools or scales do nurses use to prevent subjective opinion and initiate appropriate treatment?
- Are these tools relevant to all users? What if the individual does not speak English?
- What other ways are there to justify your choice of treatment?

50 years of age (Claster & Vichinsky 2003). There are in excess of 15,000 individuals living with sickle cell or haemoglobinopathies within the UK (Anionwu & Atkin).

Pathophysiology

Sickle cell disease results from genetic abnormalities in haemoglobin construction where a single amino acid substitution creates a cascade of events leading to the deformity of an essential component of RBCs. RBCs become misshapen, rigid and sticky, resembling a sickle. This sickling leads to an increase in blood viscosity; RBCs can adhere to the inner layer of arterial walls and literally get stuck while travelling through the capillaries, resulting in distal ischaemia and severe pain referred to as the sickle cell crisis.

The abnormal shape of the sickled cells results in dehydration due to water and potassium loss. Sickle cells also have a shorter life span (10 to 20 days) compared to that of normal RBCs. Although the body compensates for the decrease in viable RBCs, the overall count decreases resulting in anaemia, hence the term sickle cell anaemia. Common triggers include hypoxia, infection and dehydration.

With repeated attacks a chronic and progressive destruction to the internal tissues and organs occurs. Commonly affected areas include the spleen, lungs and liver.

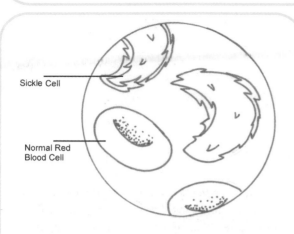

Figure 4.13 Sickle-cell disease (illustrating normal blood cells and sickle cells)

dehydration or electrolyte imbalance. Miss Ferguson was referred to a sickle cell specialist nurse with the aim of preventing further episodes.

Blood group	Antigen	Antibody
O	None	Anti A Anti B
A	A	Anti B
B	B	Anti A
AB	AB	None
Rhesus positive	D	None
Rhesus negative	D	None

Table 4.6 Blood groups and their compatibility

Treatment

Treatment initially centres on pain control, supplementary oxygenation and rehydration. An infective or ischaemic process needs to be reversed. The National Institutes of Health, National Heart, Lung, and Blood Institute (2002) have published a collaborative document focusing on developing a standard of excellence for this user group.

Analysis

Any patient with a history of pallor, lethargy, weakness and shortness of breath should have a full blood count; this simple blood test measures the number of RBCs and haemoglobin. Miss Ferguson was found to have a temporary ischaemic episode affecting her spleen. Her care involved the administration of NSAIDs to reduce inflammation and potential spasm, prophylactic administration of antibiotics in case of localised infection of the ischaemic site, and rehydration to correct any underlying

Transfusing blood and blood products

Patients require a blood transfusion for a multitude of clinical conditions ranging from chronic anaemia to acute trauma and massive blood loss. The consequences of transfusing a patient with the wrong blood type can be devastating. Despite continued improvements in the processes involved, there continue to be serious errors (McClelland 2007). Good practice centres on following a few basic principles:

- Right blood
- Right patient
- Right time
- Right place.

Applying Theory to Practice: Exercise 4.18

Over time you need to become familiar with the normal values of test results.

- Find out the normal range for haemoglobin in the blood
- Is there a difference between men and women?

Learn the normal ranges for many of the common tests performed in clinical practice and add these to your portfolio.

Applying Theory to Practice: Exercise 4.19

Identify both the blood transfusion guidelines within your placement areas and the tool used to structure the physical observations you will need to record on those that are receiving a transfusion.

There are several different blood types, with many being incompatible with each other. Table 4.6 identifies both the blood groups and their compatibility.

The early identification of incompatibility is essential. Administering incompatible blood to a patient can result

in an anaphylactic type reaction (Chapter 2). Patients with reduced renal ability or ineffective heart function may not be able to physically cope with the increased blood volume and may start to exhibit signs of cardiac failure and pulmonary oedema. It is essential to learn and follow local guidelines on blood administration. For further reading, McClelland (2007) is highly recommended.

Conclusion

With the current trend towards obesity escalating, heart disease and its prevention will play a prominent role in the foreseeable future of healthcare; therefore, the theoretical knowledge and clinical skills gained in this chapter will assist in developing a solid and dynamic approach to patient care. Gaining a solid understanding of the cardiovascular system, the fluid it carries, and its supporting system is essential to delivering expert care. Regardless of the setting or specialty in which a nurse works, they will encounter patients with both chronic and acute problems related to these systems. By anticipating both the physical and psychosocial needs of a patient, care delivery and the patient's journey can be enhanced, with potential and actual needs realised and acted upon in a partnership between the individual and the health service.

Chapter 4 Summary Quiz

1. Where can the heart's apex be easily auscultated?

A. In the fifth intercostal space in the midclavicular line to the right of the sternum
B. In the fifth intercostal space in the midclavicular line to the left of the sternum
C. In the fourth intercostal to the left of the sternum
D. Between the second and third ribs on the left side

2. The normal electrical conduction sequence of the heart can be summarised as:

A. Commencing at the atrioventricular node, travelling through the bundle of His and terminating in the atria
B. Initiating in the sinoatrial node, continuing down the bundle of His and terminating in the atrioventricular node
C. Initiating in the sinoatrial node, continuing through the bundle of His and terminating in the Perkinje fibres
D. Initiating in the sinoatrial node, continuing through the atrioventricular node, down the bundle of His and terminating in the Perkinje fibres

3. The QRS complex signifies which element of the cardiac cycle?

A. Atrial relaxation
B. Ventricular relaxation
C. Ventricular contraction
D. Atrial contraction

4. Which of the following electrical rhythms is associated with cardiac arrest?

A. Sinus tachycardia
B. First degree heart block
C. Atrial fibrillation
D. Ventricular fibrillation

5. The blood is composed of:

A. Red cells, white cells and lymphocytes
B. White cells, red cells and plasma
C. Red cells, white cells, platelets and plasma
D. Platelets, thrombocytes, white cells and plasma

6. Pernicious anaemia is caused when:

A. There is an excess of white blood cells
B. There is an inadequate number of platelets
C. There is a failure in the production of intrinsic factor in the stomach
D. Red blood cells become misshapen

7. S1 signifies which mechanical aspect of the cardiac cycle?

A. The closure of the interventricular valves
B. Opening of the interventricular valves
C. Opening of the aortic valves
D. Closure of the pulmonary and aortic valves

8. Acute myocardial infarction can be defined as:

A. The heart stops beating
B. When a clot causes occlusion of a coronary artery
C. The patient experiences chest pain
D. The patient's blood sugar being above 11

9. Which of the following is not a symptom of heart failure?

A. Shortness of breath on exertion
B. Swollen ankles
C. Pulmonary oedema
D. Pyrexia

10. Pain assessment and treatment should be focused on:

A. Both subjective and objective data in combination with a structural tool
B. The nurse's previous experience of a particular illness
C. Which medications are easily available
D. Listening solely to the patient and correlating their expression of their pain with a suitable analgesic

Further reading

Evans, C. & Tippins, E. (2007) *Foundations of Emergency Care.* Open University Press: Maidenhead.

Ghuran, A., Uren, N. & Nolan, J. (2003) *Emergency Cardiology: An Evidence-based Guide to Acute Cardiac Problems.* Arnold: London.

National Institute for Clinical Excellence (NICE) (2003) *Infection Control:. Prevention of Healthcare-associated Infection in Primary and Community Care.* Full guidelines. www.nice.org.uk.

Quinn, T. (2004) Managing acute myocardial infarction. *Emergency Nurse* 12(3): 17–19.

Resuscitation Council (UK) (2006) *Advanced Life Support,* 5th edn. RCUK: London.

http://www.britishpainsociety.org/

References

Anionwu, E. & Atkin, K. (2001) *The Politics of Sickle Cell and Thalassaemia.* Open University Press: Buckingham.

Ariyarajah, V., Asad, N., Tandar, A. & Spodick, D.H. (2005) Interatrial block: pandemic prevalence, significance, and diagnosis. *Chest* 128(2): 970–5.

British Heart Foundation (2006) *Coronary Heart Disease Statistics.* British Heart Foundation Health Promotion Research Group, Department of Public Health, University of Oxford.

British Medical Association (BMA) (2001) *Withholding or Withdrawing Life-prolonging Medical Treatment.* BMJ Books: London.

Clancy, J. & McVicar, A.J. (2002) *Physiology & Anatomy: A Homeostatic Approach,* 2nd edn. Arnold: London.

Claster, S. & Vichinsky, E.P. (2003) Managing sickle cell disease. *British Medical Journal* 327: 1151–5.

Cox, C. (2004) *Physical Assessment for Nurses.* Blackwell Publishing: Oxford.

Davies, J. & McVicar, A. (2000) Issues in effective pain control 1. Assessment and education. *International Journal of Palliative Nursing* 6(2): 58–65.

Department of Health (2000) *National Service Framework for Coronary Heart Disease.* DH: London.

Department of Health (2004) *Choosing Health: Making Healthy Choices Easier.* DH: London.

Department of Health (2005) *Shaping the Future of Public Health: Promoting Health in the NHS.* DH: London. http://www.dh.gov.uk/en/Publicationsandstatistics/Publications/PublicationsPolicyAndGuidance/DH_4116526

Department of Health (2006) *Health Challenge England – Next Steps for Choosing Health.* DH: London.

Easton, A. (1999) Intestinal worms impair child health in the Philippines. *British Medical Journal* 318: 214.

Edwards, C., Fillingham, R. & Keefe, F. (2001) Topical review. Race, ethnicity and pain. *Pain* 94: 133–7.

European Society of Cardiology Task Force for Percutaneous Coronary Interventions (2005) Guidelines for percutaneous coronary intervention. *European Heart Journal* 26: 804–47.

Evans, C. & Tippins, E. (2007) *The Foundations of Emergency Care.* Open University Press: Maidenhead.

Ezekowitz, M.D. (1999) Atrial fibrillation: the epidemic of the new millennium. *Annals of Internal Medicine* 131: 537–8.

Ghuran, A., Uren, N. & Nolan, J. (2003) *Emergency Cardiology: An Evidence-based Guide to Acute Cardiac Problems.* Arnold: London.

Gollwitzer, (1999) Implementation interventions: Strong effects of simple plans. *American Psychologist* 54: 493–503.

Hollinworth, H. & Hawkins, J. (2002) Teaching nurses psychological support of patients with wounds. *British Journal of Nursing* 11(20; Suppl 14): S8–S18.

Levine, M. & Brown, D. (2006) Heart block, second degree. *Emedicine* http://www.emedicine.com/emerg/topic234.htm (accessed 19 December 2006).

Majeed, A., Moser, K. & Carroll, K. (2001) Trends in the prevalence and management of atrial fibrillation in general practice in England and Wales, 1994-1998: analysis of data from the general practice research database. *Heart* 86: 284–8.

McClelland, D.B.L. (2007) *Handbook of Transfusion Medicine: United Kingdom Blood Services,* 4th edn. DH: London.

MINAP (2004) *How Hospitals Manage Heart Attacks: Third Public Report of the Myocardial Infarction National Audit Project. Clinical Effectiveness and Evaluation Unit.* Royal College of Physicians: London.

National Audit Office (NAO) (2000) *The Management and Control of Hospital Acquired Infection in Acute NHS Trusts in England.* National Audit Office: London.

National Institutes of Health, National Heart, Lung, and Blood Institute (2002) *The Management of Sickle Cell Disease,* 4th edn. NIH Publication: Bethesda, USA.

National Institute for Clinical Excellence (NICE) (2003) *Infection Control: Prevention of Healthcare-associated Infection in Primary and Community Care.* Full guidelines. NICE: London. www.nice.org.uk.

National Institute for Clinical Excellence (NICE) (2004) *Clopidogrel in the Treatment of Non-ST-segment-elevation Acute Coronary Syndrome.* NICE: London.

NHS Executive (2000) *Resuscitation Policy* (HSC 2000/028). DH, London; Scottish Executive Health Department (2000) *Resuscitation Policy* (HDL (2000) 22). Scottish Executive: Edinburgh.

Nurmikko, T.J., Nash, T.P. & Wiles, J.R. (1999) Control of chronic pain. *British Medical Journal.* 317: 1438–41.

Ogden, J. (2004) *Health Psychology. A Textbook.* Open University Press: Maidenhead.

Ramrakha, P. & Moore, K. (2004) *Oxford Handbook of Acute Medicine.* Oxford Medical Publications: Oxford.

Resuscitation Council (UK) (2006) *Advanced Life Support,* 5th edn. RCUK: London.

Roper, N., Logan, W. & Tierney, A. (2000) *The Roper-Logan-Tierney Model of Nursing.* Churchill Livingstone: London.

Rutter, D.R. & Quine, L. (eds) (2002) *Changing Health Behaviour: Intervention and Research with Social Cognition Models.* Open University Press: Maidenhead.

Stewart, S., Murphy, N., Walker, A., McGuire, A. & McMurray, J.J.V.

(2004) Cost of an emerging epidemic: an economic analysis of atrial fibrillation in the UK. *Heart* 90: 286–92.

Washer, P. & Joffe, H. (2006) The hospital 'superbug': social representations of MRSA. *Social Science and Medicine* 63(8): 2142–52.

World Health Organization (WHO) (1996) *WHO Guidelines: Cancer Pain Relief,* 2nd edn. WHO: Geneva.

The nervous system

Susie Scott

Chapter 5 Learning Objectives

- Build foundation knowledge and understanding of the anatomy and physiology of the nervous system
- Develop knowledge and understanding of several common conditions affecting the nervous system
- Develop the ability to apply theory to practice; understanding and recognising the physical manifestations of conditions in patients
- Gain an understanding of neurological assessment using a structured approach
- Gain insight into commonly used medications to prevent or treat disorders
- Broaden understanding and appreciation of the psychosocial impact of illnesses of the nervous system
- Rehearse a questioning approach to nursing, enabling evidence-based practice
- Construct solid evidence of professional development for your portfolio

Applying Theory to Practice: Exercise 5.1

Compose a list of the conditions that you already know that affect the nervous system, add this to your portfolio.

At the end of this chapter, reflect back on the conditions that you knew about, recognising where your knowledge and understanding has been enhanced.

Include these conditions in your portfolio. Include

Introduction

The nervous system is truly remarkable. It seems to effortlessly exert the most profound control and regulation over every aspect of life. Every thought, feeling or action reveals its fascinating activity; consequently, malfunction of the nervous system can have a devastating effect on life.

This chapter addresses the core of the nervous system, specifically the brain, the structures and systems within it, and the spinal cord. It begins with an overview of the structure and function of the brain itself, revealing anatomical features and physiological activity. The relationship between the brain and spinal cord is examined, by exploring the form and function of the cord and the integrated activity that allows the nervous system to function so eloquently. Patient scenarios are used to illustrate common disorders and diseases that affect the

nervous system and confront patients with disability and failure of a system they depend on.

Nervous system function

The nervous system is divided into the **central nervous system** (CNS), comprising the brain itself and the spinal cord, and the **peripheral nervous system** (PNS), encompassing the cranial and spinal nerves. The CNS is an integrated command centre interpreting and responding to sensory impulses. The PNS is divided into sensory (afferent, carrying towards) and motor (efferent, carrying away) divisions. The **sensory division** allows the relay of information from receptors in skin, muscles, joints and visceral organs of the body, such as the heart, so that the CNS is constantly informed of activity inside and outside the body. The **motor division** brings about a motor response; this may be for a muscle to contract or for a gland to secrete. The motor division has two main parts:

- **Somatic (voluntary) nervous system** conducting impulses to skeletal muscles only
- **Autonomic nervous system** (ANS) regulating activity of smooth muscles, cardiac muscles and glands. Its activity is involuntary, outside of our control. The ANS is functionally divided into the parasympathetic and the sympathetic branches.

The brain

Form

Isolated from the rest of the body, the brain is hidden and protected by its own bony framework, the **skull**, or cranium. The brain has the consistency of a soft-boiled egg, the wrinkled appearance of a walnut and no moving parts. This pinkish-grey structure weighs approximately 1500g and contains more than 100 billion **neurons**, the fundamental functional unit of the nervous system. The **meninges** cover, surround and protect the brain and the spinal cord. They have three layers:

- **Dura mater** is the outermost layer of the meninges. It is a tough double-layered membrane attached to the bones of the cranium, housing the veins and arteries supplying the skull.
- **Arachnoid membrane** is a thin, delicate layer loosely covering the brain. Between the dura and arachnoid membranes is the **subdural space**, below the arachnoid membrane is the much bigger **subarachnoid space**, which is filled with cerebrospinal fluid.
- **Pia mater** is the innermost layer that clings to the brain and spinal cord. It contains many blood vessels, which are important as they extend into the brain tissue.

Applying Theory to Practice: Exercise 5.2

Answer the following questions to gain insight into how theory can be applied to clinical practice:

- What conditions have you heard of that are characterised by bleeding into the spaces between the meninges of the brain?
- What are the most likely causes of such bleeding?

Cerebrospinal fluid (CSF), a clear, colourless, odourless liquid, surrounds the brain and the spinal cord. It acts as a shock absorber, floating and cushioning the brain and spinal cord from trauma. CSF is secreted from each of the four **ventricles** within the brain (Figure 5.1), specifically the **choroid plexuses**, and also provides a source of nutrients. The choroid plexuses are projections that hang from the roofs of the ventricles, and are composed of capillaries that are permeable enabling them to constantly leak CSF from their surfaces. CSF moves freely through the ventricles, a closed system continuous with the subarachnoid space of the brain and spinal cord. Most CSF is reabsorbed via the **arachnoid villi**, projections in the subarachnoid space, and then emptied into the venous sinuses.

Applying Theory to Practice: Exercise 5.3

Meningitis is inflammation of the meninges, most often caused by infection. It affects the meninges, the subarachnoid space and CSF. Most cases are caused by microorganisms, e.g. bacteria, viruses or fungi, that spread into the blood and CSF.

Meningitis is a serious condition and can lead to many complications: hearing loss, headache, hydrocephalus, seizures and reduced consciousness, to name a few.

Bacterial meningitis is a medical emergency. It requires prompt recognition and treatment with antibiotics as an absolute priority. Bacterial meningitis may cause septic shock so supportive treatment is provided to treat circulatory collapse and prevent organ dysfunction (Oh 2003).

Vaccination programmes target certain strains of bacteria that cause meningitis as a preventative strategy in those most at risk (DH 2006, Health Protection Agency 2005).

- Identify which groups within society are targeted with immunisation programmes and why.

The brain (technically known as the **encephalon**) is made up of visibly distinct regions, each of a particular shape and texture, interlocking and nestling together. The primary regions are the **cerebrum**, the brain stem and the **cerebellum** (Figure 5.2).

The cerebrum has two clear halves, known as **cerebral hemispheres**, the surface of which is convoluted. There are numerous **gyri** (convolutions), which give the brain this appearance and greatly increase the surface area. The outer layer of the hemispheres is known as the **cerebral cortex**, or **grey matter**, and is made of up billions of neurons. Underneath this lies the **white**

Figure 5.1 The cerebral ventricular system

matter containing nerve fibres and **neuroglia**. These fibres are bundled together and form **fibre tracts** within the CNS enabling the brain nerves to work together and communicate. Deep within the cerebral white matter is a group of nuclei called the **basal nuclei** or **basal gan-**

glia. These inaccessible structures are vital for complex aspects of motor function.

The cerebral hemispheres are made up of four pairs of lobes: **frontal**, **parietal**, **temporal** and **occipital** (Figure 5.3). In addition, the cerebrum also contains the **diencephalon**, which is composed of the thalamus, **hypothalamus** and **epithalamus** (Figure 5.2). The hypothalamus is connected by tissue to the **pituitary gland** (**hypophysis**) and the **pineal body**, which

Applying Theory to Practice: Exercise 5.4

The Cranial Nerves
- Name the 12 pairs of cranial nerves and identify their functions.
- During your clinical placement you may observe cranial nerve function being tested: familiarise yourself with the testing techniques used in clinical practice.
- Consider what the physiological consequences of damage to each of these cranial nerves would be and how this may manifest in a patient.

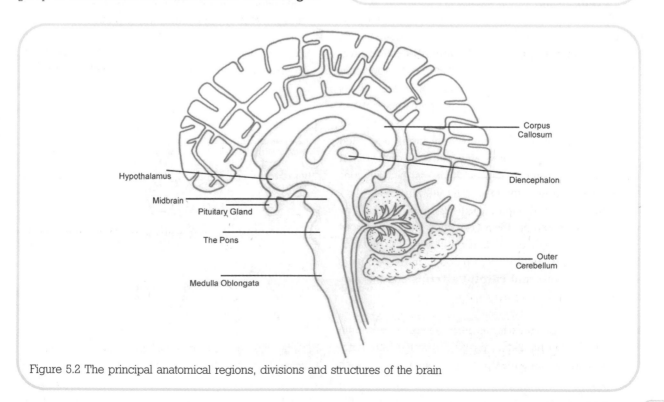

Figure 5.2 The principal anatomical regions, divisions and structures of the brain

Figure 5.3 Lateral aspect of the brain featuring the principal functional areas

extends posteriorly from the epithalamus. The diencephalon forms the central core and is surrounded by the hemispheres; the diencephalon itself encloses the third ventricle.

The cerebral hemispheres appear to sit upon a thick stalk (**brain stem**), which eventually tapers to become the spinal cord. The brain stem contains significant anatomical parts which are vital for life and are subdivided into the **midbrain**, **pons** and the **medulla oblongata**, each approximately an inch long (Figure 5.2). The brain stem is also where 10 of the 12 pairs of cranial nerves originate; they provide a pathway between the PNS and the CNS.

The cerebellum (known as the little brain) is located just below the occipital lobes and protrudes outwards. It has a distinct cauliflower-like shape, is heavily convoluted, and accounts for 11% of total brain mass.

Continuous blood supply to the brain is crucial. The brain suffers irreparably from even short periods without oxygen and is totally dependent on glucose for metabolism. The brain is supplied with blood from the two pairs of arteries: the **internal carotid arteries** and the **vertebral arteries** (Figure 5.4):

- The internal carotid arteries enter the cranium through the base of the skull, passing through the dura, eventually reaching the upper brain where they branch

off; the branches ensure blood is supplied to most of the cerebral hemispheres and the eyes.

- The vertebral arteries unite and become a single **basilar artery** at the level of the pons. The basilar artery subdivides again and supplies the cerebellum, brain stem and the posterior (occipital) part of the cerebrum.

- The anterior (carotid) circulation and the posterior (vertebrobasilar) circulation unite to become the arterial anastamosis known as the **circle of Willis**.

Figure 5.4 The circulatory system on the base of the brain, illustrating the circle of Willis

This circle of Willis is approximately 1 inch square, is located at the base of the brain and surrounds the pituitary gland. It is an important structure for the blood supply to the brain as it allows the blood pressure to be equalised, and in some circumstances provides an alternative route of circulation should an artery be occluded.

Having examined the structure of the brain and the main anatomical regions, we will now explore the matter of which the brain is composed, neurons, and how they signal to one another.

Neurons process all information and activity within the brain by conducting nerve impulses to, from and within the brain. The characteristics of each neuron depend on its function, but there are similarities in the anatomy of all neurons (Figure 5.5a).

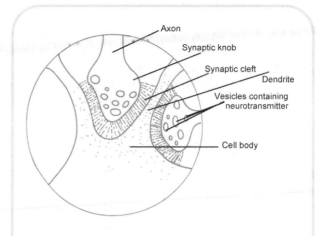

Figure 5.5b Post-synaptic neurone (synapse)

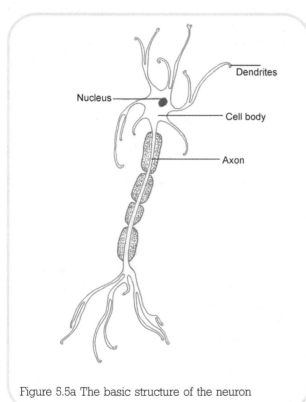

Figure 5.5a The basic structure of the neuron

All neurons have a cell body, with a nucleus, cytoplasmic material and processes extending from it. These processes are **dendrites** and **axons**. Dendrites conduct nerve impulses towards the cell body whereas axons conduct impulses away from the cell body. The numerous dendrites, associated with each cell body, create a vast surface area to receive nerve impulses. In contrast, a single neuron has a single axon. How quickly a neuron conducts a nerve impulse depends on the diameter of the axon and whether the axon is insulated with a fatty sheath known as the **myelin sheath**. The sheath is constricted at intervals. Within these intervals there are segments known as **nodes of Ranvier**, responsible for increasing the speed of nerve impulse conduction.

Anatomy and Physiology in Action: Exercise 5.5

Grey and White Matter

Within the CNS, some fibres are myelinated. These fibres form what is known as white matter and are primarily fibre tracts. The grey matter of the CNS is composed of cell bodies and unmyelinated nerve fibres.

- Which clinical conditions are synonymous with degeneration of these myelinated fibres?

Glial cells (or glue cells) are not neurons but are nonetheless plentiful in the brain, outnumbering neurons ten to one. There are various types of glial cells each with a different function. In general, their role is supportive, providing structural support, nourishment and protection for neurons.

Function

Nerve impulses occur as a result of the changes in cell membrane potential of each neuron. Alterations in the concentration of sodium and potassium on either side of

the membrane stimulate the change in membrane potential. If the change in potential is great enough, an impulse is conducted. This is known as an **action potential** and is followed by a wave of depolarisation.

Axons and dendrites of neurons do not touch. When one neuron meets another or a neuron meets an effector cell (e.g. a muscle cell) there is a junction known as a **synapse**. Chemical substances found in the CNS, known as **neurotransmitters**, act as the messenger from the **pre-synaptic terminals** over the **synaptic cleft** to the **post-synaptic membrane**. Neurotransmitters either excite, inhibit or modify the response of the adjacent cell. Over 30 different neurotransmitters have been identified; Table 5.1 illustrates some of the better known.

Acetylcholine	The neurotransmitter between neurons and skeletal muscles and within the ANS, producing predominantly an excitatory effect
Noradrenaline	The main neurotransmitter in the sympathetic nervous system, where it has a mostly excitatory effect. It is found in the brain stem and hypothalamus where it controls activity and mood
Dopamine	Found mainly in the **substantia nigra** in the mid-brain and in the basal ganglia. Its effect is the coordination of movement and control of behaviour
Serotonin	Located mainly in the brain stem, where it controls mood, sleep, body heat and appetite
Glutamate	Widespread in the CNS where it has an excitatory effect; important in learning and memory
Gamma-aminobutyric acid (GABA)	Located in the hypothalamus, cerebellum, basal ganglia and spinal cord. It is the main inhibitory neurotransmitter.

Table 5.1 Neurotransmitters

Communication between neurons and between a neuron and an effector cell occurs, in health, in an organised and purposeful manner to bring about a specific function or behaviour.

Cerebrum

The cerebral cortex governs higher mental function. It is responsible for conscious awareness, thinking, understanding and perception, language, memory, sensation and movement. However, these functions are not necessarily associated with just one location, conscious behaviour often involves the whole cortex.

The two cerebral hemispheres appear to have distinct and different roles, yet they work together in most activities dividing their responsibilities. This is known as **lateralisation**. The left and the right hemispheres communicate together using fibre tracts. In the majority of people, the left cerebral hemisphere dominates for speech, language comprehension, writing and analytical thought. The right dominates in perception, generalised thought, non-verbal and spatial perception; the more creative and insightful side. The dominance of activity between left and right sides is known as **cerebral dominance**.

The sensory and motor areas are located within the cerebral cortex, spanning the left and the right hemispheres, the motor area in the **precentral gyrus** and the sensory area in the **postcentral gyrus** (Figure 5.6a, b). The sensory area's function is to perceive sensation and the motor area's function is to control movement. The fibres controlling sensation and movement cross over, or **decussate**, from left to right, thus, perception of sensation and control of movement occur on the opposite side of the body, i.e. is contralateral. The whole body can be spatially represented in the sensory and motor cortex almost like a map (Figure 5.6). The map, commonly called the **homunculus**, illustrates the amount of cortical tissue responsible for each body part and function. In reality, specific control of functions is not neatly arranged like this but is much more functionally arranged. This allows, for example, neurons that control various muscle groups and work together to be located near one another.

Certain areas of the cortex, but not all, appear to have a correspondence with different functions; these have been summarised according to the four lobes of each hemisphere in Figure 5.3.

The **basal ganglia**, or **nuclei**, deep within the cerebral white matter, are an important group of neurons working as a system. They work with the motor cortex to provide motor control over fine movements (particularly

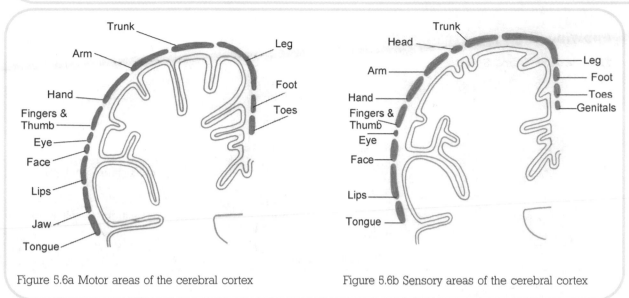

Figure 5.6a Motor areas of the cerebral cortex

Figure 5.6b Sensory areas of the cerebral cortex

the hands and lower limbs) and are the neurons responsible for preparing for movement just before it occurs.

The **thalamus**, located within the diencephalon, acts as a relay station for sensory inputs. It adjusts and directs information to the correct area of the cerebrum for it to be received and responded to. It also has a role in focusing attention and collaborates with the reticular activating system (RAS) and the limbic system. The RAS and the limbic system span the brain and cannot be localised to one area. The RAS governs the arousal of the brain and

Anatomy and Physiology in Action: Box 5.1

Summary of the Functions of the Cerebral Cortex According to the Lobes	
Frontal	Concerned with higher mental activities such as cognitive functioning, reasoning, concentration and elements of memory Prefrontal cortex exerts control over aspects of emotional expression and behaviour Motor cortex is located here along with the premotor cortex, which coordinates muscles to work together in groups. It is also associated with learnt movements Motor control of speech through the **Broca's area**
Parietal	Functions associated with movement, orientation and spatial awareness Sensory cortex is located here which works closely with the thalamus and the sensory association cortex for analysis and interpretation of inputs
Temporal	Concerned with the interpretation and comprehension of speech and sound through the **Wernicke's area**. This allows understanding of the meaning of words, both heard and expressed by oneself Components of memory that are aided by visual, auditory, olfactory and sensory inputs to help store an experience or information and facilitate learning
Occipital	Mostly concerned with processing of visual information (visual perception) along with involuntary eye movements

Applying Theory to Practice: Box 5.2

The Glasgow Coma Scale

	Eye Opening Response	
4	Spontaneous	Without any physical or verbal stimulation
3	To speech	Calling the patient's name
2	To pain	Pain should be applied centrally (in case of existing peripheral damage)
1	None	No eye opening observed or the patient has extreme swelling to eyes (C)
	Verbal Response	
5	Orientated	Full awareness of time, place and person
4	Confused	Talking in sentences, but disorientated to time, place or person
3	Inappropriate words	Unable to talk in sentences, just occasional words (often in response to stimuli)
2	Incomprehensible sounds	Groaning or grunting
1	None	No response or the patient is unable to respond due to a tracheostomy or endotracheal tube (T)
	Motor Response	
6	Obeys commands	Responds appropriately to a command such as 'stick out your tongue', 'move your hand'. Gripping the hand may be a reflex response.
5	Localizes pain	Apply central pain, preferably to the supraorbital nerve. The patient must attempt to move the pain source – the hand must be raised above chin level. May use a trapezius pinch if there is trauma.
4	Flexion to pain (withdrawal)	Bending of the elbow
3	Abnormal flexion	Bending of the elbow with rotation of the wrist (spastic flexion)
2	Extension	Extension of the elbows
1	None	No movement observed

the limbic system allows recognition and expression of emotions.

The **hypothalamus** regulates physiological drives and maintains homeostasis in many ways:

● Controls autonomic nervous system activity via the brain stem centres

● Recognises and allows expression of emotions, as a major part of the limbic system
● Regulates biological rhythms and drives such as the sleep and wake cycle and sexual arousal
● Regulates body temperature and appetite
● Regulates water metabolism and thirst via

osmoreceptors and hormone secretion of antidiuretic hormone from the pituitary gland

- Controls pituitary secretions of other hormones.

Brain stem

The brain stem encompasses the midbrain, pons and between the spinal cord, lower brain regions, cerebellum and the cerebral hemispheres. The brain stem is important in the RAS and consciousness as well as in autonomic regulation. The medulla plays a vital role in body homeostasis housing the cardiovascular and respiratory centres; it also regulates activities such as coughing, swallowing, vomiting and sneezing. The hypothalamus sends impulses (acting as messengers) to the medulla to execute an instruction.

Cerebellum

The cerebellum is responsible for smooth, precise and coordinated motor activity; it also regulates posture and balance. All sensory inputs travel via the cerebellum giving information about the body and muscle activity. Information is relayed in pathways across the brain and fed back to allow for synergy throughout the body.

Neurological assessment

Neurological assessment skills are essential in nursing practice, assessment of consciousness being the most critical. Reduced consciousness or changing levels of consciousness indicate dysfunction and alterations in the normal transmission and processing of sensory information in the CNS.

Neurological assessment should include assessment of consciousness, limb power assessment, pupillary assessment and vital signs. The Glasgow Coma Scale (GCS) (Teasdale & Jennet 1974) is used internationally to assess consciousness. The individual score for each response is plotted on a graph, with the time of the assessment, and then totalled. The minimum score of 3 would indicate a completely unconscious patient, whereas the maximum score of 15 would indicate a fully alert and orientated patient.

The eye-opening response assesses mechanisms of arousal and control of the eyes. Arousal is governed by the RAS located in the brain stem; it is possible to be awake but not necessarily aware. The verbal response assesses cerebral functioning; the patient's ability to respond verbally assesses both the processing of information as well as comprehension and the capacity to articulate. The motor response assesses global brain function; the sensory and motor processes span both cerebral hemispheres and are truly integrated within the brain. The upper limb response is assessed alone as lower limb responses may be due to spinal reflex.

Limb power assessment is also important as an alteration in power of one limb compared to another indicates focal injury to the brain. Due to **decussation**, changes in limb power usually occur on the opposite side to that of the injury. The power in all four limbs should be observed in this part of the assessment.

Questioning Clinical Practice: Exercise 5.6

Head Injuries and Associated Risks

Consider what the implications of a reduced conscious level may be for the well-being and health of a patient.

The National Institute for Health and Clinical Excellence (NICE) in 2003 published guidelines for the management of head injuries. In their guidance, they recommend that patients with a GCS less than or equal to 8 should be referred immediately for management of their airway and breathing.

Patients with a reduced consciousness level will have a significant risk of obstruction of the airway and aspiration. Their capacity to breath will also be affected.

- Using your experience of different hospital environments, consider which settings would be the most appropriate for a patient with a reduced conscious level.

Finally, pupil assessment should include the size, shape and equality of the pupils, and their reaction to light stimulus. The presence of a light reflex relies on a functioning optic nerve, intact nerve impulse transmission to the midbrain and a functioning oculomotor nerve. This is an important prognostic factor.

Epilepsy

Scenario 5.1

Status Epilepticus

Mark James, a 35-year-old man, is admitted to the emergency department by ambulance with sustained seizures. He has been continually fitting for 15 minutes. On arrival he is unconscious and displaying rhythmic jerking movements of his whole body.

Airway: a **nasopharyngeal airway** has been inserted by the paramedic crew

Breathing: respiratory rate 31, oxygen saturation 98% on 15L oxygen via a reservoir bag mask

Circulation: pulse 124 regular, blood pressure 146/89, blood sugar 9.8 mmol/l

Disability: GCS 4/15, eyes 1, verbal 2, motor 1, pupils 5mm reacting bilaterally

Environment: body temperature is recorded as 36c, there are no signs of external injury

The paramedic crew inform you that they administered 5mg of **diazepam** rectally when they arrived at the patient's house, without therapeutic effect

PMH: **epilepsy**, depression

Mr James's girlfriend informed the paramedic crew that he had not been reliably taking his usual anti-epileptic medication recently and had been feeling particularly low in mood.

Assessment and analysis of patient presentation

Mr James's presentation indicates that he is in status epilepticus. **Status epilepticus** is a term used clinically when generalised seizures occur without improvements in conscious level between seizures, or when a seizure is sustained for more than 30 minutes. At the point of presentation, the seizure had been in progress for 15 minutes. Despite intervention with the administration of diazepam (Table 5.2), the seizure had been sustained. It is rare that a single convulsive seizure, in adults, lasts longer than a few minutes and it is accepted that early diagnosis and treatment are important in this form of epilepsy. It is usual for treatment for status epilepticus to be initiated before 30 minutes elapses as this condition has a high mortality and morbidity risk; it is therefore treated as a medical emergency.

The structured clinical assessment reveals important information about Mr James's condition and will direct his treatment. Due to the seizure activity and the alteration in conscious level (GCS 4/15), Mr James's airway is compromised. This has been protected with the use of a nasopharyngeal airway as an interim measure. He is **tachypnoeic** but well oxygenated, and **tachycardic**. Seizure activity places extreme metabolic demands on the body. These demands are met by an increase in respiratory rate to keep up with the body's oxygen demand, and an increase in heart rate to deliver oxygen and glucose to the body tissues. The only sign of consciousness that Mr James displays is a grunting noise, his pupils are equal and reacting to light. The elevation in blood glucose is a sympathetic response by the liver to make more sugar available for body demands. The immediate priority of care for Mr James is to gain control of his seizure activity and stabilise his condition.

Pathophysiology

Epilepsy is characterised by a sudden abnormal burst of electrical stimulation, interrupting normal neuronal conduction and normal cerebral function. There is an imbalance between excitation and inhibition within the CNS. Seizures lead to temporary impairment of consciousness, movement, sensation and memory.

Different epilepsies differ pathophysiologically, but there are common characteristics, these include alterations of synaptic and neuron properties, changes in ion channels and increased neuronal excitability and synchronisation. The neurotransmitters, glutamate and GABA are also thought to play a role.

Any type of seizure can proceed to become status epilepticus, if there is excessive excitation or failure of the mechanisms that terminate seizures.

Classification of epilepsy

The most widely accepted classification system of epileptic seizures is that established in 1981 by the International League Against Epilepsy (ILAE).

Partial seizures originate from a focal region of the cortex and are subdivided depending on their effect on consciousness:

- **Simple partial seizures** do not affect consciousness. Symptoms may include rhythmic movements of

Applying Theory to Practice: Box 5.3

Risk Factors for Seizures	
Low anti-epileptic drug levels (poor compliance or withdrawal)	Head trauma
	Cerebrovascular disease, including stroke
Drug toxicity	Brain tumour
Alcohol withdrawal or toxicity	Neurodegenerative disorders
Hypoxia/anoxia	Unknown aetiology
Systemic or CNS infection	
Metabolic disorders (uraemia, electrolyte imbalance, hyper- or hypoglycaemia)	

(Adam & Osbourne 2005, Hickey 2003)

the contralateral face, arm or leg and possibly hallucinations involving smell, sight or hearing or feelings of fear and panic or euphoria.

- **Complex partial seizures** are the most common type of seizure in adults, commonly lasting less than three minutes. There is sometimes a warning, an aura. Conscious level is affected; a person may appear awake but will be unresponsive, motionless and be correct. Repetitive movements, known as **automatisms**, are common such as fiddling with buttons, grimacing or lip smacking. There is usually no recollection of the seizure, but patients are often sleepy and confused and may have a headache; this is known as the **post-ictal phase**.

Generalised seizures affect the whole cortex with the patient's level of consciousness usually being impaired; there is often no aura or warning. Generalised seizures have varying characteristics:

- **Typical absence seizures** are distinguished by a transient loss of consciousness and awareness of the environment with a vacant appearance, which lasts just a few seconds.

- **Atypical absence seizures** resemble typical absence seizures but last longer and are often associated with minor automatisms.
- **Myoclonic seizures** are classified by sudden muscle contractions of specific muscle groups with no loss of consciousness.
- **Tonic-clonic seizures** involve bilateral extension of limbs followed by synchronous jerking movements. There is often a cry before the seizure, a fall to the ground followed by incontinence, tongue biting, foaming at the mouth and loss of consciousness. There is a post-ictal phase and when patients wake they have muscle tenderness, transient confusion and exhaustion.
- **Clonic or tonic seizures** exhibit one phase of the tonic-clonic seizure.
- **Atonic seizures** cause loss of muscle tone and a fall to the ground, often resulting in injury; it may be so brief that the patient is unaware of the loss of consciousness.

Questioning Clinical Practice: Exercise 5.7

- Reflect on your clinical experience to date; have you observed a patient having a seizure? What characteristics of seizure could you identify?
- How confident do you now feel in your knowledge of the characteristics of seizures and your ability to recognise a seizure?

Diagnosis of epilepsy is made based on clinical signs and symptoms and a detailed description of an event, usually given by a witness. Many conditions can resemble epileptic seizures so these are fully considered and investigated during the diagnosis process. An electro-encephalogram (EEG) can be used alongside the clinical diagnosis.

The treatment of epilepsy with anti-epileptic drugs (AED) aims to control seizures and minimise side effects. NICE (2004), in their guidance on epilepsy, advise that drug choice should depend on the type of seizure the patient suffers. The patient should also have a structured treatment plan and regular follow-ups.

Applying Theory to Practice: Box 5.4

Brain Waves and EEG

The EEG records electrical activity from the brain cells just beneath the surface of the brain. This activity is known as brain waves. Electrodes are placed on the scalp and connected to the EEG. The EEG records patterns of neuronal activity in cortical areas.

In disorders such as epilepsy, where there is a surge of erratic electrical discharge, the EEG is useful in locating where damaged brain tissue lies in the cortex.

Diazepam	A sedative used for the control of seizures. In the pre-hospital setting, it is usually administered rectally or orally. In hospital, it can be administered intravenously (IV) for control of seizures.
Lorazepam or midazolam	Sedatives used in the hospital setting. Administered IV for control of seizures, including status epilepticus.
Phenytoin	Taken orally as a prophylactic. Administered IV for control of seizures, including status epilepticus, and for prevention of seizures.
Sodium valproate	Taken orally as a prophylactic. Drug choice depends on seizure type. (BMA 2007, NICE 2004)
Carbamazepine	
Lamotrigine	

Table 5.2 Summary of the Major Anti-Epileptic Drugs

The effects of epilepsy

Epilepsy affects most, if not all, aspects of a person's life. The diagnosis of epilepsy can have a profound effect on a person's self-esteem and body image. The unpredictability of seizures can limit a person's willingness and ability to socialise and form relationships. Fear of having a seizure in public, feelings of isolation and loss of control are common emotions for a person with epilepsy and can place significant restrictions and limitations on their life. Independence, employment, financial security and life insurance are all affected by the diagnosis. The nature of epilepsy also means that driving is not permitted and activities such as swimming alone and bathing are to be avoided.

It is not surprising, therefore, that there is a high incidence of anxiety and depression among people with epilepsy for which they often receive concurrent treatment.

The history of Mr James's condition indicated that he had been non-compliant with his AEDs, which increases the likelihood of seizures occurring and poses a significant risk to his health and life. Patients can find taking AEDs inconvenient and restrictive and the side-effects unpleasant. At a suitable time, it would be important for healthcare professionals to understand why Mr James has stopped taking his medication. He may need support and guidance to enable him to live safely with his condition and treatment, and enable him to have a full and active life.

Treatment of epilepsy focuses on empowering patients to manage their own condition. This includes avoiding known seizure triggers such as fatigue, sleep deprivation, stress, excess alcohol, drugs, flickering lights, certain music and low blood sugar. It also includes educating patients about their medication to encourage compliance. Support, guidance and education on how to adjust lifestyle to avoid triggers, to live with epilepsy safely and to enjoy a full and active life are important. All patients should have a thorough plan of care and have access to specialists, both nursing and medical (NICE 2004). All healthcare professionals have a responsibility to ensure that patients with epilepsy can be partners in their own care and be involved in decisions, essential for patients to feel empowered (DH 2004).

Scenario 5.2

Stroke

Eileen Applewood, a 71-year-old woman, is a patient on the acute stroke unit. She was admitted two weeks ago after suffering a stroke. This was diagnosed through history, clinical presentation and computed tomography (CT) findings.

You are looking after her today. You go to meet her, perform an initial neurological assessment and record her vital signs.

Airway – clear

Breathing – respiratory rate 18, oxygen saturation 98% on 2L oxygen via nasal cannula

Circulation – pulse 101, and irregular. Blood pressure 158/89

Disability & Neurological assessment – GCS 12/15 (E3, V3, M6)

Normal limb power to left arm and leg, no movement in right arm and severe weakness noted in right leg. Pupils equal and reacting to light (3mm)

Environment – temperature 36.7 C

PMH – coronary heart disease (CHD), atrial fibrillation

Developing and Delivering Expert Care: Exercise 5.8

Complete the following exercise to identify your current level of understanding:

- What risk factors for cerebrovascular disease and stroke do you know?
- What risk factors does Mrs Applewood have?
- Consider the nurse's role, as part of the multi-professional team in influencing the identification and management of these risks.
- How might educating patients regarding high-risk factors reduce both the morbidity and mortality rates?

Stroke

Assessment and analysis of patient presentation

From your initial assessment you identify that Mrs Applewood has a reduced GCS score indicating that her conscious level is compromised. Mrs Applewood's eye-opening response indicates an intact arousal mechanism. Her verbal response to questions is to reply with inappropriate words, indicating either a language, speech or comprehension deficit. A purposeful and intentional motor response indicates reasonable functioning of the cerebral cortex. Limb power assessment reveals a significant motor deficit, affecting the right arm and leg indicating functional damage; she has normal pupillary function.

A full examination to identify the extent of the physical, intellectual and emotional manifestations of the stroke is needed. Once this has been fully established, a thorough plan of care and rehabilitation can be implemented according to Mrs Applewood's needs.

Immediately after presentation, the nature and cause of Mrs Applewood's stroke would have been investigated and diagnosed to deliver correct treatment and to identify any remaining risk factors of a stroke reoccurring. In the Royal College of Physicians' *National Clinical Guidelines for Stroke* (CEEU 2004) a 30–43% increased risk of a secondary stroke within five years of the primary stroke is reported, as well as an increased risk of myocardial infarction. A high priority needs to be given to reduce these risks.

Pathophysiology

Stroke, also known as **cerebrovascular accident** (CVA), is defined as a sudden loss of brain function leading to a neurological deficit that lasts for 24 hours or more. Stroke occurs when blood flow to a local area of the brain is interrupted, leading to oxygen deprivation of the tissue (**ischaemia**), and eventually cell death or **infarction**. Neurons that die are irreparable, neurons that lie just outside the infarcted area, an area known as the **penumbra**, are often also damaged but these neurons may recover in time.

The causes of strokes are classified as either **ischaemic** or **haemorrhagic**:

- Ischaemic strokes account for 85% of all strokes. Cerebral blood flow is interrupted due to either an **embolus**, where a clot or atherosclerotic plaque dislodges and occludes one of the cerebral arteries, or **thrombosis**, where the vessel lumen narrows and causes ischaemia.
- Haemorrhagic strokes account for 15% of all strokes and involve rupture of a blood vessel. These are further divided into **intracerebral haemorrhage** (ICH), bleeding into brain tissue, or **subarachnoid haemorrhage** (SAH), bleeding into the subarachnoid space, often caused by an **aneurysm** or an **arteriovenous malformation**. Haemorrhagic stroke is linked closely to hypertension.

Transient ischaemic attacks (TIA) are episodes of inadequate cerebral blood flow leading to focal

neurological symptoms; these attacks are temporary, lasting less than 24 hours, but are significant as they can be a warning sign of stroke.

Every stroke is different and no two people are affected in quite the same way. The degree and form of brain injury and neurological deficit depend on the area of the brain involved and the extent of the injury.

Motor deficits

Hemiparesis (weakness) or **hemiplegia** (paralysis) is one of the most common symptoms of stroke, usually affecting one side of the body. Voluntary control of the arm or leg is affected because of damage to the upper motor neurons. As upper motor neurons decussate, damage to neurons on one side of the brain will cause disability to the limb(s) on the opposite side of the body. Other motor functions that may be affected are: difficulty with swallowing due to muscle impairment, known as **dysphagia**; and difficulty with articulation of speech due to related muscle impairment, known as **dysarthria**.

Sensory deficits

Visual disorders manifest because sensory pathways between the eye and visual cortex are disturbed. Loss of half of the visual field can occur, which usually corresponds to the side of the body with hemiparesis or hemiplegia.

Proprioception and **perception** may be disturbed, which can manifest as unilateral limb neglect, disorientation to time, place or person, and sometimes **apraxia** where a person can no longer perform purposeful actions.

Language deficits

Dysphasia and **aphasia**, where speech is defective or lost completely may occur. The left cerebral hemisphere usually dominates for speech. Damage to the Broca's area may cause expressive dysphasia due to loss of motor control, and damage to the Wernicke's area can cause receptive dysphasia as comprehension and interpretation are disrupted.

Intellectual deficits

Memory, concentration, attention and learning can be affected along with a person's ability to think, reason, and make judgments and decisions.

Emotional deficits

Depression, sadness, anger, anxiety and low self-esteem are common emotions after a stroke. Often people find it hard to control their emotions, and they may cry, swear or laugh at inappropriate times.

Other deficits

Other symptoms that may manifest include **insomnia** and **fatigue** as well as bladder and bowel dysfunction leading to urgency, frequency and incontinence.

Risk factors and preventing stroke

In England approximately 110,000 people every year will suffer a stroke, with a cost to the NHS of over £2.8 billion. It is the third biggest cause of death and the largest single cause of severe disability in the UK (DH 2007a). The government aims to reduce death by stroke (and diseases related to CHD) by at least 40% in people under 75 by the year 2010. A National Stroke Strategy is being developed by the Department of Health (DH 2007b) with the aims:

- To raise awareness stroke symptoms and risk factors
- To improve access, response and provision of stroke services

Delivering and Developing Expert Care Box 5.5

Risk Factors for Stroke

Age over 55 years	Smoking
Hypertension	Stress
Atrial fibrillation	Sedentary lifestyle
Valvular disease	Unhealthy diet
Clinical symptoms of CHD or ECG evidence	Obesity
	High alcohol intake
Diabetes mellitus	Oral contraceptive pill
Elevated blood lipids and cholesterol	
Heredity link mainly associated with hypertension and diabetes	

(Hickey 2003, Holland 2000)

- To enable high level support for stroke survivors on leaving hospital.

Prevention of cerebrovascular disease and stroke is more likely to reduce the incidence of stroke than any medical or surgical advance.

Early and accurate diagnosis of stroke is important to implement the most appropriate treatment and management. Diagnosis is made with medical history, clinical presentation and clinical examination alongside radiological diagnostic investigations such as computerised tomography (CT). A CT scan aids differentiation between an ischaemic and haemorrhagic stroke, which is vital in order to make appropriate decisions about treatment.

Mrs Applewood was diagnosed with an ischaemic embolic stroke secondary to atrial fibrillation, CHD and undiagnosed hypertension. Complete physical and neurological examination reveals that she has a right-sided hemiplegia of the arm and hemiparesis of the leg. She has expressive dysphasia and visual field disruption to the right side, along with unilateral neglect to that side.

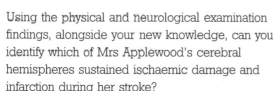

Applying Theory to Practice: Exercise 5.9

Using the physical and neurological examination findings, alongside your new knowledge, can you identify which of Mrs Applewood's cerebral hemispheres sustained ischaemic damage and infarction during her stroke?

Mrs Applewood is being cared for in an acute stroke unit. The DH (2001), in the *National Service Framework for Older People*, recommends that patients who have had a stroke should be admitted to a stroke unit in a timely manner; prompt diagnosis is crucial for this to occur. There is considerable evidence showing improved survival and functional recovery when specialist care and treatment can be provided.

Plan of care

Control and elimination of risk factors are a mainstay of care to prevent Mrs Applewood from having a secondary stroke. Specifically, this would include control of hypertension and atrial fibrillation, and lifestyle adjustments.

Alongside medical and surgical management, ongoing

neurological assessment as well as cardio-respiratory observation and physical assessment is important. Assessment findings will help the nurse identify changes in Mrs Applewood's condition, which may include extension of the stroke or the early signs of complications of immobility.

Developing and Delivering Expert Care: Exercise 5.10

- What complications of immobility do you know of and how would these manifest in a patient?

Medical and surgical treatment

Anti-thrombotic and **anti-platelet therapies**, such as **aspirin**, **clopidogrel** and **low molecular weight heparin**, may be implemented to prevent clot formation and emboli (Hickey 2003). **Thrombolysis** aims to dissolve a thrombus occluding an artery and restore cerebral circulation in the acute phase of ischaemic stroke. One drug available for this is **recombinant tissue plasminogen activator** (rTPA) (ISCTN 2007, IST-3 Thrombolysis 2007), but use of this treatment is still subject to randomised clinical trials.

Surgical management options in ischaemic stroke include **carotid endarterectomy** for atherosclerotic disease, in patients suitable for surgery, or **cerebral angioplasty** with or without **stenting**.

Treatment of haemorrhagic stroke is specific to individual cases but may involve surgery if the presence of the haemorrhage within the skull is compromising the survival and functioning of other brain tissue. For patients with SAH, a specific management strategy would be implemented.

Rehabilitation

For all survivors of stroke, an early focus on rehabilitation is crucial to optimise functional capability and recovery. Collaboration with allied health professionals is important in order to develop a plan of care to meet the patient's physical, cognitive, emotional and social needs while in hospital, but also during their transition back to the community. Physiotherapy, occupational therapy, speech and language therapy and social work support, alongside nursing care, are important in patient rehabilitation after a stroke.

Sometimes a stroke can be so extensive that a person's chance of survival is limited and subsequent possibilities for effective and meaningful rehabilitation hampered. In cases where this occurs, multi-professional opinion is sought and discussed to identify the most appropriate care management. It is important in these circumstances to also discuss the appropriateness of resuscitation, should events occur. Where possible, the patient, and those close to them, should be involved in discussions about care management and resuscitation, and their views taken into consideration. Sometimes, a stroke can be so extensive that a patient dies, and the focus of care changes to patient comfort and a peaceful, dignified death.

Parkinson's disease

Scenario 5.3

Parkinson's Disease

Wilfred Smith, a 74-year-old, is a patient on the elderly care ward. He has Parkinson's disease and was admitted to hospital by his GP three weeks ago from home.

Mr Smith has restricted and slow mobility, and regularly suffers freezing attacks. He currently has a healing laceration and bruised area on his forehead. He is frail, underweight and suffering from constipation.

It has been increasingly difficult for Mr Smith to look after himself independently and he does not have any close family to help him. In view of this, Mr Smith is now waiting for placement in a residential home, which he is looking forward to.

Assessment and analysis of patient presentation

Mr Smith's condition appears to have progressed and the manifestations of Parkinson's disease are affecting his well-being and health. He has significant mobility restrictions that are limiting his ability to perform normal daily activities independently. The bruising and laceration to Mr Smith's forehead may be indicative that he has fallen and injured himself. The weight loss and constipation may reflect poor nutrition and hydration. Multi-professional discussion and analysis of Mr Smith's con-

dition, social situation, wishes and well-being have concluded that it would be in his best interests to live in a residential home. This will mean he has help at hand for all of his needs, and the risks of harm and ill health are reduced.

Pathophysiology

Parkinson's disease is a progressive neurodegenerative condition affecting the basal ganglia, deep within the cerebral white matter. It causes loss of the melanin pigmented neurons of the **substantia nigra**, one of the structures within the basal ganglia. Loss of these neurons leads to depletion of the neurotransmitter **dopamine** (Table 5.3). These degenerative changes mean there is less thalamic stimulation of the motor cortex and the control and coordination of movement are affected. Typically this disease starts to affect people in their fifties and sixties.

Currently no diagnostic test exists for Parkinson's disease. Diagnosis is made using clinical examination and history taking, often meaning diagnosis is delayed.

There are several signs and symptoms:

- **Bradykinesia** is difficulty initiating movement and maintaining it. A patient will have a stooped posture and will move with a shuffling gait; they may lose their balance easily and fall. They can also have an expressionless face and blink infrequently.
- **Tremors** are present in the arms and hands. A characteristic tremor known as pill rolling is seen, which may be aggravated by anxiety and concentration.
- Rigidity of the muscles is seen and is associated with bradykinesia, the muscles feel stiff and are difficult to move.

There are many other manifestations making it difficult for patients to perform the usual activities of living. Fine motor control is poor, patients may be clumsy, weak and fatigue quickly. Patients momentarily freeze mid-movement, the voice weakens and drooling is not uncommon. Patients frequently have signs of depression and dementia.

Plan of care

Drug therapy is the mainstay of the medical management of Parkinson's disease, with the aim of relieving symptoms (NICE 2006). Neuro-protective drugs, aimed at halting progression of the disease, are still being developed. Some surgical treatments exist but these are

reserved for patients with severe disease who have developed complications to drug therapy. See Table 5.3.

Dopaminergic agents (levodopa)	Control of rigidity and bradykinesia
Anti-cholinergic agents	Control of tremor and rigidity
Dopaminergic agonists	Augment the effects of levodopa
(BMA 2007, NICE 2006)	

Table 5.3 Drug Therapy in Parkinson's Disease

Supportive therapy is pivotal in helping patients manage symptoms effectively and to facilitate maximal independence. The focus of care and therapy is on improving mobility, ensuring adequate nutrition, promoting good bowel function, enabling self-care and improving communication. Multi-professional teamwork is fundamental to maximising the benefits of therapy and enabling patients to live independently (NICE 2006).

Despite the progression in Mr Smith's condition, he should be encouraged to maintain as much independence as possible and his placement in residential care, rather than nursing care, reflects this. Symptom control will be essential and multi-professional advice necessary to enable excellent pharmacological and non-pharmacological management in the future.

Applying Theory to Practice: Exercise 5.11

Examples of Neurodegenerative Conditions

Alzheimer's disease
Dementia
Multiple sclerosis
Motor neuron disease

- Research the pathophysiological changes associated with these conditions; identify the clinical signs you would look for during your neurological assessment and how the care of these patients would be managed.
- Add these findings to your portfolio. You may also like to consider other acute disorders that can affect the nervous system.

Questioning Clinical Practice: Box 5.6

Stem Cell Research

Until recently, it was widely accepted that, unlike other cells in the body, neurons are not able to regenerate once damaged or destroyed. Therefore treatment has always focused on limiting the consequences of disease. However, scientific and medical advances over the last 20 years have revealed the remarkable possibilities that stem cells may offer in replacing damaged neurons.

Stem cells are very early cells that are uniquely able to divide, renew and differentiate into specialist cells, such as neuronal tissue. Stem cell therapy therefore offers new hope for the treatment of neurological disease. In the future, it is anticipated that stem cells may be used to treat conditions such as Parkinson's disease, spinal cord injury, Alzheimer's disease, multiple sclerosis, among many others (ISCR 2007, Marieb 2007).

There is a considerable controversy over stem cell research because it often relies on harvesting embryonic stem cells (other forms of stem cells originate from adults or umbilical tissue). For many people, it is unethical and unacceptable to use a human embryo for research, particularly as the embryos are eventually destroyed. People also argue that this is too close to human cloning. The British Government is supporting responsible stem cell research, of all types, believing that this offers the best opportunities for treatment of many conditions (DH 2005, ISCR 2007). This support ensures there is public and private funding for stem cell research in the future and sustains the British contribution to international debate and advances in research and medicine.

The spinal cord

Form

Protected and hidden within the vertebral column, the spinal cord is a long mass of nerve tissue with remarkable activity and responsibility. The spinal cord is continuous with the medulla oblongata and extends beyond the cranium, through the foramen magnum of the occipital lobe, into the vertebral column extending down until the level of the first or second lumbar vertebra. It is approximately 42–45cm long and 1.8cm thick, but tapers towards its end (Figure 5.7).

The spinal cord is protected by the three meningeal layers covering the brain, as well as cerebrospinal fluid and bone, in the form of vertebrae. There are seven cervical (C), twelve thoracic (T), five lumbar (L) and five sacral (S) vertebrae.

Applying Theory to Practice: Exercise 5.12

Cerebrospinal Fluid

In the spine, the subarachnoid space extends beyond the end of the spinal cord to the level of S2.

A procedure known as a **lumbar puncture** (LP) is performed to remove CSF for testing. A spinal needle is inserted between the lumbar vertebrae (L3/4 or L4/5) through the dura and into the subarachnoid space to sample the fluid. As the spinal cord is absent in this region, there is no risk of damaging the cord or nerves.

A lumbar puncture is a diagnostic procedure where both the pressure in the CSF and the contents of the CSF are examined.

- When might an LP be performed on a patient? And, what might an LP diagnose?

There are 31 pairs of spinal nerves relaying nerve impulses between the body areas they serve and the spinal cord; they establish the link between the peripheral and central nervous systems. Each nerve attaches via its root to the cord, and leaves the spinal region through openings between the vertebrae, known as intervertebral foramina. The spinal cord has two enlargements along its length, known as the cervical and lumbar enlargements. The enlargements allow innervation of the upper and lower limbs, the cervical enlargement innervating the upper limbs and the lumbar enlargement innervating the lower limbs. The lumbar and sacral nerve roots must angle sharply downwards and the nerves travel through the vertebral column to their intervertebral foramina. This is because the spinal cord itself terminates more superiorly to the exit points of these nerves (Figure 5.7).

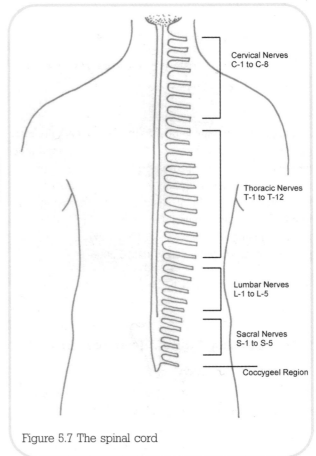

Figure 5.7 The spinal cord

Similar to brain tissue, the spinal cord is composed of grey and white matter. Unlike in the brain, the grey matter comprises the internal matter of the cord and is surrounded by the white matter. The grey matter consists of cell bodies of neurons and their projections (axons and dendrites), and the white matter consists of fibre tracts running **longitudinally**. These fibre tracts, some of which are myelinated, are either known as **ascending** or **descending tracts**. In addition to these longitudinal tracts, there are a few **transverse tracts**, relaying information across the cord. The grey matter forms a shape like the letter 'H'. The two anterior projections are known as

anterior (**ventral**) horns and the two posterior projections, the **posterior** (**dorsal**) horns. In the thoracic and superior lumbar regions, lateral horns are also present. The ventral horns carry nerve impulses to the somatic (motor) nervous system and the lateral horns to the autonomic nervous system; the dorsal horns receive afferent impulses from peripheral sensory receptors.

Function

Ascending pathways convey afferent nerve impulses from sensory regions of the body, **dermatones**, to the brain. The ascending pathways direct impulses from the dermatonal area, via the dorsal root, to one of three fibre tracts (spinothalamic, fasciculus cuneatus or gracilis and spinocerebellar), depending on the source and nature of the impulse. The impulse is sent either to the cerebellum or to the cortex via the thalamus.

The descending pathways are responsible for efferent impulses from the brain to the spinal cord and are divided into direct and indirect pathways. The pathways involve neurons referred to as upper and lower motor neurons. Upper motor neurons are located only in the CNS whereas lower motor neurons are located in both the CNS and PNS, and actually innervate skeletal muscle (Table 5.4).

The autonomic nervous system

The purpose of the autonomic nervous system (ANS) is to maintain a stable internal environment, which it does without conscious thought (Chapter 2). It is composed solely of motor neurons and governs the activity of visceral organs including cardiac muscles, glands and other smooth (involuntary) muscles. The hypothalamus is the overall control centre of the ANS sending impulses via the **medulla oblongata**.

As well as using nerve pathways, the ANS sends impulses by neurotransmitters, noradrenaline within the sympathetic nervous system, and acetylcholine within the parasympathetic (Table 5.1). The sympathetic division is activated under times of stress, known as the fright, fight or flight phenomena, leading to an increase in heart rate and blood pressure and vasoconstriction of peripheral blood vessels. The parasympathetic division is concerned with rest and relaxation, known as the feed and breed phenomena; it typically reduces heart rate and blood pressure and encourages gastrointestinal activity. Both divisions act together to maintain homeostatic balance.

Sympathetic neurons are located in the thoracic and lumbar regions of the spinal cord (T1–L2), they leave the cord via the ventral roots, travel just 1cm and join a chain of neurons, known as the **sympathetic chain**, which is located on each side of the spinal cord. These neurons are connected by longitudinal fibres and extend the whole length of the spinal cord. Eventually the nerve fibres rejoin the spinal nerves and extend to their visceral organs, glands or muscles.

Parasympathetic neurons are located in two sections: the brain stem and the sacral region of the cord. The cranial section acts via the oculomotor, facial, glossopharyngeal and vagus cranial nerves leading to constriction of the pupillary muscles and the glands of the head and mouth. The vagus nerve synapses with multiple visceral organs including the heart, lungs, stomach, liver and bowel. The sacral section innervates the bladder and bowel and is involved in emptying of the bladder and bowel. The sacral roots and the vagus nerve are connected, resulting in reflex arcs.

Spinal nerve root	Motor and sensory area
Cervical nerves C1–C8	Movement and sensation to the arms, neck and upper trunk, including the diaphragm and intercostal muscles
Thoracic nerves T1–T12	Movement and sensation to the trunk and abdomen
Lumbar and sacral nerves L1–L5, S1–S5	Movement and sensation to the legs, bladder, bowel and genitals

Table 5.4 Association between Nerve Roots and the Various Motor and Sensory Areas

Scenario 5.4

Spinal Cord Injury

David Adam, a 29-year-old man, is a patient on the neurosurgical ward. He fell from a ladder while at work two weeks ago. Anteroposterior and lateral X-rays were carried out in accident and emergency, followed by a CT scan. They confirmed that he had sustained a compression injury to his spine with a burst fracture of the vertebral body at T4 and transection of the spinal cord in this region. Mr Adam had surgical stabilisation of the fracture, with internal fixation, one week ago.

You go to meet Mr Adam, and record his vital signs:

Mr Adam is lying supine in bed. He is alert and orientated. During your initial conversation, he informs you that he has been unable to move or feel his lower body and legs since his accident.

Vital signs:
Airway: Mr Adams is freely talking
Breathing: respiratory rate 19
Circulation: pulse 65, blood pressure 125/73
Disability and neurological: GCS 15/15, patient has paraplegia
Environment: temperature 36.5C

Assessment and analysis of patient presentation

Mr Adam has a spinal cord injury with complete sensory and motor loss below the level of the injury to the cord, leaving him **paraplegic**. He complains of inability to move his body or legs, which are consistent with an injury at the level of T4. Spinal nerve roots exiting from T4 and below serve the mid-chest, the abdomen and the legs. A physical examination should reveal that Mr Adam has normal sensation and movement in his neck, shoulders and arms. Mr Adam's fracture has been stabilised meaning there is no risk of further damage to the spinal cord.

The patient's observations appear to be within normal range for a man of his age. This is an important element of the assessment, for many reasons, not least because Mr Adam's injury exposes him to potential cardiovascular instability and respiratory insufficiency. Damage to the spinal cord can affect respiratory muscle function, leading to respiratory failure and can also affect the autonomic nervous system resulting in cardiovascular instability.

Developing and Delivering Expert Care: Box 5.7

For any patient with an actual or suspected spinal cord injury, care should be taken to ensure the spine remains in anatomical alignment in order to reduce the risk of further damage to the spinal cord. This is achieved by positioning patients in a neutral anatomical position. The head and neck should be secured using a rigid collar and bolsters, sometimes called sand bags/head blocks, on either side of the head; these are then strapped to a secure point.

During moving or positioning the whole spine must be kept in the neutral position. A coordinated manoeuvre known as a **log roll** is performed using a minimum of four people. The nominated leader manages the patient's head and neck; this person will move the head through an arc as it rotates with the rest of the body, while keeping the spine in perfect alignment.

Pathophysiology

Any damage to the spinal cord, or the nerve roots, will lead to functional loss with paralysis and/or **parathesis** (sensory loss), as connection with the cerebral cortex is cut off. Most spinal cord injuries occur as a result of road traffic accidents, falls or sport; however, some are caused by disease, infection or bleeding (Spinal Injuries Association 2007). More men sustain injuries than women, with a significant proportion under the age of 30 years.

The effects of spinal cord injury depend on the type of injury and the level of injury. Lesions are described as either complete or incomplete. A **complete injury** means that there is total sensory and motor functional loss below the level of the injury. An **incomplete injury** means that there is some function below the injury; some sensory or motor fibres, or both, are undamaged.

Cervical injuries result in quadraplegia, injuries at C4 or higher may result in the inability to breathe. Patients will require a **tracheostomy** and be dependent on a ventilator. Lower cervical injuries may also have restricted respiratory function due to the functional loss of the intercostal muscles. Injuries from C5–C8 affect progressively more movement and sensation in the shoulders, upper arms and even the wrists. Dexterity and

Applying Theory to Practice: Box 5.8

Quadraplegia	An injury to the spinal cord above T1, paralysis affects all four limbs
Paraplegia	An injury to the spinal cord below T1, paralysis affects the legs only

manipulation are significantly restricted and patients require assistance with the activities of daily living.

Thoracic injuries result in paraplegia. Those with high thoracic injuries may have poor trunk control and lack abdominal muscle control, whereas with lower thoracic injuries patients have better trunk control and good use of the abdominal muscles.

Lumbar and sacral injuries result in a loss of control of the legs and hips and either complete or incomplete paraplegia depending on the level.

Paralysis also leads to loss of voluntary control of the bowel and bladder, loss of temperature control (**poikilothermia**) and the inability to sweat below the level of the injury. **Postural hypotension** may occur and the autonomic nervous system is disrupted below the injury. In men, sexual function may also be affected leading to fertility problems. It is not uncommon for patients to also suffer chronic pain.

Plan of care

Mr Adam's plan of care should be focused on recovery from his operation as well as his comprehensive needs following his injury. A multi-professional approach should be adopted to meet these needs and to facilitate maximum rehabilitation. Referral to a specialist spinal centre is a priority to ensure Mr Adam can access specialist rehabilitation in the future (Grundy & Swain 2002). Specific care should focus on encouraging and facilitating good respiratory function, as loss of abdominal muscle function means Mr Adam may not be able to cough effectively without treatment and education. He will require a regimen of care to enable good bladder and bowel function, and will need excellent nursing care to prevent any complications of immobility, of which there will be a significantly increased risk. Pain from muscle spasm is common and should be treated to ensure comfort and rest.

The devastating functional loss and disability associated with spinal cord injury are catastrophic. The nurse's role in supporting patients emotionally and psychologically should not be underestimated or dismissed in favour of a patient's physical needs. Often specialist care is required to enable patients to process events that have happened to them, to manage emotions and their reaction to the injury, and to enable patients to move forward and learn to live with their disability.

Conclusion

Developing a fundamental understanding of the form and function of the nervous system, alongside knowledge and appreciation of common disorders, is essential to nursing practice. As nurses we are empowered to use our knowledge, understanding and skill to care for patients expertly and compassionately. Irrespective of the location or specialty, a nurse will engage with patients who are living with chronic neurological disorders or who are experiencing acute problems. Having analysed and explored these disorders, the nurse will be in a better position to understand the pathophysiology, to appreciate the challenges and difficulties that a patient faces and ultimately to be insightful when caring for patients.

Chapter 5 Summary Quiz

1. The meninges consist of three layers, which is the correct order?

A. Dura mater – Pia mater – Arachnoid mater
B. Pia mater – Arachnoid mater – Dura mater
C. Dura mater – Arachnoid mater – Pia mater
D. Dura mater – Doesn't matter – Arachnoid mater

2. The primary regions of the brain are?

A. The cerebrum, the brain stem and the cerebellum
B. The cerebrum, the cortex and the cerebellum
C. The cortex, the brain stem and the cerebellum
D. The cerebrum, the brain stem and the cortex

3. How many pairs of cranial nerves are there?

A. 10
B. 21
C. 33
D. 12

4. Dopamine is a neurotransmitter, responsible for:

A. Sexual preference
B. Sexual behaviour
C. The coordination of movement and control of behaviour
D. Relaying messages, specifically regarding the mesenteric circulation

5. The lobes of the brain are:

A. The frontal, temporal, occipital and parietal
B. The Pons, and the circle of Willis
C. The frontal, temporal, occipital and parental
D. The occipital, the basal, the parietal and the temporal

6. The Glasgow Coma Scale is composed of how many sections?

A. 2
B. 3
C. 4
D. 5

7. Pupil assessment should include:

A. The size, shape and colour of the pupils, and their reaction to light
B. The shape and size of the pupil, and the colour of the iris
C. The shape, colour and equality of the pupils, and their reaction to light
D. The size, shape and equality of the pupils, and their reaction to light

8. Which risk factor is not associated with seizures?

A. Drug toxicity

B. Metabolic disorders (uraemia, electrolyte imbalance, hyper or hypoglycaemia)

C. Head trauma

D. A high pollen count

9. Which of the following is not a form of seizure?

A. Complex partial seizures

B. Simple partial seizures

C. Partial seizures

D. Total seizures

10. What are the three causes of 'stroke'?

A. An embolism, thrombotic, haemorrhagic

B. An embolism, phagocytic, haemorrhagic

C. Phagocytic, thrombotic, haemorrhage

D. A thrombus, embolism, phagocytic

Further reading

Adam, S. & Osbourne, S. (2005) *Critical Care Nursing Science and Practice*, 2nd edn. Oxford University Press: Oxford.

British Medical Association & Royal Pharmaceutical Society of Great Britain (2007) *British National Formulary* (BNF). BMJ Publishing Group: London.

Department of Health (2001) *National Service Framework for Older People*. DH: London.

Department of Health (2006) *Preventing Meningitis*. www.dh.gov.uk/en/Aboutus/MinistersandDepartmentLeaders/ChiefMedicalOfficer/ProgressOnPolicy/ProgressBrowsableDocument/DH_4102788

Department of Health (2007) *Developing a National Stroke Strategy*. www.dh.gov.uk/en/Policyandguidance/Healthandsocialcaretopics/Stroke/DH_4132138

Marieb, E. (2007) *Human Anatomy and Physiology*, 6th edn. Pearson International: San Francisco.

References

Adam, S. & Osbourne, S. (2005) *Critical Care Nursing Science and Practice*, 2nd edn. Oxford University Press: Oxford.

Department of Health (2001) *National Service Framework for Older People*. DH: London.

Department of Health (2004) *Better Information, Better Choices, Better Health: Putting Information at the Centre of Health*. www.dh.gov.uk/en/Publicationsandstatistics/Publications/PublicationsPolicyAndGuidance/DH_4098576 (accessed 26 May 2007).

Department of Health (2005) *Stem Cell Research: Medical Research with Responsibility*. www.dh.gov.uk/en/Aboutus/MinistersandDepartmentLeaders/ChiefMedicalOfficer/ProgressOnPolicy/ProgressBrowsableDocument/DH_4108203 (accessed 18 May 2007).

Department of Health (2006) *Preventing Meningitis*. www.dh.gov.uk/en/Aboutus/MinistersandDepartmentLeaders/ChiefMedicalOfficer/ProgressOnPolicy/ProgressBrowsableDocument/DH_4102788 (accessed 5 May 2007).

Department of Heath (2007a) *Stroke*. www.dh.gov.uk/en/Policyandguidance/Healthandsocialcaretopics/Stroke/index.htm (accessed 7 May 2007).

Department of Health (2007b) *Developing a National Stroke Strategy*. www.dh.gov.uk/en/Policyandguidance/Healthandsocialcaretopics/Stroke/DH_4132138 (accessed 7 May 2007).

Grundy, D. & Swain, A. (2002) *ABC of Spinal Cord Injury*, 4th edn. BMJ Books: London.

Health Protection Agency (2005) *Meningitis*. www.hpa.org.uk/infections/topics_az/meningo/backgrd.htm (accessed 25 May 2007).

Hickey, J. (2003) *The Clinical Practice of Neurological and Neurosurgical Nursing*, 5th edn. Lippincott Williams & Wilkins: Philadelphia.

Holland, W. (2000) *Stroke Past, Present and Future*. Oxford University Press: Oxford.

Institute for Stem Cell Research (ISCR) (2007) www.iscr.ed.ac.uk/outreach/FAQs_Content.php?categ=1&ques=18 (accessed online 10 May 2007).

ISRCTN (2007) *The Third International Stroke Trial (IST-3) of Thrombolysis for Acute Ischaemic Stroke*. www.controlled-trials.com/ISRCTN25765518 (accessed 27 May 2007).

IST-3 Thrombolysis (2007) *The Third International Stroke Trial (Thrombolysis)*. www.dcn.ed.ac.uk/ist3 (accessed 16 May 2007).

Marieb, E. (2007) *Human Anatomy and Physiology*, 6th edn. Pearson International: San Francisco.

National Collaborating Centre for Acute Care (2003) *Clinical Guideline 4 Head Injury: Triage, Assessment, Investigation and Early Management of Head Injury in Infants, Children and Adults*. NICE: London.

National Collaborating Centre for Chronic Conditions (2006) *Clinical Guideline 35 Parkinson's Disease: diagnosis and management in primary and secondary care*. NICE: London.

National Collaborating Centre for Primary Care (2004) *Clinical Guideline 20 The Epilepsies: Diagnosis and Management of the Epilepsies in Adults in Primary and Secondary Care*. NICE: London.

Oh, T. (2003) *Intensive Care Manual*, 5th edn. Butterworth Heinemann: London.

Royal College of Physicians Clinical Effectiveness and Evaluation Unit (CEEU) (2004) *National Clinical Guidelines for Stroke*, 2nd edn. RCP: London.

Spinal Injuries Association (2007) www.spinal.co.uk/a-05.aspx (accessed 21 May 2007).

Teasdale, G. & Jennet, B. (1974) Assessment of coma and impaired consciousness: a practical scale. *Lancet* 13: 81–4.

The renal system

Cliff Evans

Chapter 6 Learning Objectives

- Gain knowledge and insight into the anatomy and physiology related to the renal system and its components
- Gain insight into common conditions affecting the renal system
- Gain the ability to apply theory to practice by rationalising the physical manifestation of these illness in patients and instigating care
- Gain insight into commonly used medications directed at either preventing or treating relevant conditions
- Collect and assemble additional materials for your growing professional development portfolio
- Through the application of theory into practice question and critique the evidence base and effectiveness of the care you deliver

Introduction

This chapter discusses the renal, or urinary, system, which is a multifaceted, complex and vital structure. Diseases affecting this system are common, particularly infections, although failure of the system does not necessarily need to include an underlying infection as complete failure can result from many origins. Symptoms can be acute, insidious or chronic; this can make renal nursing an exciting and rewarding specialism. However, a nurse need not specialise in renal care to encounter patients experiencing renal dysfunction. During their career all nurses will be confronted by patients experiencing varying degrees of renal failure either as the patient's primary condition or as a secondary consequence. For knowledgeable practitioners with insight into the classic clinical signs and symptoms associated with an insult to renal function, the serious internal repercussions of leaving this condition untreated can be prevented.

This chapter initially focuses on providing the student with essential and relevant anatomy and physiology knowledge to enable them to understand the fundamental functioning of the renal system. Clinical signs and symptoms associated with the failure of this system are highlighted to provide the student with several prominent theoretical links to clinical practice. The chapter progresses into demonstrating some of the common illnesses associated with the renal system, highlighting the main causes of renal failure through the use of patient scenarios, which will also demonstrate many of the complexities associated with modern patient management.

Throughout the chapter the reader is asked to participate in and complete relevant exercises specifically designed to boost their developing portfolio of clinical practice and also to assist in the acquisition of essential skills associated with lifelong learning and the development of a strong and solid foundation of underpinning theoretical knowledge to their clinical practice.

Applying Theory to Practice: Exercise 6.1

Before reading on, compile two separate lists of:

Diseases you already know that affect the renal system

Potential instigators (causes) of renal failure

Add these lists to your developing portfolio. On completion of this chapter expand your portfolio by adding the new disorders you have gained knowledge on and elaborate on how these disorders affect physiological function.

Form

The renal system is composed of two **kidneys**, two **ureters**, a **bladder** and the **urethra**. The kidneys are classically described as two bean-shaped organs suspended at the rear, or posteriorly, within the abdomen (**retroperitoneal**).

Figure 6.1 Overview of the components of the renal system

- The Bowman's capsule and glomerulus
- The proximal convoluted tubule
- The loop of Henle
- The distal convoluted tubule
- The collecting duct.

Figure 6.2 The intricate workings of a nephron

- The structure of a kidney can be described in two distinct parts:
- The **cortex** on the outside
- The **medulla** on the inside leading to the **renal pelvis**.

The centre of each kidney is called the hilum, which is concave in shape. This is where the nerves, blood and lymphatic vessels enter the kidney.

Each kidney is connected to the bladder via a ureter; the ureter also enters at the hilum. The urethra connects the bladder to the external environment and therefore provides the exit point for **urine**.

A layer of fat and **fascia** enclose each kidney providing localised protection. Blood supply is delivered via the renal arteries branching off from the main body of the aorta. Interestingly, the kidneys, that comprise only around 0.4% of the total body weight (around 160g), receive approximately a quarter of the entire blood supply or cardiac output each minute. Therefore if the cardiac output is 4900ml per minute, then the kidneys receive 1225ml (Clancy & McVicar 2002). Each kidney is composed of around one million excretory units called **nephrons** measuring around 3cm, each containing an extremely intricate pathway involving several prominent points essential to optimal renal function:

The ureters

The ureters are the muscular tubes leading from the kidneys to the bladder; they measure around 30cm and are around 3mm in diameter (Clancy & McVicar 2002). The ureters travel downwards and enter the urinary bladder from the posterior sides through openings in the bladder wall. These openings close when the bladder contracts to prevent urine from flowing back into the ureter (reflux/ regurgitation).

The urinary bladder

This vital organ serves as a muscular sterile reservoir positioned on the floor of the pelvic cavity; its size is variable due to its ability to stretch depending on how much urine is stored, and this normally ranges between 600–1000ml. The bladder is composed of several layers. The inside of the bladder has a special type of lining that can stretch as the bladder fills and expands; this layer,

called the transitional epithelium, prevents urine being absorbed back into the circulation. In a relaxed or empty state the bladder's inner lining is arranged in folds (rugae), which expand as the bladder fills.

The urethra

The urethra forms the final passageway for the flow of urine; this thin-walled tube conveys urine from the floor of the urinary bladder to the outside. The opening to the outside is the external urethral orifice. The mucosal lining of the urethra is the transitional epithelium. The wall also contains smooth muscle fibres, supported by connective tissue. As the urethra leaves the urinary bladder it is initially surrounded by the internal urethral sphincter under autonomic control. The external urethral sphincter surrounds the urethra as it goes through the pelvic floor; this sphincter is under voluntary control. In females, the urethra is short, only 3–4 cm long. The external urethral orifice opens to the outside just anterior to the opening for the vagina. In males the urethra is around 20cm in length, and transports both urine and semen. The first part, next to the urinary bladder, passes through the prostate gland and is called the prostatic urethra. The second part, a short region that penetrates the pelvic floor and enters the penis, is called the membranous urethra. The third part, the spongy urethra, is the longest region. This portion of the urethra extends the entire length of the penis, and the external urethral orifice opens to the outside at the tip of the penis.

Function

Renal function centres on the kidneys, which regulate both the volume and composition of body fluids. The renal system must continually function at an optimal level due to the narrow spectrum required to maintain homeostasis. The physical processes of metabolism produce a variety of waste products that, if allowed to accumulate within the body, will cause both localised damage to the kidneys, and directly poison the affected individual. Several systems are involved in the removal of these waste products but clearance centres on the renal system. Anatomically the urinary and reproductive systems develop together in the embryo, in men, the urethra has a dual function: to provide an elimination passageway for both urine and sperm. Due to the close links between these systems many specialists will treat both urinary and reproductive complaints (genitourinary disorders). At a microscopic level kidney function centres on the ability of the nephron and its components to filter, secrete and reabsorb electrolytes.

- **Excretion** refers to a route rather than a process of removing substances derived from body fluids no longer required within the body
- **Secretion** represents the internal process of facilitating substances from one area to another generally across cell membranes
- **Filtration** is the act of filtering water and other small particles out of the circulation (Chapter 4)

As blood plasma passes through the kidneys, filtrate is formed; filtrate is of a similar composition to blood

Applying Theory to Practice: Exercise 6.2

Cystitis refers to inflammation of the bladder, generally caused by a localised infection.

- Why do you think this condition may be more common in females than males?

Scenario 6.3 discusses infections of the urinary tract.

The following links provide additional information:

http://www.netdoctor.co.uk/diseases/facts/cystitis.htm
http://www.nhsdirect.nhs.uk/articles/article.aspx?articleId=119

Applying Theory to Practice: Exercise 6.3

It has been identified that the driving force behind the formation and flow of filtrate is the pressure of blood within the capillaries. Answer the following questions to reinforce your understanding:

- What happens to the formation of filtrate when patients become hypovolaemic?
- In contrast what would happen if the distal pressure the filtrate meets increased?
- What could cause this?

Scenario 6.1 provides additional information.

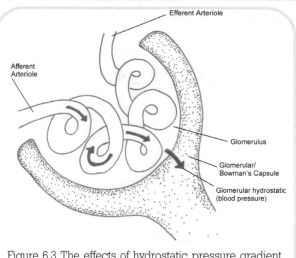

Figure 6.3 The effects of hydrostatic pressure gradient from the glomerulus to the Bowman space

Anatomy and Physiology in Action: Exercise 6.4

Classically there are seven main functions of the renal system. On completion of this chapter you should be able to identify them.

Write a short summary of what you think these seven functions are, an example is displayed below as an aid:

- A prominent function of the kidneys is the role they play in maintaining **red blood cell production**. This is achieved by producing erythropoietin, a hormone that increases the production of red blood cells within the bone marrow.
- Add this function plus the others you know or can find out about to your portfolio. A visit to the following websites may prove fruitful:
 http://www.nephrologychannel.com/anatomy.shtml
 http://kidney.niddk.nih.gov/kudiseases/pubs/yoururinary/

plasma with larger molecules and cells remaining in the blood. Each glomerulus provides a large surface area for the formation of filtrate; this takes place within the Bowman's capsule. The rate at which plasma is passed through the gromeruli is called the **glomerular filtration rate** (GFR). The driving force instigating this **hydrostatic** pressure is the pressure of blood within the capillaries.

It is estimated that the average adult has a GFR of around 180 L/day (Clancy & McVicar 2002). This rate significantly decreases with age, and it is estimated that by the age of 65 an average adult has a reduced renal function of around 30%; this figure continues to increase with each additional year of life by 1–2% (Clancy & McVicar 2002, Feest et al. 1993).

A network of **afferent** arterial capillaries almost entirely enclose the Bowman's capsule. This tubular system then continues branching into three distinct parts.

- The proximal convoluted tubule
- The loop of Henle (medullary loop)
- The distal convoluted tubule; this segment leads into the collecting duct which facilitates the final concentration of urine and transports the urine into the renal pelvis.

The collecting ducts unite and lead into the minor **calyces**.

The functioning of the renal system centres on both a secretory and excretory ability summarised in Table 6.1.

Now you have gained insight into the various functions

of the renal system you can see how complex and vital this system is. Despite its various functions, the central purpose of the renal system is the production of urine and

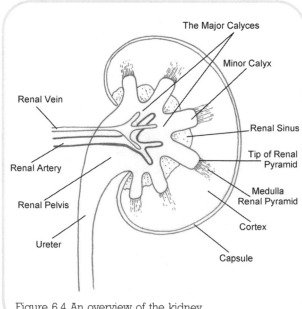

Figure 6.4 An overview of the kidney

Excretion	Secretion
Removes the waste products of cellular metabolism	Adjusts blood pressure via both the removal of urine and the release of **renin**
Concentrates or dilutes urine dependent on the current requirements of the body by removing or reabsorbing fluid	Maintains **homeostasis** through the regulation of red cell production by secreting **erythropoietin**
Regulates **pH** levels by excreting hydrogen ions (**H+**) or conserving bicarbonate ions	Standardises uptake of calcium and vitamin D
Regulates electrolyte levels	

Table 6.1 Functions of the Renal System

Anatomy and Physiology in Action: Exercise 6.5

Before continuing, write a short summary of how you think urine is formed and how this process is governed.

Add this to your portfolio. On completion of the following section insert the new information you have learnt into your portfolio.

the elimination or excretion of waste products and surplus water.

The urine

The composition of urine constantly changes depending on the current internal circumstance and regulatory requirements. Excessive amounts of any particular electrolyte can be passed within the urine; in addition electrolytes in short supply can be reabsorbed and recirculated.

The colour of urine partially reflects its concentration i.e. the lighter the urine, the less concentrated it is. It also reflects the amount of bilirubin and bile pigment present. Urine is composed of:

- 96% water
- 2% urea
- 2% chemicals, including sodium, potassium and ammonia.

It is estimated that the average adult produces 1.5 litres of urine each 24 hours, around 30–60ml per hour. It

is necessary to generate and void around 30ml of urine per hour to eliminate the waste products of cellular metabolism (Clancy & McVicar 2002).

Applying Theory to Practice: Exercise 6.6

Examination of a patient's urine can consolidate many clinical findings. It is therefore essential for nurses to understand the basic components of urine and to comprehend the significance of increasing levels of certain waste or by-products and appreciate the importance of identifying substances that should not be found within the urine.

Complete the following exercise before continuing:

- Construct a list of what you would expect to find within the urine
- There are many different types of quick and easy to use test sticks or strips that enable the user to analyse a urine sample (**urinalysis**); identify the type used on your placements and read the instruction sheet that accompanies the test strips. This will provide you with essential information regarding obtaining a correct reading and will explain which substances that particular test strip can be used to identify.
- Add the leaflet to your developing portfolio and learn the significance of each potential finding.

Many external factors can influence the results of a urinalysis; these can result in false findings, potentially leading to a wrong diagnosis. The following list identifies some classic examples:

- Menstruation (blood)
- Ascorbic acid (can cause blood, glucose and nitrate anomalies)
- L-dopa (high levels of glucose)
- Salicylates (glucose; potential false negative reading) (Dougherty & Lister 2004).

Many different drugs will alter the colour of the urine. These include commonly used antibiotics such as clarithromycin and rifampicin. Even eating beetroot can cause the colour of urine to change to a similar colour to **frank haematuria**.

Blood should not be present within the urine; a multitude of reasons can result in blood entering the urine resulting in **haematuria.** These include direct trauma to any part of the urinary tract, (kidneys, ureters, bladder or urethra), or the presence of malignant cells found in cancer-affected areas such as the prostate in men. There are also transient causes found when the kidneys temporarily receive a reduced blood supply. This can be caused by strenuous levels of exercise particularly if prolonged such as in marathon runners (Saladin 2005). In these circumstances the glomeruli deteriorate, instigating the release of blood and protein into the filtrate. Localised infection can also result in haematuria, although this is generally found under microscopic examination or via test sticks rather than by the naked eye.

When using test sticks it is paramount that the instructions are followed precisely as the potential for an incorrect result is high; this is particularly so if the test is hurried and the correct exposure times are incorrectly followed.

The process of elimination

Once the urine is formed and filtered within the kidneys, it is propelled down the ureters by peristaltic contraction of the smooth muscle of the ureteral walls. This is a continual process with urine slowly trickling into the bladder. As the bladder fills and distends, the individual is aware of the need to urinate; this is usually sensed when the bladder holds around 400 ml of urine (Waugh & Grant 2007). The elimination or passing of urine is initiated by a reflex action whereby the bladder wall begins to contract as a response to the increasing wall tension and the stimulation of stretch receptors. As the bladder continues to fill the contractions increase, resulting in the internal urethral sphincter opening, the external sphincter relaxes and urine passes out.

This appears a simple process but, due to the reliance on sphincters, and in the male the prostate gland (Chapter 9), this can be a potentially problematic process.

Developing and Delivering Expert Care: Box 6.1

Obtaining a Mid-Stream Urine Sample (MSU)

A urinalysis provides a quick and simple overview of the urine. If a potential infection is identified, a further specimen should be ascertained. This sample requires a mid-stream sample of the urine so that contaminates like bacteria that colonise around the end of the urethra are not included. The sample will be sent to a microbiology laboratory so that the bacteria can be grown and identified. The specimen is sent for micro-culture and sensitivity (MC&S), which means the identification of the bacteria (micro-culture) and what the specific bacterium is sensitive to, i.e. which antibiotic will destroy it and which antibiotics these bacteria are resistant to.

Developing and Delivering Expert Care: Exercise 6.7

Anticipating and Monitoring Urine Output

Many patients are at direct risk of experiencing acute renal failure while they are hospitalised (RCUK 2006).

Answer the following questions and expand your answers after reading the following section.

- How can you identify those at increased risk?
- What can be done to prevent acute renal failure (ARF) developing?

Scenario 6.1 discusses ARF in detail.

Acute renal failure

Acute renal failure (ARF) can be defined as an acute or rapid deterioration in renal function that is potentially reversible. The causes are varied but the result is an inability to excrete the waste products of cellular metabolism, therefore creating an internal environment

Scenario 6.1

Acute Renal Failure

Zamid Khan is a 78-year-old man of Pakistani origin. He was admitted in the early hours of the morning following a collapse at home the previous evening. Mr Khan has had type 2 diabetes for six years; this is controlled by his dietary intake and oral medications (metformin and glicazide).

You are caring for him the following morning on an acute medical ward. During your initial assessment you note the following observations:

Airway – clear, patient is talking, AVPU = A
Breathing – respiratory rate 21, regular with full inspiration
Circulation – pulse 91 regular and strong, blood pressure 109/68, blood sugar 14.2mmol. His tympanic temperature was recorded as 37.6.

On admission Mr Khan appeared dehydrated and has received two litres of physiological saline since his admission. Mr Khan has not passed any urine and is still awaiting a urinalysis as part of the investigatory process.

PMH: hypertension and type 2 diabetes.

His blood results reveal increased levels of creatinine and urea.

incompatible with the maintenance of an efficient fluid and electrolyte balance. ARF affects an estimated 0.01% of the population; this rises to around 4% of hospitalised patients and 20% of critical care admissions making iatrogenic ARF a serious concern for all hospitalised patients (Sinert & Peacock 2006).

Assessment and analysis of patient presentation

The presenting history of Mr Khan's admission elicits more questions than it provides answers. The initial assessment identifies a stable patient who is potentially physiologically compensating to maintain homeostasis, demonstrated by a raised respiratory and pulse rate. This makes sense when combined with his relative hypotension and a physical presentation suggesting dehydration. This is magnified by the increased blood sugar level, which will result in a greater internal pressure to maintain homeostasis. Mr Khan has also been found to have a slight temperature indicative of an underlying disease process; this is by far the most common cause of collapse in this age group (Evans & Tippins 2007). A urinalysis is essential as soon as possible to identify a possible infection or to identify evidence of kidney failure.

The emergency department prior to his transfer should have excluded life-threatening pathology such as cardiac disease; additionally a local tool for identifying patients at risk will have been used to provide a safe transfer to a secondary setting (PAR/MEWS). The joint presentation of

dehydration and collapse are a cause for concern when combined with a history of diabetes. Diabetes is frequently associated with the onset of acute renal failure due to the associated poor renal perfusion and reduced microcirculation to the kidneys. This is seen as a pathological cycle of events, as once the kidneys are starved of blood they initiate the release of renin, and the renin angiotensin aldosterone axis is instigated (RAAA) (Chapter 2). Mr Khan's blood has been found to contain excessive amounts of both urea and creatinine (both prominent signs of renal failure). Initial investigations will centre on identifying potentially reversible causes when renal function suddenly declines.

Pathophysiology

ARF may occur in three clinical settings:

- As an adaptive response to severe volume depletion and hypotension, with structurally and functionally intact nephrons
- In response to cytotoxic or ischaemic insults to the kidney, with structural and functional damage
- As a consequence of an obstruction to the passage of urine.

Therefore, ARF may be classified as **prerenal**, **intrinsic** and **postrenal**. While these classifications are useful in

Applying Theory to Practice: Box 6.2

Acute Renal Failure – Three Categories

Prerenal

Reduced perfusion of the kidneys results in the retention or accumulation of excessive nitrogenous compounds within the blood. Initially the kidneys are unaffected but if left untreated the GFR will be compromised, resulting in increasing prerenal uraemia directly affecting the actual kidneys. Instigating factors include:

- Dehydration
- Haemorrhage
- Burns
- Systemic Inflammatory Response Syndrome (SIRS)

Intrarenal

Damage directly affecting the kidneys:

- Acute tubular necrosis
- Acute glomerulonephritis
- Acute pyelonephritis

Postrenal

- The most common cause of postrenal failure is secondary to bladder outlet obstruction due to prostatic hypertrophy (Agraharker et al. 2006)
- Obstruction of the urethra due to calculi (Scenario 6.2), trauma or strictures
- Obstruction of the bladder due to cancer

Developing and Delivering Expert Care: Exercise 6.8

Observations for Patients Experiencing Potential Renal Failure

All patients experiencing ARF are at potential risk of fluid overload; this is particularly prominent in patients who have existing cardiac disease. Therefore close monitoring of their fluid balance is essential particularly during aggressive fluid resuscitation. Complete the following questions:

- What are the clinical signs of fluid overload?
- What changes would you be looking for in the patient's vital signs?

If suspected renal failure presents in combination with heart failure, a central line and urinary catheter are essential to monitor the patient's fluid status.

Daily weights will be used to ascertain if the patient is retaining or losing fluid:

- When are these recorded in your clinical areas?

A strict fluid input/output chart will also be employed:

- Are fluid charts known to be reliable?
- What might influence their accuracy?

establishing a differential diagnosis, many pathophysiologic features are shared among the different categories.

Mr Khan is suffering from prerenal insufficiency, a functional response of normal kidneys to acute hypoperfusion. Prerenal insufficiency accounts for approximately 70% of community-acquired cases of ARF worldwide and up to 60% of hospital-acquired cases (Devarajan 2006).

The acute phase of kidney compensation includes enhanced tubular reabsorption of salt and water initiated

Developing and Delivering Expert Care Box 6.3

Clinical Signs Associated with Acute Renal Failure

Urea is a by-product of protein metabolism commonly referred to as a nitrogenous waste; if allowed to accumulate, it will result in a physiological state referred to as **azotaemia**. This progresses into **uraemia** (excessive urea within the blood) which can be demonstrated by many clinical changes:

- Cardiac arrhythmias
- Dyspnoea
- Diarrhoea and vomiting
- Convulsions
- Coma
- Dry flaking skin
- Dimness of vision
- Weakness and lethargy

By identifying the clinical signs of impending renal failure swift action can reduce both mortality and morbidity rates (UKRC 2006).

http://www.nlm.nih.gov/medlineplus/ency/article/000471.htm

by the renin angiotensin aldosterone axis/system. In the case of Mr Khan rapid reversibility of the **oliguria** allows correction of the hypoperfusion and the re-establishment of renal perfusion. This occurs shortly after admission to the medical ward. Mr Khan was lucky: for many patients prolonged renal hypoperfusion can result in a shift from compensation to decompensation.

The physical consequences of ARF for the individual are wide-ranging and diagnostically include an excessive amount of urea and a rise in creatinine with or without a significant decrease in urine output. ARF can also be asymptomatic as significant renal dysfunction might be present even when serum creatinine is normal or only slightly abnormal, making the identification of those at risk essential to the early initiation of treatment and the prevention of the destruction of nephrons. The baseline rate of urinary protein excretion is the best single predictor of disease progression (Parmar 2002).

In the case of Mr Khan, his diabetes and history of

hypertension predispose him to the development of both acute and chronic renal failure.

Psychosocial aspects

Mr Khan is of Pakistani origin genetically predisposing him to an increased incidence of both diabetes and renal failure (DH 2000, 2006).

Questioning Clinical Practice: Exercise 6.9

Ethical Dilemma – Screening Programmes

If certain nationalities are at an increased risk of developing serious diseases, should they be identified and regularly screened for potential disease development?

- How do you think indigenous groups might react when it is surmised that 'foreigners' are receiving preferential treatment?

Although in this case scenario Mr Khan will make a full recovery due to the quick delivery of intravenous fluids and maintenance of his electrolyte balance, he will need regular blood tests to monitor his kidney function. This will generally be undertaken by his GP, who will also need to closely monitor his medications, as many modern medications taken by diabetic patients to reduce their blood pressure and cholesterol levels have been shown to adversely affect the microcirculation of the kidneys, thereby insidiously damaging the nephrons and causing renal failure (DH 2000).

Developing and Delivering Expert Care: Box 6.4

Basic Nursing Skills

A patient experiencing the clinical signs of acute renal failure and an increased level of urea may have itchy flaking skin. This should be anticipated and a skin emollient applied at an early stage to prevent skin damage.

Professional issues

Diabetes and hypertension are the two most common causes of end-stage renal failure and are associated with a high morbidity and mortality rate; individuals with pre-

existing diabetes and hypertension have an estimated 10–20 times higher mortality rate than the population at large (Parmar 2002). The current focus has, therefore, shifted to maximising the care of these patients during the phases of acute or chronic kidney disease, and before the onset of end-stage renal disease. This is particularly evident in the long-term treatment of Mr Khan, as preventing further damage to the inner workings of his kidneys is paramount to his long-term prognosis. Mr Khan must be offered information regarding the stabilisation of his diabetes. Offering him an informed choice about his chronic illness may assist him to closely monitor his blood sugars and prevent his quality of life from deteriorating. Nurses are in an ideal position for this type of health education and patient empowerment. Several government-driven targets have been identified in recently published documents directed at preventative medicine in these areas (DH 2000, 2005, NICE 2004).

Questioning Clinical Practice: Exercise 6.10

Urinary Catheterisation

- If it were suspected that Mr Khan had an underpinning urine infection but failed to pass urine, would this justify urinary catheterisation to obtain a sample?
- What would the potential risks be?
- Would they outweigh the benefits?

There are numerous clinical practices without an evidence base, carried out each day by healthcare practitioners unaware of the devastation they can cause to people they are apparently 'caring' for.

The following links provide additional information:
http://www.nhshealthquality.org/nhsqis/files/Urinary_Cath_COMPLETE.pdf

www.dh.gov.uk/prod_consum_dh/idcplg?IdcService=GET_FILE&dID=147767&Rendition=Web

Chronic renal failure (CRF)

Regardless of the underpinning aetiology of the renal injury, if left untreated, progressive destruction of the nephrons will result in the kidneys maintaining the GFR by hyperfiltration resulting in **hypertrophy** of the func-

tioning nephrons. This ability of the nephrons to adapt to meet the current requirements to maintain homeostasis allows for the continued clearance of filtrate to such an extent that substances such as urea and creatinine start to show significant increases in plasma levels only after the total GFR has decreased to 50% (Verrelli 2006). The plasma creatinine value will double with a 50% reduction in GFR. A doubling in the patient's serum creatinine baseline (potentially still within the normal range) can actually represent a loss of 50% of functioning nephrons (Sinert & Peacock 2006). Ultimately over time this innate compensatory mechanism will result in the nephrons becoming misshapen and ineffective.

Chronic renal failure is invariably a progressive process that results in end-stage renal disease and the need for dialysis or kidney transplantation (Parmar 2002).

Renal colic

Scenario 6.2

Renal Colic

Michelle Stevens, a 35-year-old Caucasian woman, is admitted to the emergency department after suffering severe right flank pain and vomiting for the past 2 hours.

On arrival she appears pale and clammy. She is unable to lie still and stands slouching over the hospital trolley.

During the initial assessment you record the following observations:

Airway – clear, patient is talking, AVPU = A
Breathing – respiratory rate 26, irregular and shallow
Circulation – pulse 129, regular and of good volume
Blood pressure 154/89
Temperature 36.4
PMH: Ms Stevens has no relevant medical history although she appears clinically obese.

Assessment and analysis of patient presentation

Michelle Stevens presents with the typical clinical signs and symptoms of renal colic; from her presenting data it can be deduced that she is suffering extreme pain. Michelle's vital signs demonstrate all too clearly the

sympathetic response to pain; her breathing rate is fast, shallow and erratic, her pulse and blood pressure are raised, she appears pale and clammy. Although flank pain accompanied by vomiting can signify many clinical conditions, the most likely condition affecting this age range is renal colic. Other serious pathology should be excluded; these include peritonitis, appendicitis, bowel obstruction, urinary tract infection, pregnancy and constipation. Michelle's stance offers invaluable information regarding her illness. Many serious pathologies affecting the abdomen cause the sufferer to lie 'doubled-up' in pain, almost resembling the fetal position, but patients attending with renal colic commonly move around trying to find a comfortable position, often slouching against a wall or other object.

Applying Theory to Practice: Exercise 6.11

Predisposing Factors Associated with Calculi Development

The term 'colic' is used in many circumstances. Answer the following questions to gain insight into this common disease process:

- What is colic?
- Renal colic is commonly described as one of the most painful disease processes; why might this be?
- What other areas are affected by 'colic'?

Renal colic is classically described as an excruciating acute pain that can occur without warning. It is usually caused by **calculi** (stones) within the kidney, renal pelvis or ureter. The pain results from the associated local inflammation, dilatation, stretching and spasms. It is estimated that renal colic has an incidence of 12% for men and 4% for women (Leslie 2006). Acute renal colic may be the most excruciatingly painful disease an individual can experience. The sudden onset of extreme and unbearable pain is often described as worse than childbirth. Renal colic affects approximately 1.2 million people each year and accounts for approximately 1% of all hospital admissions within the USA (Leslie 2006). Rapid initial treatment and symptom relief are paramount as is patient education. The risk of stones is greater in higher socioeconomic groups. The peak age of onset is 35 to 45;

presentations significantly outside this age group are often associated with a metabolic abnormality.

Pathophysiology

Calculi, otherwise known as stones, form due to an abnormal concentration of mineral salts or substances. Stones are not confined to the renal system, they are also commonly found within the biliary tract and around joints.

Anatomy and Physiology in Action: Exercise 6.12

- What increases the likelihood of developing a renal or urinary calculus?
- Do lifestyle choices affect an individual's chance of developing a renal calculi?

Add your answers to your portfolio and expand on them as you read the following section.

The classification of calculi can be separated into two main groups:

- **Small calculi**, which can pass through larger areas of the kidneys and become impacted as the pathway becomes increasingly smaller, generally within the ureters (Clancy & McVicar 2002). Although it is possible to have more than one circulating stone, commonly the obstruction occurs only on one side (unilateral). Spasmodic contraction and inflammation of the ureter ensue with the individual experiencing extreme pain on the affected side. The individual may even be able to directly pinpoint the location of the stone due to the direct localised inflammation and spasms as the urinary tract tries to force the stone down the system. Stones that are eventually forced down the pathway by ureteral contraction may be passed in the urine although it is possible for the stone to become lodged in the urethra.
- **Large calculi** can block areas proximal to the kidney resulting in occlusion within the renal pelvis and subsequent stagnation of urine and infection. Renal colic in combination with an underlying kidney infection (**pyelonephritis**) may directly lead to renal failure. Michelle is found to be apyrexial, which is considered to represent uncomplicated renal colic. If

pyrexia is present, this suggests infection and the temperature is usually very high, although this may not be the case in all presentations i.e. the elderly. Although renal colic is usually self-limiting, it does hold significant risk for those experiencing renal compromise e.g. those with a single kidney or azotaemia.

Developing and Delivering Expert Care: Exercise 6.13

Identifying Renal Stones

The initial diagnosis is based on clinical findings; definitive diagnosis can be established via various mediums. Many emergency departments will provide easy access to an intra-venous urogram (IVU) for the diagnosis of renal colic.

Many other tests exist with equal prognostic value to an IVU; helical CT scanning currently remains the gold standard (Leslie 2006).

- Identify which tests are available within your clinical areas.

By knowing which tests are available and how they are performed you will be able to inform the patient about what they are about to experience.

Many other non-specific tests exist in the identification of renal stones these include haematuria on urinalysis: stones often cause some bleeding into the renal tract resulting in a positive result for blood on stick testing, but a negative test does not exclude the diagnosis. Many studies have been undertaken to establish the reliability of urinalysis – 80–93% – therefore, the test is of some value but does not confidently confirm or refute a diagnosis (Malvinder 2004).

X-ray examination traditionally starts with visualising the kidneys, ureters and bladder (KUB). It has been estimated that around 75% of stones consist of calcium, and are therefore identifiable on X-ray examination (radio-opaque) (Leslie 2006). To increase the possible effectiveness of X-ray, an ultrasound scan can be added, an extremely easy to use tool.

Applying Theory to Practice: Box 6.5

Risk Factors Associated with Calculi Development

Many factors increase the likelihood of developing kidney stones:

- Dehydration can cause an increased reabsorption of water but does not change **solute** reabsorption, therefore resulting in a highly concentrated filtrate
- Excessive **calcium** in the urine
- Excessive **oxalate** in the urine
- Excessive **uric acid**
- Deficiency of **citrate** in the urine

Treatment and management

Pain relief must be the early priority. A pain assessment tool should be employed to guide and evaluate treatment. Non-steroidal anti-inflammatory drugs (NSAID) are usually the first-line treatment as they provide direct pain relief and may stop further pain development by reducing inflammation and spasms. Suppository administration is quick-acting and provides an easy route of administration for the typical age range associated with renal colic. If this fails to provide relief, intravenous opioids, such as diluted morphine should be titrated until pain relief is achieved, in combination with an anti-emetic to control nausea and vomiting.

Complications

- Complete obstruction of the urinary flow from a kidney decreases GFR and if left untreated may cause irreversible kidney damage.
- If infection co-exists, presentation can be life-threatening.
- Blood results may reveal a white cell count or a temperature may co-exist.

Psychosocial aspects

The association between renal colic and extreme pain is well documented; therefore, a designated plan of care should be implemented based on best practice. This usually consists of a multidisciplinary care pathway used to rationalise Michelle's care. This will expedite her

treatment and provides quick and effective pain relief as analgesics and anti-emetics will be available via a patient group direction (PGD), meaning the nurse can dispense these drugs without waiting for a written prescription.

Professional issues

Many patients will be able to be discharged once pain relief is achieved and their symptoms subside. There are cases, however, where the patient will require hospitalisation:

- Clinical signs of infection, systemic illness
- A failure to achieve adequate pain relief
- An ureteral or urethral obstruction
- An inability to maintain oral fluids
- Patients outside the normal age-range i.e. the young or old. Elderly patients may have a similar presentation to renal colic with a leaking aneurysm
- A significant history of renal failure i.e. only one kidney
- Anuria.

Analysis

Health promotion can have a powerful preventative influence if heeded. Michelle should be encouraged to maintain a good fluid intake to keep her urine dilute. Avoiding a diet high in salt or protein may prove beneficial (NICE 2004).

Urinary tract infection

Patients experiencing urinary tract infections are a common presentation within all health settings. It is estimated that between 1–3% of all consultations relate to an infection of the urinary tract (UTI) and that in hospitalised patients UTIs account for 23% of all hospital-acquired infections (Naish & Hallam 2007). In the USA, the National Institute of Diabetes and Digestive and Kidney Diseases estimate that around 8.3 million people seek medical advice related to UTIs each year (NIDDKD 2005).

Assessment and analysis of patient presentation

Despite Mrs Forbes having vital signs within normal parameters for her age she appears confused and disorientated. She does not have a temperature, which might have made the diagnosis of an infection easy, but elderly patients frequently do not demonstrate a raised temperature even with severe infection (Berman et al. 1987).

Scenario 6.3

Urinary Tract Infection

Grace Forbes, an 81-year-old Caucasian woman, was admitted to the acute medical assessment unit late last night following a fall at home. Her symptoms include slight grazing to her right arm and unsteadiness on her feet. She has been referred to the medical team for a full medical assessment including occupational and physiotherapist opinions about her needs for a safe discharge.

During the morning handover her condition is described as stable and she is awaiting a senior medical opinion before, hopefully, being discharged that afternoon.

During your initial assessment you note the following observations:

Airway – clear, patient is talking, AVPU = A
Breathing – respiratory rate 17, regular and shallow
Circulation – pulse 71 regular and strong, blood pressure 142/89
Temperature 36.4°

Mrs Forbes appears vague and disorientated; she is playing with her nightdress revealing that she is not wearing underwear. She also smells offensive and when the sheets on her bed are examined they are saturated with urine from where she has been incontinent.

PMH: hypertension. Mrs Forbes takes atenolol to control her blood pressure.

All elderly patients demonstrating confusion or a sudden reduction in their cognitive ability should have an infection screen to rule out pathology.

The most likely pathology affecting Mrs Forbes is a urinary tract infection provisionally identified by the offensive smell of the urine, confused behaviour and perhaps the incontinence. The infection was confirmed by a urinalysis revealing leukocytes and protein, both of which indicate infection. The causative bacteria will be identified when a sample of urine is obtained for micro-culture and sensitivity (MC&S).

Questioning Clinical Practice: Exercise 6.14

Stereotyping Individuals

An elderly patient being admitted to hospital in a confused state is not uncommon. Complete the following exercise adding your work to your portfolio.

There are many pathophysiologies that can result in an individual becoming acutely confused.

- Make a list of which conditions you think commonly afflict the elderly
- How can they be excluded?
- What tests would an infection screen involve?

One common example is constipation, which can cause an otherwise healthy and coherent adult to become disorientated and irrational. Visit the following link to gain further insight into this topic: http://users.ecs.soton.ac.uk/id/Omega%20dying%20decisions.pdf

Elderly people are increasingly prone to UTIs due to several physiological changes:

- Reduced bladder emptying (contractility)
- A decreased mucosal barrier
- A loss of bladder tone (Banning 2005).

Pathophysiology

Infections affecting the urinary tract can be split into four distinct classifications; although any one can occur in isolation, many infections will be transient and travel from one area of the tract to another. Infections directly affecting areas of the kidney can lead to localised necrosis and long-term kidney damage and potential failure:

- **Urethritis** – inflammation of the urethra; characterised by pain on urination (can be caused by localised inflammation/infection or linked to gonococcal infection)
- **Pyelonephritis** – infection spreading from the renal pelvis to the cortex of the kidney. Commonly linked to infections below the ureters or within the bloodstream (SIGN 2006)
- **Pyelitis** – inflammation of the renal pelvis involving **pyuria**

- **Cystitis** – inflammation of the bladder; associated with a burning sensation on urination and frequency.

The aetiology of infection can vary between men and women. Infection in males can be directly linked to prostate hypertrophy and subsequent urine stagnation within the bladder, leading to initially a localised urine infection and the potential for cystitis. Females are at particular risk of UTIs, this is possibly due to a reduced fluid intake and the close proximity between the anus and the urethra which in females can lead to the urethra becoming colonised by particular strains of bacteria such as *Escherichia coli,* otherwise known as perianal flora. Bacteria can then ascend, or migrate, up the urinary tract infecting vital structures leading to the possibility of systemic illness (SIGN 2006). See Table 6.2.

Effect on Appearance of Urine	Possible Physical Effects
Cloudy urine Offensive smelling urine	Dysuria Frequency and urgency to urinate
Haematuria (may only be microscopic)	Pyrexia
Proteinuria (may only be microscopic) Concentrated urine (dark) Pyuria (contains pus)	Possible abdominal/loin pain Cystitis – burning or discomfort on urination Confusion/collapse Shock

Table 6.2 The Signs and Symptoms of Urinary Tract Infections

Psychosocial aspects

Many women in later life are prone to urinary problems particularly after childbirth. Stress incontinence is a common and embarrassing complaint. For men a common urinary problem is an enlarged or hypertrophic prostate leading to incomplete bladder emptying, and urine stagnation, the ideal breeding ground for bacteria. Both sexes therefore have their own particular problems regarding urination. For many these problems are highly embarrassing and patients may only present for medical assistance when they have systemic reactions i.e. they collapse or become confused. Despite urinary retention

Questioning Clinical Practice: Exercise 6.15

Conflicting Information and Care Delivery

Because urinary infections in women are so common, many are treated with antibiotics only when the patient demonstrates clinical symptoms (Table 6.2). Many healthcare agencies are currently differing in their testing regimens, treatment plans and health promotion, an example being that it has been common practice to send mid-stream urine samples for further analysis to confirm appropriate antibiotic cover following diagnosis via a urine dipstick. These guidelines and articles discuss the relevance of such tests and their cost effectiveness.

● Read the following guidelines/articles and identify how you will apply them to your future practice.

Prodigy Guidance (2006) Urinary Tract Infection (Lower): Women. NHS National Library for Health, Newcastle upon Tyne. http://cks.library.nhs.uk/uti_lower_men/view_whole_guidance

Scottish Intercollegiate Guidelines Network (2006) Management of Suspected Bacterial Urinary Tract Infection in Adults: A National Clinical Guideline. SIGN. Edinburgh. http://www.sign.ac.uk/guidelines/published/index.html

Health Protection Agency (2005) Investigation of Urine. National Standard Method BSOP. 41 5. (Under review) http://www.hpa-standardmethods.org.uk/documents/bsop/pdf/bsop41.pdf

Summarise your findings for your portfolio.

being a common, highly publicised condition in men (BAEM 2007), many have failed to seek any medical help despite years of urinary problems such as leakage or dribbling. Nurses can have a profound effect on individuals by raising awareness of these conditions and positively promoting health education. An adequate intake of water, as with most urinary problems, can be extremely beneficial. Women should be informed of wiping away from the urethra after emptying their bowels as this can directly cause stool particles to migrate into the urethra and vagina promoting or directly causing infection. By actively promoting an increased awareness of these conditions in patients attending for other reasons, preventative strategies can be used to reduce both future attendances and may help to dispel taboo subjects to the benefit of those who suffer from these conditions.

Professional issues

Much of the underpinning theory related to the tests, treatment and health advice offered to patients experiencing UTIs are currently under debate. There are also various claims regarding different foods and their ability to prevent or halt urinary infections, for example, yoghurt and cranberry juice. Much of the research for these products may be driven by the companies who produce them, so be sceptical in your approach. As a future nurse you will need to continually update your practice depending on future quantitative research and the publication of definitive guidelines. Your clients will listen to your opinions, and you will potentially have a great influence over a public who place trust in you because of your position.

Analysis

Dealing with a confused elderly patient is a skill all adult nurses require. A lone elderly patient on a general medical ward lying in her own urine with her hospital gown slung to one side is a shameful sight; the patient in a time of need has lost not only mental and physical functioning but also her dignity. This patient requires caring assistance and the nurse must maintain the patient's dignity in their role of patient's advocate.

Conclusion

This chapter has discussed both the form and function of the renal system, a system which is commonly undervalued. Over the coming weeks and months apply your new understanding to the patients you meet, identify which medications they take and recall if any of these can affect kidney function, look for signs of renal disease. You can now offer patients valuable information regarding both health promotion and education. Now that you have gained insight into the basic form and function of this system, reinforce your knowledge base by working your way through the summary quiz.

Chapter 6 Summary Quiz

1. The renal system is composed of:

A. Two kidneys, two ureters, and a bladder

B. Two kidneys, a common ureter, a bladder and the urethra.

C. Two kidneys, two ureters, a bladder and the urethra

D. Two kidneys, two ureters, two bladders and a urethra

2. Each nephron contains an extremely intricate pathway involving several prominent points essential to optimal renal function. These include:

A. The collecting duct, the distal convoluted tubule, the loop of Henle, the Proximal convoluted tubule, the Boatman's capsule and glomerulus

B. The distal convoluted tubule, the loop of Henle, the Proximal convoluted tubule, the Bowman's capsule and glomerulus

C. The distal convoluted tubule, the loop of Henle, the Inferior convoluted tubule, the Bowman's capsule and glomerulus

D. The collecting duct, the distal convoluted tubule, the bundle of His, the Proximal convoluted tubule, the Bowman's capsule and glomerulus

3. Cystitis refers to:

A. A sexual disease affecting women

B. Inflammation of the bladder, generally caused by a localised infection

C. Inflammation of the kidney

D. Localised infection within the kidney

4. The following are all functions of the renal system:

A. Acid-base balance, blood pressure control, hormone production, drug removal, fluid balance, toxin removal

B. Acid-base balance, cerebral spinal fluid regulation, drug removal, fluid balance, toxin removal

C. Acid-base balance, metabolism of drugs, hormone production, fluid balance,

D. All the above

5. Pyelonephritis describes which illness?

A. Inflammation of the bladder

B. Infection spreading from the bladder to the urethra

C. Infection spreading from the renal pelvis to the cortex of the kidney

D. Inflammation of the urethra

6. What tests are commonly available for the diagnosis of renal colic?

A. IVU

B. Helical CT scanning

C. KUB

D. All the above

7. Iatrogenic means:

A. Ill health or adverse effects resulting from medical treatment

B. Medical incompetence

C. A poor knowledge related to a nurse

D. An MRSA infection

8. Which of the following diseases predisposes individuals to renal disease?

A. Glandular fever

B. Cellulitis

C. Diabetes mellitus

D. Ovarian cysts

9. The internal urethral sphincter is under:

A. Involuntary control

B. Voluntary control

C. Remote control

D. All the above

10. In males the urethra is around how many centimetres long?

A. 25

B. 20

C. 10

D. 7

Further reading

Agraharker, M., Gupta, R., Agraharkar, A. & Workeneth, B.T. (2006) *Acute Renal Failure.* http://www.emedicine.com/med/topic1595.htm

National Institute of Clinical Excellence (2003) *Infection Control: Prevention of Healthcare-associated Infection in Primary and Community Care.* NICE: London.

National Institute of Health and Clinical Excellence (NICE) (2007) *Acutely Ill Patients in Hospital: Full Guideline.* Draft. NICE: London.

Redmond, A., McDevitt, M. & Barnes, S. (2004) Acute renal failure: recognition and treatment in ward patients. *Nursing Standard.* 18(22): 46–53.

Richards, C.L. (2004) Urinary tract infections in the frail elderly: issues for diagnosis, treatment and prevention. *International Urology and Nephrology* 36(3): 457–63.

Scottish Intercollegiate Guidelines Network (SIGN) (2006) *Management of Suspected Bacterial Urinary Tract Infection in Adults: A National Clinical Guideline.* SIGN: Edinburgh.

Singri, I., Ahya, S.N. & Levin, N.L. (2003) Acute renal failure. *Journal of the American Medical Association* 289(6): 747–51. http://kidney.niddk.nih.gov/kudiseases/pubs/yourkidneys/ http://rnceus.com/renal/renalfunction.html

References

Agraharker, M., Gupta, R., Agraharkar, A. & Workeneth, B.T. (2006) *Acute Renal Failure.* http://www.emedicine.com/med/topic1595.htm (accessed 14/08/07).

Banning, M. (2005) Infections and their treatment in older people. *Nursing Older People* 17(2): 25–9.

Berman, P., Hogan, D.B. & Fox, R.A. (1987) The atypical presentation of infection in old age. *Age & Ageing* 16(4): 201–7.

British Association Emergency Medicines (BAEM) (2007) *Audit Standards for Emergency Departments.* BAEM: London. http://www.emergencymed.org.uk/BAEM/CEC/assets/Summary_of_Standards_Jan07_%282nd_draft%29.pdf

Clancy, J. & McVicar, A.J. (2002) *Physiology and Anatomy. A Homeostatic Approach*, 2nd edn. Arnold: London.

Department of Health (2000) *National Service Framework for Coronary Heart Disease.* DH: London.

Department of Health (2005) *Improving Diabetes Services - The NSF Two Years On.* DH: London.

Department of Health (2006) *Turning the Corner: Improving Diabetes Care.* DH: London.

Devarajan, P. (2006) *Oliguria.* http://www.emedicine.com/ped/topic1637.htm (accessed 14/07/07).

Dougherty, L. & Lister, S. (2004) *The Royal Marsden NHS Trust Manual of Clinical Nursing Procedures*, 6th edn. Blackwell Science: Oxford.

Evans, C. & Tippins, E. (2007) *The Foundations of Emergency Care.* Open University Press: Maidenhead.

Feest, T.G., Rounf, A. & Hamad, S. (1993) Incidence of severe acute renal failure in adults: results of a community based study. *British Medical Journal* 306(20): 481–3.

Leslie, S.W. (2006) *Nephrolithiasis: Acute Renal Colic.* http://www.emedicine.com/med/topic3437.htm (accessed 14/07/07).

Malvinder, P.S. (2004) Kidney stones. *British Medical Journal* 328: 1420–4.

Naish, W. & Hallam, M. (2007) Urinary tract infection: diagnosis and management for nurses. *Nursing Standard* 21(23): 50–7.

National Institute for Health and Clinical Excellence (2004) *Type 1 Diabetes: Diagnosis and Management of Type 1 Diabetes in Children, Young People and Adults.* NICE: London.

National Institute of Diabetes and Digestive and Kidney Diseases (NIDDKD) (2005) *Urinary Tract Infection in Adults.* United States Department of Health Services. National Institute of Health: Bethesda, MD.

Parmar, M.S. (2002) Chronic renal disease. *British Medical Journal* 325: 85–90.

Prodigy (2007) *Guidance – Renal Colic, Acute.* http://cks.liberty.nhs.uk/renal_colic_acute/view_whole_guidance (accessed 3 July 2007).

Redmond, A., McDevitt, M. & Barnes, S. (2004) Acute renal failure: recognition and treatment in ward patients. *Nursing Standard* 18(22): 46–53.

Resuscitation Council (UK) (2006) *Advanced Life Support*, 5th edn. RCUK: London.

Saladin, K. (2005) *Human Anatomy*, international edn. McGraw-Hill: London.

Scottish Intercollegiate Guidelines Network (SIGN) (2006) *Management of Suspected Bacterial Urinary Tract Infection in Adults: A National Clinical Guideline.* SIGN: Edinburgh.

Sinert, R. & Peacock, P. (2006) *Renal Failure, Acute.* http://www.emedicine.com/emerg/topic500.htm (accessed 24 May 20).

Verrelli, M. (2006) *Chronic Renal Failure.* http://www.emedicine.com/med/topic374.htm (accessed 14 July 2007).

Waugh, A. & Grant, A. (2007) *Ross and Wilson's Anatomy and Physiology in Health and Illness*, 10th edn. Churchill Livingstone: London.

The gastrointestinal system

Paul Newcombe

7

Chapter 7 Learning Objectives

- Describe essential anatomy and physiology of the digestive system
- Identify relevant anatomical landmarks and surface anatomy
- Demonstrate knowledge of common diseases and conditions which affect the digestive system
- Apply theory to practice by exploring the physical manifestation of these conditions
- Develop a thorough approach to patient assessment in relation to the digestive system
- Describe common therapies utilised in the prevention and treatment of disorders of the digestive system
- Demonstrate the ability to explore and critique the underpinning evidence-base for planned care

Applying Theory to Practice: Exercise 7.1

Before reading on:

- Compile a list of conditions which affect the digestive system.
- Add this list to your portfolio, updating it as you continue through this chapter with consideration to how these conditions affect day-to-day functioning, and the role of the nurse in their assessment and management.

Introduction

A healthy digestive system is fundamental to supporting human life. Its ability to extract nutrients from the food we eat affects our general well-being in health and our response to illness in ill-health. Disorders of the digestive system range from mild and self-limiting to severe and life-threatening, but affect everyone to some extent and at some point during their life. This chapter provides a general overview of the digestive system, and then explores its components in greater detail. Common conditions are examined through patient scenarios.

Nurses are intrinsically involved with many aspects of the digestive system during patient care, thus the NHS Modernisation Agency's (NHSMA 2003) *Essence of Care* benchmarking guidance is applied to patient scenarios where relevant. Other key nursing roles discussed in this chapter include intravenous fluid and electrolyte management.

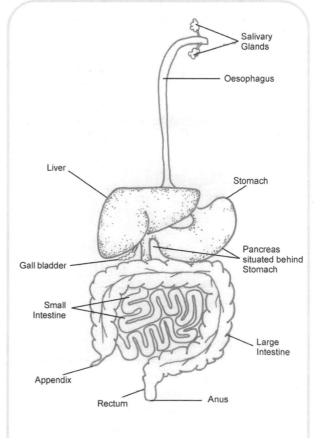

Figure 7.1 The digestive system

Overview of the digestive system

The digestive system is divided into two areas: the gastrointestinal (GI) tract (gut) and the accessory digestive organs. The GI tract is a 4.5m continuous tube (lumen) from the mouth to the anus. Between these ends it is divided into the pharynx, oesophagus, stomach, small intestine and large intestine. The walls of the GI tract have four layers: mucosa, submucosa, muscularis externa and serosa. The accessory digestive organs are exocrine glands and include the salivary glands, liver and pancreas.

The majority of the digestive system is contained within the abdominal cavity by the **peritoneum**, which has two layers. The visceral peritoneum covers the abdominal organs and is continuous with the parietal peritoneum, which lines the abdominal wall. Between these layers is a potential space called the peritoneal cavity containing serous fluid, which lubricates the organs. Some organs, such as the **pancreas**, are located behind the peritoneal cavity in the **retroperitoneum**. The peritoneum is connected by the mesentery, which secures the abdominal organs in place, provides a route for blood vessels and stores fat.

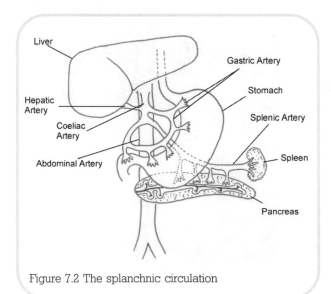

Figure 7.2 The splanchnic circulation

The digestive system is supplied by the splanchnic circulation (Figure 7.2), this conveys oxygen and nutrient-rich blood to the digestive organs allowing them to carry out their functions. However, as most of the nutrients are absorbed into the circulation via the digestive system, these blood vessels are also arranged to collect and process them effectively. The liver only receives 20% of its blood supply from the hepatic artery. The remainder

comes from the hepatic portal vein, which brings nutrient-rich blood from the gut for processing in the liver before it returns to the systemic circulation.

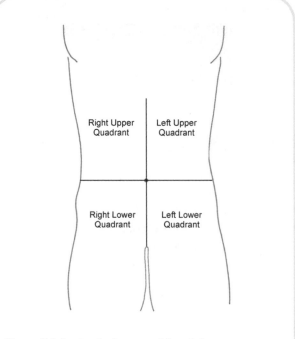

Figure 7.3 Anatomical areas of the abdomen

Anatomy and Physiology in Action: Exercise 7.2

Abdominal Surface Anatomy

- Compare Figure 7.1 with Figure 7.3 and identify which structures appear in which segment or quadrant. If possible, compare both with the abdomen of a willing companion or patient.
- Why do you think it is difficult to feel the liver?
- What happens to the abdominal contents on inspiration and expiration?

Mouth, oesophagus and stomach

Form

The mouth, or oral cavity, is usually where the digestive process begins. Some drugs are absorbed here, such as GTN, but little else. The condition of the oral cavity often reflects the health of an individual and is useful in assessment, for example, dehydration and ulceration. The mouth has several components used during digestion:

Anatomy and Physiology in Action: Box 7.1

Main Functions of the Digestive System

Ingestion – food and drink being taken into the GI tract via the mouth

Propulsion – swallowing and peristalsis

Digestion:

- Mechanical – mastication (chewing) in the mouth, churning in the stomach and mixing during peristalsis
- Chemical – breaking down of food into components suitable for absorption

Secretion – release of digestive juices for lubrication and digestion

Absorption – final components of digestion are transported across the membrane of the GI tract into the circulation

Elimination – passing of undigested material, bacteria and excreted substances as faeces, also known as defecation

- The human adult usually has 32 permanent teeth, made up of incisors and canines for cutting and tearing food, and premolars and molars for crushing and grinding food. Missing teeth can be replaced, but too few teeth or poor dental health can affect the ability to consume food.
- The tongue is a mobile, muscular structure that can change shape and position and has an important role in both eating and communication. Its dorsal surface is covered in projections of mucosa called papillae, which provide structure, texture, colour and also contain taste buds.
- There are three pairs of salivary glands: parotid, sub-mandibular and sublingual. There are also some smaller buccal glands around the oral cavity. Serous and mucous cells produce saliva, which is largely water, but also contains salivary amylase, electrolytes, protective proteins and metabolic waste.

Continuous with the back of the mouth is the muscular pharynx. This is subdivided into the nasopharynx (not involved in digestion), the oropharynx and the laryngo-pharynx. The pharynx also contains the epiglottis, which covers the trachea during swallowing. The oesophagus

Developing and Delivering Expert Care: Exercise 7.3

Oral Hygiene

There are many occasions when patients are not able to maintain their own oral hygiene. *Essence of Care* (NHSMA 2003) sets benchmarks for providing and monitoring standards of personal care, including oral hygiene:

- Individualised assessment (using a validated tool)
- Care planning, negotiated with client and/or carer
- Provision and evaluation of evidence-based mouth care.

For details of evidence-based mouth care, download guidelines from the British Society for Disability and Oral Health at: http://www.bsdh.org.uk/guidelines.html

joins the pharynx to the stomach via the thoracic cavity. It connects to the stomach at the cardiac sphincter which is surrounded by the diaphragm. Mucus is secreted by oesophageal glands for lubrication.

The **stomach** (Figure 7.4) is an expandable storage sac between the **oesophagus** and the **duodenum**. It is located below the diaphragm, in the left upper quadrant/epigastrium. There are three layers of muscle that contract to mix food and facilitate distension for storage. When the stomach is empty, the mucosal lining is folded into **rugae**. This lining is covered with a protective, tight layer of epithelial cells which produce mucus and alkaline fluid to prevent damage by stomach acid. Gastric juice is secreted by exocrine gastric glands which lie in deep gastric pits. The cellular composition of the gastric glands and the type of secretions differ between locations in the stomach:

- Parietal cells secrete hydrochloric acid (HCl) and intrinsic factor (facilitates absorption of vitamin B_{12} – essential for RBC production)
- Chief (or peptic) cells secrete pepsinogen – the inactive form of pepsin
- G cells secrete gastrin
- Enteroendocrine cells secrete chemical mediators, such as histamine which stimulates secretion of HCl.

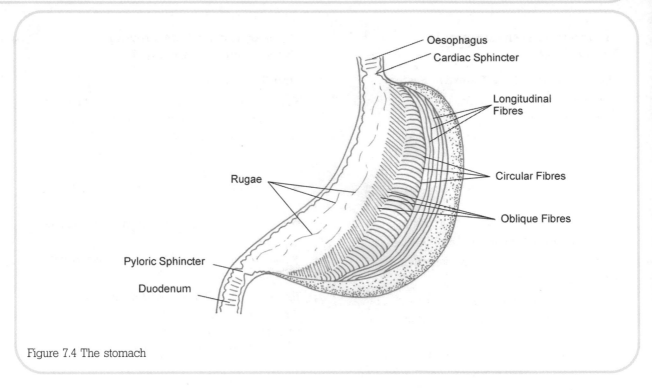

Figure 7.4 The stomach

Function

When food enters the mouth, salivation increases to hydrate and lubricate the food with mucus. Mechanical digestion commences with mastication which is partly voluntary and partly reflexive. The tongue forces food against the hard palate and mixes it with saliva, softening it and forming a **bolus**. Chemical digestion begins with the breakdown of starch by salivary amylase into smaller glucose molecules.

Once in the stomach, the food bolus is subjected to further mechanical digestion by muscular contractions which churn the bolus, breaking it up and mixing it with gastric juices to form a liquid called **chyme**. Chemical digestion is largely restricted to the initiation of protein

Anatomy and Physiology in Action: Exercise 7.4

Swallowing (Deglutition)

Three phases:

- Voluntary phase – initiated by the tongue which pushes the food bolus posteriorly into the pharynx.
- Pharyngeal phase – involuntary and commences with the activation of pressure receptors in the pharynx by the bolus. Respiration is paused and alternative routes are closed: the soft palate rises to seal the nasopharynx and the epiglottis and glottis seal the trachea. The upper oesophageal sphincter opens to allow the bolus into the oesophagus and closes again.
- Oesophageal phase – involves a peristaltic wave of contracting circular muscle. Gravity is helpful but this process also works upside down. As the peristaltic wave reaches the end of the oesophagus, the cardiac sphincter opens to allow the bolus into the stomach and then closes again, preventing regurgitation.

Dysphagia is the name for difficulty in swallowing and is common.

- What are the causes of dysphagia?
- What are the issues for a dysphagic patient?

digestion. The main substances absorbed in the stomach are aspirin and alcohol (both of which are gastric irritants).

Stomach acid denatures dietary protein to facilitate enzyme activity. HCl acid also activates the transformation of pepsinogen into pepsin. This enzyme, which works best in the acidic environment, hydrolyses (splits) denatured protein into polypeptides (shorter amino acid chains). These will undergo further digestion in the small intestine. In infants, renin is also secreted in the stomach to digest milk protein.

Gastric secretion and motility are controlled by nerves and hormones, such as gastrin and has three phases:

- The cephalic phase is initiated by the thought, sight, taste or smell of food.
- The gastric phase lasts three to four hours and commences when food enters the stomach.
- The intestinal phase begins when chyme leaves the stomach and enters the duodenum. Peristaltic contractions in the pylorus expel chyme through the normally relaxed pyloric sphincter and then close it.

Anatomy and Physiology in Action: Box 7.2

Vomiting

Vomiting, or emesis, is a reflex mechanism which protects the digestive system from toxins. Vomiting is controlled by the vomiting, or emetic, centre in the brain, and is precipitated by many peripheral and central causes, including:

- Over-distension of the stomach or intestine
- Irritation of the GI tract by drugs, chemicals, bacteria, blood, etc.
- Stimulation of the gag reflex
- Motion sickness
- Severe headaches and rising intracranial pressure
- Stimulation of the vomiting centre by drugs such as opiates and cytotoxics
- Electrolyte disturbances
- Particular sights, smells or emotions
- Painful stimulation of visceral organs such as the heart, bladder and testicles
- Increased hormone levels such as oestrogen in pregnancy
- Circulatory collapse.

Vomiting is usually preceded and accompanied by a feeling of nausea, pallor, salivation, sweating, increased heart rate and a fall in blood pressure. Just prior to vomiting deep inspiration occurs, the glottis closes to protect the trachea and the soft palate is elevated to close the nasopharynx. The diaphragm and abdominal muscles contract, the cardiac sphincter relaxes and the stomach contents are forced up through the upper oesophageal sphincter and out through the mouth. Contractions of the duodenum causes the vomiting of bile.

Developing and Delivering Expert Care: Box 7.3

Nausea and Vomiting

Caring for a patient who is experiencing nausea and vomiting is common. Excessive vomiting results in dehydration and electrolyte disturbances. There are many therapies used in the management of nausea and vomiting, and the appropriate treatment will depend on the exact cause. The NHS National Library for Health produces guidance for the management of nausea and vomiting in pregnancy (Prodigy 2007a) and palliative care (Prodigy 2007b). Commonly used drugs include:

- Cyclizine
- Metoclopramide
- Domperidone
- Prochlorperazine
- Ondansetron (JFC 2007).

Scenario 7.1

Gastrointestinal Bleeding

Steven Jenkins is a 33-year-old man who is rushed to hospital after an episode of haematemesis.

On arrival, an initial assessment shows:

Airway – clear, complaining of epigastric pain
Breathing – RR 28/min, pulse oximetry 97% on air
Circulation – radial pulse 124/min, regular but weak and thready, CRT 3 seconds, BP 92/65, pale and clammy
Disability – alert
Exposure – skin cool
PMH – takes non-steroidal anti-inflammatory drugs (NSAIDs) for an old knee injury. 15-year smoking history. Drinks 25 units of alcohol a week.

Haematemesis	Vomiting blood associated with an upper GI bleed. Fresh blood is bright red and old brown blood is termed 'coffee grounds' (not to be confused with haemoptysis which describes the coughing-up of blood).
Melaena	Black, tarry stool due to digested blood and usually associated with an upper GI bleed.
Haematochezia	Fresh blood passed per rectum usually associated with lower GI bleeding.

Table 7.1 GI Bleeding Terminology

Assessment and analysis of patient presentation

Mr Jenkins has presented with an upper GI bleed, a common medical emergency. He is displaying signs of hypovolaemic shock such as tachypnoea, tachycardia and hypotension. It is important to determine the cause of bleeding following initial resuscitation as management differs for particular causes, such as oesophageal varices (discussed later).

Pathophysiology

Peptic ulcer disease (PUD) is the commonest cause of GI bleeding and Mr Jenkins has many risk factors. Peptic ulcers occur in the stomach, but more frequently in the duodenum. Gastric (stomach) ulcers (GU) form when acid and pepsin erode the lining of the stomach where the protective mucosa is already damaged (due to NSAIDs, for example). Duodenal ulcers (DU) occur due to abnormally high levels of acid and pepsinogen in chyme leaving the

Applying Theory to Practice: Box 7.4

Causes of Acute Upper GI Bleeding (adapted from BSGEC 2002)

Diagnosis	Approx. %
Peptic ulcer	35–50
Gastroduodenal erosions	8–15
Oesophagitis	5–15
Varices	5–10

- What risk factors are associated with peptic ulcer disease?

stomach. If damage is severe enough or involves a blood vessel, GI bleeding occurs.

PUD is also the second commonest cause of dyspepsia, which patients describe as indigestion, reflux or heartburn. Dyspepsia is an imprecise term which encompasses epigastric or retrosternal pain, with or without other GI symptoms, and has a prevalence of about 40% in the UK. Dyspepsia is most often caused by the reflux of stomach acid into the oesophagus due to an incompetent cardiac sphincter or hiatus hernia which causes burning (Logan & Delaney 2002). Dyspeptic symptoms can be misleading as cardiac pain may be described as indigestion.

The plan of care

The priority for Mr Jenkins's care is immediate resuscitation in an appropriate environment. Mr Jenkins is currently alert and maintaining his own airway, but the risk of a decreasing level of consciousness and subsequent aspiration is high. Airway equipment should, therefore, be close at hand, particularly suction, and there should be a low threshold for calling an anaesthetist. High concentration oxygen should be applied via a reservoir bag mask at 10–15 L/min. A minimum of two large-bore cannulae should be sited in the antecubital fossae and fluid resuscitation commenced. Blood samples should be taken for full blood count (FBC), urea and electrolytes (U&E), liver function tests (LFT), clotting and a cross-match. Continuous cardiac and pulse oximetry monitoring should be implemented. Additionally more invasive monitoring may be necessary, such as urinary and central venous catheters.

Investigation and treatment

As Mr Jenkins has experienced a severe GI bleed he should be transferred urgently for an endoscopy once stable. An endoscope is a fibre-optic camera which is passed into the upper GI tract via the mouth, usually under sedation. This allows the clinician to directly visualise the GI tract, identify the source of bleeding and make a diagnosis. If the ulcer is still bleeding or at high risk of re-bleeding, then endoscopic therapy can be administered. This may include:

- Injection with epinephrine (adrenaline)
- Thermal haemostasis
- Mechanical clips.

In the minority of cases where one or more of these therapies are unsuccessful, surgical repair is indicated (BSGEC 2002). Following appropriate drug therapy patients with a gastric ulcer usually have a follow-up endoscopy after 6–8 weeks (NICE 2004).

Applying Theory to Practice: Box 7.5

Helicobacter pylori infection

Helicobacter pylori is a bacterium commonly found in the human stomach. Most infected people are asymptomatic, but *H pylori* is acknowledged to be the principal cause of PUD and gastric cancer.

- *H pylori* colonisation causes inflammation and damage to the mucosa and also increases acid production.
- *H pylori* is diagnosed invasively, or via non-invasive investigations such as a breath, stool or blood tests.
- The decision to test for and/or treat *H pylori* is made by following protocols for the management of GI bleeding (BSGEC 2002) and dyspepsia (NICE 2004).
- Eradication usually includes a course of a proton-pump inhibitor, such as omeprazole, and two antibiotics, such as clarithromycin and amoxicillin or metronidazole – 'triple therapy'.

Developing and Delivering Expert Care: Box 7.6

Fluid Resuscitation

Intravenous fluid therapy is targeted at replacing intravascular (IV) and/or extracellular (EC) fluid volume deficits (Chapter 2). An intravascular fluid volume (IVFV) deficit usually occurs as the result of blood loss, whereas extracellular fluid volume (ECFV) deficits are associated with other forms of fluid loss, such as dehydration. There are two main types of IV fluid available: crystalloids and colloids. Theoretically, IVFV losses should be replaced with colloids and ECFV losses should be replaced with crystalloids (Zander 2006). However, there is great debate about the use and efficacy of each fluid type, and a meta-analysis of studies in this area concluded that colloids had no advantage over crystalloids (Roberts et al. 2004). Crystalloids are cheaper than colloids and as a result they are used far more frequently for all fluid losses (Table 7.2).

The best fluid for the replacement of blood loss is blood itself. This is the only fluid which contains the oxygen-carrying component – haemoglobin. However, as blood transfusion is expensive, time-consuming and has many inherent risks, the decision to transfuse is made by experienced clinicians (Chapter 4).

Electrolyte replacement is also usually considered alongside fluid replacement, particularly with crystalloids (Table 7.2).

	Crystalloid	**Colloid**
Composition	Water and small molecules such as electrolytes and glucose	Water and large molecules such as starch (+/- electrolytes)
Movement	Diffuse freely from IV to EC spaces (some also reach intracellular space)	Starch molecules exert oncotic force which retains fluid in IV space
Destination	EC space primarily, IV space eventually: total body hydration	Remain in IV space mainly
Volume	At least three times as much as estimated blood loss	Small volumes equivalent to estimated blood loss
Timing	Slower to give due to large volumes and slower to see change in vital signs	Quick to give due to small volumes and usually swift acting
Tonicity & Types	Mostly isotonic, e.g. 'normal' saline (0.9% sodium chloride), Hartmann's solution, 5% dextrose Hypertonic and hypotonic solutions are determined by sodium/glucose content and used for particular indications	Mostly isotonic. Examples include gelatins (Gelofusine®, Haemaccel®), starches (hetastarch, Voluven®), albumin and dextrans. Colloids are also called 'plasma expanders'
Risks	Pulmonary oedema, haemodilution and hypothermia (unless warmed)	Anaphylaxis
Cost	Cheap (and long shelf-life)	More expensive
Usage	Very common	Less common

Table 7.2 Crystalloids versus colloids

Electrolyte & range	Location & function	Altered levels	Common causes	Signs & symptoms	Treatment
Sodium (Na$^+$) 135-145 mmol/L	Main extracellular cation. Osmotic properties govern fluid distribution and movement	Hyponatraemia (low sodium)	Sweating, vomiting, diarrhoea, water retention	Cerebral oedema – confusion, headaches, coma	Isotonic/hypertonic saline depending on cause & severity
		Hypernatraemia (high sodium)	Dehydration, salt overdose	Thirst, irritability, convulsions, coma	5% dextrose or fluid restriction
Potassium (K$^+$) 3.5-5.5 mmol/L	Main intracellular cation. Important role in neuromuscular function, especially cardiac muscle	Hypokalaemia (low potassium)	Increased diuresis, diarrhoea, vomiting	Arrhythmias, confusion, vomiting	Oral or IV replacement
		Hyperkalaemia (high potassium)	Renal failure, K$^+$ overdose, acidosis, trauma, burns	Arrhythmias, ECG changes, cardiac arrest, tingling	IV calcium, insulin & glucose infusion, haemodialysis
Magnesium (Mg^{2+}) 0.7-1.0 mmol/L	Abundant in bone. Involved in cellular energy production, neuromuscular and enzyme function	Hypomagnesaemia (low magnesium)	Malabsorption, renal losses, alcoholism, diarrhoea, vomiting	Arrhythmias, ECG changes, twitching, tremor, convulsions	IV replacement
		Hypermagnesaemia (high magnesium)	Renal failure, antacid overdose	Arrhythmias, coma, cardiac arrest	IV calcium, haemodialysis
Calcium (Ca^{2+}) 2.1-2.6 mmol/L (total)	99% in bone. Roles in neuromuscular function, clotting, and hormone secretion	Hypocalcaemia (low calcium)	Renal failure, hypoparathyroidism	Tetany, convulsions, irritability, fractures	Oral or IV replacement
		Hypercalcaemia (high calcium)	Renal failure, hyperparathyroidism	Weakness, confusion, nausea and vomiting	Restrict intake, haemodialysis
Phosphate (HPO$_4^{2-}$) 0.7-1.4 mmol/L	Abundant in bone. Inverse relationship with calcium. Vital for cellular energy and metabolism	Hypophosphataemia (low phosphate)	Malabsorption, hyperparathyroidism, refeeding syndrome	Weakness, confusion, nausea and vomiting, organ failure	Oral or IV phosphate with caution. Start feeds slowly
		Hyperphosphataemia (high phosphate)	Renal failure, hypoparathyroidism	Tetany, convulsions, irritability	Treat the cause, haemodialysis
Chloride (Cl$^-$) 95-105 mmol/L	Main extracellular anion. Works with sodium to govern fluid distribution. Role in acid-base balance	Hypochloraemia (low chloride)	Dehydration, GI loss, metabolic alkalosis	Symptoms associated with fluid loss	IV fluid replacement
		Hyperchloraemia (high chloride)	Sodium chloride over-dose, renal failure, metabolic acidosis	Weakness, Kussmaul respiration	Treat the cause

Table 7.3 Management of electrolytes (adapted from Moore, 2004)

Developing and Delivering Expert Care: Box 7.7

Drug Therapy for PUD/Dyspepsia (JFC 2007)

Antacids and alginates (Maalox®, Gaviscon®)

Antisecretory drugs

- Histamine H$_2$ receptor antagonists (ranitidine, cimetidine)
- Proton pump inhibitors (PPI) (lansoprazole, omeprazole)

H pylori eradication therapy

Psychosocial aspects

Mr Jenkins will need to be given lifestyle advice prior to discharge. This should include discontinuation of NSAIDs with suggestions for an alternative analgesic; education on the warning signs of another episode (dyspeptic symptoms) and appropriate action (contact GP); smoking cessation; reducing alcohol intake; weight reduction and healthy eating; and stepwise reduction of his prescribed medication.

Liver, gall bladder and pancreas

Form

The liver (Figure 7.5) is the largest gland in the body and occupies the right upper quadrant. It is divided into the left and right lobes and is composed of hexagonal units called lobules. Each lobule contains a central vein, which drains into the vena cava. Columns of hepatocytes (liver cells) and sinusoids (channels for mixed hepatic arterial and portal venous blood) radiate out from the centre. Between the hepatocytes run tiny bile canaliculi, which

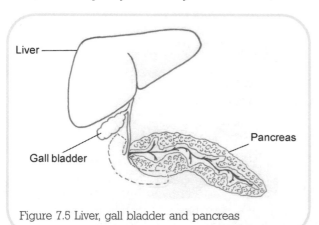

Figure 7.5 Liver, gall bladder and pancreas

drain into bile ducts. At each corner of the lobule is a portal triad – a bile duct, a branch of the hepatic artery and a branch of the hepatic portal vein. The bile ducts converge to form the common hepatic duct.

The gall bladder is a pear-shaped sac, which lies on the posterior surface of the liver and protrudes below the right lobe. The gall bladder neck opens into the cystic duct, which combines with the common hepatic duct to form the common bile duct. This is joined by the main pancreatic duct before it joins the duodenum at the sphincter of Oddi.

The pancreas is located in the epigastrium/left upper quadrant and has both exocrine and endocrine functions. The exocrine tissue is composed of acinar cells, which produce the enzymatic component of pancreatic juice. These cells drain into pancreatic ducts which converge to form the main pancreatic duct. The endocrine cells, called Islets of Langerhans, are scattered among the acinar cells and secrete insulin and glucagon (Chapter 10).

Function

The liver is one of the most important organs in the body and has the unique ability to completely regenerate itself following removal of up to 75% of its size. It has numerous functions, many of which are associated with its vital role in processing nutrient-rich blood from the GI tract. Its main digestive function, however, is the production of 1 litre of yellow/green **bile** every day. Bile contains electrolytes, bile salts, cholesterol, phospholipids, toxic waste products and bile pigments, such as bilirubin. It is an alkaline solution, which allows bile to neutralise stomach acid entering the duodenum.

Bile salts are the most important digestive component of bile. In the small intestine they emulsify (break up) fats to provide small molecules for enzymatic action, and facilitate absorption. Bile salts are reabsorbed by the small intestine and recycled by the liver. They are also the main stimulus for bile secretion.

Bilirubin is a waste product of haemoglobin recycling performed by the liver. It is metabolised in the small intestine by bacteria to form stercobilinogen, which gives faeces its brown colour. Absence of bile produces pale, fatty stools which are difficult to flush – **steatorrhoea**. Failure to excrete bilirubin causes a build-up in the blood and subsequent **jaundice**.

The gall bladder stores excess bile produced by the liver and concentrates it by removing excess water and electrolytes. The release of bile is stimulated by the arrival

Anatomy and Physiology in Action: Box 7.8

Functions of the Liver

- Production and secretion of bile
- Carbohydrate metabolism:
 - Converts monosaccarides to glucose
 - **Glycogenesis** – converts glucose to glycogen for storage
 - **Glycogenolysis** – converts glycogen back to glucose for release into blood following secretion of glucagon by the pancreas
 - **Gluconeogenesis** – manufactures new glucose from amino acids and glycerol when blood levels are low and glycogen stores are exhausted
 - **Lipogenesis** – converts excess glucose to fat for storage
- Fat metabolism:
 - Synthesis of fats (lipoproteins) for transport, storage and secretion
 - Breakdown of fatty acids to ketone bodies
- Protein metabolism:
 - Deamination of amino acids for conversion to glucose or ATP
 - Production of urea for the removal of ammonia from the body
 - Production of plasma proteins (albumin, clotting factors)
- Storage of vitamins (A, D, E, K, B_{12}), iron, glycogen, protein and fat
- Recycling of **erythrocytes**
- Detoxification of alcohol, drugs, hormones and chemicals for excretion
- Contributes to immunity by cleaning portal blood of antigens
- Body heat production

of acidic, fatty chyme entering the duodenum. This causes the muscular gall bladder to contract, the secretion of pancreatic juice and the relaxation of the sphincter of Oddi. As a result, bile and pancreatic juice enter the duodenum.

The pancreas produces up to 1.5L of pancreatic juice per day. Like bile, it is an alkaline solution, which helps neutralise acidic chyme entering the duodenum, and provides an optimum pH for enzymatic activity. Pancreatic enzymes include amylase, lipase and trypsinogen. Most are secreted in an inactive form and only become activated in the duodenum by a series of reactions.

Applying Theory to Practice: Box 7.9

Gallstones

Gallstones are very common, particularly in women, and the incidence increases with age. They are often composed of cholesterol; hence they are also associated with a high-fat diet. Gallstones cause a range of diseases:

- **Cholecystitis** (inflammation of the gall bladder) occurs when stones block the outflow of bile. The bile becomes concentrated and infected leading to a swollen and oedematous gall bladder. The patient presents with severe right upper quadrant pain, fever and occasionally jaundice. Cholecystitis can be acute or chronic and is treated by surgical removal of the gall bladder – **cholecystectomy**.
- **Pancreatitis** occurs when pancreatic enzymes become prematurely activated. Autodigestion of pancreatic tissue causes local inflammation and oedema. The activated enzymes leak into the systemic circulation causing fluid shifts, hypovolaemia and damage to other organs. The patient presents with severe epigastric pain radiating to the back and shock. Treatment is mainly supportive, but may include surgery. Acute pancreatitis can be mild and self-limiting or severe and life-threatening. There are many causes, but gallstones are the most common, followed by alcohol. Alcohol is also usually the cause of chronic pancreatitis (UKWPAP 2005).

Applying Theory to Practice: Box 7.10

Liver Function Tests

Liver functions tests (LFT) are performed to detect liver damage. The profile combines markers of function with markers of damage (liver enzymes):

- Function
 - Albumin (Alb)
 - Bilirubin (Bili)
- Liver enzymes
 - Alanine transaminase (ALT)
 - Aspartate transaminase (AST)
 - Alkaline phosphatase (ALP)
 - Gamma glutamyl transpeptidase (GGT)

Other blood tests which reflect liver function include:

- Blood glucose level
- Clotting studies

Alcohol – the facts

Millions of people enjoy drinking alcohol in moderation. However, there is an increasing minority who misuse alcohol, causing health problems for themselves and/or contributing to social problems, such as anti-social behaviour. In the UK, alcohol misuse is estimated to be responsible for:

- Costing the British tax-payer £20bn per year
- 22,000 deaths per year
- 70% of A&E admissions at peak times
- Half of all violent incidents
- One-third of all domestic violence.

These issues are attributed to two main patterns of drinking:

- Binge-drinkers – more likely to be men under 25 years old; higher risk of alcohol-related accidents, violent incidents and committing sexual assault
- Chronic drinkers – more likely to be men over the age of 30; higher risk of alcoholic liver disease, cancer, stroke and suicide.

The rate of women misusing alcohol has increased dramatically over the last 10 years, particularly binge-drinking (COSU 2004). There is evidence that moderate alcohol consumption actually has a 'protective effect' against some diseases, particularly coronary heart disease. This is estimated at 1–2 units of alcohol 2–3 times per week. However, this apparent 'protection' is lost with alcohol consumption above this level (Paton 2005).

Pathophysiology

Alcohol (ethanol) is a drug which is absorbed in the stomach and small intestine. The rate of absorption is affected by:

- Concentration of alcohol
- Aeration with carbon dioxide
- Presence of food in the stomach
- Previous exposure to alcohol
- Body size and build
- Gender.

Alcohol is distributed throughout most tissues of the body, but particularly the liver, which eliminates over 90% as water and carbon dioxide (Paton 2005b). Alcohol causes inflammation and cancer of various parts of the GI tract, for example, gastritis and PUD. Excess alcohol consumption puts stress on liver function and at least some damage is inevitable, although the changes produce few symptoms until ALD is advanced. There are three stages of ALD (BLT 2005):

Scenario 7.2 *Alcoholic Liver Disease*

Adrian Price is a 47-year-old man who is admitted for observation after sustaining a head injury while drunk. On assessment in A&E he is unkempt, abusive to staff and refuses examination. He has a superficial graze and haematoma above his right eye, but no other apparent injuries. His GCS is 12/15 overnight (E3 V4 M5).

You are allocated to look after Mr Price next morning. He is now fully orientated (GCS 15/15) and apologetic. His vital signs are: RR 16/min, pulse 110/min, BP 148/90 mmHg, temp. 36.5 °C, BM 5.0 mmol/L. He is sweaty and shaky and complains of a headache and nausea.

On the ward round the doctor takes a thorough history and Mr Price admits to being a heavy drinker for many years. This has been particularly bad over the past few months since he lost his job. On examination he has an enlarged liver, but no ascites or jaundice. Blood tests show some of his LFTs are raised. Mr Price says he wants help to stop drinking.

Developing and Delivering Expert Care: Box 7.11

Head Injury and Alcohol: A Clinical Problem

Of the one million patients who present to A&E with a head injury every year in the UK, alcohol consumption is present in 25% of all cases (Huntley and Touquet 2005). As in the case of Mr Price, these patients are notoriously difficult to assess. Aside from the potential for anti-social behaviour, the effects of alcohol and the symptoms of a head injury are very difficult to distinguish. The golden rule is to never dismiss a patient as being 'just drunk'. Regular, thorough neurological observations are paramount.

Assessment and analysis of patient presentation

Mr Price has presented to secondary care due to a common health risk associated with alcohol use – trauma. He appears to have suffered only a minor head injury although continued neurological observation is prudent. There is some evidence of the sociological effects of alcohol misuse, such as self-neglect and unemployment. Fortunately, Mr Price is honest about his situation and has the desire to begin addressing it. Unfortunately, the effects of alcohol have already started to take their toll and Mr Price is displaying the early stages of alcoholic liver disease (ALD). Mr Price also has some symptoms of alcohol withdrawal, such as shaking and nausea, which need to

be addressed. Hypoglycaemia is common and should be monitored.

- **Fatty liver** – more fat accumulates in the liver than normal. This stage may be detected by palpation of the enlarged liver. Fatty liver is common in excessive drinkers and is completely reversible with abstinence.
- **Alcoholic hepatitis** (inflammation of the liver) occurs in 20–30% of patients with fatty liver who continue to drink, and may be mild, or severe and life-threatening. LFTs are raised and the patient may be jaundiced with right upper quadrant pain and nausea. Mild alcoholic hepatitis resolves with abstinence, but severe cases need intensive care and have a 50% mortality rate from liver failure.
- **Cirrhosis** occurs in about 10% of heavy drinkers. Irreversible fibrosis (scarring) and the development of nodules severely affect liver function. LFTs are abnormal and the hard, irregular liver may be palpable. Symptoms vary but may include:
 - Lethargy
 - Anorexia
 - Nausea and vomiting
 - Weight loss
 - Jaundice
 - Itching
 - Fever and infections
 - Bruising and bleeding
 - Confusion.

Identification of the stage of ALD is confirmed by liver biopsy. One of the most significant sequels of cirrhosis is **portal hypertension** caused by resistance to blood flow

Questioning Clinical Practice: Exercise 7.5

Sensible Drinking?

- Alcohol content – one unit is equal to:
 - Half a pint of beer
 - One glass of wine
 - One measure of spirits
- Recommended daily intake should not exceed:
 - Men – four units
 - Women – three units (including two alcohol-free days a week)

Do you ever exceed these recommended limits?

If the answer is yes, how do you feel about challenging a patient's drinking behaviour? Is this hypocritical?

Developing and Delivering Expert Care: Box 7.12

Detecting Misuse: the CAGE Test (two or more correct):

- Have you ever felt you ought to cut down on your drinking?
- Have people annoyed you by criticising your drinking?
- Have you ever felt bad or guilty about your drinking?
- Have you ever had a drink first thing in the morning to steady your nerves or get rid of a hangover: eye opener?

For a more sensitive test refer to the World Health Organization's (2001) alcohol use disorders identification test (AUDIT).

through the liver due to scarring. Portal hypertension causes three serious complications of ALD:

- **Oesophageal varices** – increased portal pressure causes development of collateral circulation where blood supply bypasses the liver and is shunted mainly to veins of the lower oesophagus and stomach. Because these veins were not intended to carry such large volumes of blood they dilate and become fragile.

These vessels are prone to rupturing with catastrophic consequences and carry a 50% mortality rate. The patient presents with copious haematemesis and melaena. Bleeding is further promoted by altered clotting, which often accompanies severe ALD. Initial resuscitation is the same for any GI bleed, as often the diagnosis is not confirmed until endoscopy. However, the volume of blood, lost will mandate aggressive fluid resuscitation (avoid saline), early transfusion and correction of clotting. Definitive management includes specific pharmacological therapy (e.g. glypressin), banding, sclerotherapy, balloon tamponade and surgery (Jalan & Hayes 2000).

- **Ascites** is an accumulation of fluid in the peritoneal cavity, and is attributed to cirrhosis in 75% of cases. Its presence suggests advanced ALD and is associated with high mortality. Ascites develops due to increased portal pressure, systemic vasodilation, reduced renal blood flow and subsequent sodium retention. Ascites causes tense abdominal distension which is very uncomfortable. Complications include compression of the abdominal organs and blood vessels, and respiratory distress due to diaphragmatic splinting. The cause is determined by history, examination, blood tests and ultrasound scanning. Treatment includes low-salt diet, potassium-sparing diuretics (spironolactone) and abstinence from alcohol. Abdominal paracentesis (ascitic tap) is performed to analyse and remove fluid. Care involves weighing the patient daily, strict fluid balance and monitoring electrolyte levels (Moore & Aithal 2006).

- **Hepatic encephalopathy** is a reversible state of impaired cognitive function due to advanced liver disease. The liver is unable to detoxify the blood because of hepatocyte damage and/or blood bypassing the liver due to portal hypertension. As a result nitrogenous waste, such as ammonia, travels to the brain causing encephalopathy. Symptoms include:
 - Drowsiness
 - Confusion
 - Lack of coordination
 - Hyperactive reflexes
 - Flapping tremor
 - Coma.

In the cirrhotic patient hepatic encephalopathy is precipitated by insults such as severe GI bleeding or infection. If hepatic coma has developed, supportive care

should be provided in an appropriate specialist setting. Treatment is aimed at correcting precipitating factors, cleansing the GI tract of nitrogenous substances with lactulose, and restricting dietary protein (Krige & Beckingham 2001). Other causes need to be excluded through thorough investigation, but once ALD is implicated, early consideration should be given to liver transplantation. This is found to be successful in carefully selected patients, although six months of supervised abstinence is desirable (Devlin & O'Grady 1999).

Questioning Clinical Practice: Exercise 7.6

There is a long waiting list for liver transplants in the UK and many patients die from liver failure while waiting.

How do you feel about alcohol misusers being given the chance of liver transplantation?

Do we have the right to judge their behaviour?

Applying Theory to Practice: Box 7.13

Other Common Causes of Liver Disease
- Viral hepatitis (A, B, C, D or E)
- Drugs, for example, paracetamol overdose
- Trauma
- Cancer
- Abscesses

The plan of care

Mr Price's care will focus on facilitating alcohol detoxification while monitoring for the complications discussed above. Alcohol withdrawal produces symptoms such as agitation like those displayed by Mr Price, but can progress to delirium tremens ('DTs') which can be life-threatening. The mainstay of pharmacological therapy is a reducing dose of benzodiazepines, such as chlordiazepoxide. Monitoring for symptoms such as hallucinations, confusion and particularly seizures is essential, and emergency equipment should be available.

Alcohol misusers are often malnourished as food is replaced by alcohol, which can lead to serious problems.

Vitamin B_1 (thiamine) deficiency is common and results in Wernicke's encephalopathy (WE). Deficiencies should be replaced prophylactically with IV Pabrinex, as the symptoms of WE are difficult to distinguish from either drunkenness or withdrawal. Patients should be discharged with a course or oral vitamin supplements (RCP 2001). Early dietician referral is recommended, especially if any dietary restrictions are necessary.

Psychosocial issues

Mr Price will require support to help him address his problems. Health professionals have been found to have negative attitudes towards patients who misuse alcohol (RCP 2001), limiting the development of an effective nurse–patient relationship. A non-judgemental approach is paramount as is involvement of his significant others. Health promotion is also often dismissed by health professionals as futile for alcohol misusers, but there is evidence that even interventions lasting as little as 10 minutes can be successful in promoting abstinence. It should be emphasised to Mr Price that as he is only in the early stages of ALD, total abstinence could completely reverse the damage thus far. He should be referred to appropriate primary care services and peer support, such as Alcoholics Anonymous (Ritson 2005).

Small intestine

Form

The small intestine is a 6m tube, which extends from the pyloric sphincter of the stomach to the ileocaecal valve of the large intestine, and is divided into three sections:

- Duodenum – 25cm long and containing the sphincter of Oddi where the common bile duct joins the small intestine
- Jejunum – 2.5m long
- Ileum – 3.5m long.

The small intestine provides a massive surface area for absorption due to deep folds in the mucosa and finger-like villi covered in microvilli (Figure 7.6). Each villus contains a lymph capillary called a lacteal and a blood capillary bed. The surface is comprised of absorptive epithelial cells whose membranes contain microvilli – the brush border. These bear the digestive brush border enzymes. The mucosa also contains goblet cells, which secrete mucus, endocrine cells, and lymph nodes called Peyer's patches.

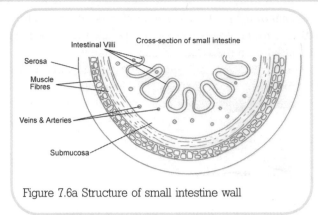

Figure 7.6a Structure of small intestine wall

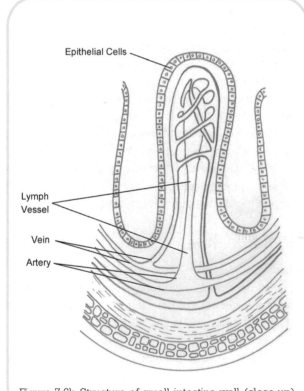

Figure 7.6b Structure of small intestine wall (close-up)

Between 1–2L of intestinal juice is secreted from Paneth cells in the crypts of Lieberkühn between the villi. This is a watery, alkaline solution containing mucus, electrolytes and antibacterial enzymes.

Function

The small intestine is the main location for digestion and absorption. The arrival of acidic chyme in the duodenum stimulates the secretion of bile, pancreatic and intestinal

juice. Rhythmic peristaltic contractions (segmentation) mix the contents and move it towards the ileocaecal valve. Chyme takes 3–6 hours to pass through the small intestine. Once each food group has been broken down into small enough molecules, they are absorbed through the small intestine lining by diffusion, passive or active transport into either the blood or lymph capillaries. Chemical digestion, absorption, utilisation and sources of each food group are summarised below:

- **Carbohydrate** digestion, started in the mouth by salivary amylase, is completed in the small intestine by pancreatic amylase and brush border enzymes. The resulting monosaccharides pass into blood capillaries via active transport and facilitated diffusion. The primary use of carbohydrates (glucose) is cellular energy production. Carbohydrates mainly come from plants, for example, fruit, vegetables, grains, sugar cane, honey and also milk. Indigestible plant carbohydrates (cellulose) provide fibre and facilitate formation of faeces.

- **Protein** digestion, started in the stomach by pepsin, is completed by proteolytic enzymes in pancreatic juice and the brush border. Resulting amino acids enter blood capillaries by active transport and diffusion. Proteins are essential for making structural tissues, such as connective tissue and muscle, and also enzymes and hormones. Excess amino acids are used for energy production. Dietary proteins come from meat, dairy products, legumes, nuts and cereals. The small intestine also digests a significant amount of secreted enzyme proteins and sloughed mucosal cells from the GI tract lining.

- **Lipids** (fats) are emulsified by bile salts in the small intestine. Resulting triglyceride molecules are broken down by pancreatic lipase into fatty acids and monoglycerides. These associate with bile salts and phospholipids to form micelles which diffuse into the mucosal epithelial cells, and are then transported into lacteals as chylomicrons. Fat is eventually transferred from the lymph to the blood stream away from the gut. It is used for cellular energy or stored as adipose tissue. Saturated fats and cholesterol come from meat and dairy products, unsaturated fats come from seeds, nuts, olive and vegetable oils. Excess intake of certain fats causes obesity and heart disease.

Applying Theory to Practice: Exercise 7.7

A Healthy Diet

The UK government regularly publishes recommendations on lifestyle choices such as healthy eating. Visit the Department of Health website (www.dh.gov.uk) and download the latest guidelines.

The small intestine is also the site for vitamin and electrolyte absorption. Fat-soluble vitamins (A, E, D and K) are transported in micelles, and water-soluble vitamins (B and C) are absorbed by diffusion, active or passive transport. Vitamins are mainly ingested in food and are essential coenzymes for utilising the main food groups. Electrolytes are absorbed along the length of the small intestine via a variety of mechanisms. They come from ingested food and GI secretions; their functions are summarised in Table 7.3. Finally, the majority of water absorption also takes place in the small intestine. Nine litres of water, predominantly as GI secretions, enters the small intestine each day. Water mainly follows sodium absorption via **osmosis**.

Scenario 7.3

Malnutrition

Ethel Higgins is a 78-year-old retired cleaner who has been readmitted by her GP for non-specific symptoms of weakness, lethargy and depression. She was discharged a month ago following a fall at home which resulted in a fractured neck of femur. She is still only able to walk short distances around her house with a Zimmer frame. Mrs Higgins lives alone, has no family, close friends or home help. On assessment Mrs Higgins is awake but withdrawn and her vital signs are within normal limits for her age. She reports no past medical history and is not taking any medication. While helping her undress you notice that she is very thin and the surgical wound on her hip is not fully healed.

Assessment and analysis of patient presentation

Mrs Higgins received seemingly appropriate treatment for her previous presenting complaint – repair of a hip fracture, but her subsequent fundamental needs have been neglected. On discharge Mrs Higgins has been unable to mobilise enough to acquire or prepare her food and as a result has become malnourished. Evidence is found in her low energy levels, underweight appearance and delayed wound healing. This is an example of where malnutrition is both a cause and consequence of ill-health.

Malnutrition – the facts

Malnutrition is a global problem affecting one in three people worldwide (BAPEN 2003). While it is often predominately associated with developing countries, it is still relatively common in the UK. Approximately 5% of the British population are considered underweight. However, the proportions are much higher in the elderly, those with chronic diseases, those in care homes, those admitted to or discharged from hospital, and the poor or socially isolated (BAPEN 2003). Malnourished patients present a significant strain on health services, with longer hospital stays and approximately 50% greater costs (Stroud et al. 2003). The consequences of malnutrition include:

- Poor immunity
- Delayed wound healing and response to illness
- Reduced muscle strength and fatigue
- Impaired respiratory and cardiovascular function
- Increased risk of hypothermia
- Apathy and depression (Lennard-Jones 1992).

Applying Theory to Practice: Exercise 7.8

Malnutrition

The causes of malnutrition in the community and hospital are complex and multi-faceted. Compile a list of barriers to gaining adequate nutrition, considering physical, mental, socio-economic and service-related issues.

- What kinds of assistance are there within the community for individuals who require assistance with some of the activities of living?
- Who funds these services?

Pathophysiology

Malnutrition (or under-nutrition) occurs when the body's energy intake is less than the energy expenditure. During the processing of a meal, the body is in the absorptive state. Blood levels of nutrients such as glucose and lipids are high, and a proportion is delivered to body tissues for immediate metabolic needs. The rest is stored in the liver and muscles (as glycogen) and adipose tissue (fat). Between meals the body changes over to the post-absorptive state. Glucose levels are maintained by glycogenolysis and gluconeogenesis, and cells begin to utilise other sources of energy, such as fatty acids. As a result, in prolonged under-nutrition the body's stores of fat and muscle become slowly depleted (Smith and Morton 2001). Additionally, the reduced consumption of protein and micronutrients, such as vitamins and minerals, impair cell replication and the production of immune molecules (Strobel and Ferguson 2005).

The plan of care

Mrs Higgins's care will focus upon excluding other causes for her symptoms through history and examination. This should include blood tests to assess for electrolyte disturbances, and anaemia, etc. The extent of malnutrition should be measured objectively by nutritional assessment using a validated tool. She will then require appropriate nutritional support under the guidance of a dietician. Of paramount importance is the assessment of Mrs Higgins's social situation and the introduction of appropriate services to ensure the situation doesn't recur on discharge.

Nutritional assessment

All patients should be screened for malnutrition by an appropriately trained healthcare professional. This should occur on admission to hospital or a care home, on initial registration with a GP, on a first outpatient appointment or when there is clinical concern. Screening should be repeated weekly for inpatients (NCCAC 2006). General questions should be posed to patients and carers (Lennard-Jones 1992):

● Has food intake been reduced?
● If yes, why?
● Has weight loss been noticed?
● If yes, over what time period?
● Has there been a reduction in activity due to fatigue?

There are many nutritional assessment tools available.

One example (Figure 7.7) is the 'Malnutrition Universal Screening Tool' (MUST) (BAPEN 2003). Height and weight measurements are used to calculate the body mass index (BMI). The MUST also takes account of recent unplanned weight loss and the effect of acute illness. The score establishes the overall risk of malnutrition and guides the user in planning appropriate care. Other tools also use further anthropometric measurements such as skin fold thickness. Ongoing assessment includes the use of food charts to document intake.

Developing and Delivering Expert Care: Exercise 7.9

Nutrition

BMI is calculated using:

$$\frac{\text{Weight (kg)}}{\text{Height (m)}^2}$$

● Calculate your own BMI and compare it to the chart in Figure 7.8
● Utilise the MUST in practice and compare the results with local tools
● Download Essence of Care (NHSMA 2003) and find out what the benchmarks are for food and nutrition: http://www.dh.gov.uk/en/Publicationsandstatistics/Publications/Publications PolicyAndGuidance/DH_4005475

Nutritional support

Nutritional support should be considered in all patients who are malnourished. The continuum includes:

● Oral nutritional interventions
 ● Advice on food choices
 ● Provision of nutritious and appetising food
 ● Provision of an environment conducive to eating
 ● Help with eating
● Oral nutritional supplements
● Artificial nutritional support
 ● Enteral feeding (NG, PEG)
 ● Parenteral feeding (IV) (BAPEN 2003)

Nutritional requirements should take account of:

● Energy, protein, fluid, electrolyte, mineral, micronutrient and fibre needs
● Activity levels and underlying clinical conditions

Figure 7.7 Malnutrition Universal Screening Tool (MUST) http://www.bapen.org.uk/must_tool.html

- Gastrointestinal tolerance and risk of re-feeding syndrome
- Likely duration of nutritional support (NCCAC 2006).

Large intestine

Form

The large intestine (colon) extends from the ileocaecal valve to the anus. It is 1.5m in length, but has a larger diameter than the small intestine. Its mucosa contains many mucus-secreting goblet cells, but no villi, and is colonised by a wide variety of bacterial flora. Subdivisions include the caecum, ascending colon, transverse colon, descending colon, sigmoid colon, rectum and anal canal. The caecum is a sac in the right iliac fossa below the ileocaecal valve, onto which the appendix is attached. This is an 8cm blind tube with no known function, but which readily collects debris and becomes inflamed. **Appendicitis** is one of the commonest reasons for abdominal surgery. The anal canal contains the internal and external sphincters.

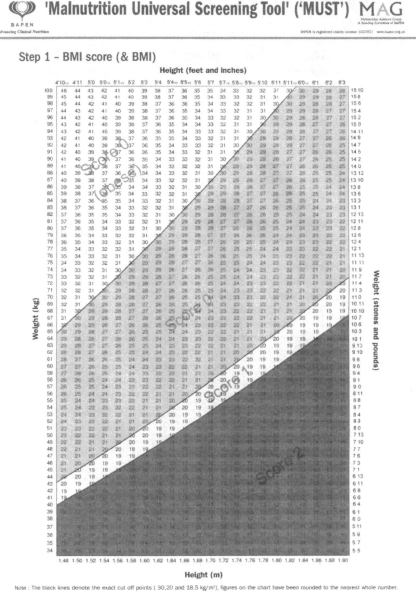

Figure 7.8 BMI chart (www.bapen.org.uk/pdfs/must/must_full.pdf)

Function

Main functions of the colon are absorption of remaining water, storage and elimination of faeces. Arrival of chyme in the caecum causes the ileocaecal valve to close preventing reflux of bacterial flora into the ileum. Peristaltic movements are slow and infrequent, and as a result contents take 12–24 hours to pass through the colon. The only digestion occurring is minimal further breakdown by bacterial flora. Water and electrolytes pass through the colon wall via the same processes described above. The resultant faeces is comprised of a small amount of water, undigested food residues, mucus, bacteria and sloughed mucosal cells. Arrival of faeces in the rectum initiates the defecation reflex, which provides the urge to defecate. This causes the sigmoid colon and rectum to contract, and the internal anal sphincter to relax forcing faeces towards the external anal sphincter. Opening of this is under voluntary control, and defecation is aided by

Developing and Delivering Expert Care: Box 7.14

Enteral Tube Feeding (Stroud et al. 2003)

Enteral tube feeding should be considered if oral intake is likely to be absent for more than five days. This may be due to surgery, unconsciousness, or dysphagia, for example. Specially formulated feeds are infused into the stomach or small intestine, usually via a **nasogastric** (NG) tube or percutaneous endoscopic gastrostomy (PEG) tube. Insertion of an NG tube is an important skill for nurses to develop. There are many inherent risks associated with their usage, such as aspiration.

Re-feeding syndrome is a risk in patients who have recently starved. Introduction of nutritional support can cause sudden fluid and electrolyte disturbances and can be life-threatening. For this reason feeds are initially started at very low levels and the patient is closely monitored.

Questioning Clinical Practice: Exercise 7.10

Food is medicine and the same ethical principles that apply to the giving, withholding and withdrawing of medicine also apply to food.

Apply what you know about ethics to nutritional support. Consider duty of care, informed consent, the competent adult and the Mental Health Act.

contraction of the abdominal muscles against a closed glottis. Gases are also present in the colon and are released in varying amounts as flatus. Most gas is from swallowed air, but it is also derived from bacterial fermentation.

Scenario 7.4

Diverticulitis

Janet Day is a 66-year-old charity worker who is admitted with severe left iliac fossa pain. She has not felt like eating and now feels nauseous. She also complains of fevers and loose stools.

On arrival her vital signs are:

Airway – clear, talking
Breathing – RR 24/min
Circulation – pulse 108/min, BP 132/84
Disability – alert
Exposure – temperature 38.2°C
PMH – constipation.

Assessment and analysis of patient presentation

Ms Day has presented with a common complaint – abdominal pain. The causes of abdominal pain are numerous, but when severe the phenomenon is termed the 'acute abdomen', and is often accompanied by a range of other symptoms. Ms Day's presentation is typical for acute diverticulitis, although she will require thorough assessment to confirm this and negate other potential diagnoses.

Applying Theory to Practice: Box 7.15

Causes of Acute Abdomen

- Appendicitis
- Cholecystitis
- Bowel obstruction
- Pancreatitis
- Peritonitis
- Renal colic
- Abdominal aortic obstruction
- Ectopic pregnancy

Diverticulitis – the facts

Diverticular disease is very common, and although some people can develop acute diverticulitis, most remain asymptomatic. Diverticula are herniations of mucosa through the wall of the colon. They are commonest in the sigmoid colon, and occur alone or in their hundreds. They are thought to be caused by increased pressure, weakening of the bowel wall and low dietary fibre. As a result, prevalence increases with age and it is considered to be a

Developing and Delivering Expert Care: Box 7.16

Assessment of an Acute Abdomen (Newcombe 2007)

PQRST mnemonic:

Precipitating factors – 'What were you doing when the pain started?'

Quality – 'What does the pain feel like?'

- **Visceral pain** originates from stretching or inflammation of an organ. It is poorly localised, intermittent and described as dull or crampy
- **Parietal (somatic) pain** is caused by inflammation of parietal peritoneum. It is easily localised, constant and described as sharp or stabbing. It is also exacerbated by movement.

Region and **R**adiation – 'Where is the pain?' 'Does it radiate elsewhere?'

- **Radiating (referred) pain** occurs because organs share nervous pathways with another area and pain is felt at a distance from the source – can you think of any common examples?

Severity and other **S**ymptoms – 'How bad is the pain?' (use a tool)

Other symptoms include:

- Nausea and vomiting (including haematemesis)
- Anorexia/weight loss
- Dyspepsia
- Constipation/diarrhoea/melaena/wind
- Distension
- Dysuria
- Fever

Timing and **T**reatment – 'When did the pain begin?' 'Does it come and go?' 'Have you taken anything for it?' 'Did it help?'

PMH – previous operations, GI or gynaecological problems?

Is the patient taking any drugs which affect the GI system?

Does the patient drink alcohol or smoke? Is there a recent history of foreign travel? Is there any family history, such as cancer?

Vital signs may show shock or an inflammatory process

An experienced clinician will perform a physical examination, including:

- Inspection
- Auscultation
- Palpation
- Percussion
- Digital rectal examination (DRE)

Further investigations may be indicated, such as blood tests, BM, ECG, urinalysis and radiography.

Western disease. Patients often have a history of constipation. Asymptomatic diverticula are usually found incidentally during screening.

Pathophysiology

Diverticulitis is acute inflammation of one or more diverticula and occurs in 10–25% of cases. Similar to appendicitis the small pouch is vulnerable to blockage with faeces. Due to local irritation, proliferation of bacteria, and ischaemia, the area becomes inflamed. Ms Day's pain is felt in the left iliac fossa due to the location of diverticula in the sigmoid colon. Associated symptoms include fever, tachycardia, nausea, anorexia and diarrhoea. Complications include abscess and fistula formation, obstruction, perforation, peritonitis and haemorrhage. Diagnosis is usually by history and examination, but further investigations may include chest and abdominal X-ray, contrast enema, CT or ultrasound scan.

Due to the location, differential diagnoses include Crohn's disease, cancer or gynaecological causes (Stollman and Raskin 2004).

The plan of care

Ms Day's care will focus on supportive treatment and observation. Most patients respond to conservative treatment within a few days. Ms Day may be allowed to drink clear fluids, but if she is nil by mouth (NBM) she will need IV fluids to maintain hydration. Broad-spectrum IV antibiotics will be given, followed by a course of oral antibiotics. She will need regular appropriate analgesia guided by an objective pain assessment tool. Cooling measures are controversial and the fever should reduce as she improves. Likewise her diarrhoea should resolve as the inflammation subsides, but she will require education on the prevention of constipation. Surgery will be required by 15–30% of patients for persistent symptoms, peritonitis or local abscesses, and may involve temporary formation of a **stoma** (Jones 1999).

Applying Theory to Practice: Exercise 7.11

Temporary or permanent formation of a stoma, such as a colostomy, may be necessary in many conditions. They present patients with significant physical and psychological issues to overcome. Nurses play an important part in assisting patients to care for their stoma and to overcome the initial psychological trauma.

- Find out about the features and management of stomas.
- How are patients assisted in overcoming this life-altering surgery?

Bowel care

In practice you will encounter bowel care in many settings, and it is a key feature of Essence of Care (NHSMA 2003).

Developing and Delivering Expert Care: Box 7.17

Bowel Assessment

There is a diverse range of 'normal' bowel habits – try to determine if there is a change from their normal. Most people open their bowels once a day, but some go several times a day and others may go for several days between bowel movements. Useful questions to ask include (Irwin 2003):

- How often do you normally open your bowels?
- When were your bowels last opened (BLO)?
- Have you had any difficulty opening your bowels?
- Are you passing wind?
- Have you had any diarrhoea?
- What is the stool consistency? (Figure 7.9)
- Have you had any incontinence?
- Is there any blood or mucus in the stool?

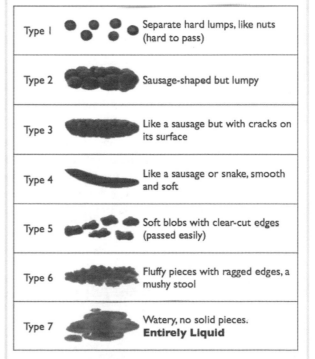

Figure 7.9 Bristol Stool Chart

Constipation is very common, particularly in the elderly, and is characterised by infrequent bowel movements, hard stools and straining at defecation. Causes include:

- Low fibre diet
- Poor fluid intake
- Reduced mobility
- Drugs (opiates)
- Neurological disorders
- Depression
- Bowel obstruction.

Management of constipation follows a stepped-care approach:

- Identify and treat underlying cause
- Change medication where appropriate
- Lifestyle changes, such as increasing fibre and fluid intake and exercise
- Consider laxatives:
 - Bulk-forming agents (ispaghula, methylcellulose)
 - Stimulant laxatives (senna, bisacodyl)
 - Osmotic laxatives (lactulose)
 - Faecal softeners (docusate sodium, liquid paraffin)
- Consider suppositories and enemas (Prodigy 2007c)

Diarrhoea is defined as the abnormal passage of loose or liquid stools more than three times per day (Thomas et al. 2003). Causes include:

- Bacteria
- Toxins
- Food
- Allergy
- Anxiety
- Over-use of laxatives
- Disorders such as inflammatory bowel disease.

Acute infective diarrhoea is a common cause of death in developing countries, particularly in children. Complications occur due to dehydration and electrolyte disturbances. Management is aimed at replacing fluids and treating the underlying cause, if appropriate. Antibiotics are only used for specific indications. Meticulous hygiene is essential as pathogens are spread via the faecal-oral route.

Faecal incontinence is distressing and embarrassing. Causes include:

- Sphincter weakness
- Neurological disorders
- Impaction
- Diarrhoea.

Careful assessment and identification of the underlying cause lead to effective treatment. Nurses have a key role in providing practical and emotional care.

Conclusion

Application of digestive anatomy and physiology is vital for understanding normal human function. Analysis of a range of disorders affecting the digestive system has illustrated patient assessment, pathophysiology and evidence-based management. Gaining knowledge of the role nutrition plays in both health and illness and the development of a range of skills reflecting the *Essence of Care* is essential for nursing practice.

Chapter 7 Summary Quiz

1. The digestive system is supplied by which circulation?

A. Portal circulation
B. Splanchnic circulation
C. Circle of Willis
D. Momentum artery

2. The main functions of the digestive system do not include:

A. Ingestion
B. Ovulation
C. Secretion
D. Elimination

3. The human adult usually has how many permanent teeth?

A. 60
B. 50
C. 42
D. 32

4. Vomiting is controlled by the vomiting, or emetic, centre in the brain, and is precipitated by many peripheral and central causes, including:

A. Stimulation of the gag reflex
B. Electrolyte disturbances
C. Particular sights, smells or emotions
D. Over-excitation of the sinoatrial node

5. Which of the following is not an-anti-emetic?

A. Metoclopramide
B. Cyclizine
C. Digoxin
D. Domperidone

6. Common medications used to treat peptic ulcers include:

A. Antacids and alginates
B. Histamine H_2 receptor antagonists
C. Proton pump inhibitors
D. All answers are correct

7. Which disease process is not a consequence of portal hypertension and ALD?

A. Oesophageal varices
B. Hepatic encephalopathy
C. Basal cell carcinomas
D. Ascites

8. The small intestine is composed of:

A. Duodenum, jejunum, ileum

B. Ileum, jejunum, oesophagus

C. Duodenum, appendix, jejunum

D. Ileum, appendix, duodenum

9. MUST stands for:

A. Malnutrition Underweight Sensitivity Tool

B. Malnutrition Universal Screening Tool

C. Minimal Underweight Selective Thinking

D. Malnutrition Universal Selection Training

10. Which of the following is not a cause of an acute abdomen?

A. Appendicitis

B. Pancreatitis

C. Peritonitis

D. Heart failure

Further reading

British Liver Trust (BLT) (2005) *Alcohol and Liver Disease.* http://www.britishlivertrust.org.uk/content/diseases/alcohol.asp (accessed 27 May 2007).

Cabinet Office Strategy Unit (COSU) (2004) *Alcohol Harm Reduction Strategy for England.* http://www.cabinetoffice.gov.uk/strategy/downloads/su/alcohol/pdf/CabOffce%20AlcoholHar.pdf

Irwin, K. (2003) Back to basics 1: Assessment of bowel dysfunction. *Journal of Community Nursing* 17(11): 26–32.

Lewis, S.J. & Heaton, K.W. (1997) Stool form scale as a useful guide to intestinal transit time. *Scandinavian Journal of Gastroenterology* 32(9): 920–4.

Moore, T. (2004) Fluid and electrolyte disturbances. In: Moore, T. & and Woodrow, P. (eds) *High Dependency Nursing Care: Observation, Intervention and Support.* Routledge: London.

Newcombe, P. (2007) Acute surgical emergencies. In: Evans, C. & Tippins, E. (eds) *The Foundations of Emergency Care.* Open University Press: Maidenhead.

References

British Association for Parenteral and Enteral Nutrition (BAPEN) (2003) *The 'MUST' Explanatory Booklet: A Guide to the 'Malnutrition Universal Screening Tool' ('MUST') for Adults.* http://www.bapen.org.uk/must_notes.html (accessed 27 May 2007).

British Liver Trust (BLT) (2005) *Alcohol and Liver Disease.* http://www.britishlivertrust.org.uk/content/diseases/alcohol.asp (accessed 27 May 2007).

British Society of Gastroenterology Endoscopy Committee (BSGEC) (2002) Non-vertical upper gastrointestinal haemorrhage: guidelines. *Gut* 51(Suppl IV): iv1–iv6.

Cabinet Office Strategy Unit (COSU) (2004) *Alcohol Harm Reduction Strategy for England.* http://www.cabinetoffice.gov.uk/strategy/downloads/su/alcohol/pdf/CabOffce%20AlcoholHar.pdf (accessed 27 May 2007).

Devlin, J. & O'Grady, J. (1999) Indications for referral and assessment in adult liver transplantation: a clinical guideline. *Gut* 45(Suppl VI): vi1–vi22.

Huntley, J. & Touquet, R. (2005) Surgical problems. In: Paton, A. & Touquet, R. (eds) *ABC of Alcohol*, 4th edn. Blackwell Publishing: Oxford.

Irwin, K. (2003) Back to basics 1: Assessment of bowel dysfunction, *Journal of Community Nursing* 17(11): 26–32.

Jalan, R. & Hayes, P.C. (2000) UK guidelines on the management of variceal haemorrhage in cirrhotic patients. *Gut* 46(Suppl III): iii1–iii15.

Joint Formulary Committee (JFC) (2007) *British National Formulary*, 53rd edn. http://www.bnf.org/bnf/index.htm (accessed 27 May 2007).

Jones, D.J. (1999) Diverticular disease. In: Jones, D.J. (ed.) *ABC of Colorectal Diseases*, 2nd edn. BMJ Books: London.

Krige, J.E.J. & Beckingham, I.J. (2001) Portal hypertension – 2. Ascites, encephalopathy, and other conditions. In: Beckingham I.J. (ed.) *ABC of Liver, Pancreas and Gall Bladder.* BMJ Books: London.

Lennard-Jones, J.E. (1992) *A Positive Approach to Nutrition as Treatment.* http://www.bapen.org.uk/pdfs/bapen_pubs/pub_kings_fund.pdf (accessed 27 May 2007).

Logan, R.P.H. & Delaney, B. (2002) Implications of dyspepsia for the NHS. In: Logan, R.P.H., Harris, A., Misiewicz, J.J. & Baron,

J.H. (eds) *ABC of the Upper Gastrointestinal Tract*. BMJ Books: London.

Moore, K.P. & Aithal, G.P. (2006) Guidelines on the management of ascites in cirrhosis. *Gut* 55(Suppl VI): vi1–vi12.

National Collaborating Centre for Acute Care (NCCAC) (2006) *Nutrition Support in Adults: Oral Nutrition Support, Enteral Tube Feeding and Parenteral Nutrition*. http://www.rcseng.ac.uk/publications/docs/nutrition_support_guidelines.html (accessed 27 May 2007).

National Health Service Modernisation Agency (NHSMA) (2003) *Essence of Care: Patient-focused Benchmarks for Clinical Governance*. http://www.dh.gov.uk/en/Publicationsandstatistics/Publications/PublicationsPolicyAndGuidance/DH_4005475 (accessed 27 May 2007).

National Institute for Clinical Excellence (NICE) (2004) *Dyspepsia: Managing Dyspepsia in Adults in Primary Care*. http://guidance.nice.org.uk/CG17 (accessed 27 May 2007).

Newcombe, P. (2007) Acute surgical emergencies. In Evans, C. & Tippins, E. (eds) *The Foundations of Emergency Care*. Open University Press: Maidenhead.

Paton, A. (2005a) Medical problems. In: Paton, A. & Touquet, R. (eds) *ABC of Alcohol*, 4th edn. Blackwell Publishing: Oxford.

Paton, A. (2005b) Alcohol in the body. In: Paton, A. & Touquet, R. (eds) *ABC of Alcohol*, 4th edn. Blackwell Publishing: Oxford.

Prodigy (2007a) *Nausea and Vomiting in Pregnancy (PRODIGY Guidance)*. Clinical Knowledge Summaries. http://cks.library.nhs.uk/nausea_vomiting_in_pregnancy (accessed 27 May 2007).

Prodigy (2007b) *Palliative Care – Nausea/Vomiting/Malignant Bowel Obstruction (PRODIGY Guidance)*. Clinical Knowledge Summaries. http://cks.library.nhs.uk/palliative_care_nausea_vomit (accessed 27 May 2007).

Prodigy (2007c) *Constipation (PRODIGY Guidance)*. Clinical Knowledge Summaries. http://cks.library.nhs.uk/constipation (accessed 27 May 2007).

Royal College of Physicians (RCP) (2001) *Alcohol – Can the NHS Afford It? Recommendations for a Coherent Alcohol Strategy for Hospitals*. http://www.rcplondon.ac.uk/pubs/brochure.aspx?e=9 (accessed 27 May 2007).

Ritson, B. (2005) Advice and counselling. In: Paton, A. & Touquet, R. (eds) *ABC of Alcohol*, 4th edn. Blackwell Publishing: Oxford.

Roberts, I., Alderson, P., Bunn, F., et al. (2004) Colloids versus crystalloids for fluid resuscitation in critically ill patients. *Cochrane Database of Systematic Reviews*. 4: CD000567.

Smith, M.E. & Morton, D.G. (2001) *The Digestive System*. Elsevier Churchill Livingstone: Edinburgh.

Stollman, N. & Raskin, J.B. (2004) Diverticular disease of the colon. *Lancet* 363: 631–9.

Strobel, S. & Ferguson, A. (2005) Immune function, food allergies and food intolerance. In: Geissler, C. & Powers, H. (eds) *Human Nutrition*, 11th edn. Elsevier Churchill Livingstone: Edinburgh.

Stroud, M., Duncan, H. & Nightingale, J. (2003) Guidelines for enteral feeding in adult hospital patients. *Gut* 52(suppl. VII): vii1–vii12.

Thomas, P.D., Forbes, A., Green, J., et al. (2003) Guidelines for the investigation of chronic diarrhoea, 2nd edition. *Gut* 52(Suppl V): v1–v15.

UK Working Party on Acute Pancreatitis (UKWPAP) (2005) UK guidelines for the management of acute pancreatitis. *Gut* 54(Suppl III): iii1–iii9.

World Health Organization (WHO) (2001) *The Alcohol Use Disorders Identification Test (AUDIT): Guidelines for Use in Primary Care*, 2nd edn. http://whqlibdoc.who.int/hq/2001/WHO_MSD_MSB_01.6a.pdf (accessed 27 May 2007).

Zander, R. (2006) *Fluid Management*. Bibliomed: Melsungen, Germany.

The musculoskeletal system

Karen Chivers

Chapter 8 Learning Objectives

- To gain knowledge and insight into the different components which comprise the musculoskeletal system
- To gain insight into both chronic and acute conditions related to these systems
- To apply theory to practice by gaining insight into the complexities of clinical assessment in relation to musculoskeletal problems
- To gain a solid understanding of the needs of patients when they are compromised by physical disability
- To construct solid evidence of professional development for your growing portfolio
- Continue to develop the ability to question and critique the evidence-base and effectiveness of a plan of care

Introduction

In order to fully appreciate the function and purpose of the musculoskeletal system, it is important that the reader fully understands the components which constitute this large and initially complex subject. Consideration needs to be given to the soft connective tissues of the musculoskeletal system, which comprise tendons, cartilage, ligaments and fascia, in combination with muscles and the joints. Each of these areas and their functioning will be discussed to provide the reader with a succinct overview of form and function. The chapter will then progress to identifying disorders/diseases that affect each area, highlighting the impact that injury and disease can have on the individual. Relevant treatments will be discussed thereby assisting inexperienced nurses in gaining the essential knowledge base and clinical skills necessary to provide effective evidence-based treatment for those placed in their care. The second part of the chapter will focus on how to assess individuals who present with an acute injury, using a systematic format.

Most injuries involving this system will be minor and will not significantly impact on the individual or their life. However, major injuries to this system can have an impact, therefore one of the scenarios will take an in-depth look at how major trauma can disrupt both an individual's physical health and ability to function within society, and how this can have an enormous psychological impact resulting in long-term consequences for the person affected and those close to them.

Applying Theory to Practice: Exercise 8.1

Before commencing this chapter:

- Compose a list of the diseases/injuries you already know that affect the musculoskeletal system (you may find this easier if you divide up the systems e.g. skeletal, muscular, joints etc.).

Add this list to your developing portfolio and on completion of this chapter expand your portfolio by writing a brief description of the new disorders you have gained knowledge on, elaborating on how these disorders affect physiological function and how to recognise a patient with them.

The skeleton

What is the skeleton?

There are 206 bones that form the framework of the adult skeleton (Figure 8.1). These bones support and protect the muscles and organs of the body. In children not all the bones are fully formed and develop gradually over years. The skeleton is predominantly divided into two parts: the axial and appendicular skeleton.

- The **axial** skeleton consists of 80 bones that support the head, neck and torso. It comprises the skull, vertebral column, ribs and sternum.

Figure 8.1 The adult skeleton

The **appendicular** skeleton consists of 126 bones and supports the appendages, or limbs, attaching them to the rest of the body. It comprises the shoulder girdle – scapula, clavicle, upper limbs, pelvic girdle – the innominate bones and the lower limbs.

Functions of the skeleton

The skeleton provides seven main functions listed below:

- It provides shape and support for the body
- It provides a framework for all structures of the body
- It provides levers that are essential for movement
- It forms attachment points for muscles that move the joints, which in turn allows movement
- It provides protection for vital internal organs e.g. the cranium protects the brain, while the pelvic girdle protects the reproductive organs, bladder and intestines
- Red bone marrow within the bones manufacture blood cells
- The skeleton stores minerals, calcium and phosphorus.

Types of bone

There are two main types of bone tissue, **compact** and **cancellous**. Bone tissues varies in density and compactness. Most bones have a central cavity, containing marrow, a tissue that is the source of most of the cells within the blood and also a site for the storage of fats.

Bone is the hardest connective tissue in the body. It is composed of 25% water, 30% organic material – which includes cells, blood vessels, connective tissue and bone marrow – and 45% inorganic substances, such as calcium, phosphorus and salt.

Compact

The outer layer of bone is called compact bone. It appears solid, but on closer inspection it is made up of structures called **Haversian canals**. These run longitudinally through compact bone and contain blood, lymph capillaries and nerves. The larger the canal, the less dense and compact the bones.

Cancellous

The inner layer of bone is called cancellous bone. It is also commonly known as spongy bone. This is because it looks like a sponge and contains many holes. The structure of cancellous bone is like a latticework of bony spikes called **trabeculae**. These are arranged along lines of greatest pressure or stress, which in turn makes bones both strong and light.

Cancellous bone is filled with red bone marrow, which produces blood cells. In mature long bones the cancellous bone loses its ability to produce blood cells and red bone marrow changes to yellow bone marrow, which is fatty tissue.

Periosteum

The blood supply to bone is delivered via the periosteum. This is a tough membrane of fibrous tissue, which contains blood vessels and covers the surface of the bone wherever it is not covered by articular cartilage. It is essential for bone growth, repair and nutrition. It also serves as a point of attachment for ligaments and tendons.

Classification of bone types

Long bones

These are longer that they are wide, and function as levers to allow movement in limbs, e.g. the humerus, femur, tibia, clavicle, metacarpals and metatarsals.

Short bones

These are constructed predominantly of cancellous bone, with a covering of compact bone. These are very strong and subject to pressure type force. Their normal shape is cuboid or trapezoid and can be found in the ankle and wrist.

Flat bones

These are protective and have broad flat surfaces for muscle attachment, e.g. cranium, scapular, sternum.

Irregular bones

These are bones that do not fit into other categories, for example, most facial bones and vertebrae.

Sesamoid bones

These are bones that develop within a tendon, occurring in regions affected by significant pressure. There are only two in the body: the patella and hyoid bone.

Bone growth

The replacement of old bone with new bone is called remodelling. Bone tissue constantly renews itself throughout life; the bone redistributes its matrix along lines of mechanical stress. Special bone cells called **osteoclasts** and **osteoblasts** are intrinsic to this process. Osteoclasts destroy old or injured bone tissue and are responsible for the reabsorption of bone tissue. Osteoblasts constantly secrete new bone matrix in its place. There are certain vitamins and minerals which are essential for bone remodelling; these are highlighted in the following section. It is important to remember that a deficiency in some of these vitamins or minerals will have an effect on the healing process, and this must be considered in the hospitalised patient, or the patient presenting with a known deficiency. Hormones largely control the mineral concentrations within the blood.

Vitamins

Vitamin A helps to control the distribution and activities of osteoblasts and osteoclasts; deficiency or excess may cause small stature. **Vitamin C** is essential for collagen synthesis, which is required for the matrix. Any deficiency hinders fracture repair and also interferes with bone growth.

Minerals

Calcium and **phosphorus** are the primary components of the salts that make the bone matrix hard. **Magnesium** is needed to stimulate the activity of osteoclasts. **Boron** inhibits calcium loss and increases oestrogen levels. A deficiency of **manganese** will inhibit the laying down of new bone tissue.

Hormones

It is important to consider the role of hormones, which contribute to normal bone tissue activity.

Parathyroid hormone (PTH) helps to increase blood calcium levels. It stimulates the release of calcium from bone and inhibits calcium excretion by kidneys, which in turn helps to ensure more is maintained in the blood. It also stimulates the formation of calcitrol, which is a hormone that also promotes the absorption of calcium by the intestines. PTH is the most important hormone that regulates calcium exchange between bone and blood in the body.

Calcitonin is secreted by the thyroid gland and reduces the blood calcium levels. It inhibits the release of calcium from bone and stimulates calcium excretion by the kidneys.

Human growth hormone is released by the anterior pituitary gland and is responsible for the general growth of all tissues of the body. It helps to stimulate the growth of epiphyseal cartilage and stimulates calcium excretion by the kidneys and calcium absorption by the intestines.

The sex hormones (**oestrogen** and **testosterone**) stimulate bone formation and cause degeneration of cartilage in epiphyseal plates. Oestrogen prevents osteoporosis, which is possibly by a direct effect on osteoblasts.

Insulin increases bone formation when functioning at normal levels. Consider diabetic patients when reflecting on bone remodelling following a fracture.

Glucocorticoids, both **cortisol** and **aldosterone**, are produced in the adrenal cortex and reduce blood calcium levels.

The thyroid hormones, **thyroxine** and **triiodothyronine**, help to increase the blood calcium levels.

Diseases and disorders of the skeletal system

Paget's disease (osteitis deformans)

Paget's disease is a disorder of bone remodelling; excessive re-absorption occurs with a subsequent compensatory increase in new bone formation (Kumar and Clark 1998). The new bone is structurally abnormal resulting in a fundamental weakness within its structure. Paget's disease is a disorder that seldom affects men and women before the age of 40 (Adams 1986). There are often no symptoms and the condition is discovered incidentally during a radiology examination. It is possible that 60–80% of patients with Paget's disease are asymptomatic (Adams 1986) there appears to be a significant genetic component. There are increased numbers of osteoclasts containing an increased number of nuclei. Bone resorption does not occur in a uniform pattern with collagen fibres tending to be random, leading to a woven bone formation, which is weaker than unaffected bone. Paget's disease does not spread and so unaffected bone remains normal. The most common sites that are affected are the femur, pelvis, tibia, skull and the lumbosacral spine.

When patients are symptomatic (it is important to note that many patients do not experience symptoms and are diagnosed accidentally), their symptoms may include:

- Bone pain
- Deformities, most common in the skull or bowed tibia
- Joint pain, when bone close to a joint is affected, leading to cartilage damage and osteoarthritis.

Treatment

This depends on the presenting symptoms. Pain being the usual indicator, this is treated with analgesics and non-steroidal anti-inflammatory drugs (NSAID), which are normally adequate. Patients who are asymptomatic require no treatment.

Some patients can require further treatment, for example with oral bisphosphates. Kumar and Clark (1998) note that responses to bisphosphates are long-lasting with approximately a 50–70% reduction in serum alkaline phosphatase activity. When new bone is formed, it is lamellar rather than woven.

Osteoporosis

Osteoporosis is a condition of **porous** bones, and it occurs when bone resorption is quicker than bone deposition (Tortora 2001). The bone mass becomes depleted, and the mechanical stresses placed on the skeleton by everyday living are not tolerated. It is a disorder that affects mainly middle-aged and elderly women, although it can affect men too. It is mostly seen in the female population due to oestrogen levels falling rapidly

in women after the **menopause**. The decline in testosterone in men is more gradual and therefore they suffer less osteoporosis. In osteoporotic bones the mineral density is decreased. Patients who are suffering from osteoporosis are more likely to suffer fracture of bones more frequently and to a greater degree than those not affected. The treatment is focused on prevention rather than cure.

Treatment

Preventative measures include adequate calcium intake and exercise earlier in life rather than reliance on drugs and calcium supplements at menopausal age. In postmenopausal women osteoporosis can be treated with hormone replacement therapy (HRT). HRT is the treatment of choice although the potential side-effects of HRT remain controversial, but the risk of side-effects is less than that of experiencing fractures without HRT (Kumar and Clarke 1998).

Applying Theory to Practice: Exercise 8.2

Over recent years there as been much debate surrounding the use of HRT. Complete the following exercise to gain insight.

- What are the possible side effects of HRT?
- What 'life-style' choices have been implicated in the development of osteoporosis?

Osteoarthritis

Osteoarthritis can be limited to only a single joint and can be triggered by localised wear and tear. Joint degeneration may be hastened by congenital defect, injury, infection or obesity. **Articular cartilage** begins to break down and become thinner and roughened. Bone beneath the cartilage eventually erodes so that the bone surfaces rub against one another causing discomfort. Commonly affected areas include weight-bearing joints like knees, feet and the back. Osteoarthritis in the spine is extremely common in the elderly population, although quite often it can be asymptomatic and may be discovered coincidentally when the individual is being treated for another complaint (McRae 2004).

Treatment

Unfortunately drugs cannot repair damaged bone and cartilage and their sole role is to reduce any inflammation and control pain. By acting in this way they can help to maintain joint mobility and minimise deformity to the affected areas. NSAIDs are prescribed primarily as long as they are not contraindicated in each individual case by any predisposing illness. Occasionally, injections of corticosteroid drugs are used for severely inflamed joints.

Osteomalacia

This condition differs from osteoporosis in that there is no loss of the bone's protein matrix; in osteomalacia bones are weakened by the loss of calcium and phosphorus. The bone calcification fails; as a consequence, the bones become soft and rubbery and are easily deformed. In children this is called rickets. A primary cause is a shortage of vitamin D, essential to enable the body to deal with calcium and phosphorus. Inadequate sunlight can also reduce vitamin D synthesis (Chapter 10).

Brittle bone syndrome (osteogenesis imperfecta)

This is an inherited disorder and there are four different types, notable by their varying clinical picture.

- Death in perinatal period (type 2)
- Severe bone deformity (type 3)
- Normal life span (types 1 and 4) (Kumar & Clark 1998).

The main clinical signs are very fragile and brittle bones that fracture frequently. It is important to note that other collagen-containing tissues can also be affected such as tendons, skin and eyes.

Type 1 sufferers present with mild bony deformities, but will experience other oddities such as blue sclerae, defective dentine, early onset deafness and heart valve disorders. It is these factors that assist the medical personnel in making a diagnosis.

The more severe forms present with multiple fractures and gross deformities. The severity of the disease will dictate the prognosis.

Treatment

Early recognition of the condition is vital for correct management. All fractures would be treated individually as they present to the emergency department.

Postural deformities

The spine has two natural curves: in the lumbar region there is an inward curve, and in the thoracic region an outward curve (Figure 8.2).

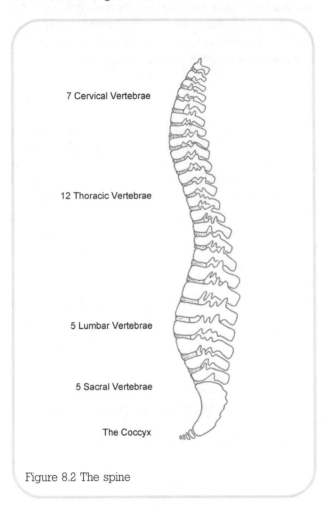

Figure 8.2 The spine

The spine is also known as the **vertebral column** and consists of 33 vertebrae; some of these bones are fused, so there are actually 26 individual bones, which are divided into cervical vertebrae, thoracic vertebrae, lumbar vertebrae, the sacrum and the coccyx. There are three main functions of the vertebral column:

- Allowing movement
- Protecting and enclosing the spinal cord
- Acting as a point of attachment for the ribs and muscles of the back.

There are a number of reasons why the natural curves of the spinal cord may become disrupted leading to pos-

tural deformities. The three main reasons why a postural deformity occurs are: following a traumatic event such as an accident; a congenital or heredity deformity present at birth; and environmental factors such as sitting and standing incorrectly resulting in long-term damage.

Types of postural deformity

Figure 8.3 Postural deformities

Kyphosis–A
Kyphosis is an exaggerated outward curvature of the upper part of the back below the neck. It is usually obvious when the patient is viewed from the side. It generally affects the thoracic spine with several vertebrae being affected.

Scoliosis–C
Scoliosis is a sideways (lateral) curvature of the spine; there are two types, structural and non-structural. Structural scoliosis is the term used when there is a change in the shape and mobility of the vertebrae and the deformity cannot be altered by a change in posture. Structural scoliosis can be congenital. In non-structural scoliosis the deformity can occur from tilting of the pelvis and therefore becomes compensatory.

The prognosis of a patient with scoliosis is dependent on the age of onset, level of spine affected, the size and number of the primary curves and the type of structural scoliosis (McRae 2004). It is thought that when the skeleton has matured, deterioration stops, but it can continue due to disc degeneration and subluxation of the vertebrae; generally the higher the level of spine involved and the

younger the patient, the worse the prognosis (McRae 2004). Scoliosis can be treated by the use of braces or fusion of the entire primary curve can be considered.

Lordosis–B

Lordosis is an exaggerated inward curvature of the spine, and can often result in a tip of the pelvis. The extent of postural deformity and the effect on life will depend on the treatment required. Some patients may need surgery to correct the deformity; others may just live with the deformity for life. Each case is assessed on an individual basis.

Spina bifida

Spina bifida is a congenital defect of the vertebral column, in which the laminae fail to unite at the midline (Tortora 2001). It can cause partial or complete paralysis, and absence of reflexes, and occurs when there is protrusion of the meninges around the spinal cord. It is often diagnosed on early pregnancy scans, and there appears to be documented evidence that it is associated with low levels of folic acid (Tortora 2001). This is why women are encouraged to commence folic acid prior to becoming pregnant and for the first three months of pregnancy, by which stage the vertebrae have formed.

Fractures

There are a number of different types of fracture and this text does not endeavour to go into great detail about the description of fractures and their treatment. The figures, however, help to demonstrate the text. A fracture is described as a bone that has broken either due to injury or disease. There are many different types of fracture.

Simple (sometimes called closed)

This is when a bone is broken in one place and has not damaged the tissue around it (Figure 8.4).

Figure 8.4 Simple fracture

Compound (sometimes called open fracture)

This is a fracture in which the fractured bone ends pierce the skin and communicate through the surface of skin through an open wound (Figure 8.5). As the skin is open over the fracture, or the bone has protruded through the skin, there is a high risk of infection. These types of fracture are covered promptly and treated with antibiotics to minimise risk of infection.

Figure 8.5 Compound fracture

Comminuted

The bone is broken in several places and is therefore fragmented (Figure 8.6). Injuries of this kind are normally caused by a direct force, and sometimes by a crush injury.

Figure 8.6 Comminuted fracture

Greenstick

This is an incomplete fracture of a long bone (Figure 8.7). It only affects the cortex on one side of the bone while the other side remains intact; common in soft and flexible bones, therefore, these are often seen in children.

Figure 8.7 Greenstick fracture

Buckle

This is where there is a small bulge in the outline of the bone. There is minimal damage to the periosteum and soft tissues. These type of injuries heal quickly, again common in children (Figure 8.8).

Figure 8.8 Buckle fracture

Impacted

This is a fracture that results in the broken ends being driven together by force (a good example is like one car shunting into the back of another), this type of fracture is often seen as a Colles fracture (Figure 8.9) and results as a direct fall onto an outstretched wrist. It can be associated with shortening, displacement and angulation.

Figure 8.9 Colles fracture

Spiral

This type of fracture is the result of a twisting force and causes an obliquely angled spiral fracture. As the broken areas are larger it allows easier union, however, the angle of broken bone may encourage slippage, angulation and shortening (Figure 8.10).

Figure 8.10 Spiral fracture

Depressed

This is a fracture where the bone has been punched out and now lies in underlying soft tissues and often occurs in the skull (Figure 8.11).

Figure 8.11 Depressed skull fracture

Crush

This occurs when a force is applied causing damage to the soft tissues and forcing the bones to crush, the commonest site is in the vertebrae (Figure 8.12).

Figure 8.12 Crush fracture

Pathological

These occur when a disease has weakened the bone, commonly seen in patients who are suffering from cancer and have metastatic bone disease (Figure 8.13).

Figure 8.13 Pathological fracture

Complications of fractures

There can be many complications of fractures:

- Infection
- Delayed union
- Malunion
- Non-union
- Avascular necrosis
- Shortening
- Injury to major blood vessels
- Injury to nerves
- Injury to tendons
- Fat embolism
- Compartment syndrome.

When a patient presents with a fracture, the key is to have an understanding of the mechanism of injury and the probability of some of the above complications. A thorough assessment and history taking will enable the nurse to be able to administer the best treatment (this is discussed in depth in the latter part of this chapter). The best treatment is to immobilise the fracture, thereby reducing the pain and discomfort for the patient and allowing natural healing to occur. The basic principle to follow will be to inform the patient that if he gets an increased level of pain in the affected area, increased swelling, numbness or coolness of the limb then he needs to seek medical advice urgently.

Scenario 8.1

Fractured Leg

Mr Robert Smith, a 34-year-old man, is brought into the emergency department by ambulance. He was a motorcyclist, involved in a road traffic accident, where his vehicle skidded on ice and he lost control of the motorbike. When he fell to the ground, the motorbike fell onto his right leg and he was unable to get up. There was a possibility that he experienced a brief loss of consciousness, although he was wearing a crash helmet. At the scene of the accident it was noted that there was an obvious deformity to his right lower leg, which the ambulance crew realigned by applying a splint to the leg after administering morphine.

The emergency department had received warning of his imminent arrival, so a trauma team were assembled and awaiting his arrival.

Vital signs on arrival
Airway & C-spine: clear, patient is talking. AVPU = A
C-Spine is immobilised with hard cervical collar, blocks and tape.
Breathing: spontaneous, respiratory rate 20/min
Circulation: pulse rate 110, regular, BP 110/70, capillary refill <2 secs
Disability: patient alert, GCS 15/15, pupils equal and reactive to light
PMH: nil of note
Medication: nil
Allergies: elastoplast

Assessment and analysis of patient presentation

With any patient involved in a trauma scenario, it is important that a structured approach is used to guide the initial assessment and management. This commonly focuses on applying the Advanced Trauma Life Support (ATLS) guidance (ACS 2004). This ensures that each system is fully assessed and that any problems can be identified early and treated accordingly. Injuries to the musculoskeletal system often look dramatic, and hospital personnel can be easily distracted by their appearance. However, they are not as life-threatening as an injury to the airway, hence the A, B, C, D, E approach. Initially the primary survey takes place and then when all life-threatening potentials are stabilised, the secondary survey follows, and this involves a top-to-toe inspection of the whole patient.

Mr Smith has no apparent airway or breathing complications although his respiratory rate is above normal. He is already receiving intravenous fluids commenced at the scene of the accident. His pulse is raised and his blood pressure within normal limits. There is the possibility of haemorrhage and potential ischaemia to the injured leg. Assessment of vital signs assists healthcare professionals in monitoring the patient's condition, but visualisation of the patient is still vitally important, as is communication with the patient. An X-ray confirms that Mr Smith has a comminuted midshaft fracture to the right tibia and fibula; there is associated swelling of the soft tissues. Mr Smith will require further immobilisation of his leg, achieved by the application of a plaster of Paris to his right leg to immobilise the fracture prior to surgery.

Treatment of fractures

The main principle of treating fractures is to immobilise them to allow the bone to remodel and repair itself so that function can be restored. If the bone ends are well opposed, then a bridging process called **union** takes place; this is a temporary state on the way to permanent healing (Purcell 2004). When the broken ends of the bone are joined, they are still not sufficiently strong enough for normal function. The time scale for this part of the healing process takes 3–4 weeks, but will be dependent on the age of patient and any predisposing medical problems.

Compartment syndrome

Compartment syndrome is one of the most serious complications of injuries sustained; this is why assessment of a limb needs to be carried out as soon as injury occurs.

Questioning Clinical Practice: Exercise 8.3

Fracture Complications

While waiting for a bed to be transferred to, Mr Smith complains of severe pain to his right lower leg.

- What conditions must be considered and how can they be treated?

Developing and Delivering Expert Care: Box 8.1

Clinical Signs Associated with Compartment Syndrome

- Severe pain
- Extremely painful movements especially on passive extension
- Limb may be cool
- Patchy pallor of limb
- Skin may look shiny, tense bulging muscle
- Sensory deficit
- Pulses might be present and gradually weaken. NB: necrosis can occur while pulses are present.

Absent pulses are a very late sign of compartment syndrome.

Vigilance of a potentially affected limb has to be paramount.

Important to note that a vascular injury can only be identified in fully conscious patients (Edwards 2004).

The temperature of the limb, sensation, pallor and pulses all need to be assessed and accurately documented on a half-hourly basis. Compartment syndrome occurs when there is significant swelling, whether caused by trauma or haemorrhage, within a muscle compartment. In Scenario 8.1 it is likely that the area affected is the anterior tibial compartment, as there is severe pain in the front of the shin; this occasionally can be associated with foot drop. The most common site of compartment syndrome is the lower leg with the anterior compartment the most frequently affected (Abramowiz and Schepsis 1994), but this would be difficult to assess as the patient's limb is

immobilised in plaster. The treatment required is that of immediate surgical decompression; this takes the form of **fasciotomy**. It is important to note that by performing a fasciotomy a closed lesion is being turned into an open wound and that heralds many complications (Fitzgerald 2000). Some of the complications that could occur include life-threatening infection, acidosis, renal failure and occasionally the loss of a limb. The reason for surgical intervention is to prevent muscle necrosis occurring. This can be a frightening experience for the patient, who is in severe pain. There is evidence to suggest that initial treatment with mannitol can decompress compartment syndrome and avoid the need for surgery (Porter & Greaves 2003).

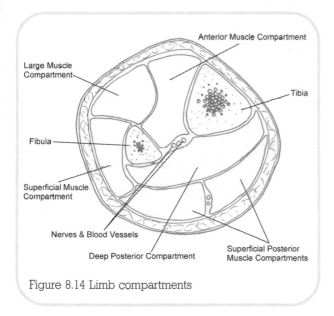

Figure 8.14 Limb compartments

Acute compartment syndrome is a common and potentially life-threatening condition that occurs in the limbs and abdomen, which requires prompt recognition and intervention (Edwards 2004).

One important consideration must be in patients pre-senting to the emergency department with fractures. Ethically should nurses advise them that compartment syndrome is a potential complication, or should the patient be informed that should they experience a sudden severe pain, numbness or coolness to the limb that they should return immediately? By taking the second course the nurse is warning them about the risks of compartment syndrome without mentioning the words. With access to the internet, patients are well informed and will often find out more information anyway.

Joints

A joint is the place where two bones meet; there are three main types of joint within the skeletal system:

- **Fixed** (also known as fibrous). These fibrous joints have no movement. An example of these is in the pelvic girdle bones.
- **Slightly movable** (also known as cartilaginous joints). An example is the white fibrocartilage between bones, e.g. vertebrae.
- **Freely movable** or **synovial**. Within this section there are five different types, which are discussed below:
 - Ball and Socket. This type of joint is the most movable and allows movement of action, for example, at the shoulder joint.
 - Hinge. This allows movement in one direction only, e.g. at the elbow where it can extend and flex. It is the simplest of joints.
 - Gliding. Here the bones glide over each other, e.g. tarsals or carpals. In these joints movement is still limited as there are strong ligaments encasing them.
 - Pivot. This allows movement around one axis, e.g. the first two vertebrae. The first vertebra, C1, known as the Atlas, allows the head to rotate and the second vertebra, C2, known as the Axis, allows the nodding action.
 - Saddle. This allows movement around two axes. It is only found between the phalanges of the thumb and metacarpal.

Conditions affecting joints

Rheumatoid arthritis

This is a form of arthritis that affects the auto-immune system. The immune system attacks the body tissues which is usually triggered by an antigen in a genetically predisposed person. The synovial membranes are attacked and they go on to degrade and malform the articular surfaces of the bones (Tucker 2005).

Rheumatoid arthritis of the wrist is common, due to thickening of the joint and related tendon sheaths, which leads to swelling, pain, stiffness and increased heat in the affected area. Many small joints are affected, for example on the hands and feet. In severe cases of rheumatoid arthritis joint spaces disappear and the angle at which the bone ends meet changes, due to ligament laxity. The bone

ends become rough, eroded and noduled, by aggregates of inflamed tissue cells collecting around the bone ends. Above the nodules the skin is thin and fragile; this in turn results in restricted movement. A diagnosis is confirmed if a blood test detects an antibody that is associated with rheumatoid arthritis.

Treatment
The use of splints can help, especially for those patients whose wrists are affected and who suffer from increased pain at night. When the individual is not experiencing acute pain and is in remission gentle exercise can help to keep the affected joints mobile.

Gout

This is a condition that is caused by an excess of uric acid in the body, which is normally excreted in urine. In gout this substance collects in the synovial fluid of a joint forming needle-like crystals, which can cause sudden and severe pain, swelling and redness in a joint. Often the joint affected is the greater toe, although it can occur in any part of the body. It is known to affect the male population more than the female.

Diagnosis can be made from measurement of the level of uric acid in the blood if the patient presents in an acute phase.

Treatment
In the acute presentation treatment will be by NSAIDs to reduce the level of discomfort in the joint. To reduce the risk in the chronic phase the drug of choice is allopurinol (300–600mg), but it is not normally indicated unless the attacks are frequent or there is associated renal impairment.

The muscular system

While the bones and joints form the framework of the body, they are unable to move the body on their own. In order to create movement of the skeletal system, motion comes from the relaxation and contraction of muscles. Muscles constitute approximately 23% of total body weight in women and 40% in men.

The next section will examine the function of muscles and how normal function can be affected; common disorders will also be discussed.

Muscle tissue

There are three types of muscular tissue: skeletal, smooth and cardiac. For the purpose of this chapter only skeletal tissue will be addressed. Skeletal muscle is striated tissue that can be made to contract and relax by conscious control. They are controlled by a part of the peripheral nervous system known as the somatic nervous system.

Functions of skeletal muscle
Through sustained contraction or alternating contraction and relaxation, muscle tissue has six main key functions:

● Contraction of muscles that produce movement. This occurs through the ability to contract and relax in a coordinated manner
● Postural muscles maintain the body in a stable position
● Both muscles and tendons help to stabilise joints
● Assists the movement of substances within the body. As skeletal muscle contraction, helps to aid the return of blood to the heart
● Aids temperature control. This occurs as muscle contraction produces heat and shivering and vasodilatation of capillaries cools the body down, while vasoconstriction helps to retain heat
● The diaphragm regulates breathing.

Structure of skeletal muscle
Muscle cells are called fibres because of their cylindrical shape and long length. Each fibre has many nuclei and myofibrils that contain both actin and myosin filaments. The muscle cells appear striped due to the actin and mysosin filaments arrangement. The fibre is surrounded by a sarcolemma, which is the plasma membrane of a muscle cell that surrounds the sarcoplasm, the cytoplasm of a skeletal muscle cell.

How muscles work
In order for muscles to move, they need to be stimulated into action by a nerve impulse. This in turn will then cause the muscle to contract creating a movement. Motor nerves cause movement and break down into many nerve endings, with each one stimulating a single muscle fibre. When the muscle contracts, the actin filaments slide between the myosin filaments causing a shortening of the fibres.

Bones act as levers for movement. When the muscle contracts, it causes a muscle action at the joint. Muscles

must cross a joint in order to cause a movement at that joint. There are many different actions for different muscles but all muscles work by contraction (Tucker 2005).

For a muscle to contract when stimulated by a nerve, its cells require oxygen and fuel in order to produce enough energy for muscle contraction to take place. For this purpose muscles use glucose and fats. Muscles have the ability to store glucose as glycogen, which is converted back to glucose when required for muscle action. Muscle burns the glucose and fats to produce energy by combining with oxygen. When a muscle is required to contract and relax over a long period of time more oxygen is required to burn the fuel. This results in heavy breathing so that an increased amount of oxygen can be obtained. If the muscle is not allowed enough time to recover, the muscle will become deprived of oxygen, causing a build-up of lactic acid, a by-product of energy production. When lactic acid builds up in a muscle it causes a burning sensation and presents in varying degrees of discomfort. Oxygen is needed to excrete lactic acid, so the individual will need to stop or slow down the activity being undertaken. Lactic acid affects the end plate of the nerve controlling the muscle and so prevents destructive overaction of the muscle.

Applying Theory to Practice: Exercise 8.4

- Compose a list of the different movements that you are aware of. Think about how you could describe these movements to a colleague.
- Why is it important to have knowledge of movements that the body can perform?
- Add this list to your developing portfolio and on completion of this chapter expand your portfolio with any new terminology that you have learnt.

Some of the movements that are created by muscles are mentioned below with brief descriptions. It is important to have an understanding of the terminology used to describe movements as it can make it easier when describing a patient's presenting condition or injury and also make documentation succinct.

- **Flexion** – bend or flex a limb inwards
- **Extension** – bend or extend a limb outwards
- **Abduction** – move a limb away from the midline

- **Adduction** – move a limb towards the midline
- **Inversion** – turning towards centre e.g. sole of foot
- **Eversion** – turning outwards from centre
- **Rotation** – rotate head at neck
- **Supination** – turn a limb to face upwards
- **Pronation** – turn a limb to face downwards
- **Dorsiflexion** – flexing/bending foot up (with toe up and heel down)
- **Plantarflexion** – flexing/bending foot down towards the ground (think of planting the foot to the ground!)
- **Opposition** – opposing the thumb to little finger

Demonstrating these movements with a colleague will help in an understanding of the different movements.

Disorders affecting the muscular system

Guillan–Barré syndrome

This normally occurs after one to three weeks following an initial infection. The cause of Guillan–Barré syndrome is often identified as campylobacter infection.

The patient may complain of muscle weakness in the distal limbs and often numbness in the same region too. Gradually this weakness and numbness progress and ascends; it can occur over several days or take up to several weeks to progress. The pattern appears to be that the weakness and numbness occur in the fingers and toes. There can be mild cases where there would be little disability before the patient recovers of their own accord, but there can be more extreme cases. In approximately 20% of cases the patient can become paralysed as their respiratory and facial muscles are affected (Kumar & Clarke 1998). These patients would need care in hospital with careful monitoring to ensure that their condition does not deteriorate and require further intervention. The diagnosis is confirmed from the clinical picture and from nerve conduction tests.

Treatment

Some cases do not require treatment and recovery seems to occur in approximately three weeks. In the more severe cases the paralysis may be severe and the patient requires assisted ventilation and the support of intensive care. Recovery from Guillan–Barré syndrome may be incomplete and there may be some residual paralysis.

Abnormal contractions of skeletal muscle

Cramp

This is a painful, spasmodic contraction, which is involuntary. The most usual cause is vigorous exercise, but it can also occur in certain metabolic disorders. For example, when there is a deficiency of sodium or water in the blood. A deficiency of calcium can also cause cramp, as can a lack of blood supplying oxygen to a certain part of the body, for example, sitting awkwardly. A common example of cramp is colic, when muscles in the stomach and other organs of the abdomen are affected.

Treatment

Most often cramp in a limb resolves spontaneously and requires no treatment, but if it is due to a metabolic disorder this will need treating accordingly.

Strain

Injury to a muscle or tendon is often caused by overexertion or overuse. Warming up before exercise is essential to prevent damage.

Treatment

Treatment depends on the severity of the sprain; the principal guidance is based on the PRICE acronym:

● Prevention
● Rest
● Ice (application in short bursts)
● Compression
● Elevation.

Myositis

Myositis is inflammation of a muscle.

Treatment

Treat with rest and NSAIDs if the condition is due to overuse of the muscle. It is rare to develop myositis spontaneously.

Ligaments

Ligaments are dense bundles of collagenous fibres that run in parallel lines. Their function is to connect bone to bone (Figure 8.15).

They are often formed from the outer layer of the joint capsule, but can also connect nearby non-articulating

Figure 8.15 Ligaments

bones. Ligaments contain numerous sensory nerve cells, which are capable of responding to speed, movement and the position of a joint, as well as to stretching or pain. The sensory neurons constantly transmit such information to the brain, which in turn sends signals to the muscles via motor neurones. In this way the body is usually able to avoid damage or undue stress to ligaments through a corrective action. Even so, excessive movements or trauma may result in spraining or a rupture of the ligaments, common in injuries sustained through sporting activities.

When damaged, ligaments are extremely painful, due to the high number of sensory nerve cells. Ligamentous damage does not repair quickly due to a limited vascular blood supply.

Function

The function of ligaments is chiefly to strengthen and stabilise the joint in a passive way. They are unlike muscles as they cannot actively contract, nor can they stretch. There are exceptions to this rule, with a few ligaments that contain a high proportion of yellow elastic fibres. Ligaments are placed under tension by certain positions of joints and slackened by others.

Injuries to or surrounding joints usually involve the tearing of a ligament, often accompanied by a muscle tear resulting in pain and varying degrees of swelling.

An ankle sprain is a common presentation to walk-in centres, minor injury units and even emergency departments. Normal history involves an inversion injury to the ankle while playing sport, but can occur with an eversion

Scenario 8.2

Right Ankle Injury

Sam Jones attends A&E with a complaint of right ankle injury. This was sustained one day previously while playing football. The injury he describes sounds like an inversion injury and he was unable to walk immediately or continue playing football. He limps into the emergency department.

On examination the ankle is swollen and bruised, this extends down to the dorsum of the foot. The skin is intact with no obvious deformity.

The ankle has a normal temperature, no excess warmth or coolness. Capillary refill is <2 seconds. Pedal pulses are present and equal.

Maximum tenderness can be felt over the lateral maleolus. There is no discomfort to the fifth metatarsal or head of the fibula.

Mr Jones is weight-bearing although in discomfort. (He has not taken any analgesia.)

Range of movement is limited, especially on dorsi and plantar flexion.

X-ray shows no bone injury. Mr Jones is diagnosed as having a sprained right ankle.

Applying Theory to Practice: Exercise 8.5

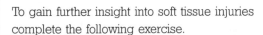

To gain further insight into soft tissue injuries complete the following exercise.

- What treatment will this patient require?
- Consider the importance of health education for this patient.
- Will a severe sprain result in long-term instability of the joint?

injury too. An appreciation of the anatomy of the ankle and the mechanism of injury can assist with the diagnosis. It is important to note that an X-ray is not always required and standard practice should be to follow the guidelines of the Ottowa Ankle Rules (Stiell et al. 1995) to avoid the necessity of an X-ray and the subsequent exposure to radiation.

Treatment

An X-ray confirms that there is no bone injury and therefore a diagnosis of sprain can be made. The treatment is to try and restore normal function as quickly as possible. RICE: Rest, Ice, Compression and Elevation are normally recommended, as the traditional method of treating soft tissue injuries. The use of tubigrip™ has generated a lot of debate in recent years. Pollard and Cronin (2005) write that sometimes compression bandaging can create swelling rather than reduce it. Sometimes patients feel that the tubigrip™ is assisting them. They should be advised on removal of the bandage at night and to continue with regular elevation.

Health education on care of the ankle following a significant injury needs to be addressed. Return to sports that involve running should be avoided until normal function is restored; this will vary on an individual basis, and should be gradual. The patient should also seek advice if function is not fully restored, as there may be a need for physiotherapy input.

Fascia

Fascia is made from white, fibrous, dense connective tissue and can be found in all parts of the body. Fascia plays an important part in the musculoskeletal system, and has different names depending on what it surrounds. Epimysium surrounds the whole muscle; perimysium surrounds the bundles/fascicles of fibres; and endomysium surrounds the muscle fibres/cells.

Superficial fascia

This is a continuous sheet of fibrous connective tissue and is found between the dermis of the skin and the deep fascia of the muscle. It is also called the subcutaneous layer when referring to the skin.

Functions

- to help the skin move over underlying structures
- To provide a passageway for nerves, blood vessels, lymph vessels
- To conserve body heat due to the presence of adipose tissue (fat)

Deep fascia

This is a sheet of dense connective tissue that is wrapped around a muscle forming an inelastic sheath to hold it in place. It is thicker in areas of the body that are unprotected.

Functions

- Assists muscle action through the tension and pressure it provides
- Provides a broad surface for muscle attachment

Tendons

These are formed from muscle and fascia combining together and extending beyond the end of muscle into flat bands or round cords. They are very strong and are not at all elastic; they have a poor blood supply and very few nerves. Tendons are made from white, fibrous, densely packed connective tissue. Under a microscope, closely packed bundles of parallel collagen fibres would be visible.

Function

To connect muscle to bone via the periosteum.

Injuries

There are two main injuries that occur to tendons:

- Rupture/division
- Acute or chronic inflammation due to overuse

Tendons tear when they are stretched to 5% or more beyond their normal length (Purcell 2004), but they can also be divided by blunt force or cut. Tendons with poor blood supply, for example, the distal part of the Achilles tendon, can be prone to rupture.

Achilles tendon injury

The Achilles tendon is the second most ruptured tendon in the body. Apart from the quadriceps, it suffers rupture more than any tendon (Ballas et al. 1998, cited in Kerr 2005). This occurs when there is sudden plantarflexion of the foot. Patients will often describe the injury as a sudden popping sensation to the ankle or as though they were kicked from behind in the leg above the heel. It is vital that these types of injuries are diagnosed promptly as misdiagnosis can have a long-term impact on the patient's everyday life. They may develop an abnormal gait or have chronic pain (Kerr 2005).

Treatment

Achilles tendon ruptures can be treated in two different ways: by surgical intervention where the ends of the tendon are reunited and surgically sewn together with sutures followed by immobilisation in a cast, with the ankle plantar flexed; or by conservative management where the leg is placed in a cast in plantar flexion held in equinus position. The objective is to enable the tendon ends to reunite by approximating them and then holding them in position to encourage healing. The cast is changed and the position of the foot gently altered over the course of treatment.

Both conservative and surgical measures have their advocates, but neither guarantees freedom from

Scenario 8.3

Limb Amputation

Boris Bulthorp-Smyth, a 38-year-old man, was brought into the emergency department three days ago following a high speed crash in which his car crashed into a ditch. His arm was crushed resulting in a comminuted compound fracture. The arm was unsalvageable and had to be amputated just below the elbow yesterday morning. He is now a patient on the orthopaedic ward where you are on placement. You are caring for him on a late shift; on assessment your findings include:

Airway clear, Mr Bulthorp-Smyth answers any questions you ask him but fails to engage in conversation. His respiratory rate is 14, pulse 71, blood pressure 131/72, temperature 38.8. You ask him to show you his dressing site as he has his arm covered by a blanket. His wound dressing is intact and there is no sign of bleeding or exudate penetrating through the layers. You notice that he has not washed or shaved and that his hair is uncombed. His dinner is still sitting on the bedside table untouched.

You complete a pain assessment and administer Mr Bulthorp-Smyth his medications, which include antibiotics and analgesics. He describes his pain score as 1 out of 4, which equals mild. You ask him if he has been undertaking his exercise plan. He states he cannot see the point, as the arm is useless. You inform him that if he fails to use his shoulder it may become frozen and that muscle wasting may ensue, resulting in poor healing of the wound and decreased focus. He states he does not care and wishes he were dead. He then turns his back towards you to end the conversation.

complications (McRae 2004). Possible complications include re-rupture, poor wound healing, infection, deep vein thrombosis from being in a cast, and chronic stiffness of the ankle. Some patients are more suitable for conservative treatment, for example the elderly or those considered a high anaesthetic risk, while the surgical route seems to be indicated in the younger, athletic patient.

Some of the common presenting complaints involving tendons include damage to extensor or flexor tendons resulting in trigger finger/mallet finger, and chronic inflammation of tendons generally through repetitive use i.e. tenosynovitis/tendonitis.

Assessment and analysis of patient presentation

Mr Bulthorp-Smyth has two immediate problems. First, he may be demonstrating signs of an acute infection; and because he has had surgery involving a major long bone there is the potential for osteomyelitis or septicaemia, both of which are life-threatening. Although Mr Bulthorp-Smyth is currently taking antibiotics, they will not necessarily be effective. His orthopaedic team need to be urgently contacted. They will visualise the wound, inspecting for any signs of infection such as heat, offensive odour, inflammation and tracking extending proximally up the arm. Increased pain is also a good indicator although complications such as compartment syndrome may cause this. The wound may have become infected during the initial surgery or during the first dressing change; the causative agent may be resistant to the antibiotics prescribed or the infection may exist in a part of the body such as the bone where this particular antibiotic is ineffective. His second problem is that he appears to be neglecting himself, demonstrated through his unkempt appearance, and is deliberately hiding the affected arm away.

Limb loss – the facts

There are many causes of an alteration in an individual's body image, these include:

- Traumatic amputations/injuries
- Cancerous growths or tumours
- Non-malignant growths
- Burn injuries
- Weight gain/loss
- The ageing process.

After the First World War it was commonplace to see young otherwise fit men using crutches due to traumatic amputations of their legs. Today, traumatic limb loss is again at an increased rate due to global conflicts such as Iraq and Afghanistan where soldiers are being physically traumatised by landmines or explosive devices. In African states such as Sierra Leone, young men have had the lower part of their arms removed with machetes due to differing political viewpoints. In the modern Western world most traumatic amputations are associated with industrial accidents or road traffic accidents. This can be devastating for the individual and end their intended career or lifestyle.

Psychosocial aspects

How an individual reacts to an acute alteration to their body image is dependent on many factors: for some the ability to overcome both the physiological and psychological trauma is almost seen as a challenge of physical and mental courage, this is clearly demonstrated by the story of Douglas Bader during the Second World War. His exploits have been immortalised in books and movies (Brickhill 2000). For others a lifetime of depression and social withdrawal are potentials.

Applying Theory to Practice: Exercise 8.6

Why do you think people react so differently when confronted by trauma or an alteration to body image?

How do you think you would react?

Would you expect others to act in the same way as you or do you accept that an individual's response will always be unique although many characteristics may be similar and happen at differing times?

Suffering a traumatic loss of a limb has been described in a similar way to the loss of a family member or friend, in that the individual must go through several stages of grief in order to regain a sense of normality and acceptance of their loss. These stages of grief are described as:

- Acceptance
- Denial (not believing/accepting the loss)
- Adjustments (getting on with ordinary life)
- Letting go.

Applying Theory to Practice: Exercise 8.7

Which of these stages do you feel Mr Bulthorp-Smyth is in?

● Do you have a duty of care to assist him with accepting the alteration to his body image or are you solely concerned with his physiological problems such as infection?

Professional issues

Nurses need to understand that the patient will have to live with an alteration of their body image for the rest of their lives and should therefore try and understand the viewpoint of the patient. Despite the wide use of the term body image, it is a poorly defined term. Atkinson (2002) describes body image as a non-static concept, developing early in life and altering at the key stages of life experience and development such as puberty, pregnancy and ageing. One definition of altered body image is a state in which personal distress indicates that the body no longer supports the individual's self-esteem, causing social dysfunction to the individual. This is caused by limited coping strategies or an overwhelming injury, disease, disability or social stigma (Price 1995). Gaining insight into the individual's feelings, showing empathy and empowering the patient to regain control of their life are essential elements to providing quality of care and assisting them to regain their long-term health and social well-being. Qualitative tools such as the Amputee Body Image Scale exist that can be used to assess or measure how a patient perceives, or feels about, his or her body disturbance (Breakely 1997).

Mr Bulthorp-Smyth is currently failing to accept the loss of his limb. His feelings probably involve anger directed at himself; these feelings can quickly be directed at others if he is pushed too far too early. This means a gentle, non-threatening approach to his care is essential; this will involve active listening skills. Encouraging the patient to eat is also essential to the physiological process of wound healing; supplements may need to be prescribed if failure to eat continues. Family support or the input from friends can provide far better outcomes than healthcare intervention alone. His friends and family will also have psychological needs, but they may be able to assist him into accepting this change and overcoming his

newfound disability. Support networks have been shown to be extremely effective to the long-term prognoses of patients. Most debilitating or disease states have national and international support networks whereby those afflicted can discuss their personal experiences and share ways of overcoming problems they may encounter. There can be many positive aspects involved in this and patients should be given information on their existence. Counselling may also be an option; many associations or help groups will have details of reputable practitioners with whom the patient may seek a consultation.

Assessment of the musculoskeletal system

To be able to fully assess and treat injuries to the musculoskeletal system it is essential that a systematic approach be applied. This part of the chapter will look at a systematic approach that can be applied to both acute and chronic disorders of the musculoskeletal system. Before beginning an assessment of the injury, establishing cause and prior problems need to be discussed with the patient, as this in turn will have an impact on the physical assessment. The general pattern for assessment of an individual with a musculoskeletal injury is the Look, Feel, Move principle, but the same principle can be applied to any person with a musculoskeletal problem whether it is chronic or acute.

Acquiring information

When assessing patients with any injury or disorder of the musculoskeletal system, it is important to take a full history. It is best to allow the patient to tell you in their own words what has happened and the reason why they have attended. The patient may be a child, a person who cannot speak English or an elderly patient who has dementia. Always look at the individual and look for non-verbal cues, as this will help you gather important data, for example, how much pain they appear to be in. As well as asking about the injury you need to acquire other information, which is listed below:

Presenting complaint (PC)

● What has happened that has made the patient seek medical assistance?

Applying Theory to Practice: Exercise 8.8

Before commencing this part of chapter:

- Compose a list of the injuries to the musculoskeletal system that you think may require emergency treatment
- Write a list of the questions you need to ask when a patient presents with an acute injury
- What information helps you to ascertain the type of injury and the correct course of treatment?

Add this list to your developing portfolio and on completion of this chapter expand your portfolio with the new disorders you have gained knowledge on and elaborate on how these disorders affect physiological function and how to recognise a patient with them.

Think of the advice you would give to a patient presenting with these problems to ensure that they have a quick recovery and can return to normal function rapidly .

History of presenting complaint (HPC)

- How did it happen?
- When did it happen?
- Why did it happen?
- What happened?
- Where did it happen?
- Past medical history
- Medication
- Allergies
- Social history

When this information has been elicited, the patient will require examination. This can be applied by structuring the assessment in the following way:

Look

If the patient is walking, observation of their gait and posture is essential as this may lead you to document postural deformity, which may be a chronic problem or may give a clear indicator of an acute injury, for example, if they are limping. If examining a limb, the principles are

the same and below are some aide-mémoires of what should be looked for and in turn documented.

Swelling

It is important to note if there is any swelling present and, if so, whether it is localised or diffuse. If the swelling is localised think of the underlying structures that therefore may be affected. This goes hand in hand with considering the mechanism of injury. Establishing this simple information can help you form a working diagnosis. If swelling is confined to a joint, it can be one of three problems:

- **Blood** (haemoarthrosis): this can occur from a recent injury, but can also occur if the patient is suffering from a blood coagulation defect. It would be unusual for a blood disorder to be discovered through an acute injury and is more likely to be an ongoing problem that the patient is aware of.
- **Effusion**: caused by excess synovial fluid. This can occur from trauma or a non-pyogenic inflammatory process. A couple of examples of the latter are rheumatoid arthritis or osteoarthritis.
- **Pus** (pyarthrosis): possibly from acute pyogenic infection (McRae 2004).

If swelling is diffuse and travels further than the joint, it can often indicate a more serious cause. This can be seen in the presentation of a patient suffering from a major infection, tumours or a problem with lymphatic and venous drainage.

Bruising

Is there any bruising present? This may be an indicator of trauma, and it is important to note whether the bruising is relatively new or if it is old; this can be apparent by the discoloration of the bruise. This is vitally important to document especially if there is any indicator of abuse, whether it be child abuse, elder abuse or if the patient is a victim of domestic violence. Potentially this could have been established from the history given of the injury by the patient.

Deformity

Is there any obvious deformity, and if there is, does it require urgent treatment to protect the integrity of the limb? Is the skin shiny and appears under pressure from the underlying bones? Patients presenting with an obvious deformity to a lower limb, often a fracture dislocation,

need urgent treatment and this should not be delayed for X-ray.

Wounds

Are there any wounds, or is the skin intact? If there is a wound, what does it look like? Is it a straight laceration or jagged? Is the wound clean or dirty? Is the wound bleeding? Is it controllable or not? Is the wound deep? Are underlying structures visible and if so to what depth? Purcell (2004) writes that the fundamental concept of wound assessment and treatment is never to close a wound unless you have seen the base. Is there any evidence of necrosis to surrounding skin edges? Most of the above questions can be addressed by observing the wound with the naked eye. However, if the wound is bleeding excessively, it may hinder the ability to observe the base.

Discoloration or oedema

This may occur due to infection or trauma. Also consider past medical history as this may give information as to a potential reason for the oedema. For example, a patient who has had a mastectomy may have lymphoedema of the arm on the affected side, which has then been injured.

Muscle wasting

This occurs in a long-term condition and is rarely seen in acute injuries, although it may depend on the time lapse before the patient presents. It often occurs because of disuse due to pain or inability to move the affected area. It can also occur from denervation of muscles (McRae 2004).

Look to see if there is any change in the posture of the patient; consider congenital abnormalities, previous injuries and past medical history. Once the look phase has been performed, the feel/palpate process can be carried out and findings documented accordingly.

Quite often you will find a diagram of the affected injury in the patient's notes. This is particularly useful when describing and demonstrating certain injuries, especially wounds.

Under the look section it is important that the affected side is compared to the non-injured side.

Feel

Often this section of examination is termed as palpation. The object of feeling the affected area is to discover a variety of different factors, which are mentioned below.

This assists in the differential diagnosis and helps to establish what might be wrong with the presenting symptoms.

Temperature

Establishing whether a limb/joint is warm or cool is important in a differential diagnosis. The information that you are looking for is whether the increase in temperature is localised or more diffuse. Generally, when the increase in temperature is localised, it suggests inflammation of underlying structures. If the warmth is more widespread, it means a larger amount of tissue is involved. If a limb is cool or cold it may indicate that for some reason the circulation is impaired.

Tenderness

Seeking where the point of maximum tenderness can be elicited is vital in trying to form a differential diagnosis. If there is generalised tenderness, it can make a diagnosis more difficult, but once again knowledge of the underlying anatomy can assist. When examining a joint it is important to examine the joint above and the joint below the affected area. Also the non-affected side should be examined and comparisons made.

Sensation

Sensation should be assessed in all patients who present with an injury, whether it is an ankle injury or a wound. Assessing sensation is vitally important as it may indicate areas of paraesthesia, which could direct you to a nerve injury. Sensation is assessed for both light touch and pin prick and there are a variety of different methods to assist in this assessment. If sensation is normal then this should be documented.

Perfusion

Assessing the capillary refill, which should be less than 2 seconds, is a key indicator of damage to the affected area. If there is a delayed capillary refill it should be reported on and acted on accordingly. Assessment of distal pulses should be assessed and documented. Any absent pulses need to be reported immediately, but beware that in the feet they can be difficult to find in the first place.

Movement

Generally, acute injuries that affect a limb will be associated with some restriction of movement within the

related joint. Assessment of movement takes two forms: active movement and passive movement. Patient compliance is vital in order to be able to fully assess the range of movement of the injured part. First, the patient should be asked if they can perform a range of movements and any restriction documented. Once again it is essential that the good side be compared to the bad. The range of movements assessed will be dependent on the presenting complaint. This is also pertinent in the patient with a chronic condition or injury.

Once attempted active movement has been assessed the examiner will try and put the affected limb through a range of passive movements. Movement can be restricted due to an injury; also consider if the patient is in pain whether it is advisable to administer analgesia and then reassess the range of movement when it becomes effective. A restricted range of movement is normally always due to a mechanical cause.

Conclusion

Now that you have completed this chapter you will have gained considerable insight into both the functioning of the musculoskeletal system and the psychological and physical impact failure or alteration of the system can have. Reinforce your knowledge by continually reviewing the anatomy and physiology of the musculoskeletal system, as this is essential to adding this knowledge to your long-term memory. When you encounter new patients who have sustained injuries, imagine how these injuries or illnesses may have affected their lives. This may include minor changes, such as a reduced lifting capacity, through to the inability to play instruments or participate in their chosen career. By empathising with a patient's situation and understanding the inner workings of the body, nurses can have a significant impact on the future well-being of patients within their care.

Chapter 8 Summary Quiz

1. The skeleton is described as being predominantly divided into two parts:

A. The axial and appendicular skeleton
B. The limbs and the torso
C. The legs, arms and trunk
D. The torso and peripheries

2. There are two main types of bone tissue:

A. Long and flat
B. Compact and large
C. Compact and cancellous
D. Dense and superficial

3. Bones store minerals, why can this be dangerous?

A. Too much potassium can lead to the bone wasting
B. Too much calcium can lead to rickets
C. Poisonous minerals such as mercury can be accumulated leading to cancer
D. Storing minerals means the body could be in short supply

4. Common diseases affecting the bones include:

A. Osteoporosis
B. Paget's disease
C. Osteoarthritis
D. All of the above

5. Three common malformations of the spine are:

A. Scoliosis, moleosis, kyphosis
B. Lordosis, lumpyosis, kyphosis
C. Scoliosis, lordosis, kyphosis
D. Kyphosis, lumpyosis, scoliosis

6. Spina bifida is caused by:

A. A congenital deformity
B. Cancer of the spine
C. Interbreeding
D. A lack of fruit and vegetables

7. The spine consists of how many vertebrae?

A. 33
B. 31
C. 21
D. 65

8. Name the three types of muscular tissue:

A. Skeletal, rough and splenic
B. Skeletal, smooth and cardiac
C. Skeletal, smooth and cylindrical
D. Skeletal, bone and brain

9. Ligaments connect:

A. Bone to tissue
B. Bone to muscle
C. Bone to ligaments
D. Bone to bone

10. Eversion means:

A. Turning inwards
B. Twisting laterally
C. Turning outwards from centre
D. Bringing opposing bones together

Further reading

McRae, R. (2004) *Clinical Orthopaedic Examination*, 5th edn. Churchill Livingstone: Edinburgh.

Purcell, D. (2004) *Minor Injuries: A Clinical Guide*. Churchill Livingstone: Edinburgh.

Saladin, K. (2007) *Anatomy and Physiology: The Unity of Form and Function*, 4th edn. McGraw-Hill Higher Education: New York.

Tortora, G. & Grabowski, S. (2001) *Introduction to the Human Body*. John Wiley & Sons: New York.

http://orthoinfo.aaos.org/topic.cfm?topic=A00097

References

Abramowitz, A.J. & Schepsis, A.A. (1994) Chronic exertional compartment syndrome of the lower leg. *Orthopaedic Review* 23(3): 219–55.

Adams, J. (1986) *Outline of Orthopaedics*. Churchill Livingstone: Edinburgh.

American College of Surgeons (2004) *Advance Life Support for Doctors*, 7th edn. American College of Surgeons: Chicago.

Atkinson, A. (2002) Body image considerations in patients with wounds. http://www.jcn.co.uk/journal.asp?MonthNum=10&YearNum=2002&Type=backissue&ArticleID=523 (accessed 28 July 2007).

Ballas, M.T., Mytko, J. & Mannarino, F. (1998) Commonly missed orthopaedic problems. *American Family Physician* 57(2): 267–74.

Breakely, J.W. (1997) Body image: the lower-limb amputee. *Journal of Prosthetics and Orthotics* 9(2): 58–66.

Brickhill (2000) *Reach for the Sky: The Story of Douglas Bader – Hero of the Battle of Britain*. Cassell Publishing: London.

Edwards, S. (2004) Acute compartment syndrome. *Emergency Nurse* 12(3): 32–8.

Fitzgerald, A.M. (2000) Long-term sequelae of fasciotomy wounds *British Journal of Plastic Surgery* 53: 690–3.

Kerr, J. (2005) Achilles tendon injury: assessment and management in the emergency department. *Emergency Nurse* 13(2): 32–8.

Kumar, P. & Clark, M. (1998) *Clinical Medicine*, 4th edn. W.B. Saunders: Edinburgh.

McRae, R. (2004) *Clinical Orthopaedic Examination*, 5th edn. Churchill Livingstone: Edinburgh.

Pollard, A. & Cronin, G. (2005) Compression bandaging for soft tissue injury of the ankle: a literature review. *Emergency Nurse* 13(6): 20–5.

Porter, K. & Greaves, I. (2003) Crush injury and crush syndrome: a consensus statement. *Emergency Nurse* 11(6): 26–30.

Price, B. (1995) Assessing altered body image. *Journal of Psychiatric and Mental Health Nursing* 2: 169–75.

Purcell, D. (2004) *Minor Injuries: A Clinical Guide*. Churchill Livingstone: Edinburgh.

Stiell, I., Wells, G. & Laupacis, A. (1995) Multicentre trial to introduce the Ottawa ankle rules for use of radiography in acute ankle injuries. *British Medical Journal* 311(7005): 594–7.

Tortora, G. & Grabowski, S. (2001) *Introduction to the Human Body*. John Wiley & Sons: New York.

Tucker, L. (2005) *An Introductory Guide to Anatomy and Physiology*. Holistic Therapy Books: Cambridge.

The reproductive system

Lucy Tebbit

Chapter 9 Learning Objectives

- To gain knowledge and understanding of the anatomy and physiology related to the reproductive system
- To gain understanding of several conditions related to the female and male reproductive systems
- To be able to apply theory to practice by understanding the physical signs of these illnesses
- To have insight into the psychosocial aspects of these patients
- To be aware of some of the ethical dilemmas that occur within clinical practice
- To construct solid evidence of professional development for your growing portfolio
- To continue developing the ability to question and critique the evidence base and effectiveness of plans of care

Introduction

The reproductive system is one of the only systems in the body that is dimorphic, meaning it is both functionally and structurally different in males and females.

This chapter will initially focus on the anatomy and physiology of the male and female systems. The reproductive system is particularly important as it enables the human species to survive, but when it becomes diseased or illness affects this system, it can have devastating consequences, both physically and psychologically. Both systems are able to function as a response to male and female sex hormones, which are secreted by the gonads or sex glands.

This chapter will begin with an overview of the reproductive systems, identifying the anatomy and physiology of the male and female systems. Some of the common diseases associated with this system will be addressed. The effect these diseases have on the individual and their partner will also be examined; this will enable the reader to explore both the physiological components of the disease process and the associated psychological aspects.

Applying Theory to Practice: Exercise 9.1

Before reading on:

- Compose a list of diseases you already know that affect both the male and female reproductive systems.

Add this list to your developing portfolio. On completion of this chapter expand your portfolio with the new disorders you have gained knowledge on.

Function

The reproductive system enables the human species to continue and genetic material to be passed from parent cells to daughter cells. Various organs of the reproductive system are formed during the embryonic stage, but normal functioning of the reproductive system begins at puberty and for women lasts approximately thirty years until the menopause occurs. For men the decline is more gradual and slows with the ageing process. The organs can be grouped by their function: the testes and ovaries are known as gonads and their function is to produce gametes and secrete hormones. The testes produce sperm cells and the ovaries produce ova. The ducts transport and store the gametes. Finally there are the accessory sex glands, which support the gametes by producing liquid to support the semen and cervical mucus to receive the spermatozoa.

The male reproductive system is made up of testes, ducts, accessory sex glands and supporting structures, which includes the penis. The penis and scrotum, which contain the testes, are all external organs, which can make them susceptible to damage, as they are not well protected. Conversely the organs of the female

reproductive system are mainly located internally in the lower abdomen; here they are protected from physical trauma, but they can be injured or damaged by disease or infection.

The male reproductive system

Scrotum and testes

The scrotum (Figure 9.1) is a sac-like structure, which originates from the abdomen; it consists of loose skin and fascia. Its function is to support and regulate the temperature of the two testes. The scrotum is divided in two by a septum composed of superficial fascia and smooth muscle fibres, which are known as dartos muscle. This muscle allows wrinkling of the skin and is able to contract to regulate the temperature of the testes. The septum allows the testes to sit in separate sacs. Sperm can only be produced and survive if the temperature is three degrees lower than the core body temperature. The location of the scrotum and testes allows this temperature to be achieved. The cremaster muscle also helps with this regulation as it allows the testes to elevate or descend depending on the environmental temperature. When sexually aroused, the testes move closer to the pelvic cavity to enable the heat to be absorbed. The testes are located high in the abdominal wall during embryonic development; they begin to descend into the scrotum at approximately seven months' fetal development. The testes are oval glands that are approximately 5cm long and 2.5cm wide. The testis (one testicle) divides into 200–300 compartments, known as lobules. Within each lobule there are **seminiferous tubules**, where sperm are produced. The seminiferous tubules contain spermatogenic cells of varying stages of development. Those that are near maturity are known as spermatozoon; these move to the lumen of the tube where they are ready to be released into a series of ducts. They will then be stored in the **ductus epididymis** until they are needed. The youngest cells are known as spermatogonia and are found at the basement membrane, as they mature, they pass through the tubules.

Within the tubules are Sertoli cells (sustentacular cells), which are cells that aid the movement of, and provide nutrients and metabolites to the sperm cells. They also prevent blood-borne cells from reaching the sperm. This is known as the blood–testis barrier. This barrier is important as it prevents the immune system responding to the sperm, as it would be recognised as a foreign body

when in contact with blood. This would produce an immune response that would attack the sperm cells. Seminiferous tubules also contain Leydig cells; these cells secrete the male hormone testosterone. The Sertoli cells also mediate the effect testosterone and follicle-stimulating hormone (FSH) have on the process of spermatogenesis – the production of sperm.

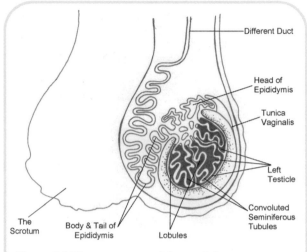

Figure 9.1 The scrotum, testicles and ducts

Scenario 9.1

Testicular Torsion

Rob Short, a 19-year-old Caucasian man, walks into to the emergency department after suffering a sudden onset of pain in his left testicle four hours before. He states that the testicle is swollen although it is not visualised at triage. He looks pale and is sweating.

His vital signs are as follows:
Respiratory rate 18, pulse 98, blood pressure 110/72, temperature 36.9
Pain score on assessment is 3 out of 4
He has no relevant medical history and no known allergies to medicines

Assessment and analysis of patient presentation

Mr Short has presented with clinical signs and symptoms of testicular pain. The most serious condition associated with the sudden onset of pain in the testicles is torsion of the testicle. His vital signs show an increased heart and

respiratory rate, and he is sweating, a sympathetic response to pain. He also says that he has a pain score of 3 out of 4, categorised as severe pain. He asks that a male doctor examine him, as he feels very embarrassed. Mr Short falls within a high-risk category for testicular torsion due to his age. Testicular torsion is more common in teenagers but can occur at any age (NHS Direct 2007). The acute onset of his pain is also another indicator of testicular torsion, a more gradual onset could be a number of other conditions listed in Applying Theory to Practice: Exercise 9.2.

Applying Theory to Practice: Exercise 9.2

Illnesses or Diseases Related to Testicular Pain

Research and record the signs and symptoms of these conditions and possible treatment options:

- Epididymitis – inflammation or infection of epididymis
- Orchitis – inflammation of testes
- Varicocele – varicose veins around testes
- Testicular cancer – tumour of the testes

Pathophysiology

A testicular torsion is the twisting of a testicle. In many cases the men have what is known as a bell clapper deformity, when the testicles are able to freely rotate and the testicles sit significantly lower in the scrotum; the patient may not be aware of this deformity. Patients with bell clapper deformity are more at risk of torsion as the testicle can move more freely enabling the spermatic cord to become twisted. The spermatic cord contains the vas deferens, autonomic nerve, testicular veins and artery. When the cord becomes twisted, it occludes the blood supply to the testicle. If the testicle is not surgically untwisted within six hours, it will infarct and the testicle will perish. If the man ignores the symptoms for more than six hours, the testicle may be unsalvageable; this may lead to an orchiectomy (removal of testicle). The fertility or sexual function of these men should not be affected as the remaining testicle can still produce testosterone and sperm. If the blood supply is restored during surgery these men will have normal sexual function and fertility too.

In conjunction with Cancer Research UK, the Department of Health (2005) produced a document entitled *A Whole New Ball Game* to encourage men to examine their testicles regularly. It was also produced to raise the awareness of testicular cancer and to make men less embarrassed about seeking help when they have problems with their testicles.

Treatment

Mr Short was categorised as 'orange' by the triage nurse in accordance with the Manchester Triage Code (1994). He was taken to the 'majors' area of the department and seen by a male doctor. Mr Short was complaining of severe pain and requested analgesia. After an initial ABC examination the doctor ordered the insertion of a cannula, blood tests and analgesia. The cannula was inserted using an aseptic technique and bloods were taken for urea and electrolytes (U&E), full blood count (FBC), clotting and cross-match. These results would indicate an electrolyte imbalance (U&E), which would be unlikely as Mr Short is normally fit and healthy, raised white cells indicative of infection, bleeding (FBC), clotting disorders, and the cross-match would ascertain his blood group and enable the doctors to access blood transfusion if required during surgery. Mr Short was given morphine sulphate 10mg titrated to his pain. This was in accordance with local protocols and he was given 1mg at a time until his pain had subsided; he was also given an anti-emetic intravenously. The anti-emetic is given prophylactically to prevent nausea and vomiting, a common side effect of morphine.

After the pain relief the doctor was able to examine the testicle. The left testicle was swollen and extremely tender. These findings, along with the acute history of this problem, were indicative of torsion of the testicle. Mr Short was referred to the on-call urologists for further management. The urologist examined Mr Short and explained his findings; some NHS Trusts offer ultrasound as a diagnostic tool. The ultrasound will identify the blood flow to the testicle (UrologyHealth.org), but it is also recognised that time is the most important factor when a patient has a testicular torsion and therefore many urologists will be led by history and clinical findings.

The urologist was keen to take Mr Short to theatre as he had suffered the pain for four hours and the testicle is only viable up to six hours. The surgeon explained the risks of the surgery, and also explained that after he had untwisted the spermatic cord he would perform testicular

fixation on both testicles. This procedure involves sutur-ing the testicles to the inner lining of the scrotum pre-venting future torsion. Mr Short had to sign a consent form for the operation; the surgeon had to explain the risks of surgery, such as infection and also the possibility of proceeding to an orchiectomy if the testicle had already infarcted. Mr Short expressed his fear of having problems with sexual activity and fertility post-operatively. The surgeon had a responsibility to reassure him that sexual function would not be affected and that, despite an orchiectomy, sperm production would continue from the other testicle. He would also explain the likelihood of having to remove the testicle as he has been treated within four hours of initial onset. Mr Short was then taken to theatre for his operation.

Applying Theory to Practice: Exercise 9.3

Blood Test Results

Review and start to learn normal blood results. In clinical placements begin to build up a portfolio of blood results, look at the patients' clinical findings against their results. Identify markers for:

- Infection
- Anaemia
- Renal impairment.

Psychosocial aspects

It is important to consider Mr Short's fears and anxiety about the operation. It is important that he is able to understand the procedure and its possible outcomes; this may help allay his fears. Mr Short was admitted for emergency surgery so was unable to seek out informa-tion; his fear may have led to slower post-operative recovery. Giving pre-operative information can influence a patient's recovery, reduce anxiety and reduce pain scores. Giving good procedural information and behavioural instructions that include how to behave after the opera-tion can result in better post-operative recovery. A further influence on the patient is the language the health pro-fessional uses to explain a procedure to them; a patient is more likely to comply and have surgery if they feel it will be of benefit to them. It is important that patients fully understand the procedure they are having. Mr Short was

worried about the long-term effects on his fertility and sexual health; the surgeon must alleviate these fears.

Conclusion

Mr Short was admitted to the surgical unit post-operatively. He recovered well from surgery. After surgery the nurse measured his vital signs and monitored the wound on his scrotum. This was to ensure that he was haemodynamically stable and that he had no haemor-rhage or infection from the wound. He was offered regular analgesia; when he accepted pain relief a pain score was taken before analgesia was given and then 30 minutes after to ensure that pain relief had taken good effect. It is important to reassess pain scores to evaluate the effect-iveness of the analgesia given. Mr Short continued to recover well post-operatively and was seen by the con-sultant two days later and discharged home. Before being discharged he was given a leaflet about caring for his sutures. He was also advised to wear a scrotal support and the nurse sat with him and spoke to him about his concerns. He was told by the nurse what to expect during his recovery and was advised to have sexual intercourse when he felt ready, but if he had any pain to stop. She also told him the signs and symptoms of infection. It is important to give the patient time to discuss any concerns they have before discharge. It is also good practice to give written information for them to refer to. Many leaflets given out by NHS trusts have a contact telephone number; this enables the patient to leave feeling confident that if

Questioning Clinical Practice: Exercise 9.4

While on clinical placement discover what type of advice is given to patients on discharge from surgical units.

- Do all patients get verbal and written information?
- Can the patient get advice following discharge? Is there a contact number?
- Is there a failed discharge policy, for patients who are readmitted within 24/48 hours?

they develop any symptoms or concerns they have access to a healthcare professional.

Epididymis, ductus (vas) deferens, ejaculatory duct and urethra

The seminiferous tubules move into the straight tubules that connect with a network of ducts known as the rete testis. The rete testis connect with the epididymis via the efferent ducts. The epididymis is an organ that is located on the posterior border of the testes. It is made up of tightly coiled tubes known as the ductus epididymis and is shaped like a comma. The epididymis is lined with pseudostratified columnar epithelium that is encircled by layers of smooth muscle. This smooth muscle helps propel the spermatozoa towards the urethra by a peristaltic action. If the spermatozoa are unused they can be stored for one month before degenerating; they are then reabsorbed by the ductus epididymis. This is possible as it also contains microvillli called **stereocilia**, which increase the surface area of the ductus epididymis, thus enabling reabsorption to occur. The main function of the ductus epididymis is to enable the maturation of the sperm. During this period the sperm increases its motility and becomes fertile.

The ductus epididymis is divided into three areas. The head is the largest portion and it joins the efferent ducts to the ductus epididymis. The body is the narrow, central portion of the epididymis and the tail the smallest area; this continues as the ductus (vas) deferens. It is a long duct that penetrates the inguinal cavity before ascending into the pelvic cavity; here it loops over the urinary bladder. It then dilates into the ampulla; this is located at the terminal end of the vas deferens. The ductus (vas) deferens is supplied with blood via a small vessel that comes from the superior vesical artery. These make up the spermatic cord.

The seminal vesicles (accessory sex gland) and the ductus (vas) deferens then unite; here they form the ejaculatory ducts. The function of the ejaculatory ducts is to eject spermatozoa into the urethra just prior to ejaculation.

The urethra is the final duct for both the urinary and reproductive system. Its function is to act as a passageway for both urine and spermatozoa and fluid known as semen. The male urethra is divided into three areas. The prostatic urethra passes through the prostate gland. As it passes through the urogenital diaphragm it becomes the membranous urethra. Finally it passes through the corpus spongiosum of the penis to the bulb of the penis, known as the spongy urethra. The angle between the membranous urethra and spongy urethra is abrupt; it is important to remember this anatomy when catheterising male patients. The spongy urethra then terminates at the external urethral meatus.

The prostate gland, seminal vesicles, and bulbourethral gland

The prostate gland, seminal vesicles and bulbourethral gland are also known as the accessory sex glands. These glands produce most of the liquid that makes up semen.

The prostate gland is a spherical-shaped gland that lies below the urinary bladder. It secretes a milky fluid that is made up of citric acid and enzymes, which include clotting enzymes and fibrinolysin, enabling the semen to clot after ejaculation; fibrinolysin then decomposes the clot. This fluid aids both the motility of the sperm and keeps it viable. The prostate gland can dramatically increase in size with advancing age (benign prostatic hypertrophy); this can result in partial obstruction of the urethra causing problems with urination.

The seminal vesicles are pouch-like structures that are located at the base of the bladder and lie laterally to the ampulla. This gland secretes alkaline fluid that contains fructose, prostaglandins and fibrinogen. The prostaglandins aid the motility of the sperm and stimulate muscular contraction within the female reproductive tract, thus enabling the sperm to be transported to the ovum. The alkaline in the fluid neutralises the acid within the female reproductive system; if it remained acidic, it would destroy the sperm.

The bulbourethral glands are found as a pair and are located beneath the prostate gland, within the urogenital diaphragm. These glands also secrete an alkaline fluid and mucus that additionally protects the sperm against the acidic environment within the urethra; the mucus acts as a lubricant.

The penis

The penis is a cylindrical structure that can also be divided into three parts: the body, the root and the glans penis (Figure 9.2).

The body has three types of tissue that are cylindrical in shape, known as the corpora cavernosa penis, which makes up two parts of the tissue mass, and the corpus spongiosum penis, which is smaller and contains the spongy urethra. The tissue is enclosed by fascia and skin; these contain erectile tissue, which enables the penis to become erect. The root of the penis is the attached part and contains the bulb of the penis. The glans penis is acorn-shaped and is located at the distal end of the penis. The external urethral meatus is the opening for urine and semen to pass through; this is located at the glans penis. The foreskin, known as the prepuce, covers the glans penis. During sexual stimulation

Figure 9.2 The penis

the arteries supplying the penis dilate and blood floods the blood sinuses. This in turn compresses the veins, trapping the blood in the penis causing an erection. While the penis is erect, ejaculation may occur. This is the forced expulsion of the semen. During ejaculation only semen is expelled as the smooth muscle sphincter located at the bladder closes to prevent urine loss, and also prevent semen entering the bladder. The function of the penis is therefore to expel urine and semen.

Scenario 9.2

Chlamydia

Billy Rodham is a 21-year-old who attends his local genitourinary medicine (GUM) clinic. He complains of a discharge from his penis. He feels otherwise well. He gives a sexual history of having unprotected sexual intercourse three weeks ago with a new partner whom he has only seen in the pub on occasions and is unsure of her name.

Vital signs: respiratory rate 10, pulse 64, blood pressure 128/68 temperature 36.4

No relevant medical history, no previous sexually transmitted infections (STIs)

No allergies

Assessment and analysis of patient presentation

Mr Rodham is physically well; all his vital observations are unremarkable. He is complaining of discharge from his penis and redness around the head of the penis, which he noticed three days ago but was too embarrassed to seek help. The nurse at the clinic establishes a sexual history from him, as this will ultimately aid diagnosis. He confirms that he had recent vaginal intercourse with her and has had unprotected vaginal intercourse twice in the last six months. He has never had a sexually transmitted infection (STI) before. Chlamydia and gonorrhoea are the two most likely causes of his complaint although the nurse feels it is most likely to be chlamydia.

Chlamydia – the facts

Genital chlamydia is the most common sexually transmitted infection (DH 2007). It is caused by the bacterium *Chlamydia trachomatis*. Prevalence is highest in sexually active women aged 16–29 and men aged 18–29 (DH 2007). The bacterium can cause an array of symptoms such as cystitis, vaginal discharge and pelvic inflammatory disease (PID). Ten to thirty per cent of women with chlamydia will go on to develop PID, a major reproductive health problem (DH 2007). PID is a major cause of infertility in women; it can also cause miscarriage and ectopic pregnancies. For men the symptoms include urethral discharge, urethritis (inflammation of the urethra) and epididymitis, and in rare cases a condition called Reiter's syndrome that affects the joints and eyes. It can also lead to impaired fertility in men. The incidence of chlamydia has risen 300% in the last 12 years. There has been a 200% rise in other STIs such as gonorrhoea, and a 300% rise in HIV (NICE 2007). It is suggested that opportunities to discuss and make a risk assessment of young people's risk of contracting an STI may arise while carrying out a consultation about contraception, cervical smears or even travel immunisations (NICE 2007). The aim is to provide one-to-one structured discussions with high-risk individuals in order to help them change their sexual behaviour. In 2002 the DH implemented ten national screening programmes for chlamydia, and by 2006 screening was available in 85 areas.

Psychosocial issues

Mr Rodham has delayed attending the GUM clinic for three days after the symptoms arose because of embarrassment. He was also having unprotected sexual intercourse with an unknown woman. This is a common

presentation of a young person with an STI; unprotected sex is still a major issue in the UK. When deciding on the use of contraception, individuals use both developmental and decision-making processes (Sheeran et al. 1991). These can be categorised into four areas: first, the background of the person – women are more likely to use contraception than men and people with higher educational aspirations are more likely to use contraception than those with lower or no aspirations; second, the interpersonal skills possessed, including a person's attitude to contraception – for example, Mr Rodham may have felt that condoms ruin the spontaneity of sex; the third factor is interpersonal factors such as peers – if Mr Rodham's peers do not use contraception, he is unlikely to. Finally there are situational factors that contribute to the use of contraception. These factors include the spontaneity of the act; the accessibility of the contraception; and finally substance misuse prior to sex may make the individual take more risks. However, it is also important to point out that it may be a problem with confidence. Bandura (1997) believes in self-efficacy, which may occur after a person has had practice at using a condom or by watching a video on how to apply a condom, or by having peer group discussions. It is therefore important that young people have access to sex education in order to have self-efficacy when in situations where contraception is needed. The DH has a policy, (NSF 2004), which aims to deliver many skills including sex education and drugs awareness to children at school.

When discussing contraception with Mr Rodham it is important that the healthcare professional recognises the individual circumstance of each person. They must also take the opportunity to give health advice and safe-sex education to the patient.

Professional issues

There are two main areas when looking at Mr Rodham's care. One is the area of health promotion and the other is the health of the woman he had sexual intercourse with. Chlamydia has increased dramatically over the years and it can affect both men's and women's fertility. It is important that healthcare professionals offer immediate care and relief from the illnesses, but it is equally important to address the health promotion aspects of their care. The Health Belief Model (Rosenstock 1966) believes that a person may be motivated to carry out preventative health behaviours when they have had a perceived threat to their health. Mr Rodham has had a

Questioning Clinical Practice: Exercise 9.5

Questioning Your Own Beliefs

Think about your own beliefs about contraception and STIs.

- Do you believe in the use of contraception?
- Do you think only promiscuous people get STIs?
- Do you think sex education and safe sex should be taught to young children?

Write down your beliefs and reflect on how this affected your own sexual behaviour and how you will deal with patients who have very different belief systems.

test for chlamydia and he may perceive this as a real threat to both the health of his fertility and his sexual health. This may make him ready to listen to and act on advice.

It is important to advise Mr Rodham to use condoms when having sex with unknown partners. Condoms are a highly effective method of barrier contraception (Guillebaud 2000). The biggest advantage is that they are the only form of contraception that reduces the risk of both pregnancy and STIs. Remembering the issues surrounding his beliefs and self-efficacy, it is important to make sure he knows how to use a condom; it may be more appropriate if he talks to a male colleague or peer.

It is also important that if the patient has a positive chlamydia result, they ensure that any sexual partners are tested. As a healthcare professional it is important that this area is not forgotten. Mr Rodham had only met his most recent partner in a pub: it is therefore important that he knows the serious effect chlamydia can have on female fertility. There may be situations where the nurse knows the patient and his or her partner; this can cause ethical dilemmas as they are bound by the NMC Code of Professional Conduct (2004) not to break confidentiality, but they also have a duty of care. In this situation the nurse must advise the person to tell the partner, as they are not able to break confidentiality, but it is important that they too understand the seriousness of chlamydia. As part of the DH national screening programme there are forms that can be used to inform partners of a positive test result; this document recommends that partners from the

last six months are contacted. This is important to convey to Mr Rodham, who may have had several partners who need to be tested. The GUM clinic may be able to help contact them.

Developing & Delivering Expert Care: Exercise 9.6

Ethical Dilemmas in Practice

- Mr Rodham is 21 years old, but what if he was 14? Ethically should you give him condoms?
- Do you have any obligation to inform his parents?
- How would your decision be supported by the code of professional conduct?

For more information about sexual health, visit www.fpa.org.uk or www.nhsdirect.nhs.uk

Treatment

Mr Rodham has presented to the GUM clinic with symptoms of chlamydia. The current test for men is a urine dipstick, which is slightly less reliable than a swab that can be taken from the opening of the urethra. This, however, is a more painful test than a urine sample. Women can also be tested by the use of urine samples or low vaginal swabs. There are also home testing kits, although these are thought to be less reliable. Mr Rodham is given the news he has chlamydia. The treatment of choice is antibiotics; the most commonly used are azithromycin and doxycycline. Azithromycin is administered as a single dose whereas doxycycline is taken twice daily for seven days. The possible side effects of diarrhoea, nausea and stomach pain are explained to Mr Rodham and he is advised to complete the course. If a patient follows advice and completes the prescribed course of antibiotics, they are likely to make a full recovery and be cured of chlamydia. He will be advised to have safe sex using a condom at least until he has completed the course. If he always uses a condom in the future he is unlikely to become re-infected with chlamydia or any other STI.

Male hormones and spermatogenesis

There are six key hormones that are relevant to male development and the reproductive system:

- Testosterone
- Dihydrotestosterone (DHT)
- Follicle-stimulating hormone (FSH)
- Luteinising hormone (LH)
- Gonadotrophin-releasing hormone (GnRH)
- Inhibin.

Testosterone can be found in the testes and is the main male sex hormone (androgen). It may be reduced and converted into another androgen known as dihydro-testosterone (DHT) in some target cells. There are several functions of testosterone. Prior to birth it stimulates the fetus to develop a male reproductive system and ensures the descent of the testes from the abdominal wall to the scrotum. During this stage of development the DHT stimulates the growth of external genitalia such as the penis. The androgens are also converted to oestrogens and this aids development of certain areas of the brain. At puberty, testosterone and DHT work to ensure the transition from child to sexually mature man. This includes growth of genitals, increased muscle mass and change in skeletal structure. It also deepens the male voice by increasing the size of the larynx. Finally it aids **spermatogenesis** (production of sperm) making the male fertile and is responsible for libido in both men and women.

The **anterior pituitary gland** secretes FSH and LH during puberty. These hormones are known as gonadotrophic hormones. The FSH is responsible for stimulating the Sertoli cells, which in turn initiates spermatogenesis. LH stimulates the Leydig cells to release testosterone. The **hypothalamus** also plays a part by secreting GnRH; this hormone is essential as it regulates the release of FSH and LH. The aim of regulating the hormones is to ensure that testosterone levels remain at a certain concentration in the blood. If the levels are too high, it inhibits the release of GnRH, which in turn reduces the release of LH, this then inhibits the release of testosterone. This is known as a negative feedback system. Finally inhibin is a hormone that regulates spermatogenesis. The hormone is located in the Sertoli cells and is released when spermatogenesis has reached an optimum level for reproduction. This in turn inhibits the secretion of FSH, which then slows the process of spermatogenesis.

Spermatogenesis is the process that occurs in order to produce spermatozoa. On average a man will produce 100 million sperm with each ejaculation. Once ejaculated, sperm have a lifespan of 48 hours in the female reproductive system, but up to 20% of these sperm are abnormal with no tails or two heads. Higher percentages of abnormal sperm or not enough sperm in the semen can lead to infertility. The process of spermatogenesis takes approximately 74 days, and has three phases: mitosis, meiosis and finally spermiogenesis.

Anatomy and Physiology in Action: Exercise 9.7

The previous section provided a basic overview, to reinforce and expand your new knowledge discover what the following terms mean:

- Oligozoospermia
- Azoospermia

Add this information to your portfolio.

The anatomy and physiology of the male reproductive system have been discussed. It is important to find out about some of the pathophysiological changes that can occur within or to this system.

Anatomy and Physiology in Action: Exercise 9.8

The Male Reproductive System

Discover what the following problems are and write a synopsis of your findings for your growing portfolio:

- Cryptorchidism epididymitis
- Inguinal hernia paraphymosis
- Benign protastic hypertrophy

Function of female hormones

In females, **oestrogens** promote the development of reproductive structures, in particular the changes in the endometrium with each cycle, development of the secondary sex characteristics, including development of breasts, voice pitch, hair pattern and the deposit of fat at the hips and abdomen. They also help maintain fluid and electrolyte balance.

Progesterone works with oestrogen to prepare the endometrium for a fertilised ovum and also prepares the mammary glands for milk secretion.

Inhibin, secreted by the corpus luteum (endocrine gland in ovary), inhibits secretion of GnRH and FSH during the uterine cycle.

Relaxin is produced in high quantities in the last trimester of pregnancy to relax the pubic symphysis and dilate the cervix during delivery.

The female reproductive system

Ovaries

The ovaries (female gonads) (Figure 9.3) lie in the pelvic cavity and are ovoid in shape. The function of the ovaries is to house and then expel ova (eggs). The ova are formed during the embryonic stages of life and remain there until puberty where they are released each month ready for fertilisation by the sperm. The ova develop into ovum by a process called oogenesis; this indicates the structural changes between being a collective within the ova and the single egg cell. This will be discussed later in this section. There are two ovaries, located either side of the uterus, and connected by the **fallopian tubes**. The ovaries are held in place by a series of ligaments: the broad ligament is part of the uterus and attaches the ovary to the mesovarium (peritoneum); the ovarian ligament attaches the ovary to the uterus, which is attached to the pelvic wall by the suspensory ligament. The ovaries are supplied with blood from the ovarian artery that is a branch of the abdominal aorta. It is made up of three layers: the epithelium, the tunica albuginea, which is connective tissue, and the stroma, which is made up of a dense outer layer known as the cortex. The cortex contains the ovarian follicles and has an inner layer called the medulla. The ovarian follicles contain oocytes that are at various stages of development. The **vesicular ovarian follicle** (graafian) contains an immature ovum, which is surrounded by fluid; it also releases oestrogens. The **corpus luteum** is a mature ovarian follicle that has ruptured releasing a secondary oocyte; this process is known as ovulation and occurs monthly once puberty has begun. More female hormones are secreted from the corpus luteum, namely oestrogen, progesterone and relaxin.

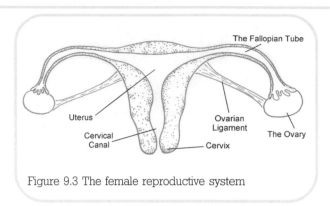

Figure 9.3 The female reproductive system

Fallopian tubes (uterine tubes)

There are two fallopian tubes (Figure 9.3), which connect the ovaries with the uterus. Their function is to propel the ova from the ovaries to the uterus. The opening near the ovary is called the **infundibulum** and is funnel-shaped; at its end there are fimbriae that are finger-like structures that move in a current-like way to allow the ova to pass with ease down the tube. The ampulla is the longest part of the tube; it is here that the ovum can be fertilised by the sperm on the day of ovulation or within 24 hours. The isthmus is the narrow part that joins the tubes to the uterus. The fallopian tubes are made up of three layers: the mucosa, the muscularis and the serosa. The mucosa can be found at the most internal point and is made up of ciliated epithelial cells, which aid the movement of the ovum. The middle layer (muscularis) is made up of an area of circular smooth muscle and an area of longitudinal smooth muscle, which along with the mucosa, aids the movement of the ovum. The serosa is the outer layer and is made up of a serous membrane.

Uterus (womb)

The uterus (Figure 9.3) is a pear-shaped structure and is located on the superior surface of the bladder. As the bladder fills, the position changes; it is then bent backwards on the **cervix** (retroflex). When examining a female abdomen, it is important to ascertain if her bladder is full or empty as this will help locate the position of the uterus. The uterus has several functions. First, it is part of the pathway for the sperm to reach the fallopian tubes, it then implants the fertilised ovum and enlarges to house the growing fetus. It is also the site of menstruation. The uterus has three areas: the fundus, the body and the cervix. The fundus is the dome-shaped structure that rises above the fallopian tubes, the body is the central area of the uterus, and the cervix is the narrow portion that

descends into the vagina. The cervix has an internal and external os. The internal os connects the cervix with the uterine cavity via a small area called the isthmus. The external os is located at the end of the cervix and opens into the vagina. The os is usually closed except when a female experiences a miscarriage or is in labour.

The uterus is made up of three layers of tissue:

- The perimetrium
- The myometrium
- The endometrium.

The perimetrium is the outer layer and is part of the peritoneum. The middle layer is the myometrium, which forms most of the uterine wall; it is made up of three types of smooth muscle, which contract in a coordinated manner in order to expel the fetus during labour. The inner layer is the endometrium which is a highly vascular area that can be divided into two layers; the stratum functionalis, located closest to the uterine cavity, shed during menstruation, and stratum basalis, the permanent layer that aids the stratum functionalis to renew after each menstrual cycle.

Vagina

The vagina (Figure 9.4) measures approximately 10cm in length. The function of the vagina is to act as a passageway for blood flow during the menstrual cycle and the fetus during childbirth, and to receive semen from the penis during penetrative intercourse. The vagina is made up of smooth muscle called muscularis, which is able to stretch to allow a penis to enter the vagina and the fetus to leave the vagina. The lower end of the vagina is called the vaginal orifice where the mucous membrane called

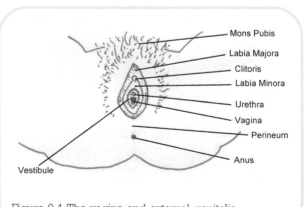

Figure 9.4 The vagina and external genitalia

the hymen is located. This partially closes the orifice but is usually torn during first sexual experience, or in some patients through sports.

External genitalia (vulva)

The external genitalia, or vulva (Figure 9.4), are made up of the following structures:

- Mons pubis – adipose tissue covered in skin and pubic hair
- Labia majora – two folds of skin either side of the vaginal entrance, which contain sebaceous and sweat glands and are covered with pubic hair
- Labia minora – two smaller folds of skin which contain sebaceous glands, not covered with pubic hair
- Clitoris – a small mass of erectile tissue and nerves, which becomes engorged with blood when sexually stimulated
- Vestibule – this area contains the vaginal orifice (opening), external urethral orifice and the para-urethral and Bartholin's glands that both secrete mucus.

Breasts/mammary glands

Before puberty male and female chests appear the same. At puberty the release of oestrogens and **progesterone** encourages breast tissue growth. At sexual maturity the

Figure 9.5 The mammary glands

ovaries secrete progesterone that continues to change the breasts until the mammary glands mature.

The breasts (Figure 9.5) are made up of adipose tissue; the amount of adipose tissue a woman has determines her breast size. The mammary glands are modified sweat glands that produce milk; each gland has 15 to 20 lobes. Each of these lobes then has smaller lobules that contain alveoli. These are milk-secreting glands that move milk into secondary tubules; from here milk enters the mammary ducts. These ducts expand into sinuses called the lactiferous sinuses to store milk. The sinuses terminate at the nipple where milk is ejected from the breast. There are 20–30 lymph nodes in the armpit, which drain fluid from the breast.

Scenario 9.3

Breast Lump

Maria Harman is a 35-year-old Caucasian woman. She is married with children. She attends her GP surgery with a pea-size lump in her right breast. She noticed it in the shower; she examines her breasts regularly. It is not painful.
PMH: mild asthma

Assessment and analysis of patient presentation

On seeing the GP Maria explains she noticed the lump yesterday; her friend has recently been diagnosed with breast cancer so she has been carrying out regular breast self-examination (BSE) in order to detect any changes early. Through regular breast examination the patient or her partner will discover 80% of lumps (breastcancercare.org.uk 2007). The GP is female so did not require a chaperone to examine Mrs Harman. First, a history was taken including dates of her LMP as changes in the breast can be due to hormonal changes around the menstrual cycle. Also relevant medical and familial history was taken; Mrs Harman has no family history of breast cancer. The GP began the examination by looking for any irregularities in the shape or colour of the breast and nipple. She then examined the breast tissue including the lymph nodes under the armpit. This is because breast lumps and cancer can be located in the lymph nodes. The GP detected a lump approximately 1.5cm in diameter in the right breast, the left breast felt normal and no lumps were detected. The GP explained her findings to Mrs Harman; she advised

her that she would be referring her to the local breast screening unit. She also informed her that it was probably a benign cyst as she did not have many risk factors, for example she had no family history of breast cancer and she was young. The GP tried to allay Mrs Harman's fears, by explaining the importance of definitive diagnosis; this would be achieved by the specialist carrying out an ultrasound and fine needle aspiration cytology (FNAC). Although the GP felt it was benign, these tests would confirm her provisional diagnosis. The waiting time for the clinic was approximately two weeks. Most clinics have a 2–10 week wait for non-urgent cases. Mrs Harman left the GP surgery and waited for the appointment to arrive.

Developing & Delivering Expert Care: Exercise 9.9

Breast Awareness

Mrs Harman was well informed about breast self-examination (BSE) as her friend had been diagnosed with cancer. BSE should be carried out several days after the menstrual cycle has finished. There are 5 steps to BSE.

- Find out how to carry out BSE.
- When on clinic placements decide if it is appropriate to offer this health education.

BSE is recommended by the Department of Health, NICE and Breast Cancer Care. Visit their websites, look at the health education advice and relevant statistics.

www.breastcancercare.org.uk www.nice.org.uk www.dh.gov.uk

Psychosocial aspects

Mrs Harman is very worried about breast cancer, as her friend has recently been diagnosed with it. When a friend or relative of similar age has been diagnosed with a disease, it can make people question their own mortality; it heightens awareness of that particular disease process. Mrs Harman's friend has taught her the importance of BSE, and also showed her the correct technique for examining the breasts. Ajzen (1991) wrote a theory of planned behaviour; from this it was noted that a person's behavioural intentions were based on how committed they were to the health belief. Mrs Harman believes that it

is important to perform regular BSE to detect abnormalities early. She is committed to the belief that early detection increases survival and also she is committed to BSE as her friend has told her how important it is. Although she believes it is right to carry out BSE, now that she has found a lump and this has been confirmed by her GP, she has a fear of being diagnosed with cancer. It is therefore important that she is given time to discuss these fears with the GP and that she is given relevant literature to read while she waits for her appointment. It is suggested that the information must be simple and that it must be repeated; this will encourage patients to be compliant with the doctor's recommendations or treatments.

One way the healthcare professional can make sure the patient has comprehended the treatment or diagnosis is by asking them to explain what they have understood. This will ensure the nurse or doctor can clarify any points that have been misunderstood; this may make the patient more compliant to the treatment. Written information is also a key part in any care given to a patient, as they are able to take the literature away from the clinical setting and study it in a less stressful environment. Therefore it is important that Mrs Harman had written information as it would increase her knowledge of the breast screening unit and allay some of her fears, as she would have advance knowledge of the procedures that will take place.

Treatment

Mrs Harman waited two weeks for her appointment. The clinic advised her to bring a friend or partner for support. On arrival at the department she was greeted by a nurse who explained the procedures to her in detail. She also gave her written information to look at while she waited to see the consultant. It is important to give patients time to listen to and then read about the procedures; this will enable them to understand what is happening and also gives them the opportunity to ask questions. Mrs Harman appeared to have understood the procedure but was anxious about the findings. It is imperative that any anxieties are recognised and addressed by the nurse and time is given to the patient.

The consultant began by taking a brief history, she also explained that she would carry out all of the procedures herself and that they should have a result from fine-needle aspiration cytology (FNAC) that afternoon. First, the consultant inspected Mrs Harman's breasts, looking for any changes in shape, puckering of the skin, colour

changes, rashes, inversion of the nipple and any discharge from the nipples. She reassured Mrs Harman that the breasts had no obvious deformities. The breasts were then examined and the lump palpated. Because of her age Mrs Harman would have an ultrasound scan. Women 35 years of age and under have an ultrasound scan as their breast tissue is more dense; over this age a mammogram is performed. The DH set up a national breast screening programme and by the mid-1990s all women over 50 years old were offered a mammogram every three years. The ultrasound confirmed a small 1.5cm lump. FNAC was performed; the consultant used a local anaesthetic and then took a small amount of aspirate for cytology. The consultant explained that the lump appeared to be a fibroadenoma, which is a benign lump but that cytology would confirm it. Fibroadenomas are common in young women and are hard moveable lumps approximately 1–3cm in diameter. They are believed to be caused by an increased sensitivity to oestrogen. Mrs Harman is told to take simple analgesia later that day as the breast may become tender or painful following the FNAC.

The results of the FNAC confirmed that Mrs Harman had a benign fibroadenoma. The consultant explained that there was no further treatment needed but if the lump grew she should see her GP again as they can be removed if they become troublesome. She was also advised to continue BSE and to encourage all her friends, relatives and colleagues to begin BSE as early diagnosis of breast cancer can reduce mortality by 24%.

Applying Theory to Practice: Exercise 9.10

Breast lumps can be malignant or benign. Below are some other causes of breast lumps:

- Ductal carcinoma in situ (DCIS)
- Lobular carcinoma in situ (LCIS)
- Phyllodes tumour

Find some possible treatments for these conditions and write your answers under the headings.

Female reproductive cycle

After puberty, women experience a monthly cycle, the length of which varies but is usually between 21–35 days.

Applying Theory to Practice: Exercise 9.11

Ethical Dilemmas

Some treatments such as perception have caused controversy, as they have not been widely available on the NHS. Find out who is allowed to be given perception by visiting www.nice.org.uk .

- How would you feel if a treatment of choice was not available in your NHS trust?
- Do you feel all patients should have equal access to treatments?

Hormones that are released by the hypothalamus, pituitary gland and ovaries control the cycle. The cycle has four phases:

- **Menstrual phase** – this lasts approximately five days. During this time a woman loses approximately 150ml of blood. The decreased levels of progesterone and oestrogen cause the uterine artery to constrict. This causes the lining of the endometrium to become ischaemic and shed via the vagina in the form of blood loss. During this phase there is a rise in FSH and primary follicles develop in the ovary; these also release small amounts of oestrogen. Towards the end of the menstrual cycle they begin to develop into secondary follicles; these contain an oocyte that continues to grow.
- **Pre-ovulatory phase** – during this phase one of the secondary follicles becomes larger than the rest; the others then degenerate. If this follicle is producing enough oestrogen to develop and grow, it is known as a **graafian** follicle or mature follicle, and is ready for ovulation. The oestrogen that is released stimulates the repair of the endometrium, so the lining becomes thick and the blood supply is improved. This is in preparation for a fertilised ovum.
- **Ovulation** – this usually occurs midway through the cycle at approximately 14 days. Some women report pain or discomfort during this time. Oestrogen stimulates the release of GnRH by the hypothalamus and LH is released by the anterior pituitary gland. The high level of LH stimulates the rupture of the graafian follicle which releases the secondary oocyte. Once this is

released, the graafian follicle collapses; this then develops into the corpus luteum.

- **Post-ovulatory phase** – the corpus luteum releases progesterone and oestrogen. The progesterone prepares the endometrium for a fertilised ovum. If a fertilised ovum is present, the corpus luteum continues to secrete hormones, maintained by the chorion, which releases the hormone human chorionic gonadotrophin (HCG). The chorion then develops into the placenta. If there is no fertilised ovum the corpus luteum degenerates and this initiates the menstrual phase.

Applying Theory to Practice: Exercise 9.12

There are many different types of pregnancy tests on the market.

- After reading the previous section, which hormonal release do you think these tests might measure?

During your placements identify which type of tests are available on the wards.

Pregnancy

Women are fertile during the years that they menstruate and they can become pregnant, if sexually active, during this time. Once the ovum has been fertilised by the sperm, the young embryo begins to develop. Pregnancy continues forty weeks from the date of the last menstrual period (LMP) to birth. The pregnancy is divided into three trimesters, which are approximately 12 weeks each. During the early stages the embryo is called a **zygote**; it develops through the mitotic division of cells. At day 6 or 7 the embryo implants itself in the uterus to ensure that the maternal blood supply feeds oxygen and nutrients to the growing embryo; the developing placenta will fulfil this role.

During the implantation stage the embryo is at risk of implanting in various sites such as the uterine tube; this is known as an **ectopic pregnancy**. Ectopic pregnancies are not viable and carry huge risks for the mother. If the pregnancy ruptures the fallopian tube, the mother can haemorrhage uncontrollably and requires urgent treatment.

Once the embryo is implanted, the cells release a hormone called human chorionic gonadotrophin (HCG), this can be detected in the mother's blood and urine. At this point the presence of HCG in the urine will result in a

positive pregnancy test. HCG stimulates the corpus luteum to grow and secrete large amounts of progesterone and oestrogen. These hormones remain at a high level throughout the pregnancy to encourage the growth of the endometrium. The oestrogen also encourages the growth of the mammary glands so that the mother will eventually produce milk. The sharp increase in hormone levels can lead to morning sickness. This normally lasts during the first trimester, although some women experience it for longer periods of time.

If the mother has released more than one ovum during ovulation, two or more zygotes may form, so that the mother is expecting more than one baby; these are known as fraternal twins and are not identical. If at the beginning of cell division the zygote divides in two, the mother will be expecting identical twins as they have the same set of genes.

During the first trimester the embryo will develop all the major organs and a fetal heartbeat can normally be seen on a scan approximately 5–6 weeks into the pregnancy. The placenta will also develop to feed nutrients to the embryo via the mother's blood supply. At the end of

Figure 9.6 Stages of pregnancy: 1

Figure 9.7 Stages of pregnancy: 2

Figure 9.8 Stages of pregnancy: 3

the first trimester the embryo is known as a fetus.

The second trimester begins in the 13th week. During this trimester the mother general feels well as the morning sickness subsides. During this trimester the fetus has all the major organs and therefore begins to develop purposeful movement. The mother can detect fetal movements at 16 weeks onwards, although first-time mothers tend to feel them later. At approximately four months the uterus begins to contract; this is known as the Braxton Hicks sign. It is not fully understood why this occurs but the mother feels a tightening of her uterus. At approximately 20 weeks most mothers will have an anomaly scan which detects any abnormalities in any of the major organs. The sex of the baby can also be determined at this scan, but the embryo has begun to determine this after the 6th week of pregnancy.

The third trimester begins at week 27 and lasts until labour begins. Delivery after 37 weeks gestation is deemed normal, although some women will give birth in the 42nd week. A few days before the mother gives birth the levels of progesterone decrease; oestrogen then begins to excite the uterine muscles and contractions begin. As the cervix begins to dilate this stimulates the hypothalamus and the posterior pituitary gland to release oxytocin. This hormone encourages the uterus to contract, thus expelling the fetus down the vagina. If a woman is having a difficult labour and her contractions are not regular and strong, the midwife can administer oxytocin to increase them. Oxytocin also helps the uterus expel the placenta after the baby has been born. Once the placenta has been expelled the breasts begin to produce small amounts of colostrum, a thick, milky fluid loaded with antibodies. Breastfeeding encourages a surge in hypothalamic release hormone for prolactin to be produced. This in turn encourages milk production.

Scenario 9.4

Threatened Miscarriage

Ruksana Ali is a 26-year-old woman who presents at her GP surgery with per vaginam (PV) bleeding. She is approximately 8 weeks (8/40) pregnant. This is her first pregnancy. She is very tearful.
Vital signs are documented as: respiratory rate 14, pulse 72, BP 114/64, temperature 36.1
Allergies: penicillin
PMH: nil

Assessment and analysis of patient presentation

The initial assessment by the GP includes monitoring of her vital signs. Her vital signs are within normal limits although her respiratory rate is slightly above normal, which may be an early indication of shock. It is therefore important that the GP takes an accurate history of her condition, including the amount of blood loss. Mrs Ali is able to give the date of her last menstrual period (LMP) as eight weeks and two days ago. She has had no problems within the first eight weeks. Today she awoke and found a small amount of blood in the gusset of her pyjama bottoms. She has been spotting ever since, has not passed any clots and the blood is dark red. This indicates to the GP that her blood loss is minimal and that the blood she describes is not a fresh bleed. Mrs Ali is not aware of her rhesus status; the GP notes this, as a blood test will need to be taken. If she is rhesus negative, she will need to have an anti-D injection to prevent complications in future pregnancies. The GP asks to examine Mrs Ali, with a nurse to chaperone him to protect both the patient and doctor from allegations of inappropriate behaviour, as he will be examining her abdomen. Each NHS trust or GP surgery has a policy on chaperones, to which staff must adhere.

On palpation of her abdomen, the GP finds her abdomen soft and non-tender, she also states she has no abdominal pain. This would indicate that an ectopic pregnancy (fetus growing outside the uterus) is unlikely as abdominal pain and tenderness are a classic sign, but until she has had an ultrasound scan, which assesses the exact location of the fetus, it cannot be completely ruled out. At this early stage of the pregnancy the uterus is still lying below the pelvis so it cannot be felt; as the pregnancy progresses, the uterus can be palpated. Many GPs will not do a vaginal examination (VE) as it is contraindicated if the patient has a possible ectopic pregnancy. However, a VE can be done if an ectopic has been ruled out; this will ascertain if the cervical os (neck of the womb) is open. The GP feels that Mrs Ali is haemodynamically stable and that it is most likely that this is a threatened miscarriage. He speaks to the early pregnancy assessment unit (EPAU) at the local hospital. They are able to see Mrs Ali within the next three hours. The GP therefore feels that a VE is not necessary as she will have an ultrasound scan and possibly VE at the hospital. The Royal College of Obstetricians and Gynaecologists (2006) recommends that EPAUs are widely available. Within this unit are facilities for ultrasound, blood tests, leaflets, referrals and algorithms for each condition that presents.

Mrs Ali is happy to visit her local EPAU later that day. The GP explains that she will need a full bladder, as this will enable the doctor to palpate the uterus more easily.

Anatomy and Physiology in Action: Exercise 9.13

There are different types of miscarriage; look up the following and write a synopsis of each. Describe what is happening physiologically. Add this to your portfolio. The Royal College of Obstetricians and Gynaecologists (RCOG) have clear explanations of each type of miscarriage:

- Threatened
- Inevitable
- Incomplete
- Complete
- Missed
- Early fetal demise.

Miscarriage – the facts

One in five pregnancies will ended in miscarriage (Miscarriage Association 1996), of these one in 100 women will have recurrent miscarriages, thus each of these women have three or more. However, 50–80% of women who have bleeding in the first trimester of pregnancy will continue to have a normal pregnancy (Allan 1995). Many miscarriages occur within the first trimester, although miscarriage can occur up to 24 weeks. If a pregnancy spontaneously aborts after this time and is delivered dead, it is classed as a stillbirth. In October 2006 the RCOG published guidelines on the management of early pregnancy loss, which examined both the physical and the psychological needs of the patient. There can be many reasons for a miscarriage, but there are four main reasons (Cecil 1996). The first cause is a genetic abnormality that is incompatible with life. Infection such as rubella (German measles) can result in miscarriage; colds and minor infections are not deemed to be associated with miscarriage. Immunological problems, for example, problems with blood vessels that supply the placenta and hormonal imbalance, may also be a cause. Finally, an anatomical abnormality in the mother, such as a weak cervix, may cause a miscarriage, as the cervix is more likely to open during pregnancy instead of remaining closed and retaining the pregnancy in the uterus.

Treatment

A midwife sees Mrs Ali in the EPAU; there is also a registrar on duty to perform the ultrasound. Initially the midwife takes a history and checks Mrs Ali's vital signs, which have remained within normal limits. The next test performed is urinalysis, which reveals that beta-HCG is present; no abnormalities are detected on urinalysis. The presence of HCG confirms that she is pregnant – the developing placenta releases this hormone. Blood may also be taken to confirm a steady rise in HCG; this is useful if they are monitoring for an ectopic pregnancy because the fetus may not have been detected. If HCG levels continue to rise, this could indicate that the fetus is growing outside the uterus. Blood samples will also be taken to ascertain her Rhesus status and her full blood count; if she were losing a large amount of blood, she might become anaemic. Mrs Ali is anxious to have the ultrasound scan, as this will give her a definitive answer about her pregnancy. The midwife explains to her that they will begin by doing an abdominal ultrasound, but if they do not get a clear view of the gestation sac, fetus and fallopian tubes, they will need to do a vaginal scan. The scan is taken by inserting a probe into the vagina; this is done in very early pregnancy and can detect smaller fetal poles. From approximately 7 weeks the fetal heart can be seen.

The registrar carries out the ultrasound, and confirms that there is a sac present in the uterus but there is no fetal heart detected. A vaginal examination confirms the os is closed and so a vaginal ultrasound is carried out; this confirms there is no fetal heart and the fetus appears small, approximately 5 weeks gestation. He explains to Mrs Ali that her dates may be wrong and that it may be too early to detect the fetal heart or it may be a delayed miscarriage; this is when the fetus has died days or weeks earlier. Mrs Ali is extremely upset by this news and needs time to understand what has been said. The midwife explains that they will repeat the scan in one week to see if the fetus has developed. During this time she may begin to bleed more heavily, which may indicate and result in a miscarriage. Mrs Ali is advised to rest and is given leaflets about miscarriage; she is also advised to return if she develops abdominal pain or heavy vaginal bleeding.

Conclusion

Mrs Ali develops abdominal pain and vaginal bleeding three days later. She is admitted to the gynaecology ward. Her vital signs are recorded and she is haemodynamically stable. The consultant carries out an ultrasound scan and confirms that she has had a miscarriage.

Applying Theory to Practice: Exercise 9.14

Mrs Ali has been given bad news. On clinical placements think about how bad news is broken.

- Does the area have a room for the patients or relatives to have privacy and time to ask questions?
- Who do you think should break bad news?

Find out about some other voluntary organisations that may be able to offer further advice and support.

www.miscarriageassociation.org.uk

Anatomy and Physiology in Action: Exercise 9.15

Pathophysiology of the Female Reproductive System

Discover what the following diseases are and write a synopsis of your findings. These can be placed in your portfolio.

- Endometriosis
- Polycystic ovary syndrome
- Fibroids
- Bartholin's cyst.

Conclusion

The male and female reproductive systems have been discussed in depth. The development of the reproductive system and the hormones involved in the male and female systems have been identified, including the changes that occur in puberty and pregnancy. The types of disorder associated with this system have been examined in the form of clinical scenarios. These scenarios have highlighted some of the most common patient presentations. It is important to update personal portfolios when new illnesses or diseases are seen in clinical placements.

Chapter 9 Summary Quiz

1. The reproductive system is one of the only systems in the body that is dimorphic, meaning it is:

A. Able to change throughout the life cycle
B. Changes during puberty
C. Functionally and structurally different in males and females
D. Functionally and structurally the same in males and females

2. Leydig cells are responsible for the production of:

A. Oestrogen
B. Testosterone
C. Progesterone
D. Adrenaline

3. Identify three functions of the vagina:

A. Acts as a passageway for both blood flow during the menstrual cycle and the fetus during childbirth, receives semen from the penis during penetrative intercourse
B. Provides a passageway for both blood flow during the menstrual cycle and for urine during urination
C. Acts as a passageway for the fetus during childbirth, acts as a temperature control mechanism
D. Provides a passageway for both blood flow during the menstrual cycle and for urine during urination, receives semen from the penis during penetrative intercourse

4. The penis is a cylindrical structure that can be described in three parts:

A. The root, the shaft and the base
B. The body, the root and the glans penis
C. The shaft, the end and the root
D. The root, the glans penis and the epididymis

5. The most common sexually transmitted infection is:

A. Syphilis
B. Genital chlamydia
C. Gonorrhoea
D. Herpes

6. A pregnancy is divided into three trimesters, which last how long?

A. Approximately 12 weeks each
B. Approximately 8 weeks each
C. Approximately 16 weeks each
D. Approximately 2 weeks each

7. There are 20–30 lymph nodes in the armpit; what is their purpose?

A. Drain fluid from the breast
B. Increase breast size
C. Act as a reservoir for milk
D. Release specific hormones that initiate the menstrual cycle

8. What percentage of pregnancies result in miscarriage?

A. 10%
B. 90%
C. 2%
D. 20%

9. What role does oxytocin play?

A. This hormone encourages the uterus to contract thus expelling the fetus down the vagina
B. This hormone allows the development of the breasts
C. This enzyme increases hair growth
D. This hormone encourages mood swings

10. The menstrual cycle can be broken down into four phases:

A. Menstrual phase, prepulsion phase, ovulation, post-ovulatory phase

B. Menstrual phase, pre-ovulatory phase, bleeding phase, post-ovulatory phase

C. Hormonal phase, pre-ovulatory phase, ovulation, post-ovulatory phase

D. Menstrual phase, pre-ovulatory phase, ovulation, post-ovulatory phase

Further reading

Government Statistics (2005/06) www.statistics.gov.uk

Miscarriage Association (2007)
www.miscarriageassociation.org.uk

NHS Direct (2007) *Health Encyclopaedia – Chlamydia.*
www.nhsdirect.nhs.uk

NICE guidelines (2007/013) NICE guidance call for more to be done to halt the rise of STIs and prevent under-18 conceptions. www.nice.org.uk

Rutter, D. & Quine, L. (2002) *Changing Health Behaviour.* Open University Press: Maidenhead.

http://www.netdoctor.co.uk/health_advice/facts/venerealdiseases.htm

http://www.nlm.nih.gov/medlineplus/pregnancy.html

References

Ajzen (1991) *Changing Health Behaviours: The Role of Implementation Intentions from Changing Health Behaviour.* Open University Press: Maidenhead.

Allan, A. (1995) cited by Washbourne, C. & Cox, C. Per vagina bleeding in early pregnancy. *Emergency Nurse* 10(8): December 2002.

Bandura, P. (1997) *Encouraging Safer-Sex Behaviours from Changing Health Behaviour.* Open University Press: Maidenhead.

Cecil, R. (1996) *The Anthropology of Pregnancy Loss: Comparative Studies in Miscarriage, Stillbirth and Neo-natal Death.* Cross-cultural Perspectives on Women. Berg Publishers: Oxford.

Department of Health (2004) *National Service Framework for Children, Young People and Maternity Services.* DH: London.

Department of Health (2007) *Chlamydia, Policy and Guidelines.* www.dh.gov.uk

Department of Health and Cancer Research UK (2005) *A Whole New Ball Game.* DH: London.

Guillebaud, j. (2000) *Contraception Today,* 4th edn. Martin Dunitz: London.

Manchester Triage Group (1994) *Manchester Triage.* BMJ Publishing Group: London.

National Institute for Health and Clinical Excellence (NICE) (2007) NICE guidance call for more to be done to halt the rise of STIs and prevent under 18 conceptions. www.nice.org.uk

NHS Direct (2007) *Health Encyclopaedia – Testicular Torsion.*www.nhsdirect.nhs.uk

Nursing and Midwifery Council (NMC) (2004) *Code of Professional Conduct: Standards for Conduct, Performance and Ethics.* NMC: London.

Rosenstock, H.B.M. (1966) *Social Cognition Model and Changing Health Behaviours from Changing Health Behaviour.* Open University Press: Maidenhead.

Royal College of Obstetricians and Gynaecologists (RCOG) (2006) *The Management of Early Pregnancy Loss.* Green-top Guideline No. 25. RCOG: London.

The immune/lymphatic and endocrine systems

Clare Culpin

Additional contribution by Cliff Evans

Chapter 10 Learning Objectives

- Gain knowledge and insight into the anatomy and physiology related to these systems
- Gain insight into several predominant conditions related to these systems
- Apply theory to practice by understanding the impact of these conditions on the individual
- Gain insight into several commonly used medications within these specialties
- Construct solid evidence of professional development for your growing portfolio
- Continue developing the ability to question and critique the evidence base and effectiveness of plans of care

Introduction

This chapter addresses two systems commonly not considered as 'dramatic' as the cardiovascular or nervous systems, and which to the uninformed may appear more complex. Both are vital in not only maintaining health and well-being, but also life, as illnesses affecting the functioning of these systems can be fatal. Two of the world's most infamous diseases relate to these systems; one is a world pandemic (HIV) (UNAIDS 2006) and the other, a potential epidemic (diabetes mellitus) (DH 2006).

The immune system in combination with the lymphatic system provides the first line of defence against the potential dangers of the outside world and provides a pivotal role in preventing disease and destroying malformations from within. This is an essential function, otherwise small injuries such as cuts and sprains would never heal. The endocrine system provides the balance for life, regulating and secreting hormones, thereby maintaining homeostasis.

This chapter will provide an overview of the function of each of these systems highlighting the essential asso-ciated anatomy and physiology. Common illnesses affecting these systems will be discussed with clinical scenarios demonstrating the devastating effects these illnesses can have on the affected individual. The scenarios will also address common professional issues that the student nurse may encounter while on placement, with learning exercises providing many opportunities to further their knowledge on various relevant issues, including current treatment regimens and evidence-based initiatives. The reader will be encouraged to explore his or her own feelings thereby aiding the process of clinical decision-making and developing the essential skill of reflective thinking.

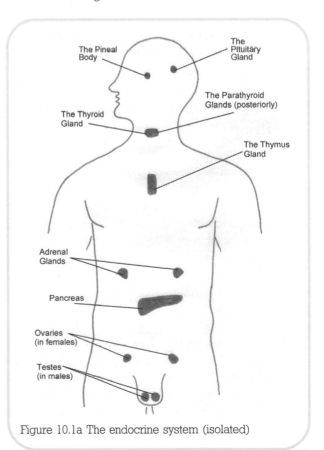

Figure 10.1a The endocrine system (isolated)

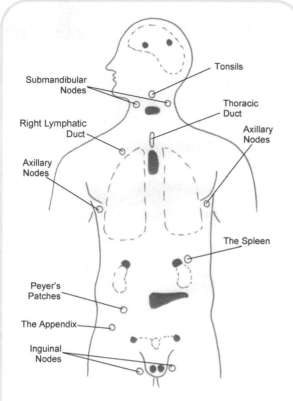

Figure 10.1b The major components of the immune/lymphatic and endocrine systems

Function

As we go about our daily lives our bodies are working hard to respond to the ever-changing internal environment, and the constant threat of foreign invaders and toxins that have the potential to lead to disease. The intricate, but fascinating, immune system is composed of two distinct functioning categories, which share many characteristics:

● Non-specific defence mechanisms
● Specific defence mechanisms.

Both categories work in partnership to provide a comprehensive defence mechanism. The skin, which provides the major component of the non-specific function of our immunity, works in partnership with the specific immune responses, involving the B and T lymphocytes, proteins produced by the plasma cells called **antibodies**, along with other chemicals including

immunoglobulins, all of which play an essential role in maintaining homeostasis. The immune system is greatly influenced by most of the other systems, in particular the lymphatic, blood, skeletal and endocrine systems. Many life factors can negatively affect the system, including the effects of ageing, poor nutrition and fluid balance, as well as the individual's emotional well-being. Many aspects need to be considered when assessing an individual's ability both to prevent and fight infection and to heal injuries.

Non-specific immunity

The skin

The most obvious physical defence barrier we have is our skin, often described as the body's largest organ (Brooker 2000), and one that we probably pay attention to for reasons other than defence. Yet this external covering has within it a number of important mechanisms and plays a major role in the first line of general defence. The skin itself consists of two layers: the epidermis, which sits superficially to the deeper layer, the dermis. Both the epidermis and the dermis are attached to underlying structures by subcutaneous and adipose tissue, which will become familiar terms when administering medications by injection.

The epidermis is the visible layer of skin, varying in thickness depending on the local requirements: it is thicker on the soles of the feet and thinner over the eyelids. The epidermis is largely formed of dead skin cells, which begin their life deeper in the skin tissue, gradually over a period of weeks working their way to the surface where eventually they flake away, through exfoliation, to be renewed by other skin cells. This process is most rapid during childhood, slowing down with the ageing process, something that needs to be considered when caring for the older adult, making them more vulnerable to pressure-related tissue damage, and influencing the rate and ability of wound healing. Stratum layers within the epidermis, containing **spinosum** (more commonly known as prickle cells) and basal cells, are responsible for the pigmentation of the skin through the production of melanin by the melanocyte cells.

The dermis, situated beneath the epidermis, is a much deeper, complex layer of the skin incorporating many structures such as sweat glands, sensory nerve endings, hair follicles each with their own muscles attached, veins, arteries, lymph vessels and connective tissue.

Anatomy and Physiology in Action: Exercise 10.1

Carcinomas affecting the skin are responsible for thousands of deaths each year. The three main types are directly related to the above-mentioned layers and cell types. Complete the following exercise to apply your anatomy and physiology knowledge to clinical practice.

- Write a short summary of the three main types of skin cancer and identify what has gone wrong with the cells to cause them; your summary should also include the possible causes.

Add this work to your portfolio.

If you encounter difficulty, the following website may prove helpful:

http://www.bad.org.uk/public/leaflets/skin_cancer.asp

http://www.nhsdirect.nhs.uk/articles/article.aspx?articleId=83

www.virtualsciencefair.org

The skin serves eight essential functions: easily remembered as **SHAPES** Very Much.

- **Secretion** – secretes sebum lubricating hair shafts and providing a natural moisturiser for the skin, acting as a barrier against bacteria
- **Heat regulation** – provides a dual function cooling or warming the body
- **Absorption** – can absorb certain substances
- **Protection** – from the effects of sunlight and harmful substances and organisms
- **Elimination** – removes waste products
- **Sensation** – the peripheral nerves 'sense' danger
- **Vitamin D** – maintaining bone density
- **Melanin** – a substance which darkens the skin resulting in increased protection for the underlying structures as radiation is absorbed

Other non-specific immunity

- Other non-specific components of the immune system are gastric juices (hydrochloric acid) found in the stomach, which destroy many organisms. In addition, vomiting rejects any unwanted food or organisms recognised as potentially harmful.

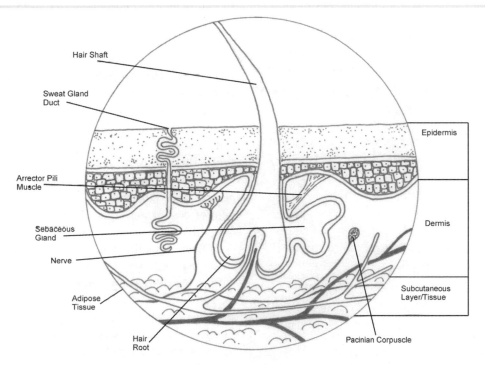

Figure 10.2 The skin, identifying its main components

Applying Theory to Practice: Exercise 10.2

Before reading on:

- Compose a list of interventions and practices carried out by the nurse which compromise the integrity of the patient's skin.
- What impact does this have on the well-being of their immunity?
- What potential problems can result from these practices?
- What can the nurse do to prevent potential problems and complications?

- Saliva in the nose and mouth contains a protein called lysozyme, also present in other body fluids (except urine and cerebrospinal fluid), which has antibacterial properties.
- Cilia are hair-like projections originating in certain types of cell within the respiratory system; they move foreign bodies and mucus away from the respiratory tract in waves (Chapter 3). Sneezing takes care of larger foreign bodies which may have escaped these defences, in the same way that coughing removes particles from the lungs or the respiratory tract.
- Villi within the gastrointestinal tract have a function similar to cilia; mucus protects the delicate lining from the effects of acid; and normal flora (micro-organisms which are found in the body) provide a barrier against pathogens in a similar way to the normal flora found in the vagina.
- Eyelashes, and the action of blinking in combination with lysozymes within the tears provide all-round protection for the eyes.

Anatomy and Physiology in Action: Exercise 10.3

A+P

Before commencing the following section write a short piece identifying the cells you know that work to prevent infection and maintain healing within the body.

Add your summary to your portfolio.

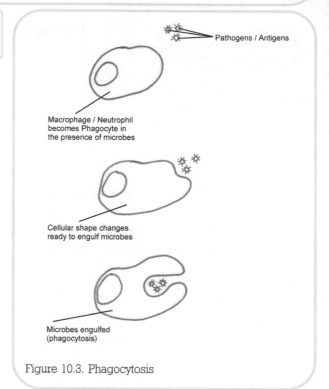

Figure 10.3. Phagocytosis

Phagocytes (eating cells)

There are a number of cells that also have a role in non-specific immunity. Phagocytes are cells which can be found in most tissues and include some leucocytes, for example, neutrophils, eosinophils, monocytes and macrophages. These phagocyte cells collaborate with chemicals called **immunoglobulins** and a substance called **complement**. Complement is a collection of specific plasma proteins, which assist in the destruction of foreign invaders or microbes. The combined action of these cells and chemicals is an elaborate process called **phagocytosis**, aimed at destroying foreign invaders (chemical or non-chemical), and dead or damaged cells. The phased process of phagocytosis commences with the identification for destruction of the foreign invaders, or damaged cells, by immune complexes i.e. antibodies. The phagocytes then engulf the cells, ingesting and absorbing them. Macrophages survive this ordeal to fight again; the leucocytes are destroyed resulting in the formation of **pus**. This process is all part of the body's natural inflammatory response. Despite this sophisticated process, it is not fail-safe and does not always work for every invasion. Some invaders are too strong to overcome and the phagocytes become victims themselves, weakening the body's defence mechanisms.

Structures	Cells and Chemicals	Actions
Skin	Epidermis Dermis	Provides a barrier when intact
Stomach	Hydrochloric acid	Destroys many organisms ingested
Stomach		Vomiting rejects any unwanted food
Nose and mouth	Lysozyme found in saliva	Antibacterial
Nose and mouth	Hair-like cilia cells and mucus	Debris attaches to the mucus and the cilia cells to move out of the nose and mouth
Respiratory tract		Coughing removes particles which may have travelled into the lungs
Gastrointestinal tract	Mucus	Protects the delicate lining from the effects of acid
Gastrointestinal tract	Normal flora	Provides a barrier against pathogens
Vagina	Normal flora	Provides a barrier against pathogens
Eyelashes		Blinking protects the eyes from particles
Eyes	Lysozyme found in tears	Antibacterial
Body tissue and blood	Phagocytes Macrophages Leucocytes ▪ Neutrophils ▪ Eosinophils ▪ Monocytes	Phagocytosis
	Immunoglobulins	
	Complement	
Body tissue and blood	Natural killer cells	Lysis (decompose)
Infected cells or T lymphocytes	Interferon	Stops the virus multiplying and stimulates macrophages and natural killer cells into action

Table 10.1 Non-specific immune function summary

Applying Theory to Practice: Exercise 10.4

The Inflammatory Response

Consider all the causes of inflammation that you are aware of.

● Write a short piece for your portfolio on how many diseases or patient presentations may have an inflammatory cause or involve inflammation.

The primary physiological effect of the inflammatory response centres on increasing blood and blood cells to an area experiencing disease or trauma. The blood vessels surrounding the affected site dilate; this allows increased blood flow to the area. Cell walls that surround the area dilate producing an increased permeability. This allows the immune cells which are larger than other cells to pass through. As a result of the increased blood flow, the immune presence is strengthened. Many different immune cells congregate at the site of inflammation, along with a large supply of proteins, which fuel the immune response. There is an increase in body heat production, which can have an antibiotic effect.

The main clinical findings associated with the inflammatory response are:

● Tissues become red and hot as a result of the increased blood flow reaching the site
● Tissues become swollen due to the congregation of blood cells, lymph and proteins
● The area is painful due the expansion of tissues, causing direct pressure on nerve cells, and also due to the presence of pain mediators such as prostaglandins.

Now that you understand this response:

● How do you think it ends?

The websites below provides a quick resource:

http://www.sumanasinc.com/webcontent/anisamples/dynamicillustrations/inflammatory.html
http://alan.kennedy.name/crohns/primer/inflresp.htm

Natural killer cells

There is another important member of the non-specific immunity team, the natural killer cell. These cells are also present in the body's tissue and blood, but work in a different way to those involved in phagocytosis. Natural killer cells recognise infected cells, or cells which have abnormal changes due to malignancy, and go on to destroy them through a process called **lysis**.

Interferons

When a virus infects a cell, the cell produces a protein called interferon. The purpose is to prevent the virus spreading to other cells, this is achieved by inhibiting the virus's ability to reproduce. Macrophages are stimulated and natural killer cells destroy the abnormal cell. Interferons will be further explored as part of the specific immune system, as T lymphocytes also produce interferon as part of their role.

Inflammatory response

Inflammation is the body's response to injury; this may be physical injury or caused by a chemical or micro-organism. The local tissue involved in the injury utilises the non-specific immunity cascade, limiting the damage, and removing the causative agents, along with dead cells that result from this process. Tissue becomes red, hot, swollen and painful; if the inflammation is gross, it may limit the movement of a limb.

Applying Theory to Practice: Exercise 10.5

The physical or clinical signs of inflammation and possible infection have been discussed, but how do you know if a patient is going through a 'normal' response?

Cells		Action
B lymphocytes	Born in the bone marrow Matured in lymph tissue When stimulated, undergo further changes which result in them becoming either a plasma cell or memory cell	Plasma cells (or effector cells) produce antibody Memory cells record the type of antibody required and store it in case it is required in future; this may involve changing its shape to become unique to the antigen (foreign invader), which may take between 2–3 weeks Memory cells may float around in the blood for some time after, waiting to be called into action Once called into action they can quickly respond to produce more antibodies
Antibody (also known as immunoglobulin)	A protein produced by the B lymphocyte	Combines with the antigen and destroys it through ● Lysis ● Stimulating and supporting phagocytosis by the macrophages ● Hampering the antigen's ability to invade other cells
T lymphocytes	Born in the bone marrow Matured in the thymus gland When stimulated, move into lymph tissue to further develop Emerge as: ● Killer T cells ● Helper T cells ● Suppressor T cells ● Memory T cells	Killer T cells attach themselves to the antigen (foreign invader) and secrete lysosome, destroying it and the antigen Helper T cells support the B cells to produce antibody, therefore the increase in T helper cells increases the effectiveness of the B lymphocytes Suppressor T cells, once the invasion has been dealt with, reduce the activity of both the B and T cells in order to prevent an overreaction, and so are important in regulating the responses of the B and T cells

Table 10.2 Specific Immunity Function Summary

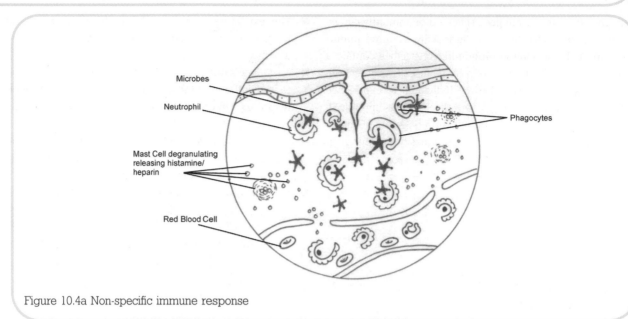

Microbes

Neutrophil

Mast Cell degranulating
releasing histamine/
heparin

Phagocytes

Red Blood Cell

Figure 10.4a Non-specific immune response

Specific immunity

Should a foreign invader move beyond the defences of the non-specific immunity, the specific immunity responses are stimulated into action. Specific immunity is also activated when an abnormal cell is detected (i.e. malignant cell), as well as transplanted cells.

Symptoms of a normal immune response

Acquired immunity

The immune response, outlined in Figure 10.4, is one of active, naturally acquired immunity, where the individual has had the disease, illness or infection. The memory cells

go on to prepare the body for further invasion by the same organism, either by knowing exactly which type of antibody to produce, or by their newly defined unique shape that

Anatomy and Physiology in Action: Box 10.1

Diseases that can be vaccinated against

United Kingdom	Other
Diphtheria	Typhoid
Tetanus	Chorea
Whooping cough	Smallpox
(pertussis)	Yellow Fever
Hib (*Haemophilus*	Rabies
influenzae) type B –	Tick-borne encephalitis
protection against some	Japanese encephalitis
types of meningitis	
Polio (oral preparation)	
Measles	
Mumps	
Rubella	
BCG (bacillus of	
Calmette–Guérin)	
protection against TB	
Hepatitis A and B	

Source: (NaTHNaC 2006)

Applying Theory to Practice: Exercise 10.6

Before reading on:

- Compose a list of all the vaccinations you have received
- Why do you think it is important for nurses to have received all their routine childhood vaccinations?
- Which vaccinations are offered to healthcare workers specifically and why?

Also refer to Exercise 10.5.

attaches itself to the antigen. This kind of immunity can be artificially produced, as active artificially acquired immunity, through vaccination programmes. Vaccines contain a weaker or slightly altered strain of the disease or infection, not strong enough to cause the individual to experience and suffer the full extent of the disease, but enough to stimulate the specific immune function and confer immunity. National vaccination programmes, beginning in childhood, have proved to be effective in controlling the spread and effects of many diseases. Travel advice now also includes vaccination to prevent disease and infections common to other continents (NaTHNaC 2006).

The effects of ageing

As we age, our cell function deteriorates due to the cells' inability to repair, renew and regenerate. In addition, some errors in the cells' renewal process can lead to abnormal cells being present and even malignancy (Farley et al. 2006). This ultimately has an impact on the effectiveness of the immune system:

- Slower to react and respond
- Unable to fight antigens due to the decline of the B and T lymphocytes
- Inefficient in removing free radicals and toxins leading to further deterioration of the cells
- Some autoimmune activity (due to the presence of some abnormal cells) means the older adult may have inflammation and swelling present most of the time (Farley et al. 2006).

Scenario 10.1

Chest Infection

Andrew Macey, a 72-year-old man, has been admitted to the acute medical ward with a severe chest infection. He has difficulty breathing and a constant productive cough, which has prevented him from sleeping and eating. As a result he has lost weight, is exhausted and weak.

Assessment and analysis of patient presentation

Mr Macey's immune system is currently very active but clearly having difficulties overcoming the cause of the infection.

- The expectorant is a result of phagocytosis in the lungs and the production of pus and mucus within the airways.
- Mr Macey's difficulties in breathing are likely to be due to the inflammation caused as part of the immune response, which is reducing the effectiveness of his airway.
- A combination of the energy demands of the immune response coupled with energy required to cough is contributing to Mr Macey's fatigue.
- Fluid used in the immune response may draw from reserves elsewhere leading to a risk of dehydration.

See Table 10.3 for a Nursing Care Plan.

Abnormal immune responses

Thus far, the immune system has been discussed based on the principle that immunity is the result of an interaction between antibodies with an antigen resulting in a comprehensive defence mechanism designed to recognise the antigen, respond and destroy it, memorise, adapt and prepare for further potential invasions. However, there are occasions when the defender becomes the attacker.

Allergic reaction

Allergic reaction can occur during the second and subsequent encounter with an allergen (an antigen causing the reaction). During their initial encounter with the allergen, the individual develops a specific antibody, immunoglobulin E that binds to the allergen. This in turn sensitises the mast cells (responsible for the release of histamine and heparin). Further exposure to the allergen stimulates the mast cells to degranulate and release histamine and heparin. The degree of reaction to an allergen can be varied, with some very mild reactions with minimal symptoms. However, when this reaction is sudden, rapid and intense in nature, and histamine and heparin are released in excess amounts, this can result in anaphylactic shock (Brooker 2000, Evans & Tippins 2005, Ross & Wilson 1990). Anaphylaxis is a life-threatening event and for a positive outcome must be dealt with immediately. It is essential, therefore, that all healthcare professionals are able to recognise anaphylaxis, and know how to respond to it (Figure 10.5).

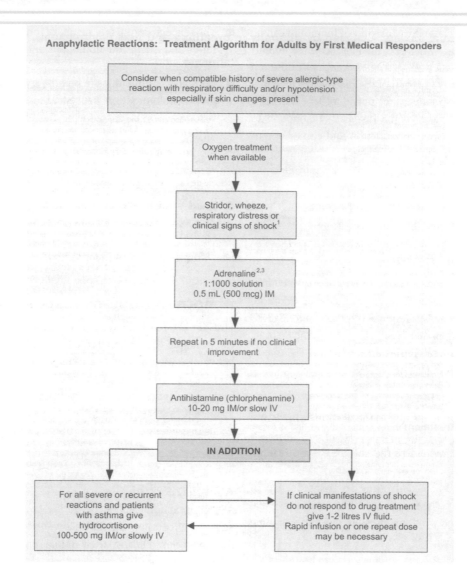

Anaphylactic Reactions: Treatment Algorithm for Adults by First Medical Responders

Consider when compatible history of severe allergic-type reaction with respiratory difficulty and/or hypotension especially if skin changes present

Oxygen treatment when available

Stridor, wheeze, respiratory distress or clinical signs of shock[1]

Adrenaline[2,3]
1:1000 solution
0.5 mL (500 mcg) IM

Repeat in 5 minutes if no clinical improvement

Antihistamine (chlorphenamine)
10-20 mg IM/or slow IV

IN ADDITION

For all severe or recurrent reactions and patients with asthma give hydrocortisone 100-500 mg IM/or slowly IV

If clinical manifestations of shock do not respond to drug treatment give 1-2 litres IV fluid. Rapid infusion or one repeat dose may be necessary

Figure 10.5 Anaphylactic reaction treatment algorithm for adults (Reproduced with permission from RC(UK) (2006)

Developing and Delivering Expert Care: Box 10.2

Signs and Symptoms of Anaphylactic Shock

Early signs and symptoms
- Urticaria
- Rhinitis
- Abdominal pain
- Vomiting
- Diarrhoea

Severe signs and symptoms
- Sense of impending doom
- Flushing/pallor
- Marked upper airway oedema
- Bronchospasm
- Stridor or wheezing

Actual and potential anxiety – caused by difficulty in breathing and new environment

Care	Rationale
Introduce yourself and the clinical team	Reduces the patient's actual and potential anxiety Supports the patient's emotional and psychological well-being
Orientate Mr Macey to his bed space and the ward environment	The patient knows where things are Reduces and relieves any actual or potential anxiety Maintains his independence where possible Promotes his dignity
Explain all procedures and care, allowing him to ask questions, answering any questions or concerns he may have	Supports Mr Macey in informed decision-making processes
Allow the patient time to talk about his concerns or ask questions	Maintains effective communication and overcomes the barriers caused by the patient's difficulty in breathing and cough

Difficulty breathing and productive cough

Care	Rationale
Help the patient position himself in an upright position	Enables more effective chest expansion to increase effectiveness of breathing and gas exchange
Administer medication as prescribed and monitor the effects	Assesses and monitors the effectiveness of medications prescribed Safe and effective administration of medication
Provide the patient with clean containers in which to expectorate, with soft tissue to help him keep a clean mouth	Maintains the patient's hygiene Maintains the patient's privacy and dignity Prevents cross-infection
Administer medication as prescribed to manage his cough	
Ensure the patient has oral fluids and mouthwashes within easy reach	Maintains the patient's fluid balance (homeostasis) Supports his oral hygiene needs Maintains his independence and privacy and dignity
Monitor and assess the patient's fluid intake and output	Prevents dehydration and maintains the patient's fluid balance (homeostasis)
Examine the patient's mouth on a regular basis	Detects and treats an adverse effect of limited fluid intake and poor appetite
Place the nurse call bell within easy reach and explain how to use it	Maintaining effective communication with your patient Maintaining the patient's safety and independence Maintaining the patient's dignity

Table 10.3 Nursing Care Plan

Weakness

Care	Rationale
Assess the patient's risk of falling with a recognised 'falls assessment tool'	Preventing and reducing the risk of fall Maintaining the patient's safety
Provide the patient with a urinal if unable to walk to the toilet	Maintaining the patient's safety and independence Maintaining the patient's dignity
Encourage gentle daily exercise	Counteracting the weakness Preventing complications of immobility
Assess the patient's risk of developing pressure tissue damage due to limited mobility and weakness with a recognised 'pressure ulcer risk assessment tool'	Preventing and reducing the risk of pressure tissue damage
Provide the patient with assistance with his personal and oral hygiene needs	Maintaining personal and oral hygiene Maintaining the patient's privacy and dignity

Poor appetite and weight loss

Care	Rationale
Weigh the patient and calculate his body mass index (Chapter 7)	Assesses and monitors the extent of the patient's weight loss
Assess the patient's nutritional status using a recognised 'risk assessment tool'	Identify possible influencing factors and the extent of risk

Table 10.3 Nursing Care Plan (continued)

Anatomy and Physiology in Action: Box 10.3

Potential allergens

Injected
- Chemicals used in vaccines
- Chemicals and substances used in injected or intravenously administered medicines/substances
- Insect bites
- Venom

Ingested
- Large molecule medicines, e.g. penicillin
- Some foods

Inhaled
- Dust
- Pollen
- Chemicals

Superficial
- Contact with chemicals
- Contact with metals

Autoimmune responses

Autoimmunity is the failure of an organism to recognise its own constituent parts as 'self', which results in an immune response against the identified cells and tissues; an autoimmune response. This can happen in the following situations:
- During transplantation of donor tissue or organs leading to rejection of the tissue or organ, only successful with supporting drugs to suppress the immune response
- During transfusion of blood products
- When the immune system wrongly identifies its own body cells as an antigen and acts to destroy them.

Immunodeficiency

Immunodeficiency is the inability or inadequacy of the immune system to respond effectively, leaving the body's defence system depleted and the individual vulnerable and susceptible to infections, diseases and malignancies (Brooker 2000). The causes of immunodeficiency can be genetic defects; acquired; due to drugs – particularly cytotoxic therapy; malnutrition or disease.

Applying Theory to Practice: Exercise 10.7

Before reading on:

- What responsibility do healthcare professionals have for preventing the spread of hospital-acquired infections (HAI)?
- What HAI are commonly transmitted between patients by healthcare professionals?
- What steps can healthcare professionals take to prevent the spread of HAI?

Diseases of the immune system

Human immunodeficiency virus (HIV) – the facts

HIV was first detected in the early 1980s when a number of homosexual men were diagnosed with a new type of pneumonia, *Pneumocystis carinii pneumonia* (PCP). Shortly after, the US Centers for Communicable Disease and Prevention recognised a global public health issue (Murray & Johnson 1996) as HIV began to be identified as a disease complex, with a whole spectrum of other associated illnesses, and the causative agent of AIDS (acquired immune deficiency syndrome).

Epidemiology

HIV infection is currently responsible for a worldwide epidemic of AIDS, with an estimated 38.6 million people infected with the virus (UNAIDS 2006). According to data produced by the Health Protection Agency (HPA 2007) 63,500 people (over the age of 15 years) were living with HIV in the UK in 2005. Approximately one-third of that population were unaware that they were HIV positive due to the fact that they may have experienced very minor, or no symptoms for a number of years (NAM 2006).

The majority of acquired HIV infection remains in the sex-between-men group and, despite focused health awareness campaigns, there remains little change over recent years in the incidence. However, the incidence of HIV among heterosexuals has risen in the past decade and more recently the incidence of heterosexually acquired HIV has overtaken the incidence of that acquired through sex between men. A large percentage of those were infected outside the UK, with the majority being acquired in Africa. Approximately one-third of individuals acquiring

HIV heterosexually are unaware of their status (HPA 2007a).

The impact on the immune system

The HIV attaches its own surface molecules (glycoprotein GP120) to receptors on the T helper cells and some phagocytes. Once attached, the HIV fuses with its host cell. The HIV goes on to convert the host cells, deoxyribonucleic acid (DNA) the 'blueprint' of the cell containing all its defining genetic material, into its own genetic material called ribonucleic acid (RNA) by using an enzyme present only in retroviruses known as reverse transcriptase. As a result the HIV has converted the host cell into one of its own. Therefore, once triggered to reproduce, it no longer reproduces another T cell, but instead an HIV.

During this initial stage, referred to as **seroconversion**, which can last 1–6 weeks (Gilson 1996), individuals infected by HIV may experience only very mild flu-like symptoms. The infected cell may remain undetected for some time until the immune system is stimulated further at a later stage. It is therefore possible for the individual to be completely symptom-free for a number of years (Gilson 1996).

When the immune system is activated, the newly infected T cells are stimulated to reproduce, believing it is to take on its usual role in the body's immune response. However, changes to the T cell DNA mean that in its place more HIV cells are born, and each T cell can be tricked into producing a considerable number of new HIV, a process more commonly known as 'budding' (Pratt 1992). The impact of this on the immune response is:

- A reduction in T cells
- A reduction in the support the T cell normally provides for the B lymphocytes in their action of producing antibodies, phagocytosis and destruction of antigens by lysis.

Overall there is a deficient and less effective immune system leading to the individual being immunodeficient, compromised and vulnerable.

AIDS-related illnesses and infections

Since AIDS was first described, the definition of AIDS has evolved as a result of more being learnt about the disease, including better testing. The Centers for Disease Control in America has redefined on a number of occasions the

Figure 10.6 HIV and T-cell infection process

factors, such as the level of CD4 T-lymphocytes in the blood, and associated illnesses caused by HIV, which lead to a diagnosis of AIDS. All of the definitions used today are a reflection of a positive HIV status combined with a number of illnesses or 'opportunistic infections' caused by the lack of the ability of the T-Cells to function (Walters 1996).

Scenario 10.2

Infectious illness

Charlie George is a 38-year-old Caucasian man who has been admitted with weight loss, lethargy, persistent cough, a sore dry mouth, a raised temperature and what he describes as ' a sore and uncomfortable chest'.

- What should you first consider when admitting Mr George to the ward environment?
- Is he an infection risk to others?
- Are others an infection risks to Mr George?

Assessment and analysis of patient presentation

Mr George clearly has the classic signs and symptoms of an infection and therefore may be infectious to others, particularly those patients with poor or compromised immune systems. It is difficult to be certain at this stage, but as you do not know the cause of the infection, isolation needs to be considered. As Mr George is quite unwell, it is important to ensure that he can be observed easily as part of monitoring his condition.

Applying Theory to Practice: Exercise 10.8

- As nurses how do we manage this situation?
- What are the local policies and guidelines to support your conclusion?

Mr George may also have a compromised immune system himself and therefore could be at risk of contracting an infection from other patients and healthcare workers.

On admission Mr George's symptoms suggest he is suffering from an acute chest infection, or pneumonia. In this situation the priority is to relieve his chest symptoms to aid his breathing, and reduce his pain and discomfort.

Clinical investigation, using chest X-ray and sputum samples will help determine the micro-organism causing the pneumonia and direct treatment plans. Mr George is also complaining of a sore, dry mouth, which, alongside his cough and lethargy, have decreased his appetite and

Agent	Illness
Virus	Cytamegalovirus (CMV) affects the eyes, gut, lungs and nervous systems and can lead to blindness if left untreated
	HIV encephalopathy, caused by the HIV virus affects the central nervous system. Can cause degrees of symptoms based on severity from changes in coordination and concentration to loss of control, mental health problems and suicidal impulses (NAM 2007)
	Hepatitis B causes liver damage and may lead to liver cancers
	Hepatitis C causes fatigue, weight loss, some food intolerance, upset stomachs with diarrhoea and swollen abdomen, jaundice, internal bleeding, nausea and vomiting. May lead to cirrhosis and liver cancers
Bacteria	MAI causes weight loss, fever and diarrhoea and can be contracted from tap water or soil
	Tuberculosis (TB) causes chest problems including pain, coughing and weight loss. TB is the leading cause of illness and death for individuals who are HIV positive
Protozoa & parasites	Toxoplasmosis contracted through raw or meat that is undercooked, causes cysts in the brain which lead to headaches, fever, fits and in serious situations, coma
Fungi & yeast	Candidiasis (thrush) affects the throat, mouth, vagina, anus and penis. Thrush can be painful
	Cryptococcal meningitis affects the lungs resulting in chest infection and may lead to meningitis
	Pneumocystis carinii pneumonia (PCP) affects the lungs causing inflammation, cough, pain and difficulty breathing. PCP can be fatal if untreated
Cancers & malignancies	Karposi's sarcoma (KS) is a cancer affecting the skin, but may also affect some organs and the gut
	Lymphoma is a cancer affecting the lymph system

Table 10.4 AIDS-related illnesses and infections

contributed to his weight loss. White plaque present inside his mouth suggests oral thrush. Administer oral antifungal therapy as prescribed, ensure you support the patient with his oral hygiene needs and promote oral fluids. Assessing his nutritional status, including body mass index (BMI) will identify if the support of the dietetic team is necessary. Either way, Mr George will need some assistance in regaining his appetite and nutritional intake, which has a vital role in supporting the immune system.

Considering the overall assessment and well-being of Mr George, and from what has been discussed so far

Applying Theory to Practice: Exercise 10.9

- What immediate strategies would you employ to address these priorities?

Consider: cough suppressants, additional oxygen therapy if required, fluids and good positioning to promote lung capacity and comfort.

about the immune system, it suggests that he has an underlying immune deficiency and it is therefore probable that clinical investigations will conclude that Mr George is suffering from *Pneumocystis carinii* pneumonia (PCP). PCP is one of the illnesses that indicate the patient is HIV positive and is also one of the AIDS-defining illnesses (Miller 1996, Mitchell 2007, NAM 2007). Mr George will thus receive two serious diagnoses at the same time.

Applying Theory to Practice: Exercise 10.10

- What are the implications of this diagnosis?
- What is your role in supporting the patient who is receiving this kind of information?
- What are key areas you will need to consider when supporting Mr George and preparing him for discharge home?

Psychosocial

Recent changes to the law ensure that it is now illegal to discriminate against an individual who is HIV positive, and yet despite this, discrimination continues to exist (NAT 2006). The main causes are thought to be largely due to lack of knowledge and ignorance of HIV and how it is transmitted (NAM 2007). Moral judgements, based on people's existing knowledge and information about how HIV is transmitted, for example sexually acquired or through injecting drugs, reinforce existing prejudices about the individuals who participate in these activities, such as gay or bisexual men. In the UK there is still a large percentage of the population who believe individuals with HIV are in some way to blame for their diagnosis (NAM 2007). These prejudices are damaging. They prevent people from using healthcare services, seeking advice or HIV testing, which may delay treatment, affect their general well-being, and contribute to feelings of isolation. National campaigns, led by HIV and AIDS foundations and groups challenge these beliefs and behaviours, and seek to remove them (NAT 2006).

Treatment of HIV

Drug therapy for HIV has developed rapidly since HIV was first recognised. Drugs are now available which target every stage of the HIV infection and reproduction sequence within the host cell, designed to:

- Prevent the HIV attaching to the T cell
- Stop the HIV and host cell fusing together
- Prohibit the HIV converting its RNA to DNA using its reverse transcriptase
- Prevent the HIV from producing enzymes to help in the process of inserting its own DNA into the host's DNA
- Stop the host cell from being used as an HIV reproduction line
- Help stop the 'budding' process of new HIV.

Since the introduction of these drugs, it is considered to be more effective if they are prescribed in combination, that way attacking the HIV at all stages. This combination of therapy is referred to as highly active antiretroviral therapy (HAART). However, none of these drugs are without side-effects and treatment is obviously necessary on a continuous basis, therefore requiring commitment from the patient to adhere to their medication regimen.

The lymphatic system

The lymphatic system plays an ancillary role supporting the cardiovascular system and an essential role as part of the immune system. As fluid circulates throughout the body, plasma leaves the circulation and bathes the cells (interstitial fluid). Plasma contains proteins that are too large to be returned via the small capillaries of the venous system, it is collected by the vessels of the lymphatic system transported to the two lymphatic ducts and returned to the venous blood through small connections to the subclavian vessels.

Form

A network of vessels, cells, tissues, and organs constitute the lymphatic system. Included in this network are:

- Lymph vessels
- Lymph nodes
- The spleen
- The appendix
- The thymus
- Lymphocytes (lymphatic cells).

Running throughout this network is a watery fluid called lymph (*lympha* means 'clear water').

Lymph

Lymph is any fluid that enters the lymph vessels. It is similar to blood plasma, containing more WBCs. Lymph circulates throughout the tissues delivering food, oxygen and water to cells, simultaneously removing waste materials. In the limbs, lymph is rich in protein, especially albumin. In the bone marrow, spleen and thymus, lymph contains higher concentrations of WBCs; in the intestines lymph contains lipids absorbed during digestion.

Lymph vessels

Lymph vessels, also called lymphatics, carry lymph in only one direction – back towards the heart. Throughout all the tissues of the body, lymph vessels form a complicated, spidery network of fine tubes. The smallest vessels, called lymph capillaries, have a closed or dead end in contrast to the cardiovascular system, forming a closed circuit. The walls of these capillaries are composed of only a single layer of flattened cells. The pressure inside these walls is lower than that of the venous capillaries making them accessible to the large molecule fragments of damaged cells and micro-organisms that they are required to filter. Lymph capillaries in the villi of the small intestine are called lacteals. These specialised capillaries transport the fat products of digestion, such as fatty acids and vitamin A.

Lymph nodes

Scattered along the pathways of lymph vessels are oval or kidney-bean-shaped masses of lymphatic tissue called lymph nodes acting as filters (Table 10.5). The smaller lymph nodes are often called lymph nodules. Lymph nodes occur in clusters or chains. The neck, armpits, chest, abdomen, pelvis and groin are areas where the nodes can be palpated. Damaged cells are taken to the lymph nodes to be destroyed. The nodes can become increasingly swollen and tender if the micro-organism is not easily destroyed, i.e. cancers.

Function

> **Scenario 10.3**
>
> ### Diseases Affecting the Lymphatic System
>
> James Nesbitt is a 19-year-old who attends his local walk-in health centre due to a two-week history of lethargy and sporadic fever.
>
> He states that he is feeling progressively weaker and just wants to sleep most of the time.
>
> His respiratory rate is 21, pulse 98 and regular, blood pressure 108/64. His temperature is recorded as 38.2.
>
> He has no relevant medical history, takes no medication and has just begun university.

Assessment and analysis of patient presentation

The physical observations suggest a slight raise in Mr Nesbitt's metabolism. This is commonly caused by an underlying infection, which is confirmed by the sporadic temperature. The presenting history of increasing lethargy and weakness are common symptoms that develop during a viral infection and can also continue for an extended period afterwards. Recently starting university may provide a clue to the source of infection and meningitis

Function	Structures
Drainage of intercellular fluid (including large proteins and microorganisms)	Lymph capillaries and vessels
Filters lymph and destroys micro-organisms (phagocytosis)	Superficial and deep lymph nodes remove micro-organisms
Manufacture of lymphocytes, monocytes and antibodies	Lymphatic tissue within the nodes, spleen, tonsils, adenoids and thymus gland in infancy
Transports digested fats after absorption	Lymph capillaries attached to the intestinal villi drain into lymphatic vessels (lacteals)
Breaks down red blood cells and platelets: pigments are distributed to the liver and iron to the bone marrow	The spleen and cells within the liver and lymph nodes

Table 10.5 The Function of the Lymphatic System

should be excluded as a serious possibility. Another common viral infection associated with communal living and close contact is glandular fever. The cause of glandular fever (infectious mononucleosis) is the Epstein–Barr virus (EBV).

Pathophysiology

The EBV is a member of the herpes family. It is an infectious illness that can result in tender swelling or enlargement of the lymph nodes as the defence system endeavours to fight the virus. The most common age to catch glandular fever is between the ages of 16 and 25 (HPA 2007b). As with most viral infections, once an individual has been exposed at a young age they acquire immunity by producing specific antibodies. The Health Protection Agency advises that young children do not need to be taken out of school or nursery when they have glandular fever (HPA 2006). This is because the infection is usually mild in young children, and the incubation period is so long that it is hard to work out the source.

Glandular fever is an infectious illness and can be passed on to family and friends, but most adults exposed to glandular fever have previously been infected with the EBV and are therefore not at risk of developing symptoms. Glandular fever is usually passed on through intimate contact between an uninfected person and someone who has the EBV but is not showing any symptoms. The EBV is normally spread via the saliva. This is most frequently seen in teenagers and young adults. It is thought to spread in a similar way to many other viruses, from saliva, and is sometimes jokingly referred to as the 'kissing disease' as it is often passed from partner to partner.

Applying Theory to Practice: Box 10.4

Signs and Symptoms of Glandular Fever

- Lethargy and weakness
- Recent flu-like symptoms
- Headache and sore throat
- Sweats and alterations to body temperature
- Enlarged lymph nodes – neck, armpits, abdomen, groin
- Pale and gaunt physical appearance
- Extensive muscular pains
- Possible splenomegaly

Glandular fever often commences with a few days of mild symptoms, including headaches and tiredness. The main symptoms then develop, lasting for up to three weeks, although post-illness lethargy can continue for an extended period (NCID 2007). The effect on the individual varies.

The plan of care

There is no specific treatment for glandular fever. Antibiotics do not combat viral infections. Anti-inflammatory analgesics may relieve some of the symptoms, due to the pain being caused by inflammation, and antipyrexials such as paracetamol will relieve the pyrexia and make him feel better. Mr Nesbitt should be encouraged to continue his normal lifestyle, take extra fluids and supplement his diet with vitamins and minerals directed at aiding his own immune system, such as zinc and vitamin C (although there is limited evidence to support this). An increasing number of antiviral medications are being developed directed at preventing viral proliferation, thereby enabling

Applying Theory to Practice: Exercise 10.11

Antivirals and Vaccines

As a student nurse you will need to develop an excellent knowledge of medications.
Complete the following exercise and add the results to your portfolio.

- Identify at least four different vaccinations.
- What are the potential side effects of these drugs?

There are many myths surrounding vaccines and what they actually contain and how the individual gains immunity from this process.

- What do vaccines really contain?
- Identify three different types of antiviral drug.

There are many complementary therapies directed at boosting the immune system. Unlike prescription medications they may not have undergone extensive research.

- What complementary therapies can you find that have a research base?

A couple of examples may include echinacea and zinc.

the immune system to eradicate the virus. Vaccines have been developed against many viral infections. A specific vaccine provides the immune system with the ability to quickly and effectively fight a particular virus.

Applying Theory to Practice: Exercise 10.12

Common Pathologies Affecting the Lymphatic System

- Lymphangitis
- Hodgkin's disease
- Lymphoedema

Research the possible physical changes resulting from these processes and identify the clinical signs you would look for during the assessment process and how the care of these patients would be managed.

Add the findings to your portfolio, which on completion of this chapter should form the foundation from which you can build an in-depth knowledge within the aforementioned areas.

The endocrine system

The endocrine system is largely concerned with regulation and therefore has a pivotal role in maintaining the body's balance. The system itself is not connected anatomically, but is a system made up of glands positioned throughout the body.

The purpose of the endocrine system is to:

- Produce and release chemicals called hormones
- Release hormones to the tissues and cells to control the body's reaction and enable it to adapt to changes thereby maintaining balance and homeostasis
- Control the body's metabolism.

Form

Abnormalities of the endocrine system are largely due to three overarching reasons; a disordered endocrine system, which may be as a result of a genetic abnormality, overproduction or underproduction of a particular hormone. One of the most common diseases of the endocrine system is **diabetes mellitus**, affecting around 180 mil-

lion of the world's population (WHO 2007) with this figure steadily rising (Holt & Hanley 2007). It is likely that you will care for patients with diabetes throughout your nursing career in all specialties.

Scenario 10.4

Diabetes

Mrs Khan is 65-year-old woman of Asian origin who is having problems with recurring urine infections.

She has been found to have a consistently high blood glucose level and has been diagnosed with type 2 diabetes.

- What care and considerations are required to ensure Mrs Khan manages her diabetes safely and effectively?

Diabetes mellitus occurs when there is a consistently raised level of glucose in the blood (hyperglycaemia), which can be detected very simply by using a small device (a glucometer) with only a tiny amount of fresh blood taken from a finger prick. Hyperglycaemia results when there is a lack of the hormone insulin, which is produced by the beta cells of the islets of Langerhans situated in the pancreas. The problem may be with the production and release of the hormone or the action of the insulin or indeed both.

There are 1.8 million people in England who have been diagnosed with diabetes and the number is increasing (DH 2003). However, if this number included all those individuals living with diabetes, but yet undiagnosed, the number would be closer to 2.4 million. This group are sometimes referred to as the 'missing million'.

There are two main types of diabetes mellitus (Table 10.7), simply called type 1 and type 2. In type 1 diabetes the body does not produce any insulin and is, therefore, completely dependent on insulin replacement therapy to survive. Out of all the people diagnosed with diabetes, type 1 accounts for 5–10% of cases (Evans & Tippins 2007). Mrs Khan has been diagnosed with type 2 diabetes. In this type of diabetes, individuals are able to produce some insulin, but often not as much as they require, or the body is resistant to the effects of insulin (Holt & Hanley 2007). This type of diabetes accounts for 85–90% of all diabetic cases (Phillips 2007).

Gland and anatomical position	Hormone	Function
Pituitary gland situated in the hypophyseal fossa of the sphenoid bone of the skull	Antidiuretic hormone	Reduces urine production in the kidneys
	Oxytocin	Produced in the hypothalamus but stored and secreted by the pituitary gland. Its role is in childbirth
	Melanocyte stimulating hormone	
	Human growth hormone	Stimulates growth of body tissue: bone, cartilage and muscle. Also influences the metabolism of fats, proteins and carbohydrates. Can be affected by exercise, emotional well-being and nutrition
	Prolactin	Stimulates lactation
	Follicle stimulating hormone	Stimulates the development and ripening of the ovum
		Stimulates spermatozoa production
	Luteinising hormone (LH)	Works with FSH to stimulate ova or spermatozoa
	Thyroid stimulating hormone (TSH)	Stimulates growth and activity of the thyroid gland to secrete thyroxin
	Adrenocorticotrophic hormone (ACTH)	
Hypothalamus situated above the pituitary gland in the brain	Thyrotrophin releasing hormone (TRH)	
	Prolactin inhibiting hormone (PIH)	Regulates the level of prolactin produced by the pituitary gland, thought to be the neurotransmitter dopamine
	Prolactin releasing hormone (PRH)	Stimulates the production of prolactin by the pituitary gland
	Gonadotrophin releasing hormone (GnRH)	Secreted at puberty to mature the gonads
	Somastostatin	Inhibits the release of glucagons and insulin

Table 10.6 Endocrine system – Form & Function

Thyroid gland situated in the neck in front of the larynx and trachea	Thyroxine	Regulates metabolic rate and the metabolism of carbohydrates. Also regulates growth and development and functioning of the reproductive system and nervous system
	Calcitonin	Regulates calcium in the blood
Parathyroid gland situated on the posterior wall of the thyroid gland	Parathyroid hormone (PTH)	Regulates serum calcium levels
Adrenal and suprarenal glands situated above the kidneys	Epinephrine	
	Glucocorticoids including hydrocortisone, corticosterone and cortisone	Control metabolism of glucose and how they are stored and released from the liver. Also influence fatty acids, sodium and water levels. Regulate some aspects of the immune system, i.e. gastric juices, enzymes and inflammatory response and allergy
	Aldosterone	Regulates haemostasis
Islets of Langerhans situated in the pancreas	Insulin	Reduces the level of glucose in the blood and stimulates the tissues to absorb
	Glucagon	Increases the level of sugars in the blood
Pineal gland situated under the brain	Melatonin	Poorly understood, but thought to be involved in puberty. Also thought to influence mood in relation to light levels
Ovaries	Oestrogen	Sex hormones
Testes	Testosterone	Sex hormones
	Dihydrotestosterone	

Table 10.6 Endocrine system – Form & Function (continued)

The treatment of Mrs Khan's diabetes, as with all patients, is individualised to her, with medication, which may be a combination of therapies (NICE 2002) being prescribed alongside consideration of her current lifestyle such as diet and weight management, which may be having an impact on her diabetes and general well-being. As most patients who are diagnosed with type 2 diabetes are overweight at the point of diagnosis (IDF 2005), it is possible that Mrs Khan will need support and advice about how to manage her weight effectively. As well as affecting her body's metabolism, being overweight can increase her resistance to insulin (Lowey 2005), and increase her risk of developing hypertension and high cholesterol, both of which can lead to cardiovascular disease. Cardiovascular disease is said to be responsible for approximately 75% of deaths in patients with diabetes (Lowey 2005).

It is vital that patients with diabetes, like Mrs Khan, learn not only to control their blood glucose levels, but also have a good understanding of how to maintain their

Type 1 – insulin-dependent diabetes	Type 2 – non-insulin-dependent diabetes
Sudden destruction of insulin-secreting cells leads to acute hyperglycaemic episodes characterised by insulin deficiency and ketosis resulting in gastric stasis, coma and death if left untreated	Insidious onset characterised by increasingly defective ability to secrete and utilise insulin, eventually leading to hyperglycaemia
Accounts for 10–15% of cases (DH 2001b)	Not traditionally associated with ketosis, results in many associated disease processes being present when disease is first diagnosed
Results early in life as a consequence of an autoimmune reaction (presentation <25) with destruction of pancreatic islet beta cells	Accounts for 85% of cases (DH 2001b)
Daily insulin injections needed to sustain life	Traditionally associated with middle age onset (>40)
Insulin requirements, physical levels of activity and diet need correlation	Increasing teenage/young adult onset: direct correlation with increasing levels of obesity (DH 2001)
Potential for hypoglycaemia high	Considered a preventable disease
Can be idiopathic	Commonly associated with high fat/calorie diet, lack of exercise and obesity (ADA 2005)
Life expectancy reduced on average by 20 years	In many cases diet and lifestyle modification may curtail symptoms and disease establishment
	Life expectancy reduced by 10 years (dependent on age of onset)

Prolonged exposure to hyperglycaemia causes widespread tissue damage. Commonly affected areas include the eyes, kidneys and feet.

Diabetes is the leading cause of renal failure and blindness (in working age) and the second commonest cause of limb amputation.

Diabetes accounts for 5% of total NHS resources. It is estimated that 10% of inpatient services are used by those with diabetes.

Table 10.7 Presentation, Classification and Pathophysiology

general health and well-being to prevent associated illnesses. However, managing weight loss may not be as straightforward for some patients. The older adult may have other illnesses or conditions which limit their mobility, and so developing an exercise programme may be more challenging (IDF 2005).

Religious and cultural differences may have an impact on any weight loss plan and need to be carefully considered. It may be necessary for patients to develop a whole new approach to food, meal preparation and mealtimes, which can be greatly influenced by whether or not the patient is dependent on others. It is also therefore necessary to not only educate Mrs Khan, but also her family and carers, which may require enlisting the support of a range of professionals and agencies.

It is possible for patients with type 2 diabetes to adequately manage their disease by making the necessary adjustments to their diet and lifestyle. However, it may

Applying Theory to Practice: Exercise 10.13

Consider the impact of diabetes for the older adult who may:

- be less able to exercise due to other illnesses and conditions
- not have access to equipment or support, such as a gymnasium
- be less able to prepare fresh meals
- rely on others for their food shopping
- have a decline in their cognitive function
- have poor visibility.

also mean that Mrs Khan will require medication, such as anti-diabetic drugs as outlined in Table 10.8. It is also

Group of drugs	Action	Drugs
Sulphonylureas	Stimulate the release of insulin from the pancreas Only effective if the patient has some beta – cells functioning Drugs in this category are wide-ranging in the length of time they remain active in the body and range between 4–30 hours	Gliclazide Glibenclamide
Biguanides		Metformin
Alpha-glycosidase inhibitors	Support the breakdown of carbohydrates in the intestine preventing absorption	Acarbose
Rapid-acting insulin secretagogues	Target post-meal blood glucose control	Repaglinide Nateglinide
Glitazones	Combat insulin resistance	Rosiglitazone

Table 10.8 Drug treatment of diabetes

possible that she will require insulin injections at a later date in the disease trajectory (IDF 2005, NICE 2002, Wallymahmed 2006).

Adherence to a medication regimen is important for Mrs Khan to ensure safe and effective management of her disease. This will also require a degree of education.

The Department of Health, alongside the National Diabetes Team, advocates structured education programmes for patients diagnosed with diabetes. This would be essential for Mrs Khan to gain a good understanding of her disease management, but her individual needs should also be considered. Information should be provided in a language and manner that she understands, and is able to retain and relate to her own disease management. Patient participation is vital if you are to ensure independence and self-management of long-term conditions such as diabetes, and has now been recognised as the key to preventing complications.

One of the complications of diabetes is nephropathy. Nephropathy is damage to the kidneys and it is estimated that 25% of all patients with diabetes experience nephropathy after 25 years (Lowey 2005). Mrs Khan therefore requires further investigation into her recurring urine infections beyond the influence of hyperglycaemia. Another complication of diabetes is retinopathy. It is suggested that more than half of patients with type 2 diabetes will have some degree of retinopathy, damage to the retina, after 20 years (Watkins 2003). Neuropathy, damage to the nerves, is also associated with diabetes, particularly where blood glucose levels are poorly managed or controlled and can lead to a number of symptoms such as numbness to the extremities and peripheries, particularly the legs and feet, as well as pain, which can lead to the patient developing ulcers.

Diabetes – the facts

The Government has clearly recognised the need to ensure that patients have access to effective healthcare, irrespective of where they live, and has outlined national standards for the provision of diabetes care in the *National Service Framework for Diabetes* (DH 2001) and the follow-up *Delivery Strategy* (DH 2003). In addition, the National Diabetes Support Team has produced guidance and best evidence-based practice initiatives to support healthcare teams and organisations to develop and achieve excellence in diabetes care.

The NSF emphasises the need to ensure that individuals at risk of developing diabetes are given advice and education to prevent development of the disease. It is

estimated that the majority of diabetes cases are preventable, that is about two-thirds of all cases.

Risk factors

- Environmental
- Diet
- Obesity
- Ageing population
- Decrease in levels of exercise and physical activity.

In addition, the 'missing million' are provided with access to a diagnosis and treatment to prevent further complications of the disease.

Professional issues

Nurses have an important role to play in educating patients in living healthier lifestyles through a balanced diet, exercise and avoidance of obesity:

- Routine screening of urinalysis and blood glucose levels
- Empowering patients diagnosed with diabetes to be self-caring in managing this long-term condition for the optimum health and quality of life.

Resources and guidance to help you understand how services have been developed for patients with diabetes in the UK

- *National Standards, Local Action – health and social care standards and planning framework 2005/6–2007/8* (2004) Department of Health, London. www.dh.gov.uk.

This document outlines key targets for improving the health of the nation, supporting patients with long-term conditions and engaging patients in their healthcare.

- *Commissioning Framework for Health and Well-being* (2007) Department of Health, London. www.dh.gov.uk. Builds on the above guidance by providing a framework designed to help commissioners create services that deliver the choices identified by patients, underpinned by quality and access, thereby reducing inequalities in healthcare. This document emphasises the need for collaboration between service providers.
- The National Diabetes Support Team (NDST) established in 2003 with the purpose of providing guidance and support to ensure the effective implementation of the NSF. The team produce some excellent guidance documents that have been the basis for services and care provided to patients with diabetes. Provides clear and concise information that supports healthcare professionals to deliver and share good practice. The NDST produce briefings, updates and newsletters with links to resources and information websites. www.diabetes.nhs.uk
 National Diabetes Audit (NDA). www.icservices.nhs.uk

Conclusion

This chapter has provided an overview of the immune/lymphatic and endocrine systems and described common diseases that can affect these systems. Neither of these systems works autonomously and many of the diseases described will be affected or have an impact on other systems outlined in other chapters of this book. It is important to be able make these links in order to fully understand these complex systems.

Chapter 10 Summary Quiz

1. Which of the following are fundamental roles of the skin?

A. Protection, sensation, heat regulation

B. Protection, reproduction absorption

C. Insulin secretion, elimination, vitamin D production

D. Heat regulation, secretion, urea regulation

2. What drugs may be given to combat an anaphylactic reaction?

A. Norepinephrine, aspirin, digoxin

B. Norepinephrine, antihistamines, salbutamol

C. Epinephrine, salbutamol, steroids

D. Paracetamol, epinephrine, steroids

3. Which of the following are both antiviral drugs?

A. Abacavir, zidovudine

B. Didanosine, amoxycillin

C. Abacavir, ciprofloxacin

D. Prednisolone, enfuvirtide

4. The endocrine system consists of which components?

A. Liver, heart, kidneys

B. Spleen, liver, gall bladder

C. Lungs, trachea, bronchioles

D. Hypothalamus, parathyroid gland, adrenal glands

5. Which cells play a major role in immunity?

A. Mast cells, neutrophils

B. Beta cells, basophils

C. Thrombocytes, leucocytes

D. Mast cells, red blood cells

6. Which common disease processes are associated with diabetes mellitus?

A. Heart disease, lymphatic cancer, foot ulcers

B. Kidney disease, heart disease, retinopathy

C. Retinopathy, foot ulcers, diverticulitis

D. Erectile dysfunction, foot ulcers, pathological fractures

7. What clinical signs frequently accompany anaphylaxis?

A. Marked upper airway oedema, intense thirst

B. Bronchospasm, urticaria

C. Constipation, expiratory wheezing

D. Seizures, headache

8. The lymphatic system contains:

A. The spleen

B. The liver

C. The kidneys

D. The brain

9. How many people are estimated to be living with HIV in the UK?

A. 2,000

B. 100,000

C. 1,000,000

D. 63,000

10. Which acts undertaken by healthcare professionals compromise the integrity of the patient's skin and therefore predispose the patient to infection?

A. Venous cannulation

B. Applying oxygen therapy

C. Assisting a patient to wash

D. Recording a temperature

Further reading

Brooker, C. (2000) *Human Structure and Function: Nursing Applications in Clinical Practice.* Mosby: London.

Department of Health (2006) *Turning the Corner: Improving Diabetes Care.* DH: London.

Farley, A., McLafferty, E. & Hendry, C. (2006) The physiological effects of ageing on the activities of living. *Nursing Standard* 20(45): 46–52.

Health Protection Agency (HPA) (2007) *Epidemiology – HIV and AIDS.* www.hpa.co.uk

National AIDS Trust (2006) *Stigma and Discrimination.* www.nat.co.uk (accessed 16 October 2007).

http://pathmicro.med.sc.edu/book/immunol-sta.htm

References

American Diabetes Association (ADA) (2005) Standards of medical care in diabetes. *Diabetes Care.* 28: Suppl I.

Brooker, C. (2000) *Human Structure and Function: Nursing Applications in Clinical Practice.* Mosby: London.

Department of Health (2001) *The Expert Patient: A New Approach to Chronic Disease Management for the 21st Century.* DH: London.

Department of Health (2003) *National Service Framework for Diabetes: Delivery Strategy.* DH: London.

Department of Health (2006) *Turning the Corner: Improving Diabetes Care.* DH: London.

East Berkshire Diabetic Network 2006–2009 (2006) *East Berkshire Diabetes Strategy.* King Edward Vii Hospital: Windsor, Berkshire.

Evans, C. & Tippins, E. (2005) Emergency treatment of anaphylaxis. *Accident and Emergency Nursing* 13(4): 232–7.

Evans, C. & Tippins, E. (2007) *The Foundations of Emergency Care.* Open University Press: Maidenhead.

Farley, A. McLafferty, E. & Hendry, C. (2006) The physiological effects of ageing on the activities of living. *Nursing Standard* 20(45): 46–52.

Gilson, R.J.C. (1996) Hepatitis B and admission to medical school. *British Medical School* 313: 830–1.

Health Protection Agency (HPA) (2007a) *Epidemiology – HIV and AIDS.* www.hpa.co.uk (accessed 14 November 2007).

Health Protection Agency (HPA) (2007b) *Factsheet on Glandular Fever.* HPA: London.

Holt, R. & Hanley, N. (2007) Overview of diabetes. In: *Essential Endocrinology and Diabetes*, 5th edn. Blackwell Publishing: Oxford.

International Diabetes Federation (IDF) (2005) *Global Guideline for Type 2 Diabetes.* IDF: Brussels. www.idf.org

Lowey, A. (2005) Drug treatment in type 2 diabetes in adults. *Nursing Standard* 20(11): 55–61.

Miller, R. (1996) Respiratory manifestations of AIDS. In: Mindel, A. & Miller, R. (eds) *AIDS: A Pocket Book of Diagnosis and Management*, 2nd edn. Arnold: London.

Mitchell, B. (2007) A background and critical analysis of the treatment of *Pneumocystis carinii* pneumonia (PCP) and HIV/AIDS. *Australian Nursing Journal* 14(9): 20–3.

NAM (2007) Lincoln House, London. www.aidsmap.com (accessed 16/10/07).

National AIDS Trust (NAT) (2006) *Stigma and Discrimination.* www.nat.co.uk (accessed 16/10/07).

National Centre for Infectious Diseases (2007) *Epstein-Barr Virus and Infectious Mononucleosis.* www.cdc.gov/ncidod/diseases/ebv.htm (accessed 17 July 2007).

National Institute for Health and Clinical Excellence (NICE) (2006). *Obesity.* NICE: London.

National Travel Health Network & Centre (NaTHNaC) (2006) *Annual Report 2005–2006.* DH: London.

Phillips, A. (2007) Starting patients on insulin therapy: diabetes nurse specialist views. *Nursing Standard* 21(30): 35–40.

Pratt, R. (1992) *AIDS: A Strategy for Nursing Care*, 3rd edn. Edward Arnold: London.

Resuscitation Council (UK) (2006) *Advanced Life Support*, 5th edn. RCUK: London.

Ross, J. & Wilson, K. (1990) *Anatomy and Physiology in Health and Illness*, 7th edn. Churchill Livingstone: Edinburgh.

UNAIDS (2006) *AIDS Epidemic Update.* http://www.aidsmap.com/en/news/B600B47A-0B6A-4FE8-BC75-5BBE13CC7D24.asp (accessed 13 November 2007).

Wallymahmed, M. (2006) Insulin therapy in the management of type 1 and type 2 diabetes. *Nursing Standard* 18(6): 50–6.

Walters, S. (1996) Paediatric aspects of HIV infection. In: Mindel, A. & Miller, R. (eds) *AIDS: A Pocket Book of Diagnosis and Management*, 2nd edn. Arnold: London.

Watkins, P. (2003) ABC of diabetes – retinopathy. *British Medical Journal* 326: 924–6.

World Health Organization (2007) *Guidance on Provider-initiated HIV Testing and Counselling in Health Facilities.* WHO Department of HIV/AIDS. http://www.who.int/hiv/pub/guidelines/9789241595568_en.pdf

The senses

Cliff Evans and Emma Tippins

Introduction

This chapter focuses on several organs that collectively provide the individual with their insight into the outside world. The ability to 'sense' is a primitive function developed through thousands of years of evolutionary change. The senses are taken for granted by those with a fully functioning ability, but for many a combination of congenital, degenerative and acute pathologies results in a decreased ability in one or more of these functions. This can have major effects on the individual's ability to function, their mental health and the way they are perceived and treated by the society they live in. The chapter is divided into sections describing the form and functioning of each component. A clinical scenario is used to address and discuss many of the issues nurses will meet in their everyday duties. Common pathologies, their recognition, possible treatment and the effects on the individual will all be discussed. Several further learning opportunities will provide the reader with the ability to gain extensive materials for their developing portfolio as well as offering the opportunity to work in combination with others and share thoughts, feelings and knowledge for mutual benefit.

Anatomy and Physiology in Action: Exercise 11.1

Before continuing, complete the following exercise:

- Write a list identifying all the organs of sense.
- What diseases can you think of that affect each of them?
- Are any of the diseases hereditary or congenital?

The eye (sight)

Form

When you think about the ability to see, the immediate focus centres on the eyes, but the eyes are only one of a number of structures involved in achieving the sense of vision, others include:

- The eyelids
- The lacrimal glands
- The extrinsic muscles of eye movement.

The eyelids are composed of very fine skin and muscle (the thinnest skin area on the body), connective tissue containing oil-secreting sebaceous glands and the conjunctiva, a mucous membrane that lines the inner surface of the eyelids and extends onto the anterior surface of the eyeball. The lacrimal gland is anatomically located laterally and superiorly within the eye orbit. This gland works in unison with glandular cells to lubricate and moisten the eye.

The eye consists of three prime components forming a spherical ball-shaped body, around 24mm in diameter.

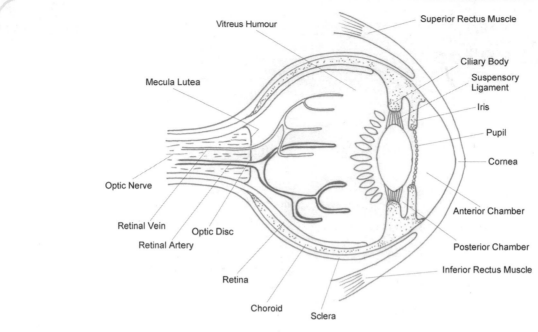

Figure 11.1 Lateral view of the eye and its components

The tunics consist of three layers:

- An outer fibrous layer consisting of the sclera (the white of the eye), which forms the transparent cornea at the front of the eye. The cornea is surrounded by a thin layer of modified skin extending from the eyelids, called the conjunctiva
- The uvea, the middle or vascular layer containing the choroids, the ciliary body and the iris
- The retina, which lines the posterior two-thirds of the eyeball thereby forming the inner layer.

The **optical components** consist of:

- The lens, composed of lens fibres, suspended behind the pupil by a fibrous ring called the suspensory ligament stabilised by its attachment to the ciliary body
- A serous fluid called aqueous humour, which fills the space between the iris and the lens called the posterior chamber. It continues into the space between the cornea and the iris called the anterior chamber. This fluid is drained out via the scleral venous sinus
- A transparent jelly called the vitreous body or vitreous humour, which fills the large space behind the lens.

Nerve supply
Many nerves combine to control a full range of eye movement. The main nerves are the oculomotor and trochlear nerves that stimulate muscles that control eye opening and rotation or movement. The optic nerve fuses with the sclera at the rear of the eye where nerve fibres from the retina become part of the optic nerve.

- The retina (located in the eye's inner layer): a complex structure consisting of many distinct layers, which are thin and delicate. The light-sensitive layer consists of rods and cones
- The optic disc: a small area of the retina where the optic nerve leaves the eye.

Anatomy and Physiology in Action: Exercise 11.2

Rods and cones are the eyes' visual receptors.

Complete the following exercise to enhance your understanding on the eyes' anatomy and function:

- What particular function do rods play?
- Does the eye contain more rods or cones?

Figure 11.2 Anterior photograph of the eye

Function

The function of the eyes centres on providing the individual with vision. Vision consists of several vital concurrent functions, the properties of which include brightness and colour. When vision is normal, seeing is so effortless that the individual functions that comprise vision are imperceptible.

Vision is composed of three distinct perceptions:

- Forms
- Colours
- Movement.

Thus, we have form perception, colour perception and motion perception.

Overview

The cornea receives light as it enters the eye. The light particles continue through the lens eventually disseminating into the receptor cells of the retina. The retina contains an area called the fovea, which is densely populated by cone cells and limited numbers of rod cells. The central point of our vision is focused on the fovea for high definition, colour and clarity (Clancy & McVicar 2002). Due to the small size of the receptor cells, light particles may enter some and not others thereby enabling an increased ability to distinguish particular details. This ability to perceive detail is called visual acuity. The visual field is a term used to describe the breadth of vision; this results from a combination of the iris aperture, the lens and the cornea. Due to the curvature of the cornea, vision extends beyond 180 degrees.

When light fragments enter the retina, the signals are relayed to the optic nerve. These signals are now converted into electrical activity for transmission and interpretation within the brain. The right side of the brain interprets signals from the left side of the retina and the left side of the brain vice versa. This process facilitates depth of vision as both eyes provide varying data to the brain.

Central interpretation

The occipital lobe, areas of both the frontal and motor cortex and the brain stem are all involved in the central act of visual perception.

To maintain vision the eyes must continually adapt to meet the external environment. In bright daylight the eye uses photopic vision, the scientific term for human colour vision under normal lighting conditions during the day. Colours are varied and easily distinguishable due to the action of three different types of cone cells that culminate to sense three respective bands of colour. In very dim light, scotopic vision is the primary source of vision; since cone cells are nonfunctional in low light, scotopic vision is produced exclusively through rod cells which only respond to luminance differences, therefore there is no colour perception; vision is purely centred on varying shades of grey. In twilight, when both rod and cone cells function, we have mesopic vision; a combination of photopic and scotopic vision. This combination effect results in an inaccurate visual acuity and colour discrimination with a resulting higher total sensitivity for the blue range of colours.

Lubrication

Keeping the eye moist is an essential function as without lubrication the eye is placed at a greater risk of infection and will become increasingly painful. The lachrymal glands (referred to as the tear glands) (Figure 11.3) provide secretions for the cornea. The secretions then drain out via the nasal cavity and the lacrymal duct. Tears continually irrigate dust and foreign particles out of the eye.

Visual defects

The cornea at the front surface of the eye acts as a lens. In perfect sight, the image is brought into sharp focus at the back surface of the eye on the retina. Problems with vision occur when the image is not accurately focused on the retina and the vision becomes blurred. This distortion to

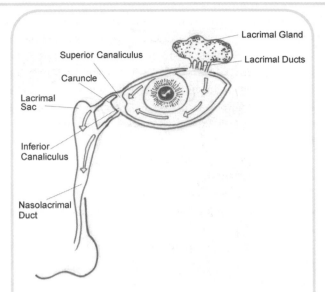

Figure 11.3 The eye and lachrymal gland demonstrating the flow of secretions

normal vision can be corrected with glasses or contact lenses.

Short sight (myopia)

Short sight is hereditary and develops through the teens, affecting approximately 20% of the population (James et al. 2004). The focusing power of the eyes is too strong. Objects at a distance appear blurred with close vision clear. Glasses will make things look smaller when held at arm's length. Laser surgery reduces the thickness of the cornea in the central zone, reducing its focusing ability. Images are then brought into correct focus. Treatment for myopia is very simple and effective and centres on three different corrective actions:

● Optical devices (glasses and contact lenses)
● Corneal refractive procedures (photorefractive surgery/laser therapy)
● Intraocular procedures (the insertion of clear plastic implants into the cornea, an interventional procedure aiming to restore eyesight in short-sightedness) (NICE 2007).

Long sight (hyperopia)

The term hyperopia refers to an inability of the focusing power of the eyes resulting in long-sightedness. Objects are more comfortably viewed at a distance rather than close up (less than 6 feet). Corrective treatment centres on

magnification. In severe cases vision is not clear at any distance. Treatment is still considered experimental by many ophthalmic surgeons (James et al. 2004).

Visual tests

There are many different tests that can be used individually or that can be combined to build a constructive view of an individual's vision. These include:

● Visual acuity
● Visual field
● Contrast sensitivity
● Colour vision
● Visual adaptation.

Questioning Clinical Practice: Exercise 11.3

The tests listed above represent only a handful of several delicate and qualitative tests currently available to healthcare professionals to enable them to assemble an informative overview of an individual's sight ability.

Complete the following exercise to gain further insight and knowledge into this fascinating topic, add your findings to your portfolio:

● Identify the tests available within your placement areas.
● Are any of these tests used to identify insidious diseases that can affect eyesight rather than an actual eye problem (primary vs secondary cause)?
● Think back to when you commenced nursing. Did you have your eyes tested?
● Which test was this, and what was the rationale?

Drugs affecting the eyes

Many drugs can affect the eyes' ability to function normally even when very low or therapeutic doses are given. Most of these drugs either dilate the pupil, known as mydriatics, or constrict the pupil, known as miotics.

Mydriatics

Drugs that have a mydriatic effect simply result in a dilated pupil. They can be used to examine the eye as they prevent muscle around the eye contracting the pupil; therefore, the pupil remains dilated. Within clinical practice atropine is commonly administered as an eye drop to dilate the pupil for examination of the retina/optic disc. Drugs do not necessarily need to be administered directly to the eye to have a dilatory effect, for example, atropine given intravenously for heart conditions will also result in dilated pupils; this dilatory affect can last for hours resulting in temporary blurred vision.

Applying Theory to Practice: Exercise 11.4

Overdoses of many drugs will also result in pupillary changes, which can mean the patient attends hospital with a good clinical indicator of the underlying cause of their problem.

- Make a short list of any drugs, legal or illegal, that affect the size of the pupil.

Read the next section and add to your current knowledge base.

Miotics

Miotics result in a constriction of the pupil by constricting muscles that surround the eye. Constriction of the eye can also be caused by metabolic disorders; these include renal failure (Chapter 6).

Scenario 11.1

Acute Conjunctivitis

Gabrielle Downing, a 29-year-old mother of two young children, arrives at the GP surgery where you are on placement. Gabrielle has an emergency appointment with the practice nurse. Her presenting complaint is a two-day history of a red, inflamed and painful right eye. This morning her eyelids were stuck together and she has a sensation of grit in her eye. On examination her vital signs are normal for her age and she is apyrexial.

Ms Downing has no relevant medical history and is allergic to penicillin.

Assessment and analysis of patient presentation

Ms Downing is presenting with the classic clinical symptoms of conjunctivitis. This centres on the physical presentation of an acute and non-traumatic red eye. Conjunctivitis can be defined as inflammation of the conjunctiva, the transparent membrane that covers the inner surface of the eyelid and most of the anterior surface of the eyeball. Because the conjunctiva has such an excellent nerve and blood supply it can become extremely swollen and painful when irritated. The cause can vary from localised infections through to allergic reactions.

Applying Theory to Practice: Exercise 11.5

There are many conditions that can result in a red and itchy or painful eye. Classically described as bloodshot, this umbrella term for several clinical conditions results in 35% of ocular attendances within primary care each year within the UK (MHRA 2004). Recent changes have now allowed the main drug used in its treatment being sold without a prescription within the UK. This is an interesting change, as many causes of a red eye are not related to an infection caused by bacteria.

Complete the following exercise to gain further understanding of acute eye conditions:

- Identify at least six different conditions that can result in the conjunctiva becoming inflamed and painful.
- What tests are available to assess the extent of damage to the affected eye/eyes?
- Could any of these acute conditions result in long-term blindness?

To help you research these questions the following sites are recommended:

http://www.eye-care.org.uk/information_listing.php?content_id=4

http://www.gpnotebook.co.uk/simplepage.cfm?ID=818937918

Conjunctivitis – the facts

Conjunctivitis is an extremely common presentation to all acute healthcare services (MHRA 2004). It is characterised by either unilateral or bilateral symptoms. These include:

- Swollen eyelids
- Inflamed inner eyelids
- Red watery eyes
- Purulent discharge resulting in sticky eyes and crust-like formations around the lids.

There are two main types of conjunctivitis:

- **Allergic**. An antigen stimulates the inflammatory response; this can be self-limiting or can continue as a hypersensitivity reaction. Causative agents include pollen and make-up.
- **Infective**. Caused by viruses or bacteria infecting the eye. The immune system is stimulated by the invading pathogen and begins trying to halt the pathogen's proliferation.

Infection is the most common cause of conjunctivitis. This condition is generally considered self-limiting. It is however, very uncomfortable and unpleasant. In infective conjunctivitis, as part of the inflammatory response to rid the disease, a rapid increase in mucus production is common. This mucus contains many white cells emanating from the blood supply. The end result is pus formation (a collection of white immune cells and destroyed bacteria). The purulent fluid clumps on the eyelashes making them stick together. The common cold can cause conjunctivitis, spreading from the patient's mouth or nose to their eyes. Infection of the eyes with chlamydia or herpes can be far more severe and take longer to treat (Watkins 2004). However, conjunctivitis caused by the common cold is very infectious and can spread rapidly between people. Various primary healthcare practitioners frequently prescribe antibiotics; the most common form, chloramphenicol, can now be obtained without a prescription.

Pathophysiology

Conjunctivitis can be caused by a multitude of organisms or varying stimuli. The most common presentation is bacterial infection caused by colonisation of the conjunctiva by pathogens such as *Haemophilus influenzae*, *Streptococcus pneumoniae* and staphylococcus (Prodigy 2007). Infective conjunctivitis is associated with many underlying causes; these include anything that can result in superficial damage to the eye, such as foreign bodies, scratches and direct entry through localised contamination, for example, rubbing the eye with dirty fingers.

Clinically it is problematic to differentiate between a bacterial or viral cause; therefore the treatment centres on eradicating bacteria so that even if the infection is caused by a virus, the administration of antibiotics will stop opportunistic bacterial proliferation.

Allergic conjunctivitis is increasingly prevalent in the spring and summer months with many cases being attributed to a hypersensitivity reaction to pollen. When the patient's clinical symptoms also include a runny nose (rhinitis), this is termed hay fever (Watkins 2004). In allergic conjunctivitis, both eyes are usually affected at the same time. Pollen irritates the eyes and causes the conjunctiva to swell; excessive mucus is produced to irrigate and cleanse the conjunctiva of the causative agent (Table 11.1). The mucus or watery discharge is clear and uninfected. In infective conjunctivitis, the infection may start in one eye, but can spread to both. The discharge is usually purulent and greenish in appearance.

Allergic	Infective
Pollen	Bacteria
Cat and other animal hairs	Viral
Make-up	Fungal
Chemicals	
Contact lenses	

Table 11.1 Causes of Conjunctivitis

Psychosocial aspects

Pain or discomfort are the main reasons for people to seek healthcare (DH 2001). It is therefore essential to treat these symptoms before detailed examination and diagnosis.

Possibly the greatest fear patients associate with disorders affecting the eyes is blindness (Evans et al. 2005). Blindness has several causes, from congenital abnormalities and ageing-related macular degeneration through to localised disease and trauma. Blindness does not mean a complete inability to see or perceive light; in the UK the statutory definition of blindness refers to persons who are so blind as to be unable to perform any work for which eyesight is essential. The causes of blindness can be categorised into three classifications or collective groups:

- Childbirth to adolescence: In the developed world

Developing and Delivering Expert Care: Box 11.1

As previously discussed, the local application of antibiotics is the main treatment plan for conjunctivitis; however, there are many adjuncts to treatment that may limit further episodes and improve the overall quality of care, these include:

- When the presenting history and symptoms suggest an allergic cause and the patient wears contact lenses, advise them to seek the advice of their supplier in case the lenses are a contributing factor, particularly outside of the summer months
- The application of cold compresses may soothe irritation and assist in reducing oedema
- Antihistamines will prevent further swelling by antagonising the further release of histamine
- Eye specialists may prescribe steroid drops to reduce inflammation
- Topical anti-inflammatory preparations including sodium cromoglicate may halt localised inflammation
- The concurrent use of NSAIDs will reduce pain and assist in reducing inflammation

In infective conjunctivitis:

- Bathe the affected eye/eyes with clean warm water frequently each day
- Avoid cross-infection with an unaffected eye
- Avoid spreading the causative agent with members of the same family by sharing towels and flannels
- Always complete a cause of antibiotics to avoid recurrence and future resistance; even if symptoms stop, the antibiotics must be completed
- Avoid wearing contact lenses until symptoms resolve
- If symptoms persist or proliferate, specialist advice should be sought particularly if there is a possibility of herpes infection

blindness at this age is usually due to genetic disease and birth trauma

- Adulthood to 60 years: Largely caused by diseases of the retina, and the secondary effects of diseases such as diabetes and hypertension that result in retinopathy
- Over 60 years: Macular degeneration. Glaucoma and cataracts are increasingly prevalent (Galloway & Amoaku 1999).

The psychological impact of receiving a diagnosis of impending blindness or a sudden traumatic loss of sight can be devastating. Jackson et al. (1998) describe several stages of emotional transition or progression that individuals go through in the search of inner understanding and acceptance of their condition or prognosis. Breaking bad news can be both distressing and uncomfortable for many nurses (York 1980). Many of these feelings can be explored through the formation of regular peer support groups or informal clinical supervision sessions. These sessions provide a forum for group discussion where individual staff members can discuss their feelings and explore ways

of dealing with difficult case scenarios in the future. Reflective practice and the ability to critique current and previous methods of practice are paramount to professional development and these sessions are pivotal to achieving good practice. In practice, mandatory sessions for manual handling, basic life support, and other clinical issues leave little time to explore feelings but sessions based around clinical supervision are just as, if not more, important.

Macular degeneration

Age-related macular degeneration (AMD) is the number one cause of registration for sight impairment within the UK (Bembridge 2005). This is due to degeneration of the small area of retina at the rear of the eye called the macula. Early symptoms include small distortions in the individual's vision; as the degeneration continues they may lose their central vision, inhibiting their ability to read, define colours and drive. The inability to drive can be a life-altering event for many sufferers for whom it may mean a loss of their independence (Hartry 2007).

Applying Theory to Practice: Exercise 11.6

Within clinical practice many issues are frequently discussed with those that are perceived most distressing normally taking precedence.

Complete the following research on your clinical placements. This may provide you with the information necessary to choose an area that you feel would be supportive when you begin work as a newly qualified nurse.

- Does the clinical area facilitate regular staff forums?
- How is the information gathered used to change practice or working conditions?
- Are debriefing sessions held after conflicts or following clinical incidents, cardiac arrests or deaths?

Professional issues

Applying Theory to Practice: Exercise 11.7

There are several disease processes that can lead to blindness or a severe compromise of an individual's vision.

- Make a list of any diseases that can lead to blindness you already know.
- Identify any other common eye conditions that you can think of.

Read the following sections on common eye disorders and add a brief summary to your portfolio.

Glaucoma

Glaucoma is a collective term used to describe diseases that damage the optic nerve caused by the effects of raised ocular pressure. The intraocular pressure needs to remain within a narrow spectrum. This equilibrium is maintained by the production and removal of aqueous humour.

Cataracts

A cataract is an opacification of the lens of the eye and the commonest cause of treatable blindness in the world (James et al. 2004). Most cataracts result from cumulative exposure to environmental influences e.g. UV radiation, smoke, chemicals (Galloway 1999).

Figure 11.4 The Snellen chart

Patient confidentiality

During the educational course you are undertaking to become a nurse you will have many discussions on confidentiality and how important it is to any healthcare profession. Patients consenting to healthcare usually disclose personal information to professionals with the expectation that this information will be used to provide effective healthcare. Sometimes healthcare professionals can find themselves in a compromising situation with the patient's rights on one hand and the beliefs or expectations of society on the other. One example is demonstrated in Scenario 11.2.

Developing and Delivering Expert Care: Box 11.2

The Snellen Test

Recording visual acuity in a patient attending for a eye-related problem is essential in establishing a basic insight into their ability to see.

The Snellen chart is used as a quick and effective method of testing for acuity of distance vision. It usually consists of a wall-mounted chart with an identified line drawn 6 metres away from where the reader or patient will be asked to stand and identify the letters, numbers or symbols placed on the chart (Figure 11.4).

In clinical practice, due to space constraints, the chart can be 3 metres away, with the size of the chart correspondingly reduced. Each row is individually numbered to represent the distance at which an individual could read that line with standard vision, in combination with the distance the patient was placed at and the individual row they were able to complete, so that a score represents both the distance and the particular line.

The first number given in the result of a Snellen test is the distance in metres from the chart and then the row number e.g. a reading of 6/36 would imply the patient had completed the line numbered 36, while standing 6 metres away.

To qualify for a driving licence within the UK the applicant is required to read a number plate from a specified distance (20.5m), equivalent to a reading of 6/12 on the Snellen chart.

Unaided visual acuity is the term used to denote vision without glasses; best corrected visual acuity means vision with glasses. Normal or standard vision is equivalent to 6/6 on the Snellen chart.

Scenario 11.2

Macular Degeneration

A 76-year-old man presents with a slight infection of his right eye. While having his visual acuity tested it is noted that the sight in both his eyes is poor. He states that it has been deteriorating over the last few years and that he now has problems reading newspapers. You know that he drove to the walk-in centre because he is unaccompanied and came in asking for change for the car park. He is given chloramphenicol for his conjunctivitis and provided with information about cross-infection and additional methods of eradicating the infection. You ask him how he is going to get home and he states he has no problem driving and that is what he intends to do. You inform him that this may be extremely dangerous and that in your opinion he is unable to drive. He calls you ageist and leaves heading for his car.

Assessment and analysis of patient presentation

Once informed that their eyesight ability does not reach the minimum standard, it is the individual's responsibility to inform the Driver and Vehicle Licensing Agency (DVLA). In this case scenario the driver refuses to do so and is about to drive, resulting in the patient's right to confidentiality conflicting with the greater public interest (NMC 2005). Although the patient's wishes need to be considered, protecting the public is paramount. This scenario could end with the patient leaving the department and due to his failing eyesight running through a zebra crossing and killing several schoolchildren on their way home. A relationship based on trust is essential to delivering effective healthcare, because patients must divulge potentially sensitive information to their healthcare provider to obtain a diagnosis and subsequent treatment. Nurses are answerable for all actions and omissions and, just like all citizens, must uphold the law. If the nurse reports the patient to the DVLA, there will be an established breach of patient confidentiality. The NMC (2004) state that if nurses decide to release personal information they must obtain consent; this further complicates the issue rather than offering assistance in decision making. Exceptional communication skills are vital in

Questioning Clinical Practice: Exercise 11.8

Scenario 11.2 provides all the essential information to create an interesting debate. Try discussing these issues with either some of your colleagues or your class.

- What would you do when placed in this situation?
- Do you have an obligation to protect the public or is your sole concern to maintain your patient's confidentiality?

Compare the class's attitudes and then complete the following section.

- Did you and your colleagues raise the issues identified?

establishing both a good rapport with patients and delivering effective care.

In this case scenario utmost attempts should be used to alert the patient to the potential danger to himself and the public at large. If this fails to persuade him to change his mind, it should be clearly documented that he has refused to be reasonable and he should be informed that this information will be released with or without his agreement. The appropriate authorities should then be contacted and the facts documented in the patient's notes. The documentation process is imperative as the patient's notes may be requested in the future as evidence of your actions. It is generally recommended that a breach of confidentiality should only take place in exceptional circumstances (DH 2003, NMC 2005); regrettably they both fail to provide a definition of 'exceptional'. Therefore each time you encounter a potentially serious ethical dilemma it is best to compose yourself and explore several avenues before committing to an action. Seek advice from senior colleagues but remember their opinions may differ from yours and it is you who are accountable for patients placed within your care.

The Public Interest Disclosure Act 1998 cited in Hartry (2007) identifies six circumstances where disclosing confidential information can be justified:

- Where a criminal offence has been, is or is likely to be, committed

- That a person has, is or is likely to fail to comply with any legal obligation to which he is subject
- That a miscarriage of justice has, is or is likely to occur
- That the health or safety of any individual has been, is or is likely to be, endangered
- That the environment has been, is or is likely to be, damaged
- That information tending to show any matter falling within any one of the preceding paragraphs has been, is, or is likely to be, concealed.

These guidelines simplify the nurse's decision making due to their broad nature. Almost any breach of confidentiality could be included within these six areas regardless of how trivial or complex the issue was as long as the information was disclosed to an appropriate source and not the press or media.

Questioning Clinical Practice: Box 11.3

Ethical Considerations

Professional judgements and sound clinical decision making are key to delivering quality care that is seen to be beneficial to both patients and society. It is therefore essential that you place as much emphasis on professional issues as on disease. The following texts are highly recommended to provide the reader with a solid knowledge base in the ethical dilemmas they will encounter throughout their clinical practice:

Tingle, J. & Cribb, A. (2002) *Nursing Law and Ethics.* Blackwell Science: Oxford.
Dimond, B. (2005) *Legal Aspects of Nursing*, 4th edition. Pearson Education: New York.

The ears (hearing)

Form

The ears are composed of three distinct sections:

- Outer ear
- Middle ear
- Inner ear.

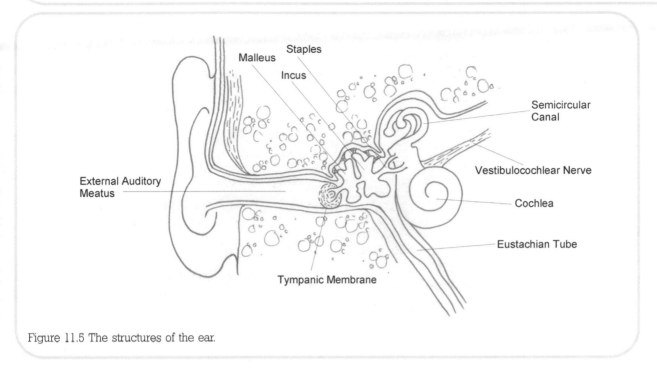

Figure 11.5 The structures of the ear.

Outer ear

The flexible external ear consists of the pinna, the external auditory meatus, the auditory canal and the lateral surface of the eardrum – the tympanic membrane. The outer ear canal is cartilaginous in its outer third and bony in its inner two-thirds. The outer third of this canal has a bony framework (Figure 11.5).

Middle ear

The tympanic membrane separates the outer and middle ear. This pearl-grey structure consists of three layers:

- Skin
- Fibrous tissue
- Mucous membrane.

The middle ear consists of the medial surface of the tympanic membrane, the tympanic cavity, the Eustachian tube and the mastoid air cells. Within the tympanic cavity are the three auditory ossicles – these transmit and amplify sound from the external ear and tympanic membrane to the inner ear. The Eustachian tube serves to equalise the air pressure between the middle ear and the atmosphere. It also connects the ear's sterile area to the nasopharynx. Upper respiratory tract infections can affect the tube by obstructing drainage from the middle ear causing otitis media or effusion.

Inner ear

The inner ear consists of closed, fluid-filled spaces within the temporal bone. It contains the bony labyrinth, which includes three connected structures: the vestibule, the semicircular canals and the cochlea. The vestibular part of the inner ear is concerned with balance; the cochlea is concerned with hearing (Figure 11.5).

Function

The ear has two main functions: hearing and balance.

Hearing

When sound waves reach the outer ear, structures transmit the waves through the auditory canal to the tympanic membrane, and onto the structures of the middle and inner ear. The cochlea branch of the acoustic nerve (cranial nerve VIII) transmits the vibrations to the temporal lobe of the cerebral cortex, where the brain interprets the sound.

Balance

Structures in the middle and inner ear control balance. The semicircular canals of the inner ear contain cristae, hair-like structures, which respond to body movement. Endolymph fluid bathes the cristae. Movement causes the cristae to bend, releasing impulses through the vestibular portion of the acoustic nerve to the brain, which controls

balance. When a person is stationary, nerve impulses to the brain orientate them to their position; the pressure of gravity on the inner ear helps maintain balance.

Overview

There are 8,945,000 deaf or hard of hearing people in the United Kingdom (Royal National Institute for the Deaf (RNID) 2007). The term deaf is used in a general way to refer to people with all degrees of deafness. There are four levels of deafness, defined according to the quietest sound that can be heard:

- Mild deafness – some difficulty following speech mainly in noisy situations, quietest sounds heard are 25–39 decibels
- Moderate deafness – difficulty following speech without a hearing aid, quietest sounds heard 40–69 decibels
- Severe deafness – heavy reliance on lip reading, even with a hearing aid, quietest sounds heard 70–94 decibels
- Profound deafness – British Sign Language (BSL) is usually the first or preferred language, or reliance on lip reading, quietest sounds heard 95 decibels or more.

Hard of hearing is the term used to describe people with a mild to severe hearing loss, usually people who have lost their hearing gradually. People who were born with the ability to hear and become severely or profoundly deaf after learning to speak are often described as deafened. This can happen suddenly or gradually.

Communication

When communicating with patients who have a degree of deafness it is important to consider non-verbal skills of communication so that we maximise our interaction without being perceived in a negative way. BSL is the most widely used method of signed communication, but there are thought to be only 50,000 BSL users (RNID 2007). Many deaf people can, to varying degrees, lip read; some people find it more difficult than others. How people speak can affect how well the person can lip read, many people do not speak clearly and lip reading an unfamiliar accent may make the skill more difficult. When communicating with a patient who is lip reading, it is important to speak in as usual as way as possible; overemphasising certain letters or syllables may lead to confusion. It is also

not necessary to shout at a deaf or hard of hearing person, as when people shout they distort their voices and make it more difficult for words to be identified. Instead of shouting, or speaking too slowly or exaggerating lip movements, it is important to speak clearly. Words should be formed properly and normal volume maintained.

Scenario 11.3

Otitis Media

John McNamara is an 18-year-old mechanic who had a sudden onset of right-sided ear pain two days ago. He took analgesia for this with good effect but the pain has continued. When John awoke this morning he noticed some discharge from his ear on the pillow and as he arose he realised his hearing was muffled. He does not have any problems walking and is not experiencing any loss of balance. John has attended the health clinic where you are on placement and is assessed by you under the guidance of a practice nurse.

John's vital signs are recorded as: respiratory rate 16 and regular, pulse rate 89 strong and regular, blood pressure 118/72, temperature 37.6.

When inspected through otoscopy it is noted that the ear canal is inflamed and there is evidence of a dried discharge. The tympanic membrane is intact, although bulging.

John has no previous medical history or allergies. He has recently suffered from what he calls flu-like symptoms and still has nasal congestion and a sore throat.

Assessment and analysis of patient presentation

John McNamara is presenting with the classic signs and symptoms of an infection affecting the middle ear. His recent history of a possible viral infection affecting the upper respiratory tract is a frequent finding (Browning 1998). Mr McNamara's vital signs exclude systemic sepsis and indicate a localised infection. There are several different classifications of ear infection dependent on the particular area of the ear affected (Applying Theory to Practice: Exercise 11.9). John has mild pyrexia demonstrating his immunologic response; this is also demonstrated through the purulent discharge he has

experienced. Hearing loss or the loss of certain frequencies is a common finding.

Applying Theory to Practice: Exercise 11.9

Infections Affecting the Ear

- Otitis media – affecting the middle ear
- Otitis externa – affecting the outer ear

Read the information provided by NHS Direct to gain further information: http://www.nhsdirect.nhs.uk/articles/article.aspx?articleID=609

The facts

Acute otitis media is an infection of the middle ear mucosa resulting in localised inflammation, pain and pyrexia. It is usually of rapid onset and short duration. It is associated with fluid accumulation in the middle ear producing the signs and symptoms of ear infection. These include a bulging eardrum, which can become perforated, the production of pus, and fever. Chronic otitis media involves persistent inflammation of the middle ear following an acute infection. Fluid referred to as an effusion is present; this fluid accumulation is far more prevalent in children and not always associated with a recent infection (glue ear). Chronic otitis media can cause damage to the middle ear and eardrum, continuing ear pressure, a subtle loss of hearing and a popping noise can be persistent for months.

Professional issues

Although Mr McNamara's presentation signifies a mild localised infection, it is extremely painful and uncomfortable. He will require a quick pain assessment and then the administration of appropriate analgesics will be the immediate priority. Antibiotics are not always prescribed as infections can be self-limiting and resolve after 2–3 days. If his eardrum had perforated he would require a follow-up appointment at the health clinic. He should be told to return if the symptoms fail to ease, or increase.

Pathophysiology

The middle ear sits in the small space behind the eardrum and is normally filled with air. It connects to the back of the throat via a small channel called the Eustachian tube. The most important factor in middle ear disease is

Questioning Clinical Practice: Exercise 11.10

Recording and Requesting Appropriate Data

When initially assessing a patient, nurses have an exhaustive array of tests and data they could collect. It is paramount that only essential or relevant tests are made as gathering and waiting for irrelevant tests can be time-consuming and have significant cost implications. The possibility of gathering wrong test results also increases.

- Which tests would you perform on Mr McNamara and why?

Write down each individual test and rationalise why this particular test would assist in establishing his illness or excluding a differential diagnosis.

Eustachian tube dysfunction whereby the mucosa at the pharyngeal end of the Eustachian tube is part of the mucociliary system of the middle ear. Negative pressure or oedema can facilitate direct entry of infectious agents such as viruses or bacteria into the middle ear causing inflammation. Therefore this space can fill with mucus as a consequence of a viral infection such as a cold.

Psychosocial aspects

Showing empathy for the clinical symptoms such as pain that the patient is suffering is fundamental to a perceived caring profession. Empathy not only has to encompass physical signs but also has to extend into psychological elements such as the concerns Mr McNamara may be experiencing regarding the temporary loss of areas of his hearing. Hearing loss, even if temporary, can have an enormous psychological impact on an individual. No two individuals will have the same reaction to a potentially life altering event. Hearing loss can make interaction with the outside world difficult and at times impossible. Experiencing a loss of hearing has been described as an invisible physical disability, especially in the social realm. Helen Keller once said that deafness cuts one off from people, whereas blindness cuts one off from things (Kaland & Salvatore 2002).

Common presentations

The most common ear complaints are hearing loss, tinnitus, pain, discharge and dizziness. Hearing loss and

tinnitus are usually caused by long-term problems; diabetes can cause hearing loss and hypertension can cause high-pitched tinnitus. If a patient has a chronic disorder it is important to establish treatment and medications; certain antibiotics and other medications can cause hearing loss.

Questioning Clinical Practice Exercise 11.11

A toxic reaction to a drug can cause a rapid loss of hearing. Drugs that may affect hearing include some NSAIDs, loop diuretics, aminoglycosides and several chemotherapeutic agents.

- Look these drug types up and familiarise yourself with specific names of drugs that can affect hearing.
- What would you do if a patient in your care, who was taking one of these drugs, reported hearing loss to you?

Pain, discharge and dizziness usually result from short-term conditions. Serous otitis media, inflammation of the middle ear, is common in people with environmental or seasonal allergies. Otitis externa, inflammation of the outer ear, can be caused by allergic reactions to personal care products, for example shampoos, hair dyes.

The olfactory sense (smell)

General overview

Smell is referred to as one of the chemical senses; this is because the sense of smell is an evolutionary skill developed to gain insight into the world and its inhabitants. All organic substances are composed of, and emit chemicals which, depending on the particular sensitivity skills of the individual or species, can be interpreted or sensed.

An advanced ability to smell potential dangers or locate food sources is associated with animals such as wolves. Humans, however, do have an incredibly acute ability to identify danger. A good example is demonstrated by the involuntary act of breathing (Chapter 3). Without being consciously aware, we are continuously testing the consistency of the air we breathe; we can sense potential dangers such as smoke or toxic gases, e.g. methane. For humans to interpret the chemicals surrounding us, our

sensory systems need to contain certain properties. Odour molecules must be small enough to be volatile (less than 300–400 relative molecular mass) so that they can vaporise, reach the nose and then dissolve in the mucus. This tells us that smell can travel over long distances thereby creating an early warning device. This innate ability to detect noxious substances begins in childhood, and develops to include an experiential component throughout life. There are suggestions that smell can influence mood, memory, emotions, mate choice, the immune system and the endocrine system (hormones). We can communicate by smell – without knowing it. In fact the sense of smell could be said to be at the mind–body interface.

Function and form

The nose is more than the sensory organ of smell; it also plays a vital role in the respiratory system by filtering, warming, and humidifying inhaled air.

Air entering the nose passes through the vestibule, which is lined with coarse hair that helps to filter dust. Olfactory receptors lie above the vestibule in the roof of the nasal cavity and the upper third of the septum. This area, the olfactory region, is rich in capillaries and mucus-producing goblet cells that help warm, moisten and clean inhaled air.

Figure 11.6 The olfactory system

The lower two-thirds of the external nose consist of flexible cartilage, and the upper third is rigid bone. Posteriorly, the internal nose merges with the pharynx and anteriorly with the external nose. The internal and external nose is divided vertically by the nasal septum. In the

roof of each nostril is a region called the nasal mucosa. This region contains the sensory or olfactory epithelium covered by mucus. The epithelium contains both sensory cells and Bowman's glands, which produce the secretion that bathes the surface of the receptors. The nasal epithelium contains an estimated 10 million receptor cells.

Four pairs of paranasal sinuses open into the internal nose:

- Maxillary sinuses – located on the cheeks below the eyes
- Frontal sinuses – located above the eyebrows
- Ethmoidal and sphenoidal sinuses – located behind the eyes and nose.

The sinuses serve as resonators for sound production and mucus secretion. Because the opening between the sinuses and the nasal cavity is lined with mucous membranes that can become inflamed and swollen, they can easily become blocked.

Common presentations

The most common complaints of the nose are: epistaxis (bleeding nose), blocked nose, runny nose, deformity (usually due to an injury), and non-smelling nose. Nasal and paranasal disorders may also present with regional symptoms such as headache, facial pain, excessive tear production, double vision, bulging eyes and orbital pain.

The most common site of nosebleeds is in the Kiesselbach's area, located in the anterior portion of the septum. They are usually caused by an injury, although can occur spontaneously. Mechanical abnormalities, for example, a deviated septum or nasal polyp, will usually cause a constant obstruction, whereas the nasal cycle and seasonal allergic rhinitis are usually intermittent, the former alternating between nostrils.

A diminished sense of smell (hyposmia) or no sense of smell (anosmia) can occur as a result of trauma or following a viral infection. Sudden loss of smell may result following a head injury, although this would need to be severe in order to tear the olfactory fibres that emerge through the cruciform plate. Some patients may report a loss in their sense of smell following an upper respiratory tract infection, known as post-influenza neuritis. In many patients who suffer from hyposmia or anosmia, however, the cause will remain unknown.

The gustatory sense (taste)

Function

The tongue is a large, mobile organ comprising several muscles and covered by a mucous membrane. The base of the tongue is bound laterally by the anterior and posterior tonsillar pillars between which, and on either side, lie the tonsils. The parotid, submandibular and sublingual salivary glands secrete saliva into the oral cavity keeping it moist and aiding the first stage of swallowing. Food entering the mouth is chewed and mixed with saliva to facilitate swallowing. As well as being an important organ of speech and taste, the tongue has a role in both the mixing of a food bolus and in propelling the bolus towards the pharynx.

Like the olfactory system, taste is a chemical sense that requires a substance to be dissolved before it can be tasted. Odours from food pass upwards into the nasopharynx and nasal cavity to stimulate olfactory receptors. Much of our interpretation of taste is actually gained through the sense of smell. A given concentration of a substance will stimulate the olfactory system thousands of times more strongly than it stimulates the gustatory system.

Form

The receptors for taste are located in the taste buds. Of the nearly 10,000 taste buds in a young adult the majority are found on the tongue, with some also on the soft palate, larynx and pharynx. The sense of taste deteriorates with age as the number of taste buds decline.

Each taste bud, which is oval is shape, consists of three kinds of epithelial cell:

- Supporting cells
- Gustatory cells
- Basal cells.

The supporting cells form a capsule, which contains approximately 50 gustatory (taste) receptor cells. Each of these receptor cells has a single gustatory hair projecting through an opening in the taste bud, called the taste pore. The gustatory hairs make contact with taste stimuli through the taste pore. At the periphery of the taste bud, near the connective tissue, are the basal cells. Taste buds occur in elevations on the tongue called papillae; these give the tongue its rough appearance. There are four

Figure 11.7 The gustatory system

primary taste sensations: sour, salty, bitter and sweet. All tastes are combinations of these four, modified by accompanying olfactory sensations. Some individual gustatory receptors may respond to more than one of the four primary tastes, but receptors in certain regions of the tongue react more strongly than others to the primary taste (Figure 11.8).

Questioning Clinical Practice Exercise 11.12

One of the functions of the tongue is to facilitate swallowing.

● Identify some clinical conditions that can affect a patient's ability to swallow.
● How can the nutritional demands of these patients be met?

Figure 11.8 Gustatory receptors

Conclusion

The senses facilitate many essential roles to maintain homeostasis and to allow an individual to experience the outside world. These include the ability to perceive and communicate. Through every moment of life an individual will be using at least one of their five senses. These five senses culminate to allow the brain to adapt to differing environments and to make higher levels of decision making. A loss of one or more of these functions is life-altering and can have a massive impact on an individual and their ability to perform within society. Complete the following quiz to reinforce your developing knowledge base within this area.

Chapter 11 Summary Quiz

1. Vision is composed of three distant perceptions:

A. Forms, colours, movement
B. Colours, light, movement
C. Light, forms, colours
D. Movement, forms, light

2. Short sight is referred to as:

A. Myopia
B. Utopia
C. Antropia
D. Mytopia

3. Which of the following is not a visual test?

A. Visual acuity
B. Visual field
C. Visual displacement
D. Colour vision

4. Miotic drugs:

A. Result in a constriction of the pupil
B. Result in a constriction of the iris
C. Result in a dilation of the pupil iris
D. Result in a dilation of the pupil

5. Conjunctivitis is not associated with:

A. Purulent discharge resulting in sticky eyes and crust-like formations around the lids
B. Swollen eyelids
C. Red watery eyes
D. Double vision

6. Causes of conjunctivitis do not include:

A. Pollen
B. Viral
C. Bacteria
D. Wearing glasses

7. The number one cause of registration for sight impairment within the UK is:

A. Conjunctivitis
B. Age-related macular degeneration
C. Diabetes mellitus
D. Hypertension

8. Glaucoma is a collective term used to describe diseases that damage:

A. The pupil
B. The optic nerve
C. The oculomotor nerve
D. The iris

9. The ears are composed of three distinct sections. Which of the following is not one of them?

A. Middle ear
B. Outer ear
C. Central ear
D. Inner ear

10. There are four primary taste sensations; which of the following is not one?

A. Sour
B. Sweet
C. Nasty
D. Salty

Further reading

Davis, G. (2006) Anatomy of the eye in relation to common drug therapies. *Nurse Prescribing* 4(7): 274–8.

Department of Health (2003) *Confidentiality. NHS Code of Practice*. DH: London.

Dimond, B. (2005) *Legal Aspects of Nursing*, 4th edn. Pearson Education: New York.

Nursing and Midwifery Council (2005) *Confidentiality*. NMC: London.

http://www.rnid.org.uk/

http://www.cc.gatech.edu/classes/cs6751_97_winter/Topics/human-cap/senses.html

References

Bembridge, T. (2005) Caring for those with age-related impaired sight. *Nursing & Residential Care* 7(11): 507–9.

Browning, G.G. (1998) *Clinical Otology and Audiology*, 2nd edn. Butterworth Heinemann: Oxford.

Clancy, J. & McVicar, A.J. (2002) *Physiology and Anatomy. A Homeostatic Approach*, 2nd edn. Arnold: London.

Department of Health (2001) *Reforming Emergency Care*. DH: London.

Department of Health (2003) *Confidentiality*. NHS Code of Practice. DH: London.

Dimond, B. (2005) *Legal Aspects of Nursing*, 4th edn. Pearson Education: New York.

Evans, J., Fletcher, A. & Wormald, P. (2005) 28000 cases of age related macular degeneration causing visual loss in people aged 75 years and above in the United Kingdom may be

attributable to smoking. *British Journal of Ophthalmology* 89: 550–3.

Galloway, N.R. & Amoaku, W.M.K. (1999) *Common Eye Diseases and their Management*, 2nd edn. Springer: London.

Hartry, N. (2007) Visually impaired drivers and public protection vs confidentiality. *British Journal of Nursing* 16(4): 226–30.

Jackson, W.T., Taylor, R.E., Palmatier, A.D., Elliott, T.R. & Elliott, J.L. (1998) Negotiating the reality of visual impairment: hope, coping, and functional ability. *Journal of Clinical Psychology in Medical Settings* 5(2): 173–85.

James, B., Chew, C. & Bron, A. (2004) *Lecture Notes on Ophthalmology*, 9th edn. Blackwell Publishing: Oxford.

Kaland, J. & Salvatore, L. (2002) The Psychology of Hearing Loss. www.asha.org/about/publications/leader-online/archives/2002/q1/020319d.htm (accessed 20 November 2007).

Medicines and Healthcare Products Regulatory Agency (MRHA) (2004) Consultation Document: ARM 25 *Request to Reclassify a Product from POM to P.* MHRA: London.

National Institute for Health and Clinical Excellence (NICE) (2007) IPG209; *Implantation of Accommodating Intraocular Lenses during Cataract Surgery.* Guidance. NICE: London.

Nursing and Midwifery Council (NMC) (2004) *The Code of Professional Conduct, Standards and Ethics.* NMC: London.

Nursing and Midwifery Council (NMC) (2005) *Confidentiality.* NMC: London.

Prodigy (2007) *Conjunctivitis – Infective.* http://cks.library.nhs.uk/conjunctivitis_infective (accessed 15/11/07).

Royal National institute for the Deaf (RNID) (2007) http://rnid.org.uk/information_resources/aboutdeafnessstatistics/ (accessed 24 jULY 2007).

Watkins, J. (2004) The recognition and treatment of the red eye. *Practice Nursing* 15(8): 405–8.

York, C. (1980) Some comments on the psychoanalytic treatment of patients with physical disabilities. *International Journal of Psycho-Analysis.* 61: 187–93.

Part 3
Nursing in practice

The child and the Children Act

Steve Campbell

Introduction

The registered nurse needs knowledge of children whether they are practising in a specialist children's area or not. The reasons for this vary, but can be exemplified by two examples: the nurse working in the emergency department, and the nurse caring for an adult patient who has been subject to violence in the home.

The first example is, perhaps, easy to understand; such nurses will care for child patients, especially when there is no designated paediatric emergency department. The nurse will need to understand how children differ from adults. Some of the reasons are a matter of physical and physiological importance (e.g. drug dosages), others are about the support systems for children at different ages when growing up. Children cannot cope with trauma in the same manner as adults, and need the psychological support of parents and prime carers. Since the 1950s changes in the way children are cared for away from the home have led to children being less 'scarred' by the

process, and systems of care have been developed in hospital and primary care that are sensitive to these needs, such as family-centred care or family nursing.

The second example is both technical and obvious. If there has been violence in the home where a child lives, then, on whomever this violence has been perpetrated, the police must carry out investigations. This is a technical issue because the law has only recently been changed to require this action, but it is also obvious because of the potential impact upon the development of a child caused by living in a violent home. Other recent changes have made it everybody's business to contribute to child safety, so the nurse caring for a patient who has been subject to violence is now required, as is every other professional, to ensure that this child, and its circumstances, are reported to the child protection team. Previously, the fact that the patient was an adult and, say, an inpatient on an adult admission ward, would have led to the presumption that such matters were the business of others.

These two examples provide a framework for this chapter as they lead to areas of necessary knowledge for the registered nurse practising within the UK. These areas are:

- What is a child?
- What is childhood?
- Where do infants and adolescents fit in?
- Why are children different – psychosocially and physiologically?
- What are the systems that promote the normal development of children when they come in contact with services in the NHS?
- How do all professionals contribute to child protection?

Childhood: infants and adolescents

There are various definitions of childhood, some of which are driven by age, and others by events in development. They are important in finding the right environment for

the child. A general definition in terms of time might be from birth until adulthood. This is rather broad, and includes babies all the way up to adolescents, who may not appreciate being referred to as a child, let alone being admitted to a children's ward. Other definitions use the period of time from infancy to the onset of puberty. Within most contemporary definitions of childhood, there is reference to this period as being one of nurturing by parents or equivalent to allow the child to become an individual and to reach full potential.

There is therefore a need to have some notion of what an infant is. Again, some view this as set by a clear time period: from birth up to 24 months of age. Interestingly, the word infant is derived from Latin *infans*, which means not to speak or speechless. This definition was based on developmental milestones with the Romans taking a view that speech for children would arrive at about two years, and those that could not speak were infants. In current times a child who could not speak at two years would be seem as unusual and in the UK would probably be referred to a speech therapist for investigation.

A medically directed definition of adolescence might be the period of physical and psychological development from the onset of puberty to maturity. However, both the start and finish of this period are very difficult to define. Some young girls show signs of puberty at 9 or 10. It is difficult to interpret them as being adolescents in the general public's notion of the word. Similarly for maturity, a young person might regard him or herself as mature, but his or her parents might not agree. Such matters become important around, for instance, informed consent for procedures. There is not the opportunity to deal with this issue in depth here, but while 16 years might be regarded as the legal age of consent, such issues as Frazer competence have meant that due consideration needs to be given to the views of the young person. While EU law might have superseded Frazer competence, most practitioners would wish to have the consent of the young person as well as the parent/guardian.

The Canadian Pediatric Society (2003) produced a paper that considered age limits and adolescents. They did so for a number of reasons, but the 'automatic' movement of young people to adult services at a certain age might not be the most appropriate action. Their definition of adolescence was:

Adolescence begins with the onset of physiologically normal puberty, and ends when an adult's identity and behaviour are accepted. This period of development

corresponds roughly to the period between the ages of 10 and 19 years, which is consistent with the World Health Organization's definition of adolescence. Those responsible for providing healthcare to adolescents must allow sufficient flexibility in this age span to encompass special situations such as the emancipated minor or the young person with a chronic condition leading to delayed development or prolonged dependency.

In other words, some young people might be so mature that keeping them in children's areas is inappropriate, in the same way as other children, despite their chronological age, might not be mature enough to cope in an adult environment, and so should stay in the child's or young person's environment. Definitions are difficult, but helpful in opening up certain debates. In this section, the term 'young person' has been used. The expression is in common use, but has not settled down to a clear and consistent definition. Some use it as an alternative to adolescent; it seems more friendly and less medically or socially laden. Others use it in a wider fashion to indicate anybody over age ten and late teens, even early twenties.

Most of the physical and mental development of a human being takes place in childhood. It is the important period when an individual can develop strong coping skills, which will be essential in later life. It is also a period when good habits such as partaking in exercise and understanding nutritional needs are established; these can transmit into adult life.

By the age of 7, most of the motor control mechanisms are present and the child rapidly develops physical motor skills. During the dominant growth periods (for girls between the ages of 9 and 12 years, and for boys between 11 and 14 years) general exercise promotes growth of muscles, tendons and bones, but too much activity can damage bones and joints. The dangers of excessive exercise are not just physical but also mental.

Why are children different?

Children, from babies through to adolescents, differ from adults, as they are vulnerable outside their normal environment, as they are still growing and developing. As such, they have special needs that health services, including preventative health services, need to be aware of. The modern history of childcare has been described many times, but continues to be central to understanding why children's acute healthcare is designed in its current

form. In the UK, during the Second World War, the removal of children from dangerous areas of big cities during periods of bombing, to the safety of the countryside, was seen at the time as being idyllic and good for the children. Without their parents, however, these children were vulnerable, and some of them showed the psychological effects of this for the rest of their lives. There was no malice in this process; indeed it fitted the current knowledge of child development at the time. Children's hospitals were run in similar ways; children would be taken to the children's hospital for planned surgery and passed to the nurses, with parents only allowed to visit at very limited occasions during the week. If the child got upset during this period, this was seen as a sign of how inappropriate it was to allow parents to visit. In the 1950s, various researchers changed the view of childcare, most notably John Bowlby and the Robertsons. The latter's work included the filming of toddlers in an orphanage showing the effect of removing the regular carer from the child. For most people who have seen this film and the reaction of this child, the image remains, and, while 'traumatic', serves as a genuine reminder of the importance of a prime and consistent carer. John Bowlby's book *Child Care and the Growth of Love* made it even clearer that children needed, according to the expertise of the time, to be with their mothers. As a result, a slow process of change began, children's wards in general hospitals and children's hospitals changed their practice. The Platt Report (MoH 1959) was pivotal, but even in the 1980s some of the recommendations of this government report still had not been enacted consistently across the country. The key issues were the admission of the mother/parent/ prime carer with the child, and caring for children in different environments from adult patients with similar diagnoses. Parents, who previously had very restricted visiting of their sick child were now allowed open access to their child and indeed the care of the child developed into a partnership between parents, child, the nursing team and the general care team in hospital. There are a number of terms used for this kind of care; some refer to it as family-centred care and others as family nursing (Campbell & Summersgill 1993; Campbell et al. 1993).

For the acutely ill child and their family there have been many changes in the last few years. Medical technology has improved the prognosis of many seriously ill children; however, this has also meant that families have had to deal with prolonged and open-ended periods of care. It remains a challenge to understand the ways in

Applying Theory to Practice: Exercise 12.1

- What behaviour would you expect from a young child separated from his/her parent without notice?
- How would you avoid this happening when this young child is admitted to a children's ward?
- What would you want the parent to tell the child about the reason for his or her admission?
- What would you want the parent to tell the brothers and sisters about the reason for the sibling's admission?

which families deal with serious illness. Approaches to care, such as family-centred care, emphasise the importance of the family, but the family processes to cope are not well known and, therefore, not as well supported by care professionals (Rennick 1995; Haines 2005). In practical terms, in the UK the Labour Government has adopted many of the principles of family-centred care within its National Service Framework, and this is discussed later in this chapter.

The above systems concentrate on ill health. The vast majority of children will only have one admission to a hospital, and this will probably only be overnight or a visit to the emergency department. Normal development including healthy development takes place in the home and school, with little input from health professionals in terms of time spent with individuals. One way to view the world of children is via Bronfenbrenner's ecological model (1979), which has a series of concentric circles, with the child at the centre. Early in infancy the mother is closest, but as the child progresses towards adolescence, the child's peers have the greatest influence on development. The roles of health visitors, school nurses, and the services of general practitioners remain important in health educational and health promotional terms (Lloyd et al. 2007).

Physical differences in children – physiological and anatomical

One of the most obvious differences between adults and children is that children are smaller than adults. This seems a blindingly obvious statement, but treating children as mini-adults is not appropriate.

Applying Theory to Practice: Exercise 12.2

- For an adolescent which people are most important to them?
- What proportion of time do you think adolescents spend with their friends and how much with their parents?
- When an adolescent has to attend the accident and emergency department, who do you think he/she wants to attend with him/her?
- Which other people would think that they should be there with their adolescent?
- Do friends of the adolescent and the family of the adolescent necessarily want each other present?
- How do health professionals resolve these issues, or are they not their business?

Temperature regulation

In most biology at school, children are taught that the elephant or the whale are well suited to dealing with changes in temperature as they have a low surface area to volume ratio. Conversely children have a high surface to area ratio and can become hypo- and hyperthermic very quickly. This, combined with young children having an immature temperature control system, leaves them vulnerable to the effects of high and low temperatures. When young children acquire infections and are pyrexial, this is a concern and opens up the potential for febrile convulsions. This is why health professionals are diligent with young children about giving anti-pyretic drugs, such as paracetamol (acetaminophen) and ibuprofen; these can be administered in combination with removal of outer layers of clothing to keep the child cool. Other more extreme practices such as cold baths can quickly induce the potential of making the child hypothermic; this is a clear example of why children are not mini-adults.

Airway

Children have much smaller airways, thus the potential for airway obstruction increases. Infants breathe through their nose only up until the age of six months. In children, the cricoid ring is the narrowest part of the upper airway; in adults it is the larynx.

Breathing

Children have a higher metabolic rate and accompanying oxygen demand, contributing to a higher respiratory rate than in adults. Initially children compensate well for a mild breathing difficulty but due to immature muscle development and, in the infant, diaphragmatic breathing they are more prone to muscle fatigue and sudden respiratory failure.

Circulation

Children have a comparatively smaller stroke volume (Chapter 2), and a higher cardiac output than adults; this is facilitated by relative tachycardia. The stroke volume increases with age; consequently heart rate falls as the child matures. Children do not possess the cardiac reserve of an adult, therefore when confronted with severe blood or fluid loss a child will quickly become critically ill.

Age (years)	<1	2–5	5–12	>12
Pulse (BPM)	110–160	95–140	80–120	60–100
Respiration	30–40	25–30	20–25	15–20
Systolic BP (mmHg)	70–90	80–100	90–110	100–120

Table 12.1 Normal Ranges of Vital Signs for Age of Child

Other considerations

Glycogen stores in the liver are limited and hypoglycaemia can be present in any paediatric patient who has been too ill to feed or subjected to high metabolic demands because of illness.

With respect to drugs, the dosage for children will, in most cases, be less than the adult dose, but the dose for children will also vary dependent upon the way in which children absorb and metabolise the drug. In recent years it has been recognised that the drug industry has failed to investigate fully the physiological behaviour of drugs in children and are now being required to do so with new drugs. Studies with adults have previously been extrapolated theoretically to children. Paediatricians and children's nurses are aware of the different ways of calculating the correct dose of a drug for children of different ages and developmental stages. Registered nurses administering drugs to children have a similar

professional responsibility to be aware of the expected drug dose, i.e. is this in the right general level? If you are not sure it is right, then do not give it. Getting the dose correct for the child can also be challenging. This might require a calculation (Applying Theory to Practice: Box 12.1). (See Chapter 16 for more on pharmacology.)

Applying Theory to Practice: Box 12.1

For instance:

Case 1. The child is prescribed 125mg of an antibiotic that is contained in a solution of 250mg in 5ml.

The simple formula that most children's nurses use is:

$$\frac{\text{What you want}}{\text{What you've got}} \quad \text{multiplied by what the solution comes in}$$

In Case 1: What you want is 125mg multiplied by 5ml = 125 X 5 = 2.5ml.

What you have is 250mg.

You can use the same formula for tablets/capsules if you are able to halve them (if they are scored for this purpose).

Until you become competent and confident at this method of calculation, administering medications to children can be dangerous and should be left to those competent at this skill.

Getting a child to take a medicine is a different matter; this includes how to deal with the toddler who dribbles some of it out, thereby not getting the full prescribed dose.

Various other differences are important in relation to drugs and children. Registered nurses are not expected to know all of these, but should be aware that there are many factors beyond the obvious that have to be taken into account when dispensing and administering drugs to children. High surface to area ratio in children, especially young children, means that for topical drugs there is greater potential for absorption into the general metabolic system. A topical steroid would be a good example, although these are used with great caution with children as they can damage the young skin; gastrointestinal

Applying Theory to Practice: Exercise 12.3

Have a look at some children's medication in two ways. Ask a friend or relative who has small children whether they have any medicines that they give to their children, such as liquid paracetamol.

- Ask them what dose range they are meant to give to their child.
- Now use the calculation format in Exercise 12.3 to calculate the quantity required for yourself.
- Ask them how they actually administer the medicine to the child.

Repeat the same exercise when on a children's area, but working with a qualified member of staff with access to the drugs and the drug prescriptions for different children.

effects are also important. Neonates have a slightly different stomach pH, so some drugs that are pH dependent can be made less effective in neonates. Similarly, neonates have slow emptying of the stomach compared with adults, and so the dosage and efficacy of drugs in young children are unclear when given by the oral route (Johnson 2007). As a result, many drugs are given via the intravenous route (or less commonly intramuscularly for the same reason), and this requires particular care of small vessels and skilled splintage and support around the IV site, especially in the very young, and toddlers and children too young to understand the importance of the intervention.

Applying Theory to Practice: Exercise 12.4

- List some physical differences between children and adults.
- Identify three physical differences and explain why these are important in the care of children.
- Why would young children and babies receive some drugs intravenously when adults would normally receive the equivalent by mouth?

The National Service Framework for Children, Young People and Maternity Service Standards for Hospital Services

The *Standards for Hospital Services* was published in advance of the full *National Service Framework for Children* in response to the concerns raised in the Kennedy Report. This report focused on the management of the care of children receiving complex cardiac surgical services at the Bristol Royal Infirmary between 1984 and 1995.

The recommendations of the Kennedy Report used the following guiding principles:

- The complexity of the NHS as an organisation must be recognised
- Patients must be at the centre of the NHS, and thus the patient's perspective must be included in the policies, planning and delivery of services at every level

- The dedication and commitment of NHS staff are and must remain at the core of the service
- The quality of healthcare must include all aspects of care: clinical and non-clinical
- Patients' safety must be the foundation of quality
- Systems of care, and facilities, as well as individuals, affect the quality of healthcare
- Learning from error, rather than seeking someone to blame, must be the priority in order to improve safety and quality
- Openness and transparency are as crucial to the development of trust between healthcare professional and patient, as they are to the trust between the NHS and the public
- The particular needs of children's healthcare services must be addressed

The final guiding principle links directly to the content of the NSF, but the other principles are clearly present throughout. The NSF was also a reaction to the

Developing and Delivering Expert Care: Box 12.2

The Principles of the Children's NSF

In *Building a Strategy for Children and Young People*, a set of principles was put forward, and these are at the forefront of the children's NSF, which maintains that all policies and services for children and young people should be:

- *Centred on the needs of the young person:* the best interests of the child should be paramount, taking into account their wishes and feelings
- *High quality:* policies and services should aspire to and reach high standards of quality for the benefit of their customers
- *Family orientated:* full recognition must be given to family members who contribute to the well-being of children
- *Equitable and non-discriminatory:* all children should have access to and be able to participate in services that they need, when they need them, in a way that respects diversity and their individual needs
- *Inclusive:* policies and services should be sensitive to the individual needs and aspirations of every child
- *Empowering:* children should have opportunities to play an effective role in the design and delivery of policies and services
- *Results orientated and evidence-based:* high quality research, evaluation, monitoring and review should ensure that decisions that affect children are well informed
- *Coherent in design and delivery:* services should be woven together in a coherent, integrated and cross-sector form
- *Supportive and respectful:* policies and services should be delivered in as manner that is respectful and supportive of children and ambitious for the future
- *Community enhancing:* communities should be empowered to make positive changes for their children so improvements can be owned and sustained locally.

recommendations of the Victoria Climbié Inquiry (Laming 2003) (discussed in relation to child protection in this chapter), which advocates services being designed and delivered geared to the needs of users of services, through:

- Interagency partnerships
- Involving children and families in choices about their care
- Seamless care pathways of care
- Robust clinical governance arrangements
- Child-friendly environments.

The Hospital Standard of the children's NSF has three main aims:

- Improving services: ensuring services are of high quality, appropriate and accessible, and provided in a modern environment. This includes providing sustainable improvements in services and training and development for staff. Ultimately, all services will be child- family-friendly, including those for pregnant women.
- Tackling inequalities: working alongside initiatives designed to reduce poverty, health services for children will have a commitment to reducing health inequalities, including reducing the infant mortality rate by 10% by 2010. The importance of social inclusion is implicit within this aim, and children in special circumstances and with disabilities are specifically targeted.
- Enhance partnerships: coordination of partnership working between services to reduce the duplications that children and families experience is a key aim. Developments within strategic planning frameworks, including the Preventative Strategy, will help achieve this aim.

The Standard for Hospital Services for Children

The NSF's overarching aim is to deliver hospital services that meet the needs of children, young people and their families and provide effective and safe care through appropriately trained and skilled staff working in suitable, child-friendly and safe environments.

The standard applies to every department and service within a hospital that delivers care to children and young people.

The standard has three parts, reflecting the three dimensions of quality that a hospital needs to get right if it is to provide the service that children deserve:

Part 1: Child-centred hospital services
Part 2: Quality and safety of care provided
Part 3: Quality of setting and environment

The contents of these parts are summarised below:

Part 1: Child-centred hospital services

Children should receive care that is integrated and coordinated to their particular needs, and the needs of their family. They and their parents should be treated with respect, given the support and information they need to understand and cope with the illness or injury, and treatment required. They should be encouraged to be active partners in decisions about their health and care and where possible, be able to exercise choice.

Children, young people and their parents will participate in designing NHS and social care services that:

- Are readily accessible
- Are respectful
- Are empowering
- Follow best practice in obtaining consent
- Provide effective response to their needs.

Child-centred hospital services will:

- Consider the 'whole child', and not simply the illness being treated
- Treat children as children and young people as young people
- Be concerned with the overall experience for the child and family
- Treat children, young people and parents as partners in care
- Integrate and coordinate services around the child and the family's particular needs
- Graduate smoothly into adult services at the right time
- Work in partnership with children, young people and parents to plan and shape services and to develop the workforce.

Part 2: Quality and safety of care provided

Children and young people should receive appropriate high quality, evidence-based hospital care, developed

through clinical governance and delivered by staff that have the right set of skills.

This means:

- Clinical governance systems that give proper and explicit focus to the different needs of children and young people
- State treating and caring for children having the education, training, knowledge and skills to provide high quality care.

Part 3: *Quality of setting and environment*

Care will be provided in an appropriate location and in an environment that is safe and well suited to the age and state of development of the child or young person.

That is:

- Child-friendly hospitals
- Hospitals that are safe and healthy places for children.

Applying Theory to Practice: Exercise 12.5

- State the three aims that govern the NSF for children and young people in hospital.
- What are the three principal parts of *The Standard for Hospital Services for Children*?
- What will the results be for children, young people and their parents participating in designing NHS and social care services?
- What are the characteristics of child-centred hospital services?

Child protection

This section will provide aspiring nurses with the essential information, relevant knowledge, history and policies to enable them to gain an understanding of child protection. This will be achieved through the following sections:

- An understanding of child abuse and neglect
- Roles and responsibilities in child protection
- What to do if you are concerned about a child
- How to access advice, guidance and support.

The Laming Report (2003) reported on the events that

led to the death of Victoria Climbié in London and changes to systems that needed to be developed to avoid any recurrence in the future. This inquiry was not the first of its kind; each generation seems to have its own example. In 1984, Maria Colwell's death at the hands of her stepfather highlighted a similarly serious lack of coordination among services responsible for child welfare. As a result the Laming Report took seriously the previous history of failed coordination and made a series of recommendations (DH 2003):

- The creation of a children and families board chaired by a senior government minister to coordinate policies and initiatives that have a bearing on the well-being of children and families
- A national agency for children and families, led by a children's commissioner, should be established to ensure local services meet national standards for child protection and implement reforms
- Committees for children and families should be established by councils, with members drawn from social services, education, housing, the NHS and the police
- New local management boards – chaired by council chief executives with members from the police, health, social services, education, housing and the probation service – should be set up. The boards would appoint a local director of children and family services to monitor effective interagency working on child welfare and protection
- The creation of a national children's database that keeps a record of every contact a child has with a member of staff from the police, health and local authorities.

Everybody's business

All those who come into contact with children and families in their everyday work, including practitioners who do not have a specific role in relation to child protection, have a duty to safeguard and promote the welfare of children.

(DH 2003)

This is an important principle for child protection, because it makes explicit the role of every professional. In the past, non-children's specialists shied clear of child protection, understandably, as it is a challenging area of practice. Current legislation makes it everybody's business.

The legislative context

While there have been many Acts that have defined child protection processes in this country, the current situation can be sourced to the Children Act 1989. In this Act two issues were established: key principles in keeping children safe, and the welfare of the child as the paramount consideration. This was confirmed and reinforced in the Children Act 2004. Concurrently the Human Rights Act was published in 1998 to which the UK was a signatory. Included in this Act was Article 19 which identified protection (of children) from abuse and neglect.

What is safeguarding and promoting the welfare of children?

- Protecting children from maltreatment
- Preventing impairment of children's health or development
- Ensuring that children are growing up in circumstances consistent with the provision of safe and effective care; and undertaking that role so as to enable those children to have optimum life chances and to enter adulthood successfully.

These statements seem self-evident, but there are problems or have been problems, for instance, in defining the failure to thrive of an infant as a result of maltreatment, or impairing the child's health and development.

Section 31(9) of the Children Act 1989 (as amended by the Adoption and Children Act 2002) defines 'harm' as ill-treatment or the impairment of health or development, including, for example, impairment suffered from seeing or hearing the ill treatment of another; 'development' is defined as physical, intellectual, emotional, social, or behavioural development; 'health' means physical or mental health; and 'ill treatment' includes sexual abuse and forms of ill treatment which are not physical.

Under Section 31(10) of the Children Act 1989, where the question of whether harm suffered by the child affects the child's health and development, his health or development shall be compared with that which could reasonably be expected of a similar child. This is particularly helpful for the example of a toddler who is failing to thrive, as harm can be identified by a significant difference from normal development. Physical development uses 'normograms' that show growth ranges of children and so sets definitions as to what is 'normal'.

What is abuse and neglect?

Abuse and neglect are forms of maltreatment of a child. Somebody may abuse or neglect a child by inflicting harm, or by failing to act to prevent harm. Children may be abused in a family or in an institutional or community setting; by those known to them or, more rarely, by a stranger. They may be abused by an adult or adults or another child or children.

(DH 2006)

Categories of abuse

There are many forms of abuse and they have been categorised in the flowing manner:

- Physical abuse
- Neglect
- Emotional abuse
- Sexual abuse.

It is important for all professionals to have a clear notion of what constitutes abuse in order to know whether they need to act in line with the legislation.

Physical abuse

Physical abuse may involve hitting, shaking, throwing, poisoning, burning or scalding, drowning, suffocating or otherwise causing physical harm to a child. Physical harm may also be caused when a parent or carer fabricates the symptoms of, or deliberately induces illness in a child.

(DH 2006)

Neglect

... the persistent failure to meet a child's basic physical and/or psychological needs, likely to result in the serious impairment of the child's health or development. Neglect may occur during pregnancy as a result of maternal substance misuse. Once a child is born, neglect may involve a parent or carer failing to provide adequate food and clothing, shelter including exclusion from home or abandonment, failing to protect a child from physical and emotional harm or danger, failure to ensure adequate supervision including the use of inadequate care-takers, or the failure to ensure access to appropriate medical care or treatment. It may also include neglect of, or unresponsiveness to, a child's basic emotional needs.

(DH 2006)

Emotional abuse

Emotional abuse is the persistent emotional mal-treatment of a child such as to cause severe and persistent adverse effects on the child's emotional development. It may involve conveying to the child they are worthless or unloved, inadequate, or valued only insofar as they meet the needs of another person. It may feature age or developmentally inappropriate expectations being imposed on children. These may include interactions that are beyond the child's developmental capability, as well as overprotection and limitation of exploration and learning, or preventing the child participating in normal social interaction. It may involve seeing or hearing the ill treatment of another. It may involve serious bullying causing children frequently to feel frightened or in danger, or the exploitation or corruption of children. Some level of emotional abuse is involved in all types of maltreatment of a child, though it may occur alone.

(DH 2006)

Sexual abuse

Sexual abuse involves forcing or enticing a child or young person to take part in sexual activities, including prostitution, whether or not the child is aware of what is happening. The activities may involve physical contact, including penetrative or non-penetrative acts. They may include non-contact activities, such as involving children in looking at, or in the production of pornographic material or watching sexual activities, or encouraging children to behave in sexually inappropriate ways.

(DH 2006)

There are internationally identified indicators of risk and vulnerability. The factors give some notion of increased risk of potential harm and abuse taking place in the family. It must be stressed that they do not mean that abuse is taking place. There are families who have most of the indicators but provide a highly supportive and nurturing family environment. Evidence of harm and abuse must be literally that: evidence of harm and abuse.

Indicators of risk and vulnerability to the child in parents and families

- Lonely and socially isolated
- Childhood was deprived

> **Applying Theory to Practice: Exercise 12.6**
>
> - What is meant by safeguarding and promoting the welfare of children?
> - What are the four forms of abuse and maltreatment of children?
>
> Define each of these and add your summary to your expanding portfolio.

- History of being abused themselves
- First baby before 20 years of age
- Failure to attend antenatal appointments or prepare for baby
- Young, immature parents
- Jealousy and rivalry towards child
- Unreal expectations of the child
- Unable to cope with the child and life in general
- Unstable or violent adult relationship
- Not parent of the child
- Frequent and different relationships
- Antagonistic to authority
- Problems of drug or alcohol abuse
- Mental illness or learning difficulties
- Aggressive behaviour
- History of violence and strict disciplinarian, previous abuse
- Rejection and negative attitude
- Asking for child to be removed

Indicators of risk and vulnerability to the child in the child

- Premature
- Neonatal problems (bonding)
- Unwanted
- Different in some way
- Difficult or slow feeder
- Cries a lot
- Unresponsive
- Fearful
- Role reversal i.e. the child cares for the parent

Roles and responsibilities in the health services

Health professionals have a key role to play in actively promoting the health and well-being of children. Health

professionals working directly with children need to ensure that safeguarding and promoting the welfare of those children form an integral part of the care they offer. Other healthcare professionals who come into contact with children in the course of their work, including when they are not directly responsible for the care of the child, also need to be aware of their responsibility to safeguard and promote the welfare of children. In cases of suspected abuse, the duty of care that a health professional owes to a child as his or her patient will take precedence over any obligation to the parent who may be suspected of abuse. The National Service Framework for Children, Young People and Maternity Services sets out a ten-year programme for improving the quality of services for children, young people and pregnant mothers. Safeguarding children is a theme throughout the National Service Framework and one of its eleven standards deals with safeguarding and promoting the welfare of children.

The involvement of health professionals in safeguarding and promoting the welfare of children is important at all stages of work with children and families:

- Recognising children in need of support and/or safeguarding, and parents who may need extra help in bringing up their children, and referral where appropriate
- Contributing to enquiries about a child and family
- Assessing the needs of children and the capacity of parents/carers to meet their children's needs
- Planning and providing support to children and families, particularly those who are vulnerable
- Participating in child protection conferences, family group conferences and strategy meetings
- Planning support for children at risk of significant harm
- Providing therapeutic help to abused children and parents under stress (e.g. mental health problems)
- Playing a part, through the child protection plan, in safeguarding children from significant harm
- Providing ongoing preventative support and work with families contributing to serious case reviews (DH 2006)

All professionals should:

- Be alert to the indicators of abuse and neglect
- Be alert to the risks potential abusers pose to children
- Share and help analyse information to assess need

- Contribute to whatever actions needed
- Take part in regular reviews of plans
- Work cooperatively with parents – unless inconsistent with safety of child (DH 2006)

Actions for all health professionals start from when there are suspicions of abuse. These might be when you observe signs and indications of abuse, you are made aware of an allegation or report of abuse by another, someone admits to you that they are harming a child, or finally on receiving a cry for help by a child. All of these should set in motion a sequence of events in which the child's welfare is paramount. In every public organisation there is a system of advice and support in which a health professional can, for instance, discuss the basis of fact in concerns. This system takes the form of designated and named professionals, including child protection advisors. Local child protection manuals will make this clear and most organisations place these prominently on their intranet. The procedures will also be there, and these will be seen to be multi-agency; training will be similarly carried out. All health professionals have to undertake level 1 child protection in-house training as part of their mandatory training.

In summary, the nurse and any other health professional's role in safeguarding children is guided by the following:

- In all matters the child's welfare is paramount
- Be alert to signs of abuse
- Via your child protection advisor make enquiries to child protection register when appropriate
- Refer your concerns on to the correct agency
- Work together with your colleagues and professionals of all kinds to promote child welfare
- Follow the local child protection procedures as laid down in your organisation
- Share information about the child and your concerns
- Record accurately your concerns and do this contemporaneously
- Consult and get advice from senior colleagues and your designated child protection advisor.

Conclusion

This chapter has discussed something of the nature of childhood, particularly milestones, and the notion of infancy, childhood and adolescence.

The vulnerability of children has been discussed. For psychological development the need for a prime carer, particularly for the young, has been made clear. Physiological differences are numerous, but the vulnerability to temperature change and need to recalculate drug dosages for small children have been elucidated.

Normal development at home has been discussed; the systems such as family nursing and the NSF for children have also been described.

The principle of child protection has been described as well as the legislation and processes to ensure that the welfare of the child is paramount.

Further reading

Department of Health (2001) *National Service Framework for Children, Young People and Maternity Service: Change for Children – Every Child Matters*. DH/DfES: London.

Haines, C. (2005) Parents' experiences of living through their child's suffering from and surviving severe meningococcal disease. *Nursing in Critical Care* 10(2): 78–89.

Johnson, T.N. (2007) The problems in scaling adult drug doses to children. *Archives of Disease in Children*. First published online 15 March 2007. doi:10.1136/adc.2006.114835

Laming (2003) *The Victoria Climbié Inquiry: Report of an Inquiry by Lord Laming*. TSO: London.

Prot, S., Fontan, J.E., Alberti, C., et al. (2005) Drug administration errors and their determinants in pediatric in-patients. *International Journal of Quality Healthcare* 17(5): 381–9.

Rowe, C, Koren, T, & Koren, G (1998) Errors by paediatric residents in calculating drug doses. *Arch Dis Child* (79): 56–8.

http://www.dh.gov.uk/en/PolicyAndGuidance/ HealthAndSocialCareTopics/ChildrenServices/ ChildrenServicesInformation/DH_4089111

www.resus.org.uk/pages/pbls.pdf

http://www.safeguardingchildren.co.uk/procedures-main-01.html

References

Bronfenbrenner, U. (1979) *The Ecology of Human Development*. Harvard University Press: London.

Campbell, S.J., Kelly, P.J. & Summersgill, P. (1993) Putting the family first: interpreting a framework for family centred care. *Child Health* 1: 59–63.

Campbell, S.J. & Summersgill, P. (1993) Keeping it in the family: defining and developing family centred care. *Child Health* 1: 17–20.

Canadian Pediatric Society (CPS) Adolescent Health Committee (2003) Age limits and adolescents. *Pediatrics & Child Health* 8(9): 577.

Department of Health (2003) *Keeping Children Safe*. The Government's response to The Victoria Climbié Inquiry Report and Joint Chief Inspectors' Report *Safeguarding Children*. Cm 5861. TSO: London.

Department of Health (2006) *Working Together to Safeguard Children: A Guide to Safeguard and Promote the Welfare of Children*. DH: London.

Department of Health, Home Office, Department for Education and Skills, DCMS, Office of the Deputy Prime Minister and Lord Chancellor (2003) *What To Do If You're Worried A Child Is Being Abused*. DH: London (superseded by the 2006 version).

Haines, C. (2005) Parents' experiences of living through their child's suffering from and surviving severe meningococcal disease. *Nursing in Critical Care* 10(2): 78–89.

Johnson, T.N. (2007) The problems in scaling adult drug doses to children. *Arch Dis Child*. First published online 15 March 2007. doi:10.1136/adc.2006.114835

Kennedy Report (2001) *Learning from Bristol: The Report of the Public Inquiry into Children's Heart Surgery at The Bristol Royal Infirmary 1984–1995*. TSO: London. (www.bristol-inquiry.org.uk/final-report/ index.htm)

Laming (2003) *The Victoria Climbié Inquiry: Report of an Inquiry by Lord Laming*. TSO: London.

Lloyd, H., Hancock, H.C. & Campbell, S.J. (2007) *Principles of Care (Vital Notes for Nurses)*. Blackwell Publishing: Oxford.

Ministry of Health (1959) *The (Sir Harry) Platt Report (Report on the Welfare of Children in Hospital)*. HMSO: London.

Rennick, J. (1995) The changing profile of acute childhood illness: a need for the development of family nursing knowledge. *Journal of Advanced Nursing* 22(2): 258–66.

Misconceptions and the reality of mental illness

Nick Wrycraft

Chapter 13 Learning Objectives

- To consider our own preconceptions of mental illness
- To examine common preconceptions of mental illness within society
- To define mental illness
- To gain an understanding of how the law applies to mental illness
- To identify common mental health problems
- To develop knowledge of care in the community
- To gain an understanding of the *National Service Framework for Mental Health* (DH 1999)

Introduction

In all practice settings nurses will encounter patients with mental health problems. This chapter considers society's' misconceptions and encourages the reader to question and examine their own views, feelings and attitudes towards mental illness. Acquiring an awareness of the different ways that mental illness can manifest itself is essential if nurses are to work effectively and provide the most appropriate treatment for an individual. Developing empathic and non-judgemental attitudes is a central part of nursing practice, consistent with the role of advocate, stated within the professional nursing Code of Conduct (NMC 2004).

At any one time a significant number of the adult population experience mental illness and the majority live within the community (SCMH 2002). Despite being so widespread, mental illness is still frequently misunderstood and often the subject of stigma. The damage caused by negative perceptions of mental illness limits the participation of these people within society and in turn prolongs the experience of mental illness and prevents successful recovery. A goal of government policy in recent years has been to promote social inclusion of people with mental health problems (DH 2004a). Therefore, it is vital that modern nursing not only understands how mental illness affects people but also promotes positive values and non-discriminatory practice.

There are a wide range of mental illnesses, which can affect people in different ways: physically, psychologically and socially. This chapter will consider what constitutes mental illness in relation to consent and the law. The chapter progresses into providing the reader with a brief overview of common mental health problems. Care in the community will then be considered before discussing the NSF for Mental Health (DH 1999a).

Scenarios and examples of mental health problems will be presented throughout the chapter to illustrate the issues discussed and the clinical and professional complexities involved. Several exercises are included to help the reader identify areas they can develop through further research, reflecting on their own practice experience and action points that can be addressed on clinical placements to facilitate further lifelong learning.

Common misconceptions of mental illness within society

Before examining common preconceptions of mental illness that exist within society, it is important for the reader

Questioning Clinical Practice: Exercise 13.1

Write down what types of behaviour you might expect from a person with a mental illness.

- From the behaviours you have listed, which of these are negative qualities?
- Once you have read this chapter, re-examine what you have written and reflect on whether your views remain the same, or whether they have changed and in what way?

After writing down your thoughts file them in your professional portfolio.

to identify their own thoughts, feelings and attitudes towards mental illness. Exercise 13.1 will help the reader to focus their ideas.

Mental illness is a common feature of everyday life for many people. At any one time mental ill health can affect one in six people of working age (DH 1998, NIMHE 2004). It is estimated nearly half of all women and a quarter of all men will experience depression, the most frequently occurring mental health problem, before they reach 70 years of age (DH 1998; NICE 2002).

Despite being a major part of daily life for so many, mental illness is misunderstood and little known about. Often society has intolerant views, for example, people with a mental health problem are regarded as malingerers who simply ought to 'pull themselves together'. At the other extreme people who are acutely mentally ill are viewed as homicidal, crazed and unpredictable individuals who represent a danger to society (DH 1998, 1999b). These negative perceptions draw heavily on isolated high profile cases, for instance the tragic death of Jonathon Zito who was killed by Christopher Clunis.

Television, film and drama productions can also portray mentally ill people as villains and bad people, prone to violence and murderous behaviour, with few redeeming features (Sayce 2000). While this may add to the dramatic effect, there is no real evidence to suggest these distorted perceptions of mental illness have any basis in reality (University of Manchester 2006). The highly potent fear of being murdered by a person with a mental health problem who was not known to the victim or 'stranger homicide' is no more likely than the risk of being the victim of 'stranger homicide' by a person without a mental illness (BBC 2006; University of Manchester 2006). While some people with mental health problems do commit acts of violence and murder, statistics suggest the risk is no more prevalent than with any other sector of the population (University of Manchester 2006).

A recent government report concluded community care has not increased the risk to the general public (University of Manchester 2006). Furthermore the established trend that murders often occur within the family or among people known to one another extends to mental illness where the majority of violent crimes committed by people with mental health problems were against people known to the perpetrator (University of Manchester 2006). Rather than that of violence towards others, the more frequent risk factors associated with people with mental health problems is the likelihood of them committing suicide,

self-harming or being a victim of violence and abuse (DH 1998, 1999a; University of Manchester 2006).

The stigma surrounding mental illness causes discrimination and a lack of opportunities for employment, meaningful occupation and the chance for people with, or recovering from, mental illness to contribute to society (DH 1998, 1999a, 2006a). It has been suggested that, to avoid attracting disapproval, people with a mental health problem feel unable, for example, to phone in sick at work due to mental health reasons and are more likely to substitute an alternative physical reason (Sayce 2000). Other consequences of mental illness are to prevent people seeking help as they fear for job security, loss of promotion opportunities and increases in home and travel insurance (DH 2006a).

People with mental health problems frequently have low incomes and socio-economic status; these factors can exert a detrimental effect on their mental health creating a vicious cycle, which is compounded by society's negative perceptions (O'Brien et al. 2001; Singleton et al. 2001). The necessity of providing effective support in the community to those people with severe mental health problems to reduce suicides or the potential of their mental health causing a threat has been a strong focus of government mental health policy in recent years, as a result of Care in the Community (DH 1998, 2006b; Social Exclusion Unit 2004).

Defining mental illness

It is necessary to identify mental illness in order to offer appropriate specialist help for people in mental distress or who are acutely mentally ill. However, defining mental illness is complex, as it exists on a continuum with mental health (Hart 2004). Identifying physical illness is not a problem as when we are well we do not need healthcare, yet when we are unwell we receive a diagnosis and treatment for a particular problem or undergo investigations to locate the cause. In contrast mental illness covers a range of disorders with various origins; these include social, psychological, genetic, biological and chemical causes. Mental illness under the Mental Health Act 1983 is defined as including one or more of the four elements listed below:

■ Incomplete development of the mind
■ Psychopathic disorder
■ A disturbance which prevents normal development

- A mental disturbance which interferes with normal behaviour and daily life.
 (Department of Health and the Welsh Office 1999).

The Mental Health Bill of 2006 (DH 2006a) revises mental health legislation and will use one definition of mental health which instead focuses on the problems the service user is experiencing rather than diagnosis within the above criteria.

Everyone experiences some symptoms of mental ill health at some time, for example, it is perfectly normal to be anxious over a driving test or exam, or to feel very low in mood over a bereavement or significant loss. Due to the body's fight or flight instinct, heightened alertness occurs in response to a perceived threat of danger and serves a useful role in self-preservation and efficient performance of certain tasks (Hart 2004). In many circumstances these feelings, while uncomfortable, are time limited, or in response to specific events.

Applying Theory to Practice: Exercise 13.2

Consider a time in practice where you have felt anxious, for example, when being assessed carrying out a technical skill under supervision by a qualified nurse.

- What physical changes did you feel?
- What helped you to feel less anxious?

Write down your reflections and include them in your professional portfolio.

- What learning points can you translate to your practice on coping with feelings of anxiety?

Mental illness can be said to occur where the response is prolonged, is triggered by inappropriate events, or where the effects limit the person's quality of life and/or cause significant distress. Yet at what point a person is said to be mentally ill depends very much on the individual case and the circumstances. Mental illness is also prone to misinterpretation as frequently people who are mentally ill display erratic or unusual behaviour, have an inaccurate perception of reality, or express views which differ from the majority of the rest of society (Hart 2004) with the potential they can become confused with people who are simply regarded as eccentric, antisocial, deviant or criminal.

Once a person is diagnosed with a mental illness, they may require treatment; the following commonly used interventions and services are available to work with people experiencing mental illness:

- In secondary care: inpatient services, intensive community-based multidisciplinary mental health teams, community mental health teams, day hospitals and day centres
- In primary care: specialist mental health teams of trained counsellors and mental health workers, for example, graduate workers and link workers or gateway workers who provide access to secondary services
- Interventions by mental health nurses within the above services working with service users to provide support and care, and the input of the specialist roles of other mental health professionals in these teams, for example, occupational therapists, social workers and psychologists
- Psychiatric medications may be overseen by a psychiatrist but, under the new wave of prescribers, monitored and managed by mental health nurses
- Psychological therapies including cognitive behavioural therapy (CBT) as recommended by NICE (2004a, b) and other therapies, for example, psychodynamic interventions provided by trained nurse therapists and other mental health professionals such as psychologists and occupational therapists
- Independent services that often work alongside and in collaboration with statutory mental health specialist services
- Other interventions including referrals for exercise, self-help groups, advice on employment and voluntary work and complementary therapies.

Prior to providing appropriate treatment, it is necessary to gain consent, which will now be discussed in the following section.

Consent to treatment, mental health and the law

In some cases a person who is mentally ill requires treatment for a period of time in an inpatient setting. In many cases individuals agree to this and are regarded as 'informal' admissions. Yet in some instances people who are acutely mentally ill lack insight into their condition and are reluctant to accept help. Their behaviour may

jeopardise their own well-being and/or the safety of others, so it may become necessary to detain them for compulsory treatment. While mental health legislation affects a relatively small number of the population at any time, according to the Department of Health (2006b) there were 14,700 patients in England and 545 in Wales detained under the Mental Health Act 1983 at 31 March, (2005), its importance ought not to be underestimated, as the Mental Health Act is the only statute outside the criminal justice system which allows individuals to be legally detained against their will.

Under the current legislation if a person is to receive treatment against their consent, there has to be a second medical opinion recommending the treatment. Furthermore the treatment can only be carried out if it is:

- Necessary to save the person's life
- Necessary to avoid a serious, irreversible deterioration in the person's health
- Necessary to alleviate serious suffering and is not hazardous
- Necessary, not hazardous, and the minimum treatment to prevent the person harming themselves or other people (DH & Welsh Office 1999).

While people detained in hospital are defined as experiencing mental illness, the Mental Health Act 1983 does not actually present a definition. Instead mental disorder is defined within four categories: see Applying Theory to Practice: Box 13.1.

Applying Theory to Practice: Box 13.1

Types of Mental Disorder

- Mental illness
- Severe mental impairment
- Psychopathic disorder
- Mental impairment (Mitchell 2004)

The Mental Health Bill (DH 2006a) proposes replacing these areas with a single definition focused on the problem(s). The design of the legislation strives to respect the rights of the individual while safeguarding society, and as a guiding principle for treatment the least intervention necessary to address the problem is the preferred solu-

tion. Detaining someone under the Mental Health Act 1983 ought to be a choice of last resort after all other options have been exhausted (DH & Welsh Office 1999).

Under English law, consent is the voluntary permission of the person for a treatment based on having reasonable knowledge of the likely effects and purpose of the treatment, the likelihood of its success and an awareness of any risks or alternatives; the patient can also withdraw their consent at any time (DH & the Welsh Office 1999).

To be informed consent, the criteria in Applying Theory to Practice: Box 13.2 must be met.

Applying Theory to Practice: Box 13.2

Informed Consent

- The person must not be under coercion
- The person must understand the procedure to which they are consenting
- The person must be legally of an age to give consent and mentally competent, or capable of giving consent (Mitchell 2004)

There are numerous different sections of the Mental Health Act 1983 which are suitable for various aspects of patient care. Applying Theory to Practice: Box 13.3 lists a selection of those sections most commonly used.

The decision to impose a section of the Mental Health Act 1983 is often based on the action which will then need to be taken to assist the person's mental health but also respect their rights. It is a crucial consideration for nursing staff to make a person aware of their rights and the conditions of their section of the Mental Health Act 1983 by which they are being detained and explain their right to apply to a tribunal and the Mental Health Act Commission if they wish to contest the section.

Significantly, the mental health legislation is centred on the detention of the person for the purpose of treatment of their mental health. In the review of the Mental Health Act 1983 a significant issue of debate concerned the status of people with personality disorders. Personality disorders are defined as difficulties resulting from a person's character, whereby a person experiences problems due to their attitudes and behaviour, for example, difficulties with relationships, finances and employment.

Applying Theory to Practice: Box 13.3

Sections of the Mental Health Act 1983

Section 2: A compulsory admission for assessment, which lasts up to 28 days. The recommendation of two doctors is required and the person has the right to appeal within 14 days.

Section 3: An admission for treatment for six months. The section can be renewed for an additional six and then annually. The recommendation of two doctors is required and an approved social worker or the next of kin. The person can appeal at any time within the six months of the duration of the section.

Section 136: The police power to remove a person to a place of safety, preferably a hospital for assessment by a doctor and approved social worker. The section lasts for up to 72 hours.

While personality disorders are not amenable to treatment for mental health problems, nevertheless many people with personality disorders come into contact with mental health services; it is an ethical dilemma as to whether it is an acceptable interpretation of the Mental Health Act 1983 to detain a person for treatment who has a primary diagnosis of a personality disorder. Under the Mental Health Bill (DH 2006a) it is proposed that service users with a personality disorder or other problems which do not fall within the four criteria of the 1983 Act but who nevertheless have a mental health problem are eligible for treatment.

Questioning Clinical Practice: Exercise 13.3

Informed Consent

● How do you think having treatment under a section may affect an individual's future life?
● When you applied for nurse training, did you have to disclose any history of mental illness?

The first major review of the mental health legislation since the 1950s was announced in 1998 and there ensued a lengthy process of consultation and discussion with stakeholders before the Mental Health Bill finally passed through parliament in late 2006.

The Bill amends rather than replaces the 1983 Act, although a number of alterations have been made to the existing mental health legislation and it will be implemented in April 2008. There are three main areas of change and each will be discussed in more detail.

Provisions of the Mental Health Bill 2006

1. To make provision for people with serious and ongoing mental health problems to receive necessary treatment, and to maintain their safety and that of the public.

2. To widen the range of healthcare professionals able to perform roles identified in the 1983 Act to reconfigure the legislation to reflect the multidisciplinary nature of modern mental health services and allow them to act more rapidly and flexibly in response to service users' needs.

3. To protect the rights of people who do not have the capacity to provide consent and whose circumstances are not covered by the 1983 Act.

1. The Mental Health Bill 2006 proposes that the focus of the legislation is shifted to emphasise the treatment of mental health illness, as opposed to allowing access to treatment based on diagnosis, which overlooks those who do not fit neatly into a pre-existing category of mental illness (DH 2006a). It is intended to replace the four categories of mental illness outlined in the 1983 Act with one definition, which, rather than categorising specific mental illnesses, instead focuses on mental health needs, risk and the action which then ought to be taken with an emphasis on treatment (House of Commons 2007). The most controversial measure in the Mental Health Bill (DH 2006a) is supervised community treatment orders (CTO) which are based on the notion that some service users who have been compulsorily detained and received a period of inpatient treatment can receive the treatment

they need in the community, which reduces the social exclusion which might be experienced through a prolonged period of detention. CTOs are recommended for use in circumstances where service users present a risk to their own safety, or that of the public, and are intended to promote compliance with treatment and prevent relapse. CTOs do not diminish the service users' rights; an application can be made by the service user for the CTO to be withdrawn to the Mental Health Review Tribunal (discussed in more detail below); and treatment can only be provided if a service user who is capable of providing consent accepts treatment. Where treatment is refused it may be necessary to return a service user to hospital for treatment (DH 2006a).

The introduction of CTOs has been greeted with concern by some service users and independent groups because of the potential for the increased use of compulsion to infringe on the rights of service users to choose whether or not to accept treatment, when, for example in the case of some psychiatric medication there are potentially unpleasant side effects (King's Fund 2007). Furthermore, the role of the nurse as advocate for the service user has the potential to be compromised if implementing a programme of care where the service user is expected to comply with treatment, or receive the same treatment compulsorily in an inpatient setting (NMC 2004). However, it has also been argued that CTOs provide another useful treatment option as an alternative to the 'revolving door' phenomenon whereby service users are repeatedly admitted to inpatient settings through not complying with treatment (DH 2006a, King's Fund 2007). In terms of the evidence base supporting CTOs, they have been in use in a number of countries including the United States, Canada, New Zealand and Australia for some years and in Scotland since 2005, and while there are positive reports from healthcare practitioners, the research literature on the clinical effectiveness is limited (King's Fund 2007).

2. The Mental Health Bill (DH 2006a) proposes to widen the range of different healthcare professionals who can carry out functions under the 1983 Act, from approved social workers and responsible medical officers to include staff with appropriate training from disciplines including nurses, occupational therapists and social workers. Previously under the Mental Health Act 1983 mental health nurses' powers were limited to Section 5(4), which was a holding power of six hours maximum duration and

intended to allow for further assessment under the Act to be made (DH & Welsh Office 1999). Increasing the role of nurses within the mental health legislation has the potential to change the nurse's therapeutic relationship with the service user with the implication that there may be less trust, and the nurse's role within the multidisciplinary team will be more focused on managing care as opposed to its delivery.

3. Protecting the rights of service users who are not able to provide consent follows from the introduction of the Mental Capacity Act implemented in April 2007. The Mental Health Bill outlines the Bournewood provisions, which are intended to protect the rights of people whose circumstances are not otherwise accounted for in the Mental Health Act 1983.

Other aspects of the Mental Health Bill protect the rights of service users include improving access for service users to the Mental Health Review Tribunal (MHRT). The MHRT is an independent organisation which considers whether a service user ought to continue to be detained under a section of the Mental Health Act 1983 to prevent them being detained too long or inappropriately. The Mental Health Bill states that a maximum period of time will be identified, before which if a service user or someone on their behalf has not applied independently to the MHRT, the hospital managers will ensure an application is made. Furthermore, access to the MHRT not only applies to inpatient detention, as those subject to a CTO are also to be eligible to appeal to the MHRT. Finally, the nearest relative of a service user detained under a section of the Mental Health Act 1983 has a range of powers, from being able to request the service user's discharge from detention to applying for or preventing detention, requesting the detention is reviewed, and being permitted to receive particular information about the service user. The new Bill makes provision to allow service users to apply through the county court for their nearest relative to be displaced, or for the nearest relative to be displaced because they are not suitable to act in that role. Civil partners have the same rights as a husband or wife.

Types of mental health problem

In this section the broad range of different mental illnesses will be discussed and some scenarios presented of individuals who may be experiencing these problems.

Broadly speaking, mental health problems can be classified as either functional or organic.

Functional mental health problems are subdivided into psychotic disorders, which include schizophrenia, and mood disorders and other affective disorders including depression, anxiety, obsessive-compulsive disorder, phobias, anorexia nervosa and bulimia nervosa.

Organic mental health problems are due to the effects of physical causes on the action of the brain, including dementia-type illnesses, infectious causes and also alcohol and substance misuse.

Other types of mental health problems include personality disorders where a person's attitudes and choices of behaviour lead them into making chaotic life choices, for example, in relationships, employment, housing and other areas of their life.

While there are a wide range of different types of mental health problems, Applying Theory to Practice Box 13.4 identifies a succinct overview adapted from Hart's (2004) model. The types of problems listed will then be briefly discussed; but the reader ought to consult more specific texts for a more comprehensive understanding of each mental illness.

Applying Theory to Practice: Box 13.4

Types of Mental Health Problems

- Depression and anxiety
- Bipolar mood disorders
- Psychotic disorders and schizophrenia
- Psychoactive substance misuse
- Self-harm
- Eating disorders
- Dementia

Depression and anxiety

Depression and anxiety are the most common mental health conditions. In reality people more often experience a mixture of both depression and anxiety. In this chapter they are discussed separately.

Depression is evident where five or more of the symptoms listed below have been experienced for two weeks continuously:

Other symptoms may also be evident, for example, agitation and restlessness, preoccupation, loss of libido and muscular pains. Often depression can be triggered by

Applying Theory to Practice Box 13.5

Diagnostic Criteria for Depression

- Depressed mood most of the time
- Markedly reduced interest in all, or almost all, activities for the majority of the time nearly every day
- Significant unplanned weight loss (5% of total body weight within a month, or the equivalent) or weight gain occurring
- Insomnia or hypersomnia most of the time
- Psychomotor agitation or retardation most of the time
- Feelings of fatigue and a lack of energy and interest most of the time
- Feelings of worthlessness, or guilt most of the time
- Reduced and slowed down ability to think, concentrate or make decisions most of the time
- Recurrent thoughts of death or suicidal ideation most of the time

(American Psychiatric Association (APA) 1994)

an ongoing life-limiting physical condition such as diabetes, chronic obstructive pulmonary disease (COPD) or cardiac problems (Kisley & Goldberg 1996); in this type of scenario, depression is less likely to be identified and diagnosed and classified as a secondary condition. The person's wider social network, family and life situation ought not to be forgotten in assessment as people do not exist in a vacuum and their behaviour both affects and is affected by significant others.

Anxiety is evident where a person is preoccupied with heightened or exaggerated concern and attention to specific issues. The person may display a heightened level of responsiveness and be hyper-alert or vigilant. While certain levels of anxiety are a part of normal life, where this exerts a detrimental effect on the person's functioning and quality of life, they may experience a mental health problem. Typical presentations of anxiety are in the form of:

- **Panic attacks** – where physical symptoms are experienced associated with the body being highly responsive. These include palpitations, chills, hyperventilation, dizziness, chest pain, choking, nausea and

Scenario 13.1

Depression

Dave experienced a myocardial infarct approximately eighteen months ago. He is 52 and gave up smoking five years ago. Prior to this he smoked up to twenty cigarettes a day for thirty years. Previously Dave worked as a successful building contractor, which often involved living away from home for several months at a time. During these periods Dave's diet was poor and he regularly drank large amounts of alcohol as part of his social life.

After having the heart attack Dave began to feel low in mood, had difficulty sleeping, woke up early in the morning and generally lost interest in life. Dave describes himself before the heart attack as a 'happy go lucky' sociable character, but since his physical illness he has not worked, abandoned many former interests, lost contact with his friends and lacks motivation. Due to losing interest in eating Dave has become underweight and his wife is worried about his physical health. Dave feels he has lost confidence and is reluctant to leave home. Recently he has been asked to look after his 3-year-old grandson while his daughter-in-law works. Dave wants to do this as he values his family but worries he will have another heart attack while caring for his grandson. On several occasions recently Dave has had chest pain and attended the emergency department (ED) at the local hospital, but no physical problems were found. Dave experienced this pain again during a weekend when his GP was unavailable so his wife drove him to the ED.

Applying Theory to Practice: Exercise 13.4

Under the supervision of a qualified member of staff you are assigned to assess Dave's condition.

- What effect do you think his state of mind might be having on his physical condition?
- What verbal and non-verbal cues would you look for in Dave's communication?
- What questions would you ask Dave to ascertain how he feels?

Scenario 13.2

Anxiety

John is 35 years old and attending a pre-admission clinic for an arthroscopy on his left knee as a result of repeated wear and tear through playing football. You are taking John's observations. Initially he appears very positive and cheerful but then you notice he begins to appear anxious. On taking John's blood pressure his hands seem sweaty. John becomes increasingly agitated, repeatedly seeking reassurance from you that he will be all right and then confides that he is worried about dying during the surgery as an uncle some years ago underwent a routine operation but never regained consciousness.

Questioning Clinical Practice: Exercise 13.5

- How do you respond to John's concerns?

The NMC Code of Conduct (2004) identifies the role of the nurse as to advocate on behalf of the patient.

- Is it your role to reassure John and, if so, is it ethical for you to reassure him when you know that, however slight, there may be an element of risk in his undergoing surgery?

stomach churning. It has been suggested the physiological basis of panic attacks has a physical origin and is a fear response triggered in reaction to a perceived but unidentified threat (Hart 2004).

Other forms of anxiety include:

- **Phobias** – evident as focused aversions or highly reactive fears to specific phenomena, for example, fear of spiders or heights
- **Obsessive compulsive disorder** – occurs where the person experiences persistent obtrusive negative thoughts and carries out specific tasks or actions to prevent feared outcomes from occurring; examples include hand washing, checking, collecting, hoarding, touching and counting rituals. In some cases the ritualistic behaviour can be of a self-harming nature, for example, skin picking or hair pulling (trichotilomania). Frequently people experiencing obsessional thoughts are aware of the problem but due to the strongly compelling sensations are unable to resist the compulsion and break the cycle of obsessional behaviour (Hart 2004).

Bipolar mood disorders

Bipolar disorder affects mood, thinking and behaviour and is characterised by mood swings. When in a high phase the person can display grandiose behaviour and express delusions but when low they become deeply depressed and, due to the impulsive and emotion driven nature of the condition, there is a high risk of suicide. The symptoms outlined below describe a person in the elevated phase but when low the person will present as deeply depressed.

Psychotic disorders and schizophrenia

Psychosis leads the person to lose touch with reality and develop personalised or unusual interpretations to events or phenomena. The causes of psychosis can vary from a response to traumatic events or problems at a particular time in life, for example, starting university and living away from home, divorce, bereavement or redundancy, to the use of illicit substances. Frequently people can experience an episode of psychosis and fully recover.

A linked but separate mental health problem is schizophrenia. While the cause of schizophrenia is not definitely known, it is felt some physical factors are active (NHS Direct 2007a.). Schizophrenia is a fragmentation of the person's perception and grasp of objective reality, which makes it difficult for them to separate their own

Applying Theory to Practice: Box 13.6

Symptoms of Bipolar Disorder

Mood

- Elevated and expansive or euphoric
- Irritable and impatient
- Rapidly changing

Thought

- Flight of ideas
- Grandiose delusions
- Jealous or persecutory views

Speech

- Rapid delivery
- Loud in volume and expansive delivery
- Singing or rhyming words together

Behaviour

- Emotionally inappropriate and disinhibited
- Uncharacteristic actions, for example, overspending
- Unusual or colourful choices of clothing

Bodily functions

- Insomnia
- Increased activity levels
- Increased appetite
- Increased libido

Perceptions

- Illusory ideas
- Misunderstanding of other people's communication
- Jumps to conclusions
- Lack of insight and congruence with reality

(Hart 2004)

thoughts and perceptions from objective reality. Generally the onset of the illness is from late teens to early twenties for men and mid-twenties to early thirties for women (NHS Direct 2007a).

Commonly people with schizophrenia experience sensory delusions (unusual beliefs which are not shared by other people) and hallucinations (hearing, smelling or tasting something which is not real), commonly hearing voices and, due to the influence of this phenomenon, the person experiences difficulty thinking logically and acting

Applying Theory to Practice: Box 13.7

Symptoms of Schizophrenia

Delusions – abnormal beliefs that are not real

Hallucinations – the feeling of having an experience, which is not real

Disordered thoughts – which result from the delusions and hallucinations

Abnormal behaviour – which occur through responding to the delusions, hallucinations and disordered thoughts

(NHS Direct 2007a)

appropriately in social situations. Symptoms are summarised in Applying Theory to Practice: Box 13.7.

Schizophrenia is acutely distressing and life-limiting for the person and their family and significant others, yet it is the subject of much fear and stigma in the general population, which limits the opportunity for social inclusion and the meaningful participation of people with a psychotic and schizophrenia-related illness in the community.

Applying Theory to Practice: Box 13.8

Substance Misuse

- A persistent desire for, and preoccupation with, the substance
- Activities to acquire supplies of the substance
- Absence of control in taking the chosen substance
- Tolerance to the chosen substance leading to increased intake being required to achieve the same effect
- Psychological and/or physical dependence leading to difficulties with withdrawal, reduction or abstention
- Reduction in participation of other activities

Psychoactive substance misuse

Substances, which can be misused include nicotine, caffeine, alcohol, amphetamines and associated compounds,

cannabis, cocaine, opioids, hallucinogens, inhalants, sedatives, hypnotics and anxiolytics. The effects vary depending on the choice and in some cases a combination of these substances are used. Frequently people experience low mood, personality changes or impulsive behaviour or impaired judgement through using substances.

Self-harm

Self-harm frequently occurs as a method of relieving pent-up feelings of emotion or anger and is caused by low mood, depression, and feelings of self-loathing or worthlessness (NHS Direct 2007b). Other causes may be sexual, psychological or emotional abuse, neglect and bullying, or harassment and it is more prevalent in adolescence and among females than males (NHS Direct 2007b). Frequent parts of the body which are self-harmed are the wrists, upper thighs, inner arms and upper chest, although self-harm can also include skin picking and the deliberate breaking of bones (NHS Direct 2007b). The most commonly used method of self-harm is knives or blades, yet it can occur in subtle and varied forms (NHS Direct 2007b). People who self-harm tend to be ashamed of their behaviour and conceal their injuries and also therefore the means by which they carry out self-harm and so the chosen methods vary and can be very discreet (NHS Direct 2007b).

Scenario 13.3

Self-harm

Sophie is 14 years old. Her school is located near the hospital. At two o'clock she is visiting her father, John, after his arthroscopy. She is dressed in a dishevelled manner and seems preoccupied and low in mood. When you ask if she is okay, Sophie avoids eye contact, replies in an offhand way and appears to become defensive, explaining that due to a teacher being taken ill she has been granted a non-pupil afternoon and that this often happens. As you leave the bedside you notice the left-hand sleeve of her shirt is rolled up and the inside of her forearm has raised horizontal pale welts from what you think is scarring. The other sleeve is pulled down and what appear to be bloodstains have soaked through the material.

Questioning Clinical Practice: Exercise 13.6

Substance Misuse

- How would you attempt to engage with Sophie?
- Is it in accordance with the NMC Code of Conduct (2004) to ask further questions about Sophie's well-being or is that exceeding the acceptable role of the nurse?

While it may be felt self-harming behaviour is associated with suicide, no direct connection has been identified and it could be argued that relieving tension in this way prevents a build-up of negative emotion which could cause suicidal behaviour. Yet death may occur accidentally as a result of self-harm (NHS Direct 2007b).

Eating disorders

Eating disorders include a range of problems. In some cases the person does not eat because they mistakenly believe they are overweight and introduce a rigorous regime of dietary control and deprivation of food (anorexia nervosa). Another form of eating disorder is where the person binge eats large amounts of food and then purges through vomiting or using laxatives (bulimia nervosa) (NHS Direct 2007c). These conditions, while varied on presentation, share some common characteristics:

Applying Theory to Practice: Box 13.9

Eating Disorders

- An abnormal attitude towards food
- Difficulty controlling the amount which is consumed, either too much or too little
- Choices relating to food, which are harmful to health

Identifying an eating disorder can be difficult due to society's preoccupation with weight and peer pressure, especially among women, promoting certain expectations regarding body size and attitudes towards food. However, eating disorders are linked to mental health; causes include loneliness, boredom, anxiety, abuse, low self-esteem, guilt and the need to feel in control (NHS Direct 2007c).

Scenario 13.4

Eating Disorders

Ellen is a 25-year-old student nurse in your intake. She moved from her home some distance away to live in university accommodation when she began training and at the same time ended a long-term relationship with her boyfriend.

While on placement Ellen does not eat, providing the reason that shifts interrupt the usual pattern of meals. She also does not keep food in the kitchen she shares in a communal flat with other students as she lives on a bursary and enjoys spending her money on clothes and travel.

During the eighteen months of the course to date Ellen has lost a significant amount of weight and often looks pale and tired. On more than one occasion you have heard other people remark to Ellen that she appears to be underweight.

Ellen responds to these comments as compliments, stating that it is fashionable to be thin and when growing up her mother always criticised her for being overweight but that now she is able to live up to that ideal. Recently on a particularly busy shift Ellen appeared to faint and lose consciousness briefly but when recovering would not seek help. She increasingly appears to have difficulty concentrating and focusing on her work and her recent marks in assignments are lower than previously on the course.

Questioning Clinical Practice: Exercise 13.7

- Are you obliged to notify the university of your concerns about Ellen? If so, how would you describe what these concerns were and your rationale to support your observations?
- Within the scope of the NMC Code of Conduct are qualified members of staff obliged to report similar instances regarding colleagues?

Once you have answered these points, read through the Code of Conduct and see if your thoughts and feelings match the professional guidelines identified by the NMC.

Dementia

Dementia is not a disease but a group of symptoms which occur as a result of a number of different illnesses, but which all cause degenerative changes in brain tissue leading to a progressive decline in cognitive functioning. Typical changes which occur in dementia are loss of memory, confusion, and change in personality, mood and behaviour (Hart 2004). While commonly regarded as a disease of older age, dementia can affect younger people: illnesses such as Korsakoff syndrome and Creutzfeldt–Jakob disease (CJD) have affected people of all ages. Examples of dementia-type illnesses are Alzheimer's disease, Lewy body, vascular disease and Pick's disease. Cerebral haematomas or space-occupying lesions in the cerebral cortex can also produce similar symptoms to dementia.

Scenario 13.5

Dementia

George is 78 years old and was bereaved of his wife, Joan, eighteen months ago. George's daughter, Sarah, became concerned, as shortly after this event she went away with him on holiday and found that he could not remember where his room was and became very easily confused and disorientated. When he returned to his home George did not understand where he was, and recently he has not known who Sarah was. When she has asked him about this, George feels it is all a part of the ageing process. Lately, George has been forgetting to wash and eat, and has neglected his needs. Late on a Sunday evening, Sarah was phoned by a neighbour of George's who found him wandering outside his house and only partly clothed.

Sarah has brought George to the ED department; she is very tearful and when registering his details with the receptionist explained she can no longer care for her father and needs urgent help.

Care in the community

For most of the twentieth century the mental healthcare system in the UK was organised around a number of large inpatient mental health hospitals. Commonly, mental health hospitals were discreetly located just outside major towns with average patient populations of up to 2,500 per hospital (Jones 1993). There were a consistently large

Applying Theory to Practice: Exercise 13.8

- What techniques would you use in a conversation with Sarah to provide support and reassurance while also gaining suitable information to be able to effectively assess George?

number of inpatients reaching a peak of over 151,400 in 1955, which was nearly 3.4 per thousand of the total UK population (Jones 1993). There was a modest reduction of inpatients between 1954 and 1959 due to the development of outpatient treatment; but in the inpatient sector there was little development in the rehabilitation of long-stay patients, and expenditure on mental health services in the community actually decreased (Jones 1993).

Yet in March 1961 the Health Minister, Enoch Powell, in a keynote speech, surprisingly announced the Government's intention to abolish long-stay mental hospitals and reduce psychiatric inpatient bed capacity nationwide by 75,000. This would have far-reaching implications for the provision of mental health services, and, while the number of inpatient beds reduced to approximately 50,000 by 1992 (Coppock & Hopton 2000), this was not a smooth transition and took many years to fully implement. In effect this represented a complete U-turn in government policy from inpatient provision for mental health services to a community-based system. Unfortunately, there was no planned development to provide for the needs of mental health patients reprovisioned within the community and there was no introduction of mental health services that could serve these patients (Coppock & Hopton 2000). Furthermore, the change was not based on research that community care could produce better outcomes for the mentally ill.

Applying Theory to Practice: Box 13.10

Care in the Community

1. Pharmacological developments
2. Legal and organisational developments
3. Economic factors
4. Ideological and social changes

This change in policy has been attributed not just to one cause but several (Coppock & Hopton 2000).

1 **Pharmacological developments**: In 1953, there was a major breakthrough in medication, with the development of a new class of drugs called phenothiazines. Chlorpromazine (largactil) was the first of these new drugs, and they led to the availability of more effective medication to treat a range of acute mental health problems, which alleviated the distress of patients who were not amenable to other forms of therapy. The effect was to transform mental hospitals from forbidding environments designed to contain aggression and distress to institutions which permitted staff to work more proactively with patients and offer the possibility of life within the community, due to the better management of psychiatric symptoms. Yet it has been claimed the impact of this development has been overemphasised, as there was a successful recovery movement that pre-existed for many years prior to the development of this new medication (Coppock & Hopton 2000). Furthermore, while phenothiazines provided effective alleviation of symptoms, they were not a cure and there were side-effects with these drugs (Jones 1993). Bearing this in mind, it can still be stated that developments of new and effective pharmacological treatments for the acutely mentally ill were active alongside other factors in a changing environment of service provision. Today ranges of psychotropic medications have been developed to alleviate the symptoms of mental health problems from depression to acute agitation and psychotic symptoms.

2 **Legal and organizational developments**: Historically the provision of care for the mentally ill has represented a dilemma between balancing the needs and rights of the mentally ill individual with the safety of the wider community. The availability of improved medication for acute mental illnesses, together with ideological and social changes as discussed below, created a more positive view of mental illness as amenable to treatment. The introduction of the NHS in 1948 led to mental health services being aligned with health; previously they had been managed by local authorities. A review of the legal status of the mentally ill was regarded as long overdue and necessary to reflect changes in the role of the mentally ill within society. Before the Mental Health Act of 1959, magistrates determined the detention of people due to mental illness, so mental illness was regarded as a matter of public order. Yet the 1959 Mental Health Act placed the responsibility for detaining a person for reasons of their mental health under the remit of psychiatrists. Acknowledging the role of psychiatrists served to confirm their status alongside that of medical doctors and defined mental healthcare statutorily within healthcare as opposed to the criminal law (Jones 1993).

Organisationally, a consequence of these changes was to shift the emphasis of mental healthcare from containing the mentally ill to providing a health-focused service. The culture of the mental hospital system was required to undergo a momentous culture change through amalgamation with health services.

3 **Economic factors**: As a consequence of becoming part of the National Health Service it soon became apparent that the existing mental health service provision was inadequate (Coppock & Hopton 2000). Many of the buildings dated from the nineteenth-century Victorian and Edwardian eras and were in dire need of repair and maintenance. In some cases, due to overcrowding, patients slept in beds inches apart or in corridors (Jones 1993). By the mid-1950s it was clear to the Government that a programme of inestimable investment was necessary simply to maintain many of the buildings, which were antiquated and outdated for use as modern hospital buildings (Jones 1993). For the Government, scaling down the mental health inpatient provision and centring care in the community offered the prospect of financial savings.

4 **Ideological and social changes**: Before the Second World War, large-scale institutions reinforced a sense of order and equilibrium within society, which disempowered patients. In the postwar era groups and therapeutic communities were established to treat large numbers of soldiers who were psychologically traumatised by their experiences. This experimental and innovative work of Bion and Foulkes fundamentally altered mental healthcare, but was also very successful and was adopted and then further developed by psychiatrists such as Laing (1959). Mental health patients were seen as active participants in their care, by forming therapeutic relationships with their carers.

In 1961, the same year as Enoch Powell's speech (as Health Minister), three major academic works appeared which were all highly critical of mental health institutions: Erving Goffman's *Asylums* (1961); Thomas Szasz's *The Myth of Mental Illness* (1961); and Michel Foucault's

(1967) *Madness and Civilization.* All three writers came from differing academic backgrounds. Goffman was a sociologist, Szasz, a psychiatrist, and Foucault, an academic. Foucault and Goffman particularly criticised large-scale mental institutions as not only failing to work therapeutically for patients' mental well-being, but as actually exerting a detrimental and coercive effect on an individual. Despite all three texts taking radically different perspectives they were all unanimous in condemning mental health institutions, arguing they were anti-therapeutic, and these authors fundamentally questioned the biomedical model of psychiatry by claiming authority yet offering little in the way of effective treatment.

The direct influence of these writers in initiating change has been doubted; it is felt their work was more notable in capturing a prevailing trend internationally away from institutional care, which had simply become outmoded. This was due to changes in society's expectations and views of mental illness and the way therapeutic relationships were formed and conducted in the care of those with mental health problems (Coppock & Hopton 2000). The emergence of care in the community as the predominant philosophy of care for the mentally ill therefore reflected changes on a legal, organisational, ideological and social level on how care of the mentally ill ought to be organised and delivered.

The National Service Framework for Mental Health

In this section a brief outline is first presented of the background to the mental healthcare system before providing a more detailed discussion of the scope and goals of the *National Service Framework for Mental Health* (DH 1999c).

The government policy to dismantle large-scale mental hospitals was slow to take effect (Coppock & Hopton 2000). While the inpatient sector dwindled in numbers between the 1960s to the latter part of the 1980s, in spite of repeated calls for improvements, community-based services as a result of years of under-investment were not well developed nationally and a cause of much concern and criticism (Coppock & Hopton 2000).

Under pressure to act, the Government appointed Sir Roy Griffiths to produce the Griffiths Report (1988), which recommended a mixed economy of care in the community combining statutory, voluntary and private sector services; with social services leading in decisions over the

provision of community care. Following on from this, the White Paper *Caring for People* (1989) and the NHS and Community Care Act 1990 instituted fundamental change in the delivery of health and social care by:

- Introducing a market-orientated approach to services with competitive tendering
- A purchaser–provider split between the service commissioner and the service provider.
- Encouraging GP fundholding to control the purchase of care.
- Using self-governing hospital trusts and mechanisms to measure outcomes (Coppock & Hopton 2000).

While these changes reformed the infrastructure of the healthcare system to deliver care in the community more flexibly and responsively to the needs of service users, there was still concern that services for mentally ill people in the community were insufficiently developed (Coppock & Hopton 2000).

The NSF for Mental Health was the first comprehensive statement of what was expected from mental health services in England, focusing on the care of working-aged adults from 16 to 65. Mental healthcare services for children, adolescents and older adults are considered in the NSF for Children, Young People and Maternity Services (DH 2001a) and the NSF for Older People (DH 2001b).

The vision of the government contained in the NSF for Mental Health (DH 1999c) was to provide services, which are presented in Applying Theory to Practice Box 13.12.

Improving the services for people with severe and enduring mental health was the first milestone with the

Applying Theory to Practice Box 13.11

NSF for Mental Health – Principles

- **Safe** – to protect the public and care for those with mental health problems at the time care was needed
- **Sound** – to ensure service users and carers are able to access a full range of services appropriate to their need when they need it
- **Supportive** – working together with service users, their families, carers and significant others to build healthier communities

(DH 1999c)

wider implementation of the other goals envisaged to occur over the next ten years until 2009. Historically, specialist and inpatient mental health services existed separately from those in primary care with limited contact and communication. An important consideration was the necessity of establishing a more fluid continuum between primary and secondary services to improve access for service users to secondary care and enhance the level of mental health services provision available in primary care (DH 1999c).

The NSF for Mental Health lists seven standards for the mental healthcare of adults up to the age of 65 in five groups with standards 2 and 3, 4 and 5 generally being paired together as these standards relate specifically to primary care and secondary care respectively: see Applying Theory to Practice Box 13.13.

An interim report *The NSF–Five Years On* by the mental health tsar, Sir Louis Appleby, was published by the DH (2004) and provided insightful commentary on the progress up to that point in each of the seven standards:

Applying Theory to Practice Box 13.12

NSF for Mental Health Service Developments

Primary care:

- Support for GPs working with common mental health problems by employing 1000 primary care mental health specialist workers (GRADUATE workers)
- Support for primary care, ED and NHS Direct in working with mental health problems by the employment of 500 community mental health workers

Secondary care:

- The creation of 50 early intervention teams nationally to work with young people experiencing first episode psychosis
- Establishing 335 crisis resolution teams to relieve pressure on acute inpatient teams
- Developing 220 teams to support service users living in the community who are reluctant to engage

(DH 1999c)

- With regards to mental health promotion it was found that while a wide range of health promotion strategies had been carried out, the effectiveness of these measures was severely limited by a lack of expenditure. The target outlined in the NHS Plan to recruit and train staff to provide mental health interventions in primary care to support GPs was not met.

- A requirement of the NHS Plan was to develop a new gateway worker role to provide a conduit for access between primary and secondary services. In 2004 there was very limited evidence of this goal being met. Access to mental health services 24 hours a day, seven days a week has not been achieved nationally.

- The NHS Plan sought to develop teams to provide community interventions therefore reducing the demand for inpatient beds. The three areas where these teams were developed were assertive outreach, crisis resolution and early intervention. Yet in 2004 these teams were not available in sufficient numbers across the country or with enough staff to constitute a nationwide service; most areas reported the service was not adequate to meet local need.

- There were increases in the numbers of secure and psychiatric intensive care beds and an emphasis on improving the environment on mental health inpatient units generally. Acute forums for service users have been established everywhere and acute admissions were reducing.

- The suicide rate is now at its lowest recorded figure with the suicide rate among younger males reduced for the first time since the 1970s (DH 2006b).

While a number of the targets were not achieved by 2004, this does not mean the NSF for Mental Health has not been a success. Positive outcomes have included the development of a more cohesive and planned mental health service on a national basis; improved communication and liaison between primary and secondary services (DH 2004); access to mental health services in many areas for people with mental health problems in primary care who would not otherwise have received access; and new and highly innovative practice and innovations in primary care mental health (Baguley et al. 2007).

Applying Theory to Practice Box 13.13

NSF for Mental Health – Standards

Standard 1: Health and social services should promote mental health and work with individuals and the community, combat discrimination against mental health problems and promote social inclusion.

Standard 2: Service users contacting their primary healthcare team with a mental health problem which is regarded as commonly occurring in the population should receive an assessment, their mental health need(s) should be identified and they should be offered appropriate further assessment, treatment and care, or if necessary referral to specialist services.

Standard 3: Any person with a mental health problem which is regarded as commonly occurring in the population should have access to services suitable to meet their mental health needs 24 hours a day, seven days a week and NHS Direct ought to be available for first-level advice and referral to specialist help-lines or local services.

Standard 4: All mental health service users registered on the Care Programme Approach (CPA) should receive care which engages them to the optimum, and strives to reduce risk or crisis; should receive a copy of a written care plan which states the action(s) to be taken by the service user, their carer and the care coordinator in the event of a crisis and advising the GP on how to respond. The care plan should be regularly reviewed by the appointed care coordinator; and the service user ought to have access to services which are available 24 hours a day, 365 days a year.

Standard 5: Every service user who is assessed as requiring a period of care which involves them being away from their home should have access to a suitable hospital or alternative bed or place as close to their home as possible, and in the least restrictive environment to protect both the service user and the public. On their discharge, they should receive a written copy of an agreed care plan identifying the care and rehabilitation which are to be provided, the care coordinator, and the action(s) to be taken in a crisis.

Standard 6: Individuals who provide regular and significant levels of care for a person on CPA ought to receive an annual assessment of their caring and physical and mental health needs and a copy of their own written care plan which is carried out in discussion with them.

Standard 7: Local health and social care communities should prevent suicides by promoting mental health among individuals and communities (cross-referenced with Standard 1); provide effective primary mental healthcare (cross-referenced with Standard 2); ensure people with mental health problems are able to access local services through primary care team, helplines or ED (cross-referenced with Standard 3); ensure people with a severe and enduring mental illness are provided with a care plan which is specific to their needs and provides access to services 24 hours a day, 365 days a year (cross-referenced with Standard 4); provide safe hospital facilities for service users requiring inpatient admission (cross-referenced with Standard 5); facilitate the carers of people with severe mental health problems to access support to allow them to continue in the caring role (cross-referenced with Standard 6). Also to support prison staff in preventing the suicide of prisoners; ensuring staff are competent in assessing the risk of suicide and that adequate audit systems are in place to learn and implement necessary changes.

(DH 1999c)

Conclusion

Regardless of whichever setting adult nurses specialise in, mental illness will be encountered within their clinical practice. You have now gained insight into some of the many causes of mental illness and numerous clinical manifestations. You have gained insight into how governments, scientific breakthroughs and public opinion influence healthcare. The role of the nurse is pivotal in promoting positive, patient-centred care and is crucial in advocating for our patients and in supporting their recovery and optimum capacity for health.

Further reading

Boardman, J. & Parsonage, M. (2007) *Delivering the Government's Mental Health Policies: Services, Staffing and Costs.* Sainsbury Centre for Mental Health: London.

Coppock, V. & Hopton, J. (2000) *Critical Perspectives on Mental Health.* Routledge: London.

Department of Health (2004) *National Service Framework for Mental Health – Five Years On.* DH: London.

Department of Health (2006) *Action on Stigma, Promoting Mental Health, Ending Discrimination at Work.* DH: London.

Her Majesty's Government (2005) *The Mental Capacity Act.* Queen's Printer of Acts of Parliament: London.

National Institute for Clinical Excellence (NICE) (2003) *Depression: The Management of Depression in Primary and Secondary Care.* Second Consultation. NICE: London.

NIMHE (2003) *Fast Forwarding Primary Care Mental Health: Gateway Workers.* DH: London.

Norman, I. & Ryrie, I. (2004) Mental health nursing: origins and orientations. In Norman, I. & Ryrie, I. (eds) *The Art and Science of Mental Health Nursing: A Textbook of Principles and Practice.* Open University Press: Maidenhead, pp. 66–99.

Proudfoot, J., Goldberg, D., Mann, A., Everitt, B., Marks, I. & Gray, J. (2003) Computerised, interactive, multimedia cognitive-behavioural program for anxiety and depression in general practice. *Psychological Medicine* 33: 217–27.

Richards, D., Richards, A., Barkham, M., Williams, C. & Cahill, J. (2002) PHASE: a 'health technology' approach to psychological treatment in primary mental healthcare. *Primary Healthcare Research and Development* 3: 159–68.

World Health Organization (1999). *The World Health Report.* WHO: Geneva.

References

American Psychiatric Association (APA) (1994) *Practice Guideline for the Treatment of Patients with Major Depressive Disorder,* 2nd edn. APA http://www.psych.org/psych_pract/treatg/pg/MDD2e_05-15-06.pdf

Baguley, C., Duggan, A., Fisher, D., et al. (2007) *The Graduate Primary Care Mental Health Worker Programme: A View from Higher Education Training Providers.* Higher Education Academy: York.

BBC (2006) Mental health peril not spotted. BBC News, 4 December 2006. http://news.bbc.co.uk/1/hi/health/620356.stm.

http://news.bbc.co.uk/1/hi/health/620356.stm (accessed 16 February 2007).

Coppock, V. & Hopton, J. (2000) *Critical Perspectives on Mental Health.* Routledge: London.

Department of Health (1998) *Modernising Mental Health Services: Safe, Sound and Supportive.* Health Service Circular: Local Authority Circular (HSC 1998/233: LAC (98) 25 DH: London.

Department of Health (1999a) *Saving Lives: Our Healthier Nation.* DH: London.

Department of Health (1999b) *The NHS Plan: A Plan for Investment: A Plan for Reform.* DH: London.

Department of Health (1999c) *National Service Framework for Mental Health.* DH: London.

Department of Health (2001a) *National Service Framework for Children, Young People and Maternity Services: Change for Children – Every Child Matters.* DH/DfES: London.

Department of Health (2001b) *National Service Framework for Older People.* DH: London.

Department of Health (2004) *National Service Framework for Mental Health – Five Years On.* DH: London.

Department of Health (2006a) *Mental Health Bill 2006: Summary Guide.* London: DH.

Department of Health (2006b) *Action on Stigma, Promoting Mental Health, Ending Discrimination at Work.* DH: London.

Department of Health & Welsh Office (1999) *Code of Practice: Mental Health Act 1983.* HMSO: London.

Foucault, M. (1967) *Madness and Civilization: A History of Insanity in the Age of Reason.* Trans. by R. Howard. Routledge: London.

Goffman, E. (1961) *Asylums: Essays on the Social Situation of Mental Patients and Other Inmates.* Anchor/Doubleday: New York.

Griffiths, R. (1988) *Community Care: An Agenda for Action.* HMSO: London.

Hart, D.A. (2004) Common mental health problems. In Kirby, S.D., Hart, D.A., Cross, D. & Mitchell, G. (eds) *Mental Health Nursing: Competencies for Practice.* Palgrave Macmillan: Basingstoke, pp. 79–94.

House of Commons (2007) 2nd Reading House of Commons, 16 April 2007 Mental Health Bill (Lords) http://www.bps.org.uk/downloadfile.cfm?file_uuid=0010EA19-1143-DFD0-7E10-B1DECC88748B&ext=pdf (accessed 15/11/07]

Jones, K. (1993) *Asylums and After: A Revised History of the Mental Health Services from the Early 18th Century to the 1990s.* Athlone Press: London.

King's Fund (2007) *Briefing: Supervised Community Treatment.* King's Fund: London.

Kisley, S. & Goldberg, D. (1996) Physical and psychiatric comorbidity in general practice. *British Journal of Psychiatry* 169: 236–42.

Laing, R.D. (1959) *The Divided Self: An Existential Study in Sanity and Madness.* Penguin: London.

Mitchell, G. (2004) Legal and professional issues in mental health nursing practice. In Kirby, S.D., Hart, D.A., Cross, D. & Mitchell, G. (eds) *Mental Health Nursing: Competencies for Practice.* Palgrave Macmillan: Basingstoke, pp. 357–70.

NHS Direct (2007c) *Eating Disorders: Introduction.* http://www.nhsdirect.nhs.uk/articles/article.aspx?articleId=651 (accessed 15 March 2007).

National Institute for Clinical Excellence (NICE) (2002) *Computerised Cognitive Behaviour Therapy for Depression and Anxiety.* NHS R & D HTA Programme. NICE: London.

National Institute for Clinical Excellence (NICE) (2003) *Depression: Management of Depression in Primary and Secondary Care.* Second Consultation. NICE: London.

National Institute for Clinical Excellence (NICE) (2004a) *Depression: management of Depression in Primary and Secondary Care.* Clinical Guidelines. NICE: London.

National Institute for Clinical Excellence (NICE) (2004b) *Anxiety: Management of Anxiety (Panic Disorder, with or without Agoraphobia, and Generalised Anxiety Disorder) in Adults in Primary, Secondary and Community Care.* Clinical Guidelines. NICE: London.

NHS Direct (2007a) *Schizophrenia: Introduction. htttp://www.nhsdirect.nhs.uk/articles/article.aspx?articleId=329§ionId=29735 (accessed 15 March 2007).*

NHS Direct (2007b) *Self Injury: Introduction.* http://www.nhsdirect.nhs.uk/articles/article.aspx?articleId=454 (accessed 15 March 2007).

NIMHE North West Development Centre (2004) *Enhanced Services Specification for Depression under the New GP Contract.* National Primary Care Research and Development Centre & University of York in partnership with North West Development Centre of NIMHE: York.

Nursing and Midwifery Council (NMC) (2004) *The NMC Code of Professional Conduct: Standards for Conduct, Performance and Ethics.* NMC: London.

O'Brien, M., Singleton, N., Sparks, J., Meltzer, H. & Brugha, T. (2002) *Adults with a Psychotic Disorder Living in Private Households: 2000.* TSO: London.

Sayce, L. (2000) *From Psychiatric Patient to Citizen: Overcoming Discrimination and Social Exclusion.* Macmillan: Basingstoke.

SCMH (1998) *Keys to Engagement: Review of Care for People with Severe Mental Illness Who Are Hard to Engage with Services.* SCMH: London.

Singleton, N., Bumpstead, R., O'Brien, M., Lee, A. & Meltzer, H. (2001) *Psychiatric Morbidity among Adults Living in Private Households: 2000.* TSO: London.

Social Exclusion Unit (2004) *Mental Health and Social Exclusion.* Office of the Deputy Prime Minister: London.

Szasz, T.S. (1961) *The Myth of Mental Illness: Foundations of a Theory of Personal Conduct.* Dell: New York.

University of Manchester (2006) *Five Year Report of the National Confidential Inquiry into Suicide and Homicide by People with Mental Illness: Avoidable Deaths.* University of Manchester Press: Manchester.

Misconceptions and the reality of learning disabilities

Alex McClimens

Chapter 14 Learning Objectives

- To appreciate the socially constructed nature of learning disability
- To understand the historical precedents that inform current thinking
- To be aware of the wide variety of causal events, processes and circumstances that can impact on these individuals
- To learn about some of the more common syndromes and associated conditions
- To be able to distinguish between the label and the living person when they present in a clinical situation
- To see the true value of definitions when set against lived reality
- To question the representation of learning disability in popular culture
- To challenge the ethics that operate around learning disability in health and social care settings
- To understand that communication is a skill that needs to be practised

Introduction

People labelled with learning disability suffer a disproportionately higher level of ill health compared to the rest of the population; they are also more likely to die younger (DH 2001). Respiratory disease is the highest cause of death; other conditions such as epilepsy, obesity, diabetes, endocrine disorders, mental health problems, sensory impairments and gastrointestinal cancers are also prevalent (DRC 2006; NHS Scotland 2004).

From this it should be clear that healthcare professionals would be in frequent and regular contact with individuals from this particular social grouping over the course of their professional careers. Caring for someone identified as having a learning disability requires as much care and attention as a patient with a physical illness, while taking into account some discussion on causes, conditions, cultural influences, medical strategies, health economics, clinical interventions and social responses to impairment issues. It is also a matter of legislation and policy initiatives.

This chapter will be presented in six sections. The first will deal with some philosophical and theoretical issues that are fundamental to an understanding of the concept of learning disability. The rationale for this is that it can be useful to reach such an understanding before going on to care for individuals who have to live with the label. The second section will incorporate the distinction between disability and impairment and introduce what is known as the **social model of disability**. The third section will deal with the epidemiology of learning disability with reference to some basic facts and figures. The fourth section will consider the broader historical, social and cultural implications that have led to our present appreciation of what constitutes learning disability, including some discussion on disability ethics. The fifth section examines in detail two of the better-known exemplars of learning disability with emphasis on the healthcare implications for the clinician. The chapter ends with a brief discussion on recent policy initiatives of relevance to the healthcare of this patient group.

Philosophical and theoretical issues

Below is an account of what happened when a patient, J., had to go into hospital for a routine procedure:

> It said I had a learning disability on the case notes. They [the nurses] talk down to you. They explained it [the procedure] to my carer, not to me. I felt upset and kept it all bottled up.

J. is a grown woman who can articulate perfectly well but the people who were supposed to be looking after her could not see past the label and ended up treating her badly. Her colleague K. initially had the same kind of experience but he found a way to change things. He could

not understand what the consultant was saying when he was in hospital for investigations. But when he asked for an explanation in simple language the consultant was very helpful. He stopped talking in what K. calls 'medical jargon' and drew a diagram. K. was much better informed regarding his care. It is important to remember that patients with 'learning disabilities' are not stupid, they have a 'learning disability'. When communicating with someone who is identified as having a 'learning disability', remember, it is the person who is sick, not his or her label. Try talking to them first. It will not always work but some common courtesies can go a long way towards a more comfortable encounter with healthcare.

We need now to briefly mention something called **social constructionism**. This philosophy challenges preconceived notions about how the world is understood by asking us to think about the way we all invent our own version of reality. Most of the time this is shared unproblematically but now and again, as in the case of 'learning disability', the understanding that emerges is skewed. Why do you think this might be? Look at Exercise 14.1 and see if that helps your understanding.

Applying Theory to Practice: Exercise 14.1

When were teenagers invented? This may appear ridiculous but think about it for a minute ... when? One answer might be that they came into being around twelve years after our species learned to walk upright. Another way of looking at it would be to consider the social forces that have organised an age group into a collective noun. Try the same argument with the words 'nursing' or 'nurses'. Now repeat the process with 'learning disability'. And when you think you might have answered the 'when' question; try this: why?

Some would suggest that there is no such thing as 'learning disability', but what about people who have 'learning disabilities'? An example could be patients you have cared for who have Down syndrome or cerebral palsy. Some believe that these people have impairments and that is not quite the same as disability. This distinction is important, especially to anyone who is serious about a career in health and social care.

Applying Theory to Practice: Exercise 14.2

List the different definitions of an impairment and a disability.

Impairments and Learning Disabilities	
Disability	Impairment

In the left-hand column of Exercise 14.2 list a few examples of what you think counts as a disability. Now do the same for the impairment column. Not as easy as it looks, is it? Where do you put dyslexia, for example?

Think about it this way. Do YOU have any impairments? Do you, for example, wear glasses? People wear prescription glasses, or contact lenses, because of a defect or impairment to their vision. This is corrected by wearing lenses. Some people have a condition called asthma. It can be very serious or merely inconvenient. Medication is available to alleviate the condition. Asthma need not prevent anyone from living a 'normal life' although it may stop you running for the bus.

The list goes on. So, what other conditions would you add to the list of what we are now going to call 'impairments'? Jot a few more down and see if there might be any linking themes. You should find that common elements here are clustered around function, use, 'normal' and physical ability. The point to grasp is that impairment can be amenable to some form of intervention (therapy, medication, equipment) that corrects the impairment, or reduces its effects and so brings the functioning of that person closer to the established norm (e.g. 20/20 or 1.0 visual acuity, full range of movement).

The social model of disability: architecture and attitudes

A lot of talk about disability is really about impairment; impairment can be treated, but what of 'learning disability'? Think of precisely *where* you find it. For the person who needs a wheelchair to assist their mobility due to athetoid cerebral palsy occurring as a result of severe

brain damage at birth, is their 'learning disability' then in their legs?

No, there's only one place you'll ever find any variety of 'disability' and that's in someone's head. And it is not usually in the head of the person living with the label.

Disability is a concept or social construction which provokes an 'attitude', or way of behaving in those who are confronted by persons assumed to have a 'disability'. This attitude is most frequently expressed in language (e.g. he's got a 'learning disability', she's a wheelchair case, they're cripples, idiots, spastics) or by access points in the built environment.

Think of the person using a wheelchair. They can get around unimpaired until they come across a steep kerb, a flight of stairs, a selfishly parked car, some forms of public transport or any other arrangement of physical objects that defeats their immediate social purpose of getting from A to B. Disability, where it exists, is a direct result of the social organisation of contemporary life which pays insufficient heed to the immediate aspirations of those who live with a variety of impairments. Such people are effectively disenfranchised from full and active engagement with their local cultures when structural responses operate to impede their physical, social and intellectual progress.

Attitudes to limited intellectual capacity also limit social activity and generally reduce life-enhancing opportunities for inclusion and participation within anticipated norms and roles.

Some people have said that under such conditions the concept of disability is more than merely descriptive but actually presents an example of socially oppressive practices, which harm human rights.

The origins of this argument come from the Union of the Physically Impaired Against Segregation. They issued a manifesto *Fundamental Principles of Disability* in 1976 (http://www.leeds.ac.uk/disability-studies/archiveuk/UPIAS/). The world has changed since then. The division between the social and the biological is not quite so clear. This will be discussed later when we talk about phenylketonuria (PKU). People are certainly disabled by society, but they are equally disabled by their own bodies. A new version of the social model of disability needs to address this. The situation is currently vacant. But whatever definition of disability you favour, you will always find that architecture and attitudes are implicated somewhere.

Applying Theory to Practice: Exercise 14.3

You have a visitor from Mars staying with you for the summer.

■ How do you explain the term 'learning disability' to them?

Basic facts and figures

Definitions are easy to find; understanding, though, is harder to come by. Learning disability is characterised by three main components:

■ Intelligence (as defined by measurement arrived at via an I.Q. test)
■ Adaptive behaviour (as assessed by psychologists)
■ Developmental aspect (understood within a medical/biological framework), which recognises that onset should occur during childhood or certainly before eighteen years.

This is an extract from the DSM-IV, the *Diagnostic and Statistical Manual of Mental Disorders* (APA 2000). ICD-10 (The International Classification of Diseases) and the AAMR (American Association on Mental Retardation). Both use the same three main criteria for classification, as does *Valuing People* (DH 2001), which adds the proviso that a low IQ in itself is insufficient to categorise people (2001: 14).

As outlined, there are three ways to decide whether someone has a learning disability or not. But are they any good? Measuring intelligence is a highly contentious. It is generally accepted that the Wechsler scale (1998) provides a reliable tool. Clinical psychologists, to classify individuals referred to them for assessment, use this widely. As suggested earlier, the IQ on its own is not sufficient to make a judgement. Another scale is used to assess adaptive behaviour. Here a popular tool is the Vineland scale. If you have the opportunity to talk to a clinical psychologist, ask them how they feel about the process; see the viewpoint of one in Box 14.1.

The third diagnostic criterion is that onset should be before age 18 and relates to maturity of the brain and 'normal' development. The main impact here is administrative and determines whether an individual is cared for

Questioning Clinical Practice: Box 14.1

Intelligence Testing and IQ (Intelligence Quotient)

Intelligence testing and IQ (Intelligence Quotient) form one of the three criteria for being diagnosed as having a learning disability. The tests with the longest history in this area are the Wechsler Intelligence Scales. The first version was developed in 1939 as the Wechsler-Bellevue Intelligence Scale. The most recent version is the Wechsler Adult Intelligence Scale, third edition (WAIS-III) (Wechsler et al. 1998). The WAIS-III has 13 subtests, each assessing a different aspect of cognitive, e.g. spatial, ability, working memory, understanding of vocabulary. The average IQ score is 100. People with learning disabilities will score at least two standard deviations below the average score of their peer group (IQ below 70).

The WAIS-III can be of great use to psychologists. It can, usually in combination with other tests, identify a person's strengths and difficulties allowing interventions to be planned that can help that person achieve their aims. This is not done by looking at the overall IQ score but by comparing scores from different parts of the test (Crawford 2004) and by gaining qualitative information from the way the person completes the subtests.

Sadly, intelligence test scores have had a long history of being misused, not to understand people's abilities better but simply to make judgements about whether people should be excluded from or included in services. For example, a common misuse of an IQ score is the assumption that it predicts people's ability to parent (Tymchuk & Andron 1990).

In the USA the use of IQ scores has been used as a cut-off for claiming social security. This has been criticised by Folstein (1989) who cites the cases of people with Huntington's disease who because of the disease cannot work, but due to their potentially normal IQ cannot claim benefits either. IQ testing and therefore the WAIS have become tainted because of such examples.

If we have one message about the WAIS-III, it would be to alert people to its misuse. If anyone tries to tell you that they can understand a person just by looking at their IQ score, then do not believe them.

Suzie Beart & Zara Clarke

in child, transition or adult services. That is why a child with brain damage due to encephalitis, for example, gets the diagnosis of learning disability whereas an adult would be labelled with acquired brain injury.

By whatever means you categorise, classify or label people there are roughly one and a half million individuals in England who are currently described as living with some degree of learning disability. The figures provided by the Department of Health divide the population further into people with severe and profound learning disabilities, whom they estimate at just over 200,000, and those with what they term mild to moderate learning disabilities, numbering approximately 1.2 million. This gives an overall prevalence rate of around 25 per 1000 (DH 2001: 6.1).

Applying Theory to Practice: Exercise 14.4

The previous figures reveal that approximately 1.5% of the population experience a learning disability.

- How do you think these people are spread across the country?
- Would you expect to find a higher level of learning disability in cities or in rural areas?
- In economically deprived areas or affluent parts of the country?
- And what factors, if any, might influence this? What do you think?

Lies and damned lies

The word 'approximately' has been used a lot when quoting figures. That is because there are real problems here in estimating numbers, even for experts. For example, if you consider the developmental aspect of identifying learning disability in a young child, then it is clear that some cases will not become apparent perhaps for several years as the child grows and develops. Hence, all the figures you will ever read will be approximations or estimates. This is because there are no reliable official statistics concerning the number of people with learning disabilities in the UK (Emerson et al. 2001). This anomaly contributes to the difficulties of planning services, recruitment and education across a whole range of disciplines. Epidemiology, which is what we have just been discussing, is not confined to learning disability studies. It is the study of the occurrence of disease processes (and related conditions/syndromes) and as such is a very broad topic. There are some related terms you will also need to understand; they appear in Box 14.2.

Applying Theory to Practice: Box 14.2

Prevalence: the number of cases, old and new of a disease/syndrome/condition existing within a population at any given time

Incidence: the number of new cases of a disease/syndrome/condition occurring within a population over a fixed timescale

Aetiology: the study of the causes of diseases/conditions/syndromes

Causes and conditions

In combination with statistical material, the causes and conditions of learning disability must also be considered. You might think that identifying causes would be a straightforward process; this quotation from Emerson at el. (2001) suggests otherwise:

> It is now known that biological, environmental and social factors are all involved in causing learning disabilities. It used to be thought that severe learning disabilities were caused by biological factors and that mild learning disabilities were caused by social and environmental factors. Most experts, however, now believe that the picture is not quite as clear-cut as this.

A simple framework of causes can nevertheless be seen by looking at the timing of the event that results in the diagnosis of learning disability being made. This applies particularly to 'biological' causes. Social and environmental factors are harder to pinpoint. Hence there are three key times to consider: preconceptual, perinatal and postnatal.

In the case of preconceptual diagnoses, causes are heredity (parental genetics leading to diagnosis of, e.g., fragile-X syndrome) or congenital (leading to diagnosis of, e.g. Down syndrome). Also at this stage the immediate social conditions (drug misuse, extreme poverty) or the more global environment (radiation, pollution) may also damage the mother's womb resulting in brain damage in the fetus. Fetal alcohol syndrome, despite longstanding medical evidence, has only recently been acknowledged as an increasingly significant contributory factor associated with learning disability (Sreissguth 1997). At the perinatal stage a typical example is cerebral palsy (CP) caused by poor oxygenation. It should be noted that not all individuals born with CP necessarily develop any learning disability since this is determined by the extent and severity of the brain damage. Postnatal causes include infection (e.g. rubella), direct trauma (e.g. head injury) and a mix of social and/or environmental conditions. For example, being born and brought up in a war zone, or having a socially deprived childhood, may result in severe developmental problems in later life.

However, in each scenario there always remains the possibility that the specific nature of the learning disability will remain unknown, which is to say that none of the circumstances identified can be implicated sufficiently to attribute cause. It is here that the psychological impact of socio-economic factors (family circumstances, parenting skills, immediate local conditions, nutrition) could influence cognitive development (Dallison & Lobstein 1995). Yet even after taking all of this into account., some instances will remain in the category of 'unknown'.

This chapter has identified how social/environmental causes and biological factors are implicated in learning disability and has discussed them as if they were entirely separate, but it is more complex than that. To illustrate this, an example from Rothman (2002) will be used. Rothman uses phenylketonuria (PKU) to show how there

is never a case for saying that any cause is 100% environmental/social or biological.

With a prevalence of 1 in 10,000, PKU is a very rare autosomal recessive gene disorder. This means that BOTH parents need to carry the same altered gene, resulting in a 1 in 4 risk of having a child affected by the condition. The heel pinprick test performed on all newborns is for phenylalanine. Phenylalanine is an essential amino acid: essential because it cannot be synthesised from artificial sources. The amounts of these amino acids in the blood are crucial to well-being and too much phenylalanine leads to PKU. This is because during digestion phenylalanine is broken down to tyrosine (another amino acid); this does not occur in the person with PKU and it is the accumulation in the blood that causes brain damage. If left undiagnosed, the metabolic changes can lead to brain damage and result in progressive learning disability and possibly epilepsy. The effects of PKU, when diagnosed, can be readily controlled by diet. The cause of PKU then may be genetic in origin but it is entirely environmental/social in its prevention and treatment.

Culture and society

At somewhere around 1.5% of the population, it is perhaps not such a surprise to find that people labelled with 'learning disability' do not feature prominently in the media, popular culture or the entertainment industry. After all, how many of you readers have direct social, rather than professional acquaintance of someone who has a learning disability? Statistically at least the chances are slim. Because of this, much of our attitude towards all manner of disability comes second hand from our exposure to portrayals in the media in general and from our viewing habits in particular.

Soap operas, for example, are a useful barometer of socio-cultural awareness. They deal with controversial and topical social issues and generally reflect an approximation of the *Zeitgeist*. But if we consider the profile of other minority groupings, and taking age and gender into account, we see that they generally get fair representation on screen, in statistical terms at least.

When you filter out physical impairment from the equation, the presence of people with learning disabilities is significantly reduced. Paula Sage and Cara Readle are two examples. Paula has Down syndrome and Cara has cerebral palsy. Paula starred in the 2004 movie *Afterlife* and has since gone on to feature in the Scottish soap

Questioning Clinical Practice: Exercise 14.5

Attitudes Towards Disability

■ How many people with a learning disability do you routinely see on the television? Not many? Why is that?

Identify some of the reasons you can think of and add these to your portfolio.

opera *River City*. Cara is a regular in the children's show *Tracey Beaker* where she plays the character Layla. These two may be exceptional in terms of their acting talent but it is unlikely that they will graduate to presenting the news or the weather where the preference for 'hair and teeth' presenters is so entrenched. Nor are they likely to feature on *Countdown* or *15 to 1* while the quiz show template demands fast minds and faster fingers. So while disability is not necessarily a barrier to a screen career, it nevertheless limits the horizons of the actor with a disability to a severely limited range of opportunities in the light entertainment industry.

It is not just in the visual media where learning disability is ignored. When did you last read a book where the central character has a learning disability? You can go back to the classics for caricature and demonisation. Just have a look at Dickens or Shakespeare who both populated their stories with entertaining monsters. But where in contemporary popular fiction will you find a sympathetic modern-day portrait? For one possible answer read *The Incredible Adam Spark* by Alan Bissett (2005). This should be on every reading list that attempts to deal with disability issues in contemporary society.

History, ethics, eugenics and euthanasia

None of us is free of the past; how we live today is shaped by history. This is particularly true for people labelled with learning disability. In this section some short history lessons will be used to set out some of the conditions that have influenced the way our society shapes and responds to the concept of learning disability and to the people who live with the label. The medical and nursing professions are two of the major institutions to have played a role here, and in the second part of the section this will be

illustrated with reference to two common conditions and how they continue to influence attitudes to care and treatment.

The Abortion Act, which came into effect in April 1967, was a true social landmark. Its repercussions are with us still, particularly in light of the changes brought about by the 1991 Human Fertilisation and Embryology Act. Not only did this more recent piece of legislation lower the upper limit for abortion to 24 weeks, it also overruled the fetal viability clause and now permits abortion for fetal handicap right up until birth, that is *any fetus* where some impairment or abnormality is detected can legally be terminated at any point up to term even if it is deemed capable of being born alive. Tom Shakespeare's (1998) view on this was: 'Current abortion law discriminates against the impaired fetus ... The law should not discriminate between impaired and non-impaired fetuses: a common time limit should be adopted for all pregnancies.'

This debate gets to the very core of **euthanasia, eugenics** and **disability ethics**. The implicit assumption appears to be that some lives are inherently worth more than others, with the implication that a life lived with some degree of impairment will automatically be of less value. If you want to fast-forward this line of thought then it is not long before you get to a situation where a clinician may have to make a decision on allocating treatment resources. The Nuffield Council on Bioethics, for example, produced a report in 2006 which recommended that doctors do not intervene with babies born prior to 22 weeks. What are your views on this? Tough questions need to be asked and answered. For example, within a limited healthcare budget, who should get that very expensive heart operation?

One response to this comes in the shape of **QALYs and DALYs** (Jelsma et al. 2002). The argument is very persuasive if you can stick to the figures and ignore the human factor. You may want to discuss this with your colleagues during the next coffee break: but be warned, these issues can cause much distress. Under some healthcare economic calculations, for example, it is theoretically possible to be better off dead, literally. So far no one has been able to produce any empirical evidence to support this claim.

Down syndrome and cerebral palsy

This chapter will now examine in detail two conditions associated with learning disability: cerebral palsy (CP) and Down syndrome (DS). These conditions were chosen for several reasons:

- They are among the most common conditions associated with learning disability and will therefore already be 'known' to some degree by students and practitioners
- Both have very many health-related implications for the individual and are therefore of professional interest to the clinician
- Both were 'discovered' at approximately the same time with implications for our present cultural understanding
- Both have subsequently been 're-branded' for modern times with different labels now being applied to the individuals who live with the condition(s)
- Both are conditions in which the person 'looks different' with implications for how we as individuals respond to their presence within wider society
- Both highlight the divide between 'impairment' and 'disability'
- DS introduces genetics, screening and selective abortion.

In London during the 1860s two medical discoveries were made which were to have a significant impact on how we understand learning disability. John Langdon Haydon Down (1828–1896) and William Little (1810–1894) were close contemporaries. Neither man was able at that

Questioning Clinical Practice: Exercise 14.6

Ethics Decision Making

You have three candidates for cosmetic surgery but you can treat only one. Who is it going to be?

- Candidate A: 19-year-old man who wants cosmetic surgery to remove a disfiguring facial birthmark
- Candidate B: 19-year-old woman who wants breast augmentation to advance a modelling career
- Candidate C: 19-year-old person with mosaic variety Down syndrome who just wants to look 'normal'

time to correctly identify what science would later confirm. Even so, both had, through their clinical observations, begun a process of medical inquiry that would eventually establish trisomy 21 and cerebral palsy as diagnostic conditions amenable to care and treatment.

Currently, in the early 21st century, understanding of both conditions has undergone some revision. Those individuals who live with the conditions have had some battles to fight over naming rights. The scientific tradition of the nineteenth century demanded that names were attached to conditions and as such 'Little's disease' was the popular name for the variety of cerebral palsy that Little documented. Similarly Down's name became attached to the syndrome he is credited with discovering. And yet this was a much more gradual process. The original label conferred by Down was 'mongolian idiocy'. The way that individuals labelled with Down syndrome and cerebral palsy have been reinvented since the original 'naming' has gone through several revisions. Significant changes in public attitude, for example, have reshaped perceptions, just as policy and practice have altered to accommodate changes in public understanding.

Questioning Clinical Practice: Exercise 14.7

Modern Correctness

Many readers may be familiar with the name Scope from their high street shopping. Scope is the name of the charity that represents individuals labelled with cerebral palsy. Originally collectively formed by parents as The National Spastic Society in 1952, an extraordinary AGM in 1994 voted to change the name to Scope.

- Why do you think they did this?
- Why is mongolian idiocy now referred to as trisomy 21 or Down syndrome?

Down syndrome

Today Down syndrome is just one of many conditions detectable by routine prenatal screening. It is also the most common genetic cause associated with learning disability. It results from the failure of chromosome 21 to segregate normally during cell division (meiosis). This disruption produces the 'extra' chromosome; hence the scientifically accurate name for the condition is trisomy

21. The extra chromosome may be present in all or only some of the cells in the body. The risk of Down syndrome varies with maternal age from 1:1500 at age 20, 1:800 aged 30; 1:270 at 35; 1:100 at 40 to more than 1:50 at >45. Two main avenues can detect its presence: serum and ultrasound.

For serum screening a blood sample is tested for a combination of proteins and hormones. During the first trimester the combination is free beta-hCG and placenta associated plasma protein A (PAPP-A). During the second trimester the combination is more likely to be alphafetoprotein (AFP) and free beta-human chorionic gonadotrophin (beta-hCG).

An early ultrasound scan can be used to measure the thickness of fluid at the nape of the fetal neck; the nuchal translucency. An increased amount of fluid may indicate that the fetus has Down syndrome or some chromosomal abnormality. As a result the number of terminated pregnancies with Down syndrome has increased, and the prevalence of Down syndrome births has decreased from 1 in 700 to about 1 in 1000 (Roizen & Patterson 2003).

Questioning Clinical Practice: Exercise 14.8

Questioning Your Beliefs

Suppose you and your partner discover after screening that your unborn child has a high risk of being born with Down syndrome. You will automatically be offered the chance to terminate the pregnancy.

- What would you do?

There are three distinct varieties (technically genotypes) of Down syndrome:

- Mosaic 1–2%
- Translocation 4–5%
- Trisomy 21 95%.

Refer to Figure 14.1 for a graphic illustration.

These are only detectable under a microscope and not during a social encounter. All individuals, no matter what chromosomal variety they live with, share the physical characteristics to some extent. The standard variety of trisomy 21 is far more common and this is the classic

Figure 14.1 Down syndrome genotypes

presentation. The individual will have short stature, upward slanting eyes, lowered muscle tone, a small mouth (giving the appearance of a large tongue), a single crease across the palm of the hand, a significant gap between the large and second toes and fine dark hair. Some degree of learning disability will always be present.

The translocation or Robertsonian variety occurs rarely. The mechanics of this means that the extra 21st chromosome replaces some of the 14th chromosome. This very rare mosaic variety means that not all cells are affected by trisomy 21. In these cases the degree of learning disability may be much reduced and the appearance of the individual less affected.

Cerebral palsy

In a series of nine lectures delivered at the Royal Orthopaedic Hospital, William Little described the distorted postures and rigid muscle tone of some newborns on his caseload. He also noted that the condition was undocumented in medical science. By 1861, after studying the disorder for 20 years, he had tabulated over 200 cases. In a thesis before the Obstetrical Society of London he proposed that the causes of this previously overlooked disorder included asphyxia at birth, premature birth and direct mechanical injury.

The derivation of the term 'cerebral palsy' is cerebral = concerning the brain, and palsy = paralysis. This is not a single particular disease or illness. The term covers a range of physical conditions which affect movement as a result of an injury to the brain. The main clinical points to note are:

● The incidence of cerebral palsy is approximately 3 per 1000 births
● It is non-progressive (the condition remains stable throughout the life course)
● Babies born pre-term have a slightly higher incidence
● In the majority of cases the damage occurs before or during birth
● The most common cause is cerebral hypoxia (reduced oxygen supply to the brain)
● Most, but not all, affected individuals will have a degree of learning disability.

Cerebral palsy can be defined as:

the commonly used name for a group of conditions characterised by motor dysfunction due to non-progressive brain damage early in life ... The range of severity may be from total dependency and immobility to abilities of talking, independent self-care and walking, running and other skills, although with some clumsy actions (Levitt 2004).

Mobility is a big issue, and the input of physiotherapists and occupational therapists should not be underestimated as they form the core of any treatment regime.

The classification of CP can be addressed in two main ways: by affected limb(s) or by the origin of the brain damage. See Figure 14.2.

By limb the classification is as follows:

● **Tetraplegia/quadriplegia**: all four limbs equally affected
● **Diplegia**: either arms or legs are affected
● **Hemiplegia**: the arm and leg on one side of the body are affected.

By origin within the brain the taxonomy is as follows:

● **Spastic cerebral palsy** (spasticity): caused by impairment in the cerebral cortex (the outer layer) of the brain. This leads to disordered control of movement and accounts for approximately 60% of all cases.
● **Athetoid cerebral palsy** (athetosis): caused by impairment in the basal ganglia area of the brain. This causes involuntary spasms with jerky arm and leg

Figure 14.2 Cerebral palsy classification

Questioning Clinical Practice: Exercise 14.9

Questioning Beliefs and Attitudes

- Is it acceptable to make fun of people with impairments and disabilities or are some subjects taboo?
- Can comedy reduce barriers or does it draw attention to the obvious differences between people?
- If your football team, race, nation, religion or hair colour becomes the butt of jokes, what does this do for your social standing? And how should you respond?

Q: What did the guy with trisomy 21 say to his dog?
A: Down, syndrome!

- Was that funny?

Questioning your beliefs and the beliefs of those around you provides valuable insight into the 'hows' and 'whys' in modern society.

movements and accounts for approximately 20% of all cases.

- **Ataxic cerebral palsy** (ataxia): caused by impairment in the cerebellum. This causes a lack of balance and spatial awareness leading to severely affected walking/gait. This accounts for approximately 10% of all cases.
- **Mixed**: many people have a permutation of the above types.

From this it will be obvious that people with cerebral palsy will also have to live with a variety of extra impairments that are associated with the condition. The problems they experience in using and controlling muscles cause mobility problems and difficulty with all activities of daily living. The consequences of this condition are global in their application. As something like 30% of people who have CP also have epilepsy, the impact on quality of life can be severe. The ageing process also leaves them more susceptible to Alzheimer-related disorders (Holland 1999).

The comedian Laurence Clark (http://www.laurenceclark.co.uk/) has cerebral palsy. He performs a routine about trying to look macho in the local pub while sitting in a wheelchair and drinking beer from a plastic cup with a spout-lid and two handles.

Healthcare for people labelled with 'learning disability'

It is an unfortunate paradox that living with a learning disability does not provide immunity from the whole range of physical, emotional and psychological problems that beset human beings. It is often as a result of living with learning disability that the individual is even more susceptible in the first place. In this section material that illustrates the discrepancies apparent in the provision of health and social care will be discussed.

Part of the reason for people labelled with learning disability living with a lower level of general health is that their overall well-being is often compromised by associated conditions such as epilepsy and musculoskeletal problems. The National Patient Safety Agency (2004) acknowledges the difficulties people face with regard to access to treatment. Symptoms are not always diagnosed early enough, which can lead to serious health conditions deteriorating and the occurrence of avoidable deaths. Consequently 'diagnostic overshadowing' occurs when a condition is ignored or misdiagnosed because the label of 'learning disability' takes precedence. This is probably what happened to J., from earlier in the chapter, when she

was in hospital. Now take a few minutes to do the Exercise 14.10.

Applying Theory to Practice: Exercise 14.10

Think back to the last time you were in pain.

- Describe the pain.
- What made the pain better?
- What made the pain worse?
- How did being in pain affect your behaviour?
- How did being in pain affect your thinking?
- How would someone who does not know you well know you are in pain?
- How do you treat pain?

Add your findings to your growing portfolio.

Now consider the following brief scenario, what would you do?

Scenario 4.1

The Case of Sarah

Sarah approached me (psychologist) at the day service. She placed her hand rather heavily on my shoulder. She then held her tummy and I asked her if she was OK. She shook her head and said 'No'. I said I was sorry to hear that; then I walked away. When I turned away to talk to a member of staff Sarah spat at me.

Assessment and analysis of patient presentation

Sarah was a 43-year-old woman diagnosed with moderate learning disabilities. She has very limited verbal communication skills. She also has a history of behaviours that challenge services and she can be aggressive to herself and to others. There was evidence of faecal smearing and while the reasons for this were not fully understood at the time, Sarah had a history of chronic constipation. Despite considerable weight loss, her stomach was distended and she was often seen with her hand up her jumper, rocking and crying.

Was Sarah's behaviour due to her learning disability? When Sarah was referred to the chronic pain team at her

local hospital, initial investigations for gynaecological problems proved inconclusive. However, further tests revealed that Sarah had a massive gallstone, which had to be surgically removed, and type II spina bifida, which would account for her constipation. Although people with learning disabilities have conditions one would associate with pain, they are rarely referred to specialist pain services.

Questioning Clinical Practice: Exercise 4.11

Does Labelling Affect Access to Healthcare?

Endometriosis is an extremely painful condition, which affects 1 in 10 women and can occur at the onset of puberty and last until menopause. None of my colleagues can think of one woman with a learning disability having been treated for it.

Think about common elective surgical procedures.

- How often do the patients have a history of learning disability?

The benefits of people with learning disabilities accessing mainstream expertise cannot be underestimated; yet we know difficulties persist. Furthermore, they are often excluded from health promotion initiatives such as cervical screening, which raises another important issue. There is a strong argument that people with learning disabilities should be included in strategies relating to National Service Frameworks (NSF). However, as with cancer, comorbidity issues are different, and by concentrating on what is prevalent in the general population one could argue that instead of reducing inequalities, we could actually be widening the gap.

Questioning Clinical Practice: Exercise 14.12

Class Discussion

- Should people labelled with a learning disability be cared for in segregated or integrated services?
- What differences do you think it would make?

People attend clinics, surgeries, hospitals and other treatment centres for only one reason: they need some form of medical attention. This may be in the shape of therapy, investigation, medicine, surgery, screening, counselling/advice or a permutation of any of the above. It is almost certain that a nurse or allied healthcare professional will be involved somewhere along the line, and that person might be you.

People labelled with learning disability usually have their own carers, so you might feel entitled to ask why you need to get involved at all. Maintaining good health is a complex business and it frequently involves many areas of expertise; when dealing with individuals labelled with learning disability, this can get even more complicated, so some degree of inter- and intra-professional collaboration is often required.

Valuing People (DH 2001) was the first government White Paper to focus on learning disability for thirty years. As with much legislation, it was long on rhetoric but short on action. It did, however, contain some useful initiatives. Putting these into practice is often the responsibility of the community nursing teams. The focus on health in *Valuing People* has provided the impetus for community learning disability teams to further develop the process of partnership working with primary and acute care services. Mainstream health staff need to be aware of the inclusion of people labelled with learning disabilities within their services, as this is crucial to the debate on access to ordinary health services.

The strategy has emphasised that a primary role of the teams is to support access to mainstream services. More recently, the Department of Health's (2007) report *Promoting Equality* further promotes this key role as a way of 'closing the gap' of inequality for people with learning disabilities. This means in practice that learning disability nurses, and other members of the community learning disability team, work in partnership with primary and acute care services either by working on a one-to-one basis with individuals to support their understanding of their own health and so enable access to services that way, or working with the mainstream health services to develop their skills and knowledge around the health and support needs of people with learning disabilities. This is helping to provide better health outcomes for people with learning disabilities. *Valuing People* also identified health action plans and health facilitators as a way of supporting people with learning disabilities to meet their health needs. The person chooses their health facilitator who helps them to collect information about their own health and have a health screening at their GP practice.

The health facilitator does not need to be a nurse; they can be a parent, friend, support worker or key worker. However, people with more complex disabilities and medical needs may have a community learning disability nurse as their health facilitator. The facilitator then supports the person, or in the case of someone with multiple and profound disabilities, the people who know them best, to identify their health needs. They then ensure that the plan is written in a format which the person can understand. A copy of the plan is usually given to the primary care practice either with the person's consent, or for people who cannot give informed consent, by following best practice guidance, which is outlined in the Mental Capacity Act.

As well as the usual gamut of physical ailments, people labelled with learning disability are often prone to other conditions that complicate their overall health and well-being. In an introductory chapter it is impossible to cover all eventualities. This will, therefore, be limited to discussion of a cursory examination of two of the most common 'overlying' conditions, while introducing the concept of consent.

Mental health

People who are labelled with learning disability sometimes have overlying mental health problems. This may affect on estimate up to 30% of the population (Cole 2002). Sometimes referred to as 'dual diagnosis', this can be difficult to establish. Typically the potential for overlap between what is commonly known as 'challenging behaviour' and genuine mental health problems can be hard to untangle. Also there are difficulties in providing an accurate assessment for people living with severe learning disability and, to a lesser extent, to fit standard diagnostic criteria, although this has been addressed by the recent DC-LD (2001) which is a relatively new classificatory system designed for use with adults with learning disabilities and intended to be complementary to ICD-10 (WHO 1992).

Another problem arises from the fact that the figures may well be inflated by the inclusion of individuals who are somewhere on the autistic spectrum of disorders. Their place within mental health or learning disability services is highly contentious and represents an example of what Cole (2002) refers to as 'people falling between

eligibility criteria and through the net of service provision'.

Autistic spectrum disorder

As with the sub-population of individuals labelled with learning disability and the wider population of the country, the range of ability and intelligence on display within the so-called autistic spectrum is very wide. Some few individuals living with what is sometimes called high functioning Asperger's syndrome operate at extremely high IQ levels, while those more severely affected by autism may have badly affected social competence and seriously compromised intellectual ability.

There is still no definitive cause identified. Leo Kanner in America first described what we now understand as autism in 1944. Hans Asperger in Austria in the same year described the syndrome that now bears his name. Both were thought of as two sides the same coin. It was largely the work done by Wing and Gould (1979) that eventually separated the two, conceptually at least. Wing describes a 'triad of impairments' affecting communication, interaction and imagination. While textbooks are useful, sometimes another angle is necessary to approach understanding.

Consent: The Bournewood case

It is common for a doctor or a dentist to ask carers to sign a consent form for an adult with learning disabilities. This is not legally acceptable and has no basis in law (Matthews 2003). The European Court of Human Rights had to review the case of HL *v* United Kingdom – known as the 'Bournewood' case from the institution where Mr L., a 49-year-old man with autism, was an inpatient. In summary it was agreed by all concerned that Mr L. lacked capacity to consent to treatment. Since he was not detained (under the Mental Health Act 1983) but was cared for in his own 'best interests', his legal team were able to argue that he was in effect kept in hospital in contravention of Article 5 of the European Convention on Human Rights. This has led to a change to the 2005 Mental Capacity Act. Anyone in Mr L.'s position now needs to have an independent mental capacity advocate (IMCA) to represent him or her during the assessment/treatment process. The DH website (http://www.dh.gov.uk/en/index.htm) has comprehensive coverage of the legal, ethical and clinical implications of this case for practising healthcare professionals.

Conclusion

People labelled with learning disability have the same rights as the rest of the population. That includes access to health and social care services. They have higher levels of ill health, including epilepsy and mental health problems, and many have communication difficulties. They have lower income, less secure tenure, poorer education and reduced social prospects. Very few have a proper job, and intimate personal relationships are rare. Many live in accommodation not of their choosing, and are subject to ridicule and harassment in their own local communities. A small minority are subject to physical, financial and sexual abuse from the people employed to provide their care. Like the rest of us they sometimes need to access health and social care services. As a healthcare provider you can now have a direct impact on the standard of treatment they can expect and receive.

Further reading

Basford, L. & Slevin, O. (eds) (2003) *Theory and Practice of Nursing: An Integrated Approach to Caring Practice.* Nelson Thornes: Cheltenham.

Berger, P.L. & Luckmann, T. (1971) *The Social Construction of Reality: A Treatise in the Sociology of Knowledge.* Penguin: London.

Haddon, M. (2004) *The Curious Incident of the Dog in the Night Time.* Vintage: London.

Hope, T. (2004) *Medical Ethics: A Very Short Introduction.* Oxford University Press: Oxford.

Jackson, L. (2002) *Freaks, Geeks and Asperger Syndrome: A User Guide to Adolescence.* Jessica Kingsley Publishers: London.

National Patient Safety Agency (NPSA) (2004) *Listening to People with Learning Difficulties and Family Carers Talk about Patient Safety.* NPSA: London.

Sutherland, A. (1997) Black hats and twisted bodies. In Pointon, A. & Davies, C. (eds) *Framed: Interrogating Disability on the Media.* British Film Institute: London.

World Health Organization (WHO) (1992) *The ICD-10 Classification of Mental and Behavioural Disorders: Clinical Descriptions and Diagnostic Guidelines.* WHO: Geneva.

World Health Organization (WHO) (2001) *International Classification of Functioning, Disability and Health.* WHO: Geneva.

References

American Psychiatric Association (APA) (2000) *Diagnostic and Statistical Manual of Mental Disorders. DSM-IV (text revision).* APA: Washington. DC.

Bissett, A. (2005) *The Incredible Adam Spark.* Headline Review: London.

Cole, A. (2002) *Include Us Too: Developing and Improving Services to Meet the Mental Health Needs of People with Learning Disabilities.* IAHSP/King's College London: London.

Crawford, J.R. (2004) Psychometric foundations of neuropsychological assessment. In Goldstein, L.H. & McNeil, J. (eds) *Clinical Neuropsychology.* John Wiley & Sons: New Jersey, pp. 357–70.

Dallison, J. & Lobstein, T. (1995) *Poor Expectations.* London Maternity Alliance: London.

Department of Health (2001) *Valuing People: A New Strategy for Learning Disability for the 21st Century.* DH: London.

Department of Health (2007) *Promoting Equality.* DH: London.

Disability Rights Commission (DRC) (2006) *Equal Treatment: Closing the Gap.* A Formal Investigation into the Physical Health Inequalities Experienced by People with Learning Disabilities and/or Mental Health Problems. DRC: Stratford-upon-Avon.

Down, J.L.H. (1866) Observations on an ethnic classification of idiots. *London Hospital Reports* 3: 259–62.

Emerson, E., Hatton, C., Felce, D. & Murphy, G. (2001) *Learning Disabilities: The Fundamental Facts.* Foundation for People with Learning Disabilities: London.

Folstein, S.E. (1989) *Huntington's Disease.* Johns Hopkins University Press: Baltimore, MD.

Holland, A.J. (1999) Down's Syndrome. In: Janicki, M. & Dalton, A.J. (eds) *Dementia, Ageing and Intellectual Disabilities: A Handbook.* Bruner/Mazel: Philadelphia.

Jelsma, J., De Weerdt, W. & De Cock, P. (2002) Disability Adjusted Life Years (DALYs). *Rehabilitation Disability and Rehabilitation* 24(7): 378–82.

Kanner, L. (1944) Autistic disturbances of affective contact. *Nervous Child* 2: 217–50.

Levitt, S. (2004) *Treatment of Cerebral Palsy and Motor Delay.* Blackwell Publishing: Oxford.

Matthews, D. (2003) Learning Disability: Capacity and Consent. *Learning Disability Practice* 6(2): 26–7.

National Patient Safety Agency (NPSA) (2004) *Listening to People with Learning Difficulties and Family Carers Talk about Patient Safety.* NPSA: London.

NHS Scotland (2004) *Health Needs Assessment Report: People with Learning Disabilities in Scotland.* NHS Scotland: Glasgow.

Nuffield Council on Bioethics (2006) *Critical Care Decisions in Fetal and Neonatal Medicine: Ethical Issues.* Nuffield Council on Bioethics: London.

Roizen, N.J. & Patterson, D. (2003) Down's syndrome. *Lancet.*361(9365): 1281–9.

Rothman, K.J. (2002) *Epidemiology: An Introduction.* Oxford University Press: Oxford.

Shakespeare, T. (1998) Choice and rights: eugenics, genetics and disability equality. *Disability & Society* 13: 665.

Streissguth, A. (1997) *Fetal Alcohol Syndrome: A Guide for Families and Communities.* Paul Brookes Publishing: London.

Tymchuk, A.J. & Andron, L. (1990) Mothers with mental retardation who do or do not abuse or neglect their children. *Child Abuse and Neglect* 14: 313–23.

Union of the Physically Impaired Against Segregation (1976) *Fundamental Principles of Disability.* http://www.leeds.ac.uk/disability-studies/archiveuk/UPIAS/fundamental%20principles.pdf (accessed March 2007).

Wechsler, D. (1998) *Manual for the Wechsler Adult Intelligence Scale,* 3rd edn. Psychological Corporation: Sidcup.

Wing, L. & Gould, J. (1979) Severe impairments of social interaction and associated abnormalities in children: epidemiology and classification. *Journal of Autism and Childhood Schizophrenia* 9: 11–29.

World Health Organization (WHO) (1992) *The ICD-10 Classification of Mental and Behavioural Disorders: Clinical Descriptions and Diagnostic Guidelines.* WHO: Geneva.

World Health Organization (WHO) (2001) *International Classification of Functioning, Disability and Health.* WHO: Geneva.

First aid knowledge and skills

Dimple Charters and Cliff Evans

15

Chapter 15 Learning Objectives

- Gain knowledge and insight into common injuries that would benefit from immediate first aid intervention
- Gain understanding of the professional issues involved in attending accidents
- Gain insight into several commonly used first aid techniques including dressings and bandages
- Apply relevant anatomy and physiology knowledge to clinical practice by identifying potential injury patterns
- Construct solid evidence of professional development for your growing portfolio
- Continue developing the ability to question and critique your care delivery by adding essential professional regulatory information to your practice

Applying Theory to Practice: Exercise 15.1

Do pre-registration courses prepare future nurses for emergency situations?

If your friends and family know you are a nurse, they may expect you to have more than just basic first aid skills. Many nurses feel completely lost when placed outside their normal working environment. It is therefore essential that nurses gain a solid understanding of how they can apply their generalised nursing knowledge to everyday situations.

- How has your nursing course prepared you for encountering either a minor injury in the community or an emergency situation?
- Do you feel your chosen course should include aspects of first aid?

Introduction

Possessing the underpinning theoretical knowledge and skill base to enable a rapid, but thorough, initial assessment of a potentially unwell individual, and the ability to initiate treatment, are essential skills that all student and qualified nurses require (NMC 2004). The Department of Health (DH) and the Nursing and Midwifery Council (NMC) have both published documents directed at ensuring that all healthcare professionals acquire certain fundamental skills that can be translated or adapted to multiple environments (DH 2001; NMC 2004). The NMC Code of Professional Conduct, Standards and Ethics (2004): clause 8.5 states, 'In an emergency, in or outside the work setting, you have a professional duty to provide care. The care provided would be judged against what could reasonably be expected from someone with your knowledge, skills and abilities when placed in these particular circumstances.'

First aid is the care given to a sick or injured person before professional help arrives. It can come from a member of the family, a friend, or a stranger who happens to be present. The help they give can literally mean the difference between life and death. The key aims of first aid are:

- To preserve life and limb
- To prevent the injury/injuries from becoming worse
- To promote recovery.

This list can be extended to include:

- The prevention of further injury to the individual or yourself.

The most serious of injuries can leave no apparent bleeding or potential life-threatening signs; by using a structured or methodical approach to the assessment process these types of injury can be identified and life-altering damage prevented. This is achieved by applying

the airway, breathing and circulation (ABC) approach to all patient assessments.

Applying Theory to Practice: Exercise 15.2

Before reading on:

- Compose a list of common injuries you associate with requiring first aid.

Add this list to your developing portfolio. On completion of this chapter expand your developing portfolio by adding some of the many conditions contained within this chapter. This can include the immediate safety issues, the immediate assessment and your approach to maintaining both your own safety and that of the individuals you may encounter.

Applying basic life support

Basic life support (BLS) is a tried and trusted method of both assessing and, more importantly, applying basic techniques that can preserve life (RCUK 2006).

Applying Theory to Practice: Exercise 15.3

All nurses need to be proficient in the provision of BLS and this is a mandatory component of all pre-registration courses. Complete the following exercise to gain further insight and experience in this area.

Visit the Resuscitation Council (UK) website; familiarise yourself with its format and content. This site provides all the information you require!

- Identify the BLS algorithm for children; distinguish the differences between how the two age groups are treated. Why do you think there are differences?

The Resuscitation Council also provide an in-hospital approach to BLS. Familiarise yourself with this as you will certainly be performing this act sometime during your working life.
www.Resus.org.uk

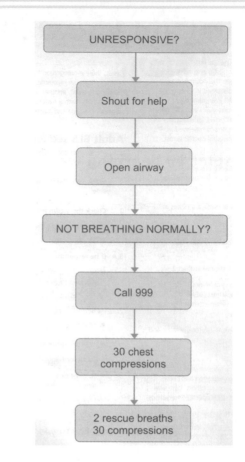

Figure 15.1 The basic life support algorithm (Source Resuscitation Council UK (2006) (Reproduced with permission)

Basic life support should consist of the following sequence of actions:

1. Make sure the casualty, any bystanders, and you are safe. When approaching any scene involving casualties the rescuers' personal safety must be your primary concern, due to two main factors: first, depending on the cause, what has affected the casualty may affect you! Secondly, many hidden dangers are faced by good Samaritans assisting those who do not appreciate help; there is also the chance of being assaulted by the casualty or other assailants. The manner in which you approach a particular incident will depend on the nature of that individual incident, although many basic principles can be universally applied. When approaching the scene of an accident or a casualty:

- Inspect for danger – ensure that injured individuals,

any onlookers, and you yourself are free from any actual or potential dangers.

- Approach all situations in a calm and collected manner, thereby instilling confidence in the injured. This will also provide you with time to collect your thoughts and structure your assessment.
- Be observant, visually assess the local environment, identify the nature of the problem.
- How many injured are there?
- If there are several injured, call for help before continuing, then approach those with what appear to be serious injuries first (triage).

2. Check the casualty for a response. If the casualty does not appear alert, assess their responsiveness, or level of consciousness, by gently shaking them, simultaneously asking in a very loud manner 'Hello, can you hear me, are you all right?' This is based on the AVPU approach applied throughout this book.

3. If the casualty responds:

- Leave them where they are and ensure that no further danger is imminent.
- Ascertain what the problem is and obtain help or alert emergency services if necessary.
- Keep the casualty warm and reassure them that the emergency services are on the way.
- Continually reassess the casualty and the safety of the situation.

4. If they do NOT respond: During your initial assessment if the patient fails to respond to both verbal stimulation and shaking, you will classify them as unresponsive. You must then move immediately into the BLS algorithm (Figure 15.1).

- Shout for help.
- Turn the casualty onto their back and then open the airway using head tilt chin lift (Figure 15.2).

5. Keeping the airway open – look, listen and feel for normal breathing.

- Look for chest movement.
- Listen at the patient's mouth for breath sounds.
- Feel for air on your cheek.

Figure 15.2 The head tilt chin lift manoeuvre

Assess for normal breathing for no more than 10 seconds; if you are in any doubt whether breathing is normal, assume it is not normal.

An alert patient may still have an underpinning problem that may lead to severe **airway** compromise. Follow these next steps to quickly assess for potential compromise:

- Has the injury involved smoke inhalation or facial burns? If so, there is a significant risk of impending airway compromise. Assess the airway and nasal passages for signs of swelling, singeing or soot and if present inform the emergency services of the immediate risk to life
- Assess the patient's **breathing** using the **look**, **listen** and **feel** approach. Remember you are looking to make sure they are breathing symmetrically, with a good inspiratory depth, and that their breathing rate is within the normal parameters (Chapter 3). You are listening for signs of difficulty in either getting air into or out of their lungs. There can be many reasons for breathing difficulties, which are discussed in Chapter 3. Feeling the patient's chest can have a dual purpose: initially you can quickly identify if the chest is moving symmetrically by placing one hand on each side of the chest wall (in the rib area); secondly, you can feel for any **crepitus**, the noise or sensation that broken pieces of bone will have as you run your hand over them. The noise is a slight cracking sound: remember if identified to take a mental note of the area and do not press any harder. The casualty may want to guard the area if conscious. If no open wound is present, applying gentle pressure over the area may result in

greater lung expansion and an increase in the effectiveness of their breathing.

6. If they are breathing normally:

- Put the casualty into the recovery position (Figure 15.3).
- Send or go for help, or call an ambulance.
- Check for continued breathing.

If the casualty is breathing and you are competent to, check for a carotid pulse at the side of the neck, simultaneously look down their body for signs of life. If you cannot feel a pulse and there are no signs of life commence BLS as described below.

If the casualty is breathing and has signs of circulation, but remains unresponsive, place them in the **recovery position**. It may be fatal to leave an unresponsive person on their back as there is a serious potential that their airway will become obstructed by either soft tissues such as the tongue falling backwards, or if they vomit they will be unable to clear the vomit, resulting in **asphyxia**.

Recovery position

Kneel beside the unresponsive casualty between the hip and shoulder. Straighten out the arms and legs. With the arm closest to you at a right angle to the body and the palmar side of the hand facing up, place the casualty's other arm across the chest with the hand across the other side of the cheek. Position your hand under their knee

(the leg that is away from you) bringing it up into a right-angle position. Remember to keep their hand pressed against their cheek. Support their head with your other hand ensuring that their airway is open and patent by lifting the head and tilting the chin. Grasp their opposing hip and roll them towards you. Adjust the upper leg that the hip and knee from a right angle to the body.

7. If they are not breathing normally:

- Ask someone to call for an ambulance or, if alone, call yourself even if you need to leave the casualty. Start chest compressions.

Delivering chest compressions

Kneel beside the patient, lean over the patient with your arms straight, place the heel of one hand on the centre of the patient's chest then place the heel of your other hand on top of the first one, keeping your fingers interlocked (Figure 15.4).

Position yourself above the patient's chest and, keeping your arms straight, press down on the sternum 4–5cm. Following each compression release all the pressure on the chest; repeat at a rate of about 100 compressions a minute (compression and release should take an equal amount of time).

Figure 15.4 Hand positioning for chest compressions

Figure 15.3 The recovery position

Combined chest compressions with rescue breaths

After 30 compressions open the airway using head tilt chin lift manoeuvre; pinch the patient's nose closed using the index finger and the thumb of the hand you had placed

on their forehead. Take a normal breath and place your mouth around the patient's mouth ensuring there is a good seal.

Blow steadily into the mouth while watching for the patient's chest to rise. It takes about a second for the chest to rise in a similar fashion to normal breathing. This is considered as an effective rescue breath. Maintain the head tilt chin lift and remove your mouth from the patient and watch for the patient's chest to fall. Take another normal breath and give another effective rescue breath – two in total. Return your hands without delay to the correct position on the sternum and give a further 30 chest compressions. Continue with chest compressions and rescue breaths in a ratio of 30:2.

However, if the rescue breaths were not sufficient to make the chest rise, you should check the following before attempting another rescue breath:

- Check the casualty's mouth for any visible obstruction and remove it (as discussed previously).
- Reassess that the degree of head tilt chin lift is sufficient. You may need to either extend or flex the neck a small amount to fully open the airway or remove soft tissues from blocking the **oropharynx**.

Chest compression only CPR

If you would prefer not to give rescue breaths, give chest compressions only; in this instance chest compressions

Developing and Delivering Expert Care: Box 15.1

You might be justifiably concerned about your own safety when delivering mouth-to-mouth ventilations. The Resuscitation Council UK recommends that chest compression only CPR may be administered in cases where the rescuer is unwilling to put their mouth in contact with the casualty's. Your local resuscitation officer (usually based in the acute hospitals) can provide you with a protective airway device that is sold within a key fob. This device has a one-way valve so that body fluids from the casualty cannot enter your mouth; the device is simply placed between your mouth and theirs. This device makes an excellent key ring and may prove invaluable one day.

should be continuous at a rate of 100 per minute. Only stop to reassess the patient if they start breathing normally.

Resuscitation should continue until:

- Further qualified help arrives
- The patient shows signs of life – reassess ABC
- The rescuer becomes exhausted.

Go back to the casualty's head and assess that the airway remains open, check breathing and again check for signs of life and a carotid pulse.

Developing and Delivering Expert Care: Box 15.2

Remember:
If You Mess, Reassess!
Meaning: if you suddenly alter the position of the casualty you may also alter their airway alignment, so always reassess and evaluate after implementing any action.

Road traffic accidents

The scene surrounding a road traffic accident can be full of actual and potential dangers: an example of an actual danger is being struck by a passing car and an example of a potential danger is an explosion due to a leaking fuel pipe. From this you can see that a quick, but thorough, examination of the surrounding area is essential. Your own safety must come first; call the emergency services and try to protect the scene from other vehicles. Approach the scene only once you have established the stability of the vehicles involved. Call out and see if there is any response from the driver or passengers (be aware that in high speed crashes occupants may have been ejected from the vehicle or there may be casualties under the vehicle). Approach the vehicle and immediately switch off any engines that are running. If there is no response from the casualty immediately apply the ABC format. Because there is a risk potential for C-spine damage the casualty's spine will need to be immobilised or stabilised at the same time as their airway is assessed; this is achieved in an unresponsive casualty slumped over the steering wheel by firmly placing one hand on either side of their neck and

Figure 15.5 Stabilising a potential C-spine injury

jaw line (Figure 15.5) and assisting them into a neutral position. Listen carefully to their airway in the neutral position for breath sounds; if absent or there are no pulse/ signs of life and you are able to remove them from the vehicle do so, and commence BLS; if the casualty is breathing maintain their position until help arrives. Their level of consciousness may increase, at this time you will need to provide psychological support for them by gently reassuring them. It will be beneficial to their long-term outlook if you to build a solid rapport with them.

Do not put the patient in the recovery position if a spinal injury is suspected. Maintain their C-spine alignment until the emergency services arrive; they will immediately fully immobilise them.

Motorcycle helmets

If the casualty is wearing a protective helmet it is best to leave it in place unless you have received specific training on removal techniques. If the casualty is unconscious, they may vomit; this is the only time you will need to turn them on their side to prevent asphyxiation and possible instant death. Try to maintain C-spine alignment, although the airway clearance must come before spine immobilisation.

First aid for epilepsy/seizures

When encountering an individual experiencing a seizure many people feel unprepared to deal with the circumstance. Seizures are not only associated with long-term conditions such as epilepsy (see Chapter 5), they are also associated with significant head trauma and in children they can be a consequence of a prolonged high temperature.

In most cases of recurring seizures the National Society for Epilepsy recommend there is no need to call an ambulance (National Society for Epilepsy 2007). Most seizures occur unexpectedly and last for a short time and usually stop by themselves (self-limiting). Many seizures can be characterised into two main types: generalised seizure or partial seizure that involves a fairly short period of absence.

Medical assistance is indicated if:

- This is the person's first seizure
- The person has injured themselves during the seizure (a dislocated shoulder or a head injury are common findings)
- The casualty experiences difficulty in breathing after the seizure
- When the seizure continues with no recovery period (tonic clonic).

Characteristics of a generalised seizure	Characteristics of a partial seizure
Person may lose consciousness	Twitching
Body stiffens, often becomes floppy	Glassy stare
High incidence involving falls	Disturbances in one of the senses i.e. taste, smell, hearing or vision
Shaking or jerky movements	Inappropriate responses to questions
Breathing might be affected and there may be a blue tinge around the mouth	Not totally aware of their surroundings
Incontinent of urine or bowels	Wandering around aimlessly
The casualty may bite their tongue resulting in blood around the mouth	Smacking of lips and chewing movements
	Agitated and fidgeting with objects

Table 15.1 Characteristics of seizures

What to do during a generalised seizure

- Stay calm
- Try and prevent further injury
- If possible, keep a record of the length of seizure
- Try and achieve a safe, comfortable environment for the individual
- Look for any medical alert bracelets
- Do not try and restrain the casualty, consider your own safety. The casualty might be agitated or be thrashing around, try and limit the local risk potential
- Do not attempt to put anything into the casualty's mouth (including medication)
- Remember and apply the ABC approach
- If the seizure is not self-limiting, call for help or dial 999

What to do during a partial seizure

- Stay calm
- Place the casualty away from danger, but do not restrain them, as they might get upset or increase the confusion
- Stay with casualty until they become fully recovered
- Reassure the casualty

Remember that after a seizure a person is at risk of vomiting so place them in the recovery position until they are fully alert. After seizures the person will awake in a confused and disorientated frame of mind; they will require reassurance and protection during this period. Stay with the patient until they recover and become orientated, if in any doubt of their well-being call for an ambulance.

First aid for a choking casualty

Applying Theory to Practice: Exercise 15.4

- If you witness someone who finds it difficult to breathe or cough due a potential obstruction in his or her throat what would you do?

By identifying your current approach you will be directly able to see how your practice could change for the benefit of those you come into contact with by applying your newly found insight.

To initiate what could be life-saving first aid you will initially need to be able to identify the underpinning problem. This is made easy with some conditions such as cuts and grazes, slightly harder when the individual can only inform you of what they are experiencing, and, depending on your knowledge base, quite difficult when their ability to communicate is lost. According to the American College of Emergency Physicians (1992) the international distress sign for someone physically choking is clinically demonstrated by them clutching at their throat.

Treating a choking conscious patient

If the person has the ability to speak, encourage them to cough. Do not interfere with their throat but encourage the victim to continue coughing and if the foreign body if visible in their mouth remove it. However, if the patient is unable to speak and the airway is compromised the initial treatment is to give five back slaps (by hitting them firmly between the shoulder blades using the heel of the palm of your hand). The effectiveness of this procedure can be increased if you bend the casualty forward (RCUK 2006).

Check the mouth after each blow for any obvious dislodged obstruction.

If choking continues, administer five abdominal thrusts.

Figure 15.6 The choking algorithm (Source: Resuscitation Council UK (2006). Reproduced with permission)

stand behind the patient's waist, with a clenched fist placed just below the xiphisternum between the navel and the bottom of the breastbone; place your other hand over the clenched fist then pull inwards and upwards approximately 6–10 times alternating with the back slaps.

Complications – pregnancy/obesity

If the casualty has a misshapen anatomy due to pregnancy or severe obesity, you will need to adapt the technique for it to be safe or effective. Chest thrusts can be substituted for abdominal thrusts: place the thumb of the left fist above the middle of the casualty's breastbone, place your right hand over your fist then compress the chest approximately four times fairly quickly. Be careful to avoid the abdomen as compressing here can lead to damage of vital organs.

If the casualty becomes unconscious

- Guide them safely to the ground
- Call for help/ambulance
- Begin BLS/CPR

Eye injuries

Most eye injuries result from foreign objects or particles entering and subsequently irritating the surface of the eye (Rosenburg & Dougherty 1996). Chapter 11 explores both the anatomy and physiology of the eye; it is therefore recommended that the reader review this chapter before continuing.

Occasionally eye injuries can be dangerous or sight-threatening. Suspicious findings include:

- A sudden loss of vision
- A feeling of increasing pressure within the eye.

Problems affecting the casualty's vision may be caused by trauma to the head or the eye/eye socket; this includes retinal detachment, a serious complication.

In these scenarios the casualty should seek immediate professional care.

Corneal abrasions

A corneal abrasion is an injury or scratch involving the outer layer of the eye, usually resulting from a superficial scratch to the surface. The cornea has multiple nerve endings under the surface, which can make a corneal abrasion very painful.

Causes of corneal abrasions

Everyday activities may lead to corneal abrasions, common causes include playing sports, rubbing or directly scratching an eye (children are frequently implicated), prolonged application of contact lenses and exposure to ultraviolet light from sun lamps or welding arcs which can result in damage to the corneal structure and should be treated as a burn injury to the eye.

Signs and symptoms

- The feeling of sand in the eye
- Blurred vision or distortion of vision
- Increased sensitivity
- Redness around the eye
- Increased watering of the affected eye
- There may be a sensation that there is something in the eye but the casualty cannot get it out.

Immediate treatment

Use clean water or a saline solution to immediately wash the eye out (irrigation). Encourage the casualty to repeatedly blink as this natural defence mechanism will remove any small dust or sand particles that might be causing irritation and damage. Gently extend the upper eyelid over the lower lid as the eyelashes can brush and remove foreign bodies from the under-surface of the eyelid.

If a foreign body appears embedded within the eye, or if the mechanism of injury suggests a high impact such as industrial injuries involving metal filings etc., do not try and remove the particle; immediately seek medical assistance. If the particle is visible, to provide stabilisation and further protection surround the particle with a rigid shield without applying pressure or keep the eye closed and seek medical assistance.

If chemicals are involved, irrigate the eye vigorously holding the eye open, call assistance and get the casualty to hospital as soon as possible.

Wounds

An accurate and quantitative assessment of a chronic or acute wound is essential to the initiation of appropriate and effective treatment. There are many types of injury that can result in damage to the skin's integrity. Remember this also means that bacteria have an entry point for colonisation, therefore all wounds have the potential for infection.

Scenario 15.1

Minor Injuries

You are out on a Sunday afternoon in the park with a friend and her 8-year-old son, when he suddenly falls and grazes his knee. He has not sustained a head injury and is crying and holding his knee. On inspection you note superficial skin loss to the wound and slight bleeding.

● What would you do?

Applying Theory to Practice: Exercise 15.5

There are various terms used to describe wounds. Read the following terms and see what your current understanding of them is by writing a short description of each.

● Abrasion
● Incision
● Puncture
● Laceration
● Avulsion
● Amputation

Compare your answers to the following section; add your findings to your portfolio for direct evidence of your new understanding.

To appreciate the potential hazards related to what are commonly termed minor injuries you will need to have an understanding of the structures involved; Figure 15.7 identifies the skin and its superficial structures and components. Chapter 8 discusses deeper structures, which should also be considered.

Abrasions are classified as a superficial injury where the epidermis is wounded from a rubbing or frictional type injury occurring against its soft outer surface. The wound can be linear in nature described as a 'scratch'. If the border is involved, for example, if a cyclist has fallen from his pushbike and skidded across the tarmac, this is described as a 'graze'. Most commonly affected areas are the elbows and knees; the resulting wounds are generally

Figure 15.8 Superficial abrasion injury

Stratum Corneum (skin surface)	
Stratum Lucidum (clear layer)	
Stratum Granulosum (granular layer)	Epidermis
Stratum Spinosum (prickle cell layer)	
Stratum Germinativum (basal layer)	
	Dermis

Figure 15.7 The skin

Figure 15.9 Incisional injury

Figure 15.11 Skin laceration

superficial although an extreme version of a graze is a degloving injury in which enough force was applied to the skin that it results in the skin being forced away from its underlying attachments.

Incisional wounds are normally smooth-edged and associated with knives or as a result of broken glass. The potential damage varies dependent on the size and depth of the incision and the exact position of the entry. Stab wounds can be classically deceiving to the inexperienced eye as the length or depth of the injury might look superficial due the muscle and skin contractility close to the wound which often obscures the actual size and extent of the wound.

Figure 15.10 Puncture wound

Puncture wounds result from a sharp, piercing object that goes through the both the epidermis and dermis. This type of injury can result in life-threatening internal damage when deeper structures or organs are involved. Puncture wounds are generally sustained from animal/human bites, nail punctures, splinters. Animal, and in particular, human bites are prone to high rates of infection. It is therefore essential to seek medical assistance for both antibiotic and tetanus prophylaxis.

Lacerations are commonly referred to as 'cuts' or 'gashes' affecting the skin. They commonly have jagged, irregular edges. Lacerations commonly occur over bony structures such as the eyebrows and knees. Lacerations can result from sharp objects or blunt trauma involving the various layers of the skin. They commonly bleed profusely.

Avulsions result in a noticeable absence of tissue, rapid bleeding and can involve a large surface area depending on the mechanism of injury.

Amputations can occur when a body part such as a toe or finger are partially or completely cut off.

Initial treatment/first aid

- Stop or control any bleeding/haemorrhage
- Prevent contamination i.e. clean and cover/dress the wound to avoid further infection potential
- Be aware that further medical assistance may be needed if the patient is demonstrating signs of haemodynamic compromise or if the mechanism of injury is significant.

Applying Theory to Practice: Box 15.3

Clinical Signs of Haemodynamic Collapse

When confronted by a casualty who is potentially seriously ill, regardless of the setting, a nurse is expected to make a quick but factual assessment of the casualty's circulation.

Many ways exist to assess circulation, the last tool you require is a DINAMAP!

These signs include:

- Increased respiratory rate and depth
- Absent or weak radial pulse
- Prolonged capillary refill time (CRT)
- Decreased level of consciousness
- Sweaty/clammy appearance
- Pale, cyanosed or mottled appearance.

Radial pulses provide an excellent indication of the patient's circulation.

Once the blood pressure has fallen to <90mmHg, the radial pulse will become progressively weaker until it is lost (Evans & Tippins 2007).

How to control bleeding

Apply direct pressure over the wound with a dressing or improvise by using material with a clean absorbent substance e.g. a rag, towel or piece of clothing. In the case of amputation, wrap the affected area in wet gauze and if possible seal in a bag with water and ice. This needs urgent medical attention.

Do not remove the bandage if the bleeding seeps through the dressing. Apply a new dressing over the previous dressing, ensuring the bleeding wound is not disturbed thereby allowing it to stop bleeding and for any clot formation not to be dislodged.

Frequently check the bandage and the circulation of the patient as it may become too tight due to swelling. Check the circulation distal to the wound by either using the CRT or if possible palpating the pulse.

If the wound is on the arm or leg and there is no suspicion of an underlying fracture, the limb should be elevated above the level of the patient's heart while direct pressure is maintained. Elevation of the wound allows gravity to reduce the flow of blood to the area.

Reassure the casualty.

If the bleeding is continuous and uncontrollable, try applying pressure over the major artery that is supplying the limb. Try and immobilise the injured part and get medical attention; if necessary call 999.

Direct pressure should not be applied if there is a:

- Protruding bone
- Potential skull fracture
- Embedded object.

Dressing of a minor wound

Once the bleeding has stopped, the wound should be cleaned and dressed to prevent infection.

Clean the area with normal tap water ensuring that the water flow is directed away from the wound.

Once the wound is cleaned and dried apply a bandage, monitor the site in case bleeding recommences. If the casualty requires no further treatment remind them to see their GP for advice on tetanus vaccination.

Types of dressing

- Gauze impregnated with petroleum jelly to aid moisture and subsequently wound healing
- Adhesive strips i.e. traditional plasters
- Non-adherent dressings
- Foams (very absorbent)
- Alginates i.e. kaltostat seaweed-based highly absorbent dressings
- Carbon-infiltrated dressings
- Hydrogels
- Hydrocolloids i.e. Duoderm, Granuflex, which promote debridement and healing.
- Transparent adhesive films/semipermeable films i.e. Biocclusive, Tegaderm that provide the ability to visualise the wound.

To aid wound closure Steristrips or tissue glue can be applied to a wound that has stopped bleeding and that has been cleaned.

Slings

The sling is probably one of the most useful pieces of equipment in first aid, with the aim of providing localised support and reducing further damage and pain. Slings are multipurpose:

- Broad arm sling
- High arm sling
- Also can be used in innovative ways: the army use improvised slings for battlefield first aid dressings that can be adapted to suit almost every circumstance

Broad arm slings are normally used in arm (wrist/elbow) injuries and can be applied to support the arm if the casualty has a suspected fracture of the clavicle (collarbone).

Application of a broad arm sling

1. Place the sling on the casualty's chest on the injured side with the shortest corner under the elbow and one point over the injured shoulder
2. Place the casualty's arm across their waist at 90 degrees
3. Bring the third end of the sling over to the uninjured side/shoulder
4. Tie at the back of the neck in a reef knot (avoiding catching hair or skin)
5. Finally fold the corner piece over the elbow and secure it with a pin or tie a small knot

Figure 15.12 Application of a broad arm sling

High arm slings provide elevation to facilitate haemostasis and the reduction of swelling. High arm slings will also provide support for the hand and forearm.

Application of a high arm sling

1. Assist the casualty to bend the injured arm and place it on the uninjured/opposing shoulder
2. Place the sling on top of the injured arm with the shortest corner over the elbow and one point at the uninjured shoulder
3. The free side/point of the sling is brought under the elbow to the side of the body and tie a knot across the back
4. Finally fold the piece over the elbow and secure it with a pin or tie a small knot

Figure 15.13 Application of a high arm sling

Splinting

The use of a sling in splinting a limb is a temporary measure and when properly applied it can aid in the immobilisation of a fracture, thereby reducing the potential for further blood loss, shearing of internal vessels or nerve damage. Immobilising an injured area will also provide pain relief.

First aid for nosebleeding (epistaxis)

Nosebleeds often appear frightening for both sufferer and onlooker. Many nosebleeds look much worse than they

really are. The application of basic first aid skills can prevent casualties requiring further medical attention.

Most nosebleeds originate from the anterior of the nose, where the vessels sit close to the surface (Evans 2005). However, some bleeds originate from the posterior of the nose; this involves larger vessels and is usually associated with older people (Corry 2005). Atherosclerosis and high blood pressure are predisposing factors. Nosebleeds originating in the posterior vessels are notoriously difficult to stop and may require further medical attention.

Causes of nosebleeds

- Nose-picking (epistaxis digitorum)
- Blowing the nose with force
- Dryness
- Use of medication e.g. aspirin, anticoagulants
- Injuries
- Allergies
- Introduction of foreign objects, most common in children
- High blood pressure
- Atherosclerosis
- Blood clotting disorders
- Use of cocaine or other inhaled drugs (amphetamines)

For most nosebleeds the application of simple first aid can usually stop the bleeding.

Applying first aid

- Regardless of the amount of blood loss, stay calm
- Sit with the casualty and loosen any tight clothing around their neck
- Assist the casualty in tilting their head slightly forward, encouraging the casualty to breathe through their mouth
- If the casualty is able to, assist them to apply their thumb and index finger over the soft portion of the nose (just under the bridge; if you apply pressure too low it will fail to be effective), and firmly squeeze the nostrils together
- Apply this pressure for at least 10 minutes; this is essential as every time you remove the localised pressure and assess for bleeding the newly formed clot may dislodge and the casualty is in the same situation as you found them. Resisting the temptation to look can prove difficult for both the rescuer and casualty

- Reassess after 10 minutes. If the bleeding does not stop continue to apply pressure for a further 10 minutes and if available apply an ice pack across the bridge of the nose or to the back of the neck. Be careful not to burn the skin.

If the bleeding stops, advise them to avoid blowing their nose for a couple of hours, avoid hot drinks and avoid picking the nose.

If the patient feels faint, lay them in the recovery position and elevate the legs if necessary. Remember to continually assess and reassess their haemodynamic status: by monitoring their respiratory rate, radial pulse, and CRT. The casualty's colour will also show obvious signs of deterioration.

If the bleeding continues for more than 20 minutes or as a result of an accident, injury to the head, or a punch to the face, seek urgent medical attention.

If this is a recurring problem, encourage the casualty to make an appointment with their general practitioner and possible follow-up in a specialist clinic with the ENT (ears, nose and throat) specialist.

Tips on preventing further nosebleeds

- Keep the nostrils moist, for example, in the winter by use of a cool mist vaporiser or humidifier in the bedroom
- Apply petroleum jelly or other nasal lubricant inside the nostril
- Avoid picking the nose
- Open the mouth when sneezing, blow gently one side at a time; this will reduce localised pressure

Assessing and managing burn injuries

According to the National Burn Care Review in 2001, in the UK it is estimated that around 250,000 people experience burn injuries annually. The causes vary and include hot surfaces and fluids, electrical sources,

Applying Theory to Practice: Exercise 15.6

Burn injuries can result in varying degrees of damage.

How do you think these are classified?

Figure 15.14 Superficial burn

chemicals and flames. Approximately 90% of these injuries can be safely treated in a primary care setting; however, there will be times when the individual will require hospitalisation and specialist treatment, due to the severe effect burn injuries can have on the individual (National

Figure 15.15 Partial thickness burn to right foot

Depth of burn	Skin structures involved	Key signs	Healing information
Superficial: i.e. sunburn, minor scalds	Epidermis	Erythema, painful	Not life-threatening, no obvious scarring, heals within a few days
	Epidermis and superficial dermis (papillary layer)	Absence of blisters, skin is dry and intact	
Superficial dermal/ partial thickness: (often a scald injury)		Painful, red and mottled in appearance, swelling and blistered areas, may have weeping, hypersensitivity to air	Should heal within 2–3 weeks if there is no infection, pressure or trauma within or on the wound. May experience hypo/ hyperpigmentation depending on the remaining intact melanocytes
Deep dermal partial thickness: (usually caused by hot liquids, steam, flames)	Epidermis, deep dermis, including the superficial parts of hair follicles, sweat and sebaceous glands		
		May be painful but generally areas are insensitive. Exposed dermis white/yellowish creamy, does not blanch, no capillary refill	
Subdermal full thickness: over a limited area (hot oil, hot materials)	Epidermis and dermis both destroyed. In cases of chemical and electrical involvement the subcutaneous tissues and deeper structures can be involved		Any period from 3–8 weeks for healing with variable degrees of scarring. Surgical intervention may be required to maximise healing and a functional recovery
Full thickness: over an extensive area		Painless, no capillary refill, generally dry	
		May appear dark (charred), grey, cherry red, leathery, waxy	
	Epidermis and dermis	white (which might be mistaken for unburnt skin)	Requires surgical repair and skin grafting

Table 15.2 Burn injury classifications

Figure 15.16 Varying depths of burn
(Reproduced with permission of Dr. Adel Aulaqi).

Burn Care Review 2001). When sustaining a serious burn, failing to seek specialist assistance can result in a reduced function of an affected limb, increased scarring of facial injuries and infection-related problems due to the loss of the skin's integument (Chapter 10).

This section provides the reader with an in-depth knowledge of the immediate treatment of burn injuries, but it is paramount that expert assistance is sought as soon as possible for burns that result in more than superficial skin damage.

According to the National Burn Care Review report (2001), of the 175,000 people that attended accident and emergency departments annually, 13,000 were admitted for further hospital treatment.

What is a minor burn?

There are a variety of definitions which describe a minor burn or scald injury, the most commonly used definition of a minor burn is a superficial burn involving less than 5% total body service area (TBSA) in adults (Fowler 1998).

Depth of the burn

In the past burns were described as first, second and third degree. However, this terminology leaves the definition open to a great deal of potential subjectivity on the assessor's part and therefore practically unreliable. It is

therefore commonplace within emergency care in the UK to describe burns by the extent of visible damage (Evans & Tippins 2007). This classification scale provides a basic descriptive tool that can be used to quickly establish the amount and severity of damage following an injury. The classification of a burn is not a life-saving act; remember ABC. Identifying the depth of damage can be undertaken after the initial assessment, i.e. ABC and secondary assessment of the casualty including an in-depth examination of patient, history of the burn/incident, cause of the burn and the first aid treatment delivered.

The severity of the burn is also judged by the amount of total body surface area (TBSA) involved. Healthcare workers commonly use the Wallace (1951) rule of nines to determine the percentage of TBSA affected. For a more detailed calculation of the burn size, the Lund & Bowder chart (1944) can also be used.

Alternatively one of the casualty's palmar surfaces with fingers closed can be used to provide a crude estimation of approximately 1% of their TBSA. This is useful for quick and early assessment of a casualty who has sustained small and multiple burns over their body (Mertens et al. 1997).

Treating burns

The initial first aid for a burn injury can be essential to the long-term prognosis. An easy to remember acronym will be applied to the initial management for burns to aid consistency in the early and essential treatment phase:

Applying Theory to Practice: Box 15.4

The Rule of Nines

Age	Adult	Child
Head	9%	18%
Chest	18%	18%
Back	18%	18%
Arm	9%	9%
Leg	18%	13.5%
Groin	1%	1%
Total	100%	100%

SCALD
Stopping the burning process
Cooling the burn
Analgesia
Last tetanus
Dressing the burn

Stopping the burning process
Remove the casualty from the heat source. If in flames the affected area should be submerged in water, or rolled on the ground to smother the flames. This can also be achieved with a blanket or coat. In the event of an electrical burn turn the electricity off at the mains before assisting the casualty. If the casualty is still in contact with a live source of electricity, call for assistance and avoid touching them, as you may well become the next casualty. Clothing should be removed as it is a source of heat and the burning process can continue, but do not remove clothing if the burns are extensive and if the material is adherent to the skin, e.g. nylon, as this could exacerbate the injury. Submerge the affected area in water. The rescuer should ensure that they do not jeopardise their own safety.

Cooling the burn
It is suggested that the affected area be cooled for a minimum of 20 minutes. This cooling process eliminates the heat and prevents further damage to the tissues. It should be noted that very cold water or the use of ice should not be used as it causes vasoconstriction with the likelihood of further tissue damage or burn progression (remember ice can burn!). Special attention should be taken when cooling large areas as this can lead to hypothermia. Recommendations vary with regard to the water temperature. Mccormack et al. (2003) suggest that temperatures between 5 and 25 degrees Celsius have been proven to be the most effective method of cooling burn wounds. Chemical burns should be treated as a normal burn, but in addition to normal treatment they may require copious amounts of irrigation to remove the offending particles (this is particularly evident in alkaline injuries involving the eyes). The exception to this rule is electrical burn injuries, where an electrical source has travelled through the body and out of an exit point. This is an interesting phenomenon as an electrical burn to the shoulder may exit at the foot resulting in internal damage to both areas.

Analgesia
In major burns with moderate to severe pain opioids are indicated for the initial pain control, but with superficial or mild burns effective first aid in the form of cooling may bring instant relief. NSAIDs such an ibuprofen or combination drugs involving paracetamol and codeine may be effective (all of which are easy to obtain).

Last tetanus booster
Check tetanus immunisation status for casualties sustaining burns, particularly those who originate from outside the UK, as they may not have had childhood immunisation.

Dressings
Initially wrap the burn with cling film or a clean plastic bag as it is non-adherent, water-resistant, keeps the wound clean, prevents air flow over the skin and is translucent for further examination. Cling film should be applied in layers to prevent a tourniquet effect. Many different nationalities have traditional remedies for burns; many involve applying toothpaste to the burnt area. Avoid putting anything on the wound other than water.

Overview: putting theory into practice
The collapsed adult or child
Although this book is directed at students undertaking the adult branch or specialty of nursing, frequent encounters requiring the provision of first aid may include children and pregnant women. This may appear daunting to the inexperienced practitioner, but, by employing a solid structure to your assessment of the situation and the individual's needs, you can and will be competent and confident to assist and potentially deliver life-saving assistance to all casualties.

What can cause a person to suddenly collapse?
The previous chapters in this book have identified many conditions or illnesses that could lead to a person collapsing. The intention of this chapter is not to make a diagnosis but to manage the care of an individual outside the protective atmosphere of modern hospitals.

The assessment process
- **A**: Airway and C-spine immobilisation
- **B**: Breathing and ventilatory support
- **C**: Circulation and haemorrhage control

- **D**: Disability and neurological assessment
- **E**: Exposure (assess full body for potential injuries) and environment (temperature control)

Recognition of airway and breathing difficulties

Look: Airway obstruction – foreign bodies within the mouth (including blood and vomit); soft tissues such as the tongue can also obstruct the airway. Count the respiratory rate; look for an increased respiratory rate although bradypnoea may develop as a preterminal sign. See if the patient is using the accessory muscles of respiration. Sweating and a clammy appearance may also be present. Hypoxic patients often become agitated and confused, this progressive state continues with the patient becoming drowsy and eventually unconscious.

Listen: For any of the following:

- Gurgling: Presence of liquid in the upper airway
- Snoring: Obstruction of the pharynx by the soft tissues or tongue
- Crowing: Laryngeal spasm
- Stridor: Upper airway obstruction (i.e. choking)
- Wheeze: Lower airway collapse during expiration; a silent chest can indicate complete airway obstruction or severe respiratory failure.

Identify if the patient can complete a sentence without stopping to gasp air.

Feel: Air movement at the mouth, adequate chest rise and fall (this can be assessed by assisting the patient to sit up). Ascertain if the patient is excessively hot (sepsis/infection) or cold (sepsis/hypothermia).

Recognition of circulatory failure

- Pale and sweaty in appearance, possible decrease in level of consciousness
- Pulse rate/rhythm/depth; tachycardia can indicate compensation although extreme bradycardia can also lead to haemodynamic collapse
- A weak barely palpable pulse when combined with blood loss is a bad sign
- Reduced capillary refill time
- Cold clammy limbs may indicate physiological shock development

Conclusion

As a trained nurse you have a duty of care and are required to assist those in need even when off duty. By gaining insight into some of the simple techniques in this chapter you may save a life one day or genuinely make a difference to someone's life. Assessment of immediate physiological needs, reassurance and the use of the recovery position are all essential first aid skills. The number one intervention remains assisting the patient to breathe when they have a reduced level of consciousness; this straightforward skill is simply put – life-saving. Always remember your own safety and when in doubt call for immediate assistance; this is what is minimally required within the NMC's Code of Conduct (NMC 2004). Possessing first aid skills can be extremely rewarding particularly when dealing with members of your own family or friends.

Chapter 15 Summary Quiz

1. What are the key aims of first aid?

A. To preserve life and limb
B. To prevent injury/injuries from becoming worse
C. All answers are correct
D. The prevention of further injury to the individual or yourself

2. What is the correct order of approach to patient assessments?

A. Breathing, Airway, Circulation
B. Airway, Breathing, Circulation
C. Circulation, Breathing, Airway
D. Breathing, Circulation, Airway

3. List three possible scenarios where medical assistance is indicated in an epileptic fit:

A. Their first seizure (ABC)
B. They have injured themselves during seizure i.e. dislocated shoulder, head injury
C. The person experiences difficulty in breathing after the seizure, compromised airway
D. When the seizure affects a known epileptic and is self-limiting

4. Which of the following is a characteristic of a partial seizure?

A. A high incidence of a fall
B. Shaking or jerky movements
C. A glassy stare
D. Incontinent of urine and bowels

5. What is the international distress sign for someone choking?

6. You are out at a restaurant when a person at the next table starts coughing and clutching his throat. They are able to speak to you. What would be your initial treatment?

A. Give 5 abdominal thrusts
B. Give the person something to drink
C. Stay calm, continue to speak to the person and encourage them to cough. If any foreign body is visible remove it
D. Give 5 backslaps

7. Which of the following is not associated with corneal abrasions?

A. Playing sport
B. Rubbing or directly scratching the eye (children are frequently indicated)
C. Prolonged application of contact lenses
D. Swimming without goggles

8. **Which of the following best describes the following: 'a superficial injury where the epidermis is wounded from rubbing or friction against the outer surface'?**

A. Abrasion

B. Avulsion

C. Laceration

D. Puncture

9. **A patient presents to an A&E department after spilling hot coffee on their hand. It is very painful and there is erythema but no loss of skin. How would you best describe the burn?**

A. Subdermal/partial thickness

B. Superficial

C. Full thickness

D. Second degree

10. **List three common causes of nosebleeds/epistaxis.**

A. Nose picking

B. Blowing the nose with force

C. High blood pressure

D. Anaphylaxis

Further reading

Department of Health (2006) *Immunisation against Infectious Disease*. The Green Book. DH: London. http://www.dh.gov.uk/en/Policyandguidance/Healthandsocialcaretopics/Greenbook/DH_4097254

Evans, J. (2005) *Epistaxis*. http://www.emedicine.com/emerg/topic806.htm

Fowler, A. (1998) Nursing management of minor burn injuries. *Emergency Nurse* 6(6): 31–7.

http://www.hse.gov.uk/firstaid/

http://www.nhsdirect.nhs.uk/articles/article.aspx?articleId=450

Historical

The Lund and Browder charts originate from the 1944 edition of *Surgery, Gynaecology and Obstetrics*, edited by C.C. Lund (American surgeon) & N.C. Browder (American paediatrician).

The Rule of Nine appeared in Wallace, A.B. (1951) The exposure treatments of burns. *Lancet* 1(9): 501–4.

References

American College of Emergency Physicians (1992) *Perform First Aid to Clear an Object Stuck in Throat of a Conscious Casualty*. www.acep.org (accessed 17/07/07).

Corry, J. (2005) Management of epistaxis. *American Family Physician* 71: 305–11, 312.

Department of Health (2001) *Comprehensive Critical Care: A Strategic Programme of Action*. DH: London.

Evans, C. & Tippins, E. (2007) *The Foundations of Emergency Care*. Open University Press: Maidenhead.

Evans, J. (2005) *Epistaxis*. http://www.emedicine.com/emerg/topic806.htm (accessed 13 October 2007).

Fowler, A. (1998) Nursing management of minor burn injuries. *Emergency Nurse* 6(6): 31–7.

McCormack, R.A. (2003) First-aid management of minor burns in children: a prospective study of children presenting to the Children's Hospital at Westmead, Sydney. *Medical Journal of Australia* 178(1): 31–3.

Mertens, D.M., Jenkins, M.E. & Warden, G.D. (1997) Outpatient burn management. *Nursing Clinics of North America* 32(2): 343–64.

National Burn Care Review Committee (2001) *National Burn Care Review*. British Association of Plastic Surgeons. www.baps.co.uk

National Society for Epilepsy (2007) *Information on Epilepsy and the National Society for Epilepsy*. www.epilepsynse.org.uk. (accessed 13/06/06).

Nursing and Midwifery Council (NMC) (2004) *The NMC Code of Professional Conduct: Standards for Conduct, Performance and Ethics*. NMC: London.

Resuscitation Council (UK) (RCUK) (2006) *Advanced Life Support*, 5th edn. RCUK: London.

Rosenburg, S.J. & Dougherty, K. (1996) *The Complete Idiot's Guide to First Aid Basics*. Alpha Books: New York.

Pharmacology and drug calculations

Andrew Frazer

Chapter 16 Learning Objectives

- Gain understanding of what is meant by the terms pharmacology, pharmacodynamics and pharmacokinetics
- Learn about the stages of absorption, distribution, metabolism and excretion of medication
- Understand the importance of careful prescribing for older patients
- Understand the importance of patient education and concordance in provision of medications
- Define an adverse drug event and learn how to avoid them
- Learn how to deliver medication safely through a variety of routes
- Learn about the major classes of drugs, with some specific examples
- Apply theory to practice by performing drug calculations related to specific medications and patients

Introduction

A large percentage of a qualified nurse's time is spent in dispensing medication and related information and advice. A sound knowledge base is required if potentially catastrophic errors are to be avoided, and medication is to have the desired effect.

A chapter of this length cannot hope to provide a comprehensive introduction to all classes of medication, but it will offer indications for further study in the practice area, and provide the basic principles for the safe provision of medication to patients.

An understanding of pharmacology requires consideration of the concepts of **pharmacokinetics** and **pharmacodynamics**. These appear to be complex terms, but are relatively simple concepts, and should be understood by anyone giving a potentially toxic substance to a patient. The potential toxicity of all medications may lead to an adverse drug event (ADE), particularly in elderly patients. Potential sources of ADEs will be examined, and strategies outlined to protect against them.

Errors in drug calculations are the cause of many ADEs, and methods of calculation, along with practical examples, will be provided to ensure the reader can effectively and safely calculate medication doses in practice.

Definitions

Pharmacology derives from the Greek *pharmakos* (drug) and *logos* (science). It is concerned with the study of how a substance interacts with an organism to produce a change. We tend to consider only pharmaceuticals (substances with medicinal properties) in relation to pharmacology, but foodstuffs may also have important effects on the organism, and are also studied pharmacologically. We may give drugs for a number of reasons, for diagnostic purposes, for prophylaxis, or for a therapeutic effect. The central concepts in pharmacology are pharmacokinetics and pharmacodynamics.

Pharmacokinetics is concerned with the study of the effects of the body on the drug, including absorption, distribution, metabolism and excretion. Pharmacodynamics, on the other hand, is concerned with the study of the effects of the drug on the body, including effective doses and response.

Absorption begins once the drug accesses the body (through the many potential routes, including oral ingestion, topical administration, intravenous injection, etc.). The rate and method of absorption affect the **bioavailability** of the drug (how much of the drug reaches its intended target, and how quickly it does so). Absorption is affected by the physical properties of the drug itself (capsule, tablet or liquid form), as well as by the physiology of the person taking the drug (e.g. how long it takes the drug to move through the digestive tract). If the drug is released too swiftly, an excessive response may occur due to high blood levels. If it is released too slowly, it may be eliminated in the faeces prior to being absorbed.

Manufacturers formulate medications to ensure specific drugs are released at the rate calculated to maximise effective absorption. This may entail delivering the drug in a capsule, which will rapidly dissolve, or in an injectable form when the drug may not survive the acidity of the stomach. An enteric coat may be provided, to protect the drug from the stomach's acidity, or the stomach itself from the harmful effect of the drug. These drugs are absorbed in the small intestine.

Crushing medications (for example, to allow them to be passed down a nasogastric tube); should only be undertaken where it can be confirmed that it is acceptable. This could fundamentally affect the absorption of the drug, particularly in the case of modified or slow release medications, which are designed to release a steady drug level over 12 or 24 hours. A large toxic dose may be provided if you crush such a tablet. If you are considering crushing a tablet, you should establish if a liquid formulation is available – this will be preferable.

Anatomy and Physiology in Action: Exercise 16.1

Examine the anatomy and physiology of the gastro-intestinal tract, and consider how alterations in its function may affect drug absorption – particularly in relation to diarrhoea, ingestion of high fibre foods, or surgical removal of parts of the GI tract.

Once the drug has accessed the body, it will generally be absorbed via passive diffusion across a cell membrane (the only exceptions to this being inhaled and intravenous medication).

Once absorption has begun to occur, and the drug enters the bloodstream, **distribution** of the drug can take place. The rate at which the drug is delivered (and the amount of drug) are determined by the rate and quantity of blood perfusing the part of the anatomy targeted. There are a number of other factors which impact on drug distribution. Water-soluble drugs remain within the blood and interstitial spaces, whereas fat-soluble drugs (lipophilic) cross cell membranes more easily.

Drugs may bind to plasma proteins within the bloodstream, being released when the plasma concentration (of 'free' drug) falls. The protein-bound portion is generally inactive, and therefore provides an effective reservoir of the drug, which is released as the level of free drug in the

plasma decreases. Problems arise with this system when a drug displaces another drug by preferentially binding with its protein sites e.g. verapamil displaces digoxin from its protein binding sites, releasing the free drug into the bloodstream with potentially toxic effect.

Applying Theory to Practice: Exercise 16.2

Warfarin is heavily bound to plasma proteins (99%), but is displaced by a number of drugs (and foodstuffs). Obtain a copy of the *British National Formulary* (BNF), and examine warfarin in the appendix on interactions.

Consider how knowledge of these interactions will affect the advice you provide to patients on warfarin.

Metabolism of a drug involves chemical alteration of the drug by the body into a metabolite. The body will attempt to metabolise what it sees as a potential toxin as fast as it can. This generally occurs in the liver, and can either activate or deactivate the drug – some drugs (termed pro-drugs) are given as inactive substances, which are then metabolised into an active form. A group of enzymes termed the cytochrome P-450 enzymes are primarily responsible for drug metabolism in the liver. This can lead to problems where several drugs compete for levels of the enzyme. Where one drug inhibits the enzyme-mediated metabolism of another drug (which would normally render it inactive), the second drug may accumulate to a toxic level. There are naturally occurring substances, which affect the P-450 enzymes, including grapefruit – patients

Applying Theory to Practice: Exercise 16.3

Look up grapefruit juice in the interaction section of the BNF.

Consider how you will obtain information on your patient's diet, and what advice you will need to provide for patients on vulnerable medication.

While you are there, look up dairy products and alcohol too.

should be advised not to take grapefruit juice if they are taking some medications.

A drug will be metabolised prior to excretion, which generally helps to make it more water-soluble, enabling elimination via the kidneys. Elimination refers to the removal of the drug from the body. Some drugs are excreted in sweat, saliva, breast milk, and in the case of inhaled anaesthetic agents, exhaled air.

Some drugs are excreted unchanged in bile, which then enters the gastrointestinal tract. The drug is then excreted in faeces, or reabsorbed and 'recycled'. This explains why such a low dose of oestrogen may be used for the oral contraceptive pill, as it is constantly recycled. Any diarrhoea may reduce this enterohepatic cycling, rendering the contraceptive pill ineffective. Women should be advised when taking antibiotics (which may cause diarrhoea through alterations in the natural gut flora) to take additional contraceptive precautions while on the antibiotics, and for one week afterwards.

The primary route for excretion is the kidney, however. Elimination via the kidneys is affected by urine flow, the rate of blood flow through the kidney, and the health of the kidneys. Patients with hypertension, diabetes, or recurrent kidney infections may have impaired ability to eliminate drugs, and will require a dose reduction. Kidney function decreases with age – a person aged 70 will have only 50% of the renal function they had at 30. This is one of the reasons why great care must be taken in prescribing for the older patient.

Drugs and the older patient

Elderly patients have a higher level of chronic disease than other patients – by their seventies, three out of four patients will have at least one chronic disease. They may be subject to polypharmacy (treatment with a number of drugs for a number of conditions), and are often given drugs to counteract the side-effects of other medications. The ability of elderly patients to eliminate drug metabolites may be significantly reduced due to poor hepatic or renal function, or in acute illness. Age-related changes affect all four pharmacokinetic stages:

● Absorption is affected in most routes of administration. Transdermal patches may not be as effective in patients with poor circulation. Increased gastric acidity, reduced intestinal motility and delayed gastric emptying may all serve to reduce the effective absorption of oral medications in the elderly patient.

● Distribution of drugs may be significantly altered in elderly patients. Altered body composition (an increase in body fat, decrease in lean muscle mass and decrease in total body water) may mean that hydrophilic drugs (such as digoxin, which normally distributes through lean body mass) may accumulate in the circulation, exceeding therapeutic levels. Lipophilic drugs, on the other hand, are stored in the larger fat tissues in the elderly patient, resulting in reduced clearance and potentially prolonged effect (e.g. benzodiazepines). Poor nutrition can reduce serum albumin levels, resulting in less protein binding, causing higher than normal levels of 'free' drug in the circulation, potentially producing undesirable effects (remember that warfarin is 99% protein bound).

● Metabolism of drugs is significantly affected by the relative health of the liver. Decline in function in the hepatic system associated with ageing may cause altered metabolism – a typical 65-year-old patient has an almost 50% reduction in hepatic blood flow compared to a 25-year-old.

● Elimination is affected by the relative health of the kidneys. A natural decline in function may be exacerbated by concomitant diseases such as hypertension and urinary tract infection.

Applying Theory to Practice: Exercise 16.4

Review the medication for a patient over 65: find a patient on five or more drugs – check the BNF to establish what they are for, and whether there are any interactions between them. Then check the appendices in the BNF on liver disease and renal impairment.

Add the findings to your portfolio.

Most doctors are aware of the dangers of overprescribing in the elderly patient, but it may be unavoidable in patients with several co-existing conditions, which require treatment. The fact that 27% of all reported adverse drug events happen in elderly patients, and 10–12% of emergency hospital admissions in the over-70s are caused by prescribed drugs (McGavock 2005), mean that

special care must be taken to ensure that patients know how to take their drugs correctly, and have the physical and mental capacity to do so. Nurses are perhaps best placed to ensure this understanding prior to the patient's discharge from hospital, or while caring for the patient in the community.

Elderly patients may have difficulty in swallowing, possibly leading to tablets dissolving in the mouth and causing ulceration. They should be advised to take their tablets with plenty of fluid. Frail or confused patients require supervision of medication, and the district nursing service may need to be mobilised to ensure that appropriate medication is taken at the right time. If patients have carers or relatives and are happy to have their medication discussed with them, this may help to ensure concordance with a medication regime.

Concordance implies an agreement to the regime by the patient; 'compliance' (which was the word previously used when discussing patients and medication) means agreeing to do what you are told. Patients are far more likely to take their medication if they understand what it is for, what the side-effects might be, and what the relative risk/benefit of the drug is to them as an individual. Investing some time in personalised drug education will ensure the patient understands why they are taking the drug, improving concordance, and efficacy of the treatment (Ryan & Chambers 2000).

Applying Theory to Practice: Exercise 16.5

Find several patients on five or more medications. For each drug, ask the patient:

- What they are for
- How they work
- What the potential side effects might be.

Devise a short education programme for each patient.

Ensuring that a patient is fully educated may help to reduce adverse drug events (ADEs). While drug interactions may cause an ADE (and the risk increases with each new drug the patient takes), we can minimise the risks to the patient by taking some elementary precautions. Ensuring that we know *all* the drugs that a patient is taking will help us to reduce potential ADEs. Asking a

patient what medications they take may elicit only a list of prescription medications from their GP. You must ask specific questions in addition, including:

- Do you take any herbal medication? (Patients on St John's Wort significantly alter the cytochrome P-450 activity of the liver.)
- Do you take any recreational drugs, including alcohol?
- Do you take any other drugs? (Patients occasionally self-medicate with their partner's medication!)

Apart from drug interactions, a major source of ADEs, and one that is particularly important to nurses, is 'medication error'.

Perhaps the best available definition of a medication error comes from the National Coordinating Council for Medication Error Reporting and Prevention in the USA (2007):

> A medication error is any preventable event that may cause or lead to inappropriate medication use or patient harm while the medication is in the control of the healthcare professional, patient, or consumer. Such events may be related to professional practice, healthcare products, procedures, and systems, including prescribing; order communication; product labelling, packaging, and nomenclature; compounding; dispensing; distribution; administration; education; monitoring; and use.

This definition provides a wide spectrum of potential error, from prescription through to education, and encompasses the system within which the medication is provided. While individuals may provide incorrect doses to wrong patients through the wrong route, there are arguments in the literature which state that the errors spring from a weak system, rather than (simply) an individual weakness. A hospital which allows its staff to keep concentrated potassium where it can be easily accessed has a much higher risk of an adverse drug event than one which stores it only in the pharmacy.

The 'five rights' of medication administration are often quoted in the literature:

- The right patient
- Should receive the right drug
- In the right dose
- At the right time

- Via the right route (NMC 2002).

Checking a patient's wristband before giving them any medication is essential. Every qualified nurse has a story about a patient who cheerfully admitted to being Mrs Smith, and taking her medication, when she was in fact Mrs Jones. Where there are two 'Mrs Smiths' on the ward, special care must be taken. Checking all details on the wristband is a good habit to adopt.

Provision of the right drug should be simple, but occasionally (often due to handwriting issues) is not. If you are not 100% sure what has been written, check it with the prescriber – if you are unable to decipher the prescription, it is unlikely a colleague will have any more luck. If something plainly incorrect has been prescribed (for example, the patient has a documented allergy to penicillin, but augmentin has been prescribed), then this should also be drawn to the prescriber's attention. Many errors of prescription are picked up by nurses and sub-sequently corrected – your vigilance should not stop at ensuring the prescription is correctly spelt, however! You should have an awareness of the appropriateness or otherwise of the drug for the patient – this means ensuring your drug knowledge is current and compre-hensive. This may be difficult initially, but noting each unfamiliar drug you are asked to give, and looking it up in the BNF, will soon ensure you have the necessary knowledge to provide safe care.

Providing the right dose is also fundamental to safe provision of medication. Moving a decimal point in error one place may involve giving 10 times the recommended dose, and mistaking micrograms for milligrams will involve an error in the magnitude of 1000 times the dose! If you find yourself drawing up several vials of a drug, or getting more that two tablets for a dose, it is worth checking to ensure you have the right dose. Always check the strength of the medication you are about to give – something with which you feel you are familiar may have a new supplier, with a different strength. There may be a national shortage of a certain drug, entailing the use of higher strength preparations, or different sizes of the preparation may have different strengths (e.g. enoxaparin, a heparin preparation for injection, has a strength of 100mg/ml in doses up to 100mg, but a strength of 150mg/ml in 120mg and 150mg doses).

Medicines that are prescribed as a weight-related dose (e.g. mg/kg) entail accurate weighing of the patient. Esti-mating weights is very difficult, especially in the prone patient – some medicines have a very narrow effective dose related to the patient's weight, and under- or over-estimating the weight may reduce their effectiveness.

Applying Theory to Practice: Exercise 16.6

Estimate the weight of a variety of your colleagues. Weigh them and check your accuracy. Try the same exercise with patients (where this can be done without causing them discomfort).

Providing medication at the right time is necessary to provide the consistent therapeutic level designed by the drug's manufacturer. Missing doses or providing them early or late may entail unwanted effects or reduced efficacy.

Medication may be given by a variety of routes:

- Oral
- Buccal
- Intravenous
- Aural
- Sublingual
- Rectal
- Nasal
- Transdermal
- Intramuscular
- Subcutaneous
- Inhaled
- Topical
- Vaginal
- Urethral
- Intrathecal.

Medicines are licensed for specific routes – giving an intramuscular injection intravenously, or vice versa, may be painful and ineffective or even deadly. If you are unsure of the correct route, check it.

Applying Theory to Practice: Exercise 16.7

Look up the terms enteral and parenteral in relation to drug administration – place each of the above-mentioned routes into one of the categories.

In addition to the five accepted 'rights' of drug administration, we should add the 'right documentation'. If the drug is not signed for, or timed or dated, there is a risk that the dose may be repeated. By the same token, if a dose is omitted, the reason should be documented and the prescriber contacted if appropriate.

Methods of administration

The correct method of administration must match the route, that is, provision of an intramuscular injection must not be given subcutaneously or intravenously, both of which may occur with incorrect technique.

Oral medication may come in a number of forms, e.g. liquids, tablets, capsules. Patients who have difficulty swallowing will benefit from a liquid formulation – do not crush tablets, or ask the patient to chew or break the tablet, unless specifically instructed to do so. Some oral medications should be taken with food; some before or after – check which one applies and follow the instructions correctly – remember that absorption may be significantly affected if you fail to do so.

Skin patches are used for a variety of sustained release preparations – any previous patches should be removed before the new one is put on. They should be applied to skin that is clean, dry, has little or no hair, and no cuts or irritation (this is why it is best not to shave an area before applying a patch). New patches should be applied in a different area from previous patches. If a patch falls off, you should not try to stick it back on – a new patch will have to be applied.

Suppositories should be inserted by the patient, if they are able to do so, after instruction. Provide the patient with a glove and lubricant. Advise them to lubricate the suppository, lie on their left side, drawing their right leg up, and push the suppository well into the rectum. If a patient is to be sent home with suppositories, they should be advised to keep them in a cool place, as they may melt in warm conditions, making them very difficult to insert. If this occurs, advise the patient to place them in the fridge for a while, where they will re-solidify.

Eye drops should be applied by the patient if they are able to do so. Separate bottles should be provided for each eye to avoid cross-contamination of infection, and labelled as left eye and right eye to avoid confusion. The container should be kept tightly closed to avoid contamination, and should not be allowed to touch the surface of the eye if possible. The patient should wash their hands, tilt back the head, and pull the lower eyelid away from the eye, dropping the required number of drops into the resulting space. They should gently close the eye and keep it closed, without blinking, for one minute. For eye ointment the same technique applies, where a thin strip of ointment is applied to the space – approximately 1cm in length – again without touching the eye, and the eye is closed for one minute.

Ear (otic) drops are applied while lying down so the ear requiring treatment is uppermost, gently pulling the earlobe up and back (down and back for children) and placing the required number of drops into the ear canal. The patient should lie in the same position for five minutes if possible, to allow the drops to fully penetrate the canal. Once again, the container should be kept tightly closed and should not make contact with the ear, to prevent contamination.

Buccal medications should be placed under the upper lip against the gum, or between the cheek and the gum. The tablet should be allowed to dissolve slowly – the patient must be advised not to chew or swallow the tablet. They should not touch it with their tongue, or drink hot fluids while using the medication, as this will increase the rate at which the tablet dissolves. If the patient has a very dry mouth, then moistening the area before placing the tablet will be helpful.

Sublingual medications should be placed under the tongue (as far back as possible) until they melt – the same advice regarding chewing or swallowing of hot fluids applies to these medicines.

Subcutaneous injections are administered into the subcutis, the layer of skin below the dermis, composed primarily of adipose tissue. The small amount of blood flow to fatty tissue means that medication given by this route is absorbed slowly, which makes it a very useful route for giving insulin. The most easily accessed sites for subcutaneous injection are the outer area of the upper arm, the upper outer thigh, or the abdomen (not the 2-inch area around the navel). Injection sites should be rotated to avoid scarring and hardening of the tissue. It is helpful to use the same relative site, however, for insulin injection – e.g. giving the morning injection in the abdomen, and the evening injection in the leg, will provide consistency of absorption for patients on long-term therapy. Grasp the skin between thumb and forefinger as shown in Figure 16.1.

Insert the needle at a 90 degree (right) angle (for people with very little subcutaneous fat, or children, a 45

When administering LMWH squeezing the fat will reduce local haematoma formation due to capillary constriction and reduce pain

Figure 16.1 Subcutaneous injection

degree angle may be used). Release the skin, pull back the plunger of the syringe to ensure you are not in a blood vessel (blood will appear in the syringe if you are – remove the needle and find another site – using a new syringe and medicine) and inject the medication at a slow steady rate.

Intravenous injections are given directly into a vein – normally through an intravenous cannula, but also through 'central' lines, where the cannula is placed in a large vein (usually superior or inferior vena cava). Infection control is extremely important for any procedure involving direct access to the bloodstream – hands should be washed and disposable non-sterile gloves worn when drawing up the injection and during its administration. The cannula site should be examined for signs of infection; if present the cannula should be removed and another one re-sited prior to administration of the medication. (Cannulae should be changed every 72 hours, irrespective of the presence of infection.) Medicines should be prepared and administered using a 'no touch' technique – this means avoiding touching critical areas, such as needles, syringe tops and infusion ports.

Intramuscular (IM) injections offer more rapid absorption than subcutaneous injections, but take effect more slowly than intravenous injections. They are generally given into either the deltoid muscle (upper outer arm, about one-third of the way down the humerus), the vastus lateralis muscle (middle outer third of the thigh muscle), or the gluteus medius muscle – also known as the ventrogluteal route. This is preferable to the better-known dorsogluteal site (the upper outer quadrant of the buttock), as it is less likely to be covered with adipose tissue, and is not near the track of the sciatic nerve. Finding the site is slightly more difficult, but comes easily with practice – place the heel of the hand (left hand for

right hip, right hand for left hip) over the greater trochanter (hip joint) of the femur with fingers pointing towards the patient's head. Place your index finger over the anterior superior iliac spine and the middle finger over the posterior iliac crest. Inject into the triangle formed by the separated fingers (Figure 16.2).

Figure 16.2 Intramuscular injection

Anatomy and Physiology in Action: Exercise 16.8

Examine the anatomy of the deltoid, vastus lateralis and gluteus medius muscles – especially the relevant landmarks for the ventrogluteal route.

Practise locating them on different people.

Prepare the skin by wiping with an alcohol swab and allowing it to dry. Hold the syringe with the thumb and forefinger of the dominant hand, piercing the skin and entering the muscle in a swift but controlled manner to lessen the patient's discomfort. If there is not much muscle mass, especially in children or older patients, you may need to pinch the muscle between finger and thumb to provide more tissue to inject into. Aspirate at the injection site in the same manner as for subcutaneous injection – if blood is aspirated, remove the needle and prepare a new injection for a different site. If no blood is aspirated, slowly inject the medication at a constant rate.

Withdraw the needle quickly to minimise patient discomfort.

Inhaled medications are given by a variety of devices, notably metered dose inhalers (MDIs), nebulisers and rotary inhalers, or other dry powder devices that do not use chemical propellants. Metered dose inhalers are the most commonly used inhalers provided to many asthmatic patients. They provide a measured dose with each triggering, but require a specific technique – the patient must be taught to breathe in as the inhaler is triggered. This is imperative if the medication is to reach the lower airways. Ensuring a patient is able to use their inhaler properly is very important, even if they have been using them for some time – studies show that approximately half of patients with asthma do not use their inhalers correctly (BTS 2005). MDIs can be used with a spacer (Figure 16.3), which allows the patient to simply breathe in and out normally, while still allowing the active medication to access the lungs. This makes it particularly useful for children, who may not comply with an ordinary inhaler.

Nebulisers deliver a fine mist of medication which the patient breathes in through a mask or mouthpiece. They can be driven by oxygen or air – the prescription should make it clear if they are to be air driven, which is sometimes required in patients with long-standing lung disease. These routes can be used to deliver all the major classes of drugs. There is insufficient space in one chapter to review the very large number of medications available, but it is instructive to examine some of the major subdivisions, looking at some of the pitfalls associated with their administration.

Medications

Antibiotics

Antibiotics can be subdivided into bacteriostatic and bacteriocidal medicines. Bacteriostatic medicines do not destroy the invading organism. They work by inhibiting reproduction of the bacteria, allowing the host's natural defences to eventually overcome them. Many organisms are becoming resistant to antibacterial drugs – this may entail modification of treatment, the most important being not using antibiotics where there is no indication for them.

Prior to giving antibiotics it is very important to ask about previous drug reactions – patients may state they are allergic to penicillin, when what they have experienced is a mild sensitisation rash. If a patient reports a previous allergy, however, they should not be given penicillin without discussion with the prescriber, as it can (on rare occasions) cause a rapid and severe anaphylactic reaction. Ideally the patient should be observed for at least 30 minutes after a penicillin injection, especially if there is a history of allergies to drugs or foodstuffs.

Gentamicin is an effective antibiotic when maintained at the correct blood levels. The dose may need to be adjusted based on a 'gentamicin level' which is a blood test usually measured every 48 hours. Gentamicin is

Figure 16.3 Spacer devices

Applying Theory to Practice: Exercise 16.9

Look up the definitions of anaphylactoid and anaphylactic reactions, and the treatment thereof.

Establish how you would provide that treatment in your current practice area.

eliminated via the kidneys, whose function may worsen in acute illness, leading to significant toxicity (Chapter 6). If giving gentamicin, you need to establish that levels have been measured and the dose adjusted as required.

It is very important that patients are advised to take their antibiotics at the recommended intervals and for the full duration of the treatment. Failure to do so may render them ineffective, or worse, may encourage the development of resistant strains of the bacteria – the treatment of these resistant strains may prove to be one of the most significant challenges in medicine over the next 50 years.

Analgesics

Analgesic agents are used to relieve pain. They work at various sites. Opioid drugs work at the level of the brain or spinal cord to reduce the perception of pain. They have powerful central nervous system (CNS) and respiratory depressant effects, potentially producing significant drowsiness. These effects, if severe, may be reversed with the opioid antagonist naloxone, which competes for the opioid binding sites and has a rapid effect – it is often used for patients with a suspected heroin overdose.

Although long-term use of opioid analgesics may encourage dependency, this is not a reason to avoid their use in the short term for patients in pain – patients may need to be reassured that they will not instantly become addicted to morphine from one dose! Morphine is often given intravenously for severe pain. It is generally given as a 1mg/ml injection (10mg made up to 10ml with water for injection) and titrated to the patient's pain – i.e. small amounts are given until the patient's pain is relieved. The results are dependent on the size of the patient and the relative pain – a 100kg man with a partially amputated leg may require significantly more than a 55kg woman with a pretibial laceration! Morphine can precipitate vomiting, and an anti-emetic is often given concurrently (most commonly metoclopramide 10mg IV).

Codeine is a derivative of morphine, with approximately one-seventh of the potency – it is often given combined with paracetamol as a mild oral analgesic. It shares similar properties to morphine and has a significantly constipating effect.

Non-steroidal anti-inflammatory drugs (NSAIDs) are used in the treatment of less severe pain. The term encompasses a large number of drugs, the common feature being suppression of prostaglandins, substances which arise due to cell damage and inflammation, and cause swelling and pain.

Anatomy and Physiology in Action: Exercise 16.10

To gain further insight into common concepts identify the following terms:

- The gate control theory of pain
- Prostaglandin formation

The NSAIDs have analgesic, anti-inflammatory and anti-pyretic properties. Paracetamol has virtually no anti-inflammatory action, but, unlike the other NSAIDs, it does not cause indigestion or gastric bleeding. This is because most NSAIDs block enzymes concerned with the production of prostaglandins cyclooxygenase 1 (COX 1) and cyclooxygenase 2 (COX 2). Prostaglandins produced by COX 2 cause pain and inflammation, but those normally produced by COX 2 have a protective effect on the gastric lining. Giving NSAIDs blocks this protective effect, and may leave the patient susceptible to peptic ulceration, not through the local irritant effect on the stomach lining – giving these drugs via the rectal route can still have the same effects on the stomach. NSAIDs should be cautiously used in the elderly or those patients on warfarin, or with a history of peptic ulceration or bleeding disorders.

Paracetamol, while safe and effective at normal dosage, has a relative low margin of safety (the ratio of drug needed to give adverse effects against therapeutic effects), with only 2–3 times the normal dose potentially precipitating liver damage. Patients who are given a course of paracetamol must be advised to check any other medication they may take to ensure it does not contain paracetamol – many cough, cold and 'flu' remedies contain it.

Applying Theory to Practice: Exercise 16.11

Look up the emergency treatment of poisoning in the BNF; look at both the non-opioid and opioid sections.

Cardiac drugs

An understanding of how cardiac drugs work requires knowledge of the normal cardiac cycle.

Anatomy and Physiology in Action: Exercise 16.12

Study the factors that determine cardiac output, and the causes and consequences of cardiac failure (Chapter 4). Pay attention to the renin-angiotensin mechanism.

Diuretics

Diuretics, no matter what their class, work by decreasing re-absorption of water and electrolytes by the renal tubules. The various classes are: osmotic diuretics, loop diuretics, thiazide diuretics and potassium-sparing diuretics.

Applying Theory to Practice: Exercise 16.13

Look up diuretics in the BNF. Examine the different classes – look at the physiology of the kidneys (Chapter 6) to establish the mechanism for potassium loss with diuretics.

Diuretics are often discontinued by patients because of the need to go more frequently to the toilet, which may be more difficult for patients with infirmities. You should establish the patient's ability to reach the toilet, especially at night, and it may be necessary to provide a commode for the patient's use at home. If the patient develops diarrhoea or vomiting, the diuretic should be temporarily discontinued, to minimise fluid and electrolyte loss.

Digoxin

Digoxin has two effects that make it a useful cardiac drug – it has a positive inotropic effect (this means it strengthens the heart), and it slows the heart through its effect on the parasympathetic nervous system. In order to obtain a rapid effect, digoxin is often given with a loading dose, which serves to obtain an effective level of the circulating drug as quickly as possible. The patient's apical heart rate (Chapter 4) should always be checked before giving digoxin – if less than 60, you should withhold the drug and discuss with the prescriber.

Antihypertensives

There are a number of classes of antihypertensive drugs:

- Vasodilators act on the smooth muscle cells of blood vessels to decrease peripheral resistance to blood flow.
- Sympathetic blocking drugs also decrease peripheral resistance by blocking vasoconstrictor nerve supply to small arteries and arterioles.
- Angiotensin-converting enzyme (ACE) inhibitors work by inhibiting the conversion of angiotensin 1 to angiotensin 2, which inhibits the release of aldosterone, further reducing sodium retention. Since water follows sodium, the effect is to reduce the circulating volume, and consequently the blood pressure falls.

Applying Theory to Practice: Exercise 16.14

Find the section on hypertension in the BNF.

- Find an example of each of the classes of drug
- Write a short description of each class

This knowledge or insight will gain you respect from clinical mentors.

In addition to providing medication, you should give patients advice on diet, lifestyle and smoking cessation. If antihypertensives are ineffective, it should be established that they are being taken appropriately. Patients sometimes stop medications because of the troublesome side-effects from these drugs (e.g. persistent dry cough with ACE inhibitors, syncope).

Whatever drug you are giving, the correct dose is critical. A significant source of ADEs is the provision of a wrong dose (DoH 2004). While the majority of these are not fatal, they are never acceptable, and the practitioners responsible may feel that the subsequent problem far outweighs the small amount of trouble required to ensure a correct dose.

Drug calculations

In order to perform drug calculations correctly, you must be able to manipulate the values of the accepted international scale of weight (kilogram, kg) and volume (litre, L) the *système internationale* or SI units. Understanding the sizes of the relevant units and how they relate to each other is fundamental to correctly calculating doses.

Various other units are used to denote sizes that are smaller than the standard unit, e.g. 1 kg is 1000 grams (g). Rather than writing 0.75kg, it is conventional to use the smaller unit for clarity, i.e. 750g, unless the larger unit is exceeded, e.g. 1300g = 1.3kg. Weight equivalents are:

- 1 kilogram (kg) = 1000 grams (g)
- 1 gram (g) = 1000 milligrams (mg)
- 1 milligram (mg) = 1000 micrograms (should not be abbreviated)
- 1 microgram = 1000 nanograms (should not be abbreviated)
- 1 nanogram = 1000 picograms (should not be abbreviated).

The only volume equivalent you will probably require in practice is 1 litre (L) = 1000 millilitres (mL), (1000 microlitres = 1 mL). The capital 'L' is often used to denote litres, as the small 'l' is easily mistaken for a figure 1.

In order to convert from a larger unit to a smaller unit, you therefore simply need to multiply by multiples of 1000 (e.g. 1mg = 1000 micrograms, but also 1,000,000 nanograms (1000 x 1000). In contrast, to convert from a smaller to larger unit, you need to divide by multiples of 1000 (e.g. 1500mL = 1.5L). Conversions between units can be made by simply by moving the decimal point three places to the left to divide by 1000 (e.g. 1750 mL = 1.75L)

Applying Theory to Practice: Exercise 16.15

Convert the following units:
A) 0.066g to milligrams
B) 1.35mg to micrograms
C) 4.4 Litres to millilitres
D) 0.06g to micrograms (careful with this one – check your units)
E) 1600 micrograms to milligrams
F) 2200 mg to kilograms (check your units again!)

Answers are found in Answers to Box 16.11.

or three places to the right to multiply by 1000 (e.g. 3g = 3000mg).

Medicines can also be expressed as a weight contained in a given volume – e.g. epinephrine is often prescribed as either 1 in 1000 or 1 in 10,000. While this may appear confusing, if you understand that the first figure relates to the weight in grams, and the second to the volume in ml, it becomes clearer – 1 in 1000 means there is 1g of epinephrine in 1000mL, whereas 1 in 10,000 means there is 1g in 10,000mL. Further subdivision enables us to obtain a realistic dose – if 1000mL contains 1g, it also contains 1000mg (1g = 1000mg), giving us a strength of 1mg in 1mL. In contrast, 1mL of 1 in 10,000 will contain only 100 micrograms.

You may also see moles or millimoles mentioned on some medication doses – e.g. 10mL of 10% calcium chloride (the dose given in cardiac arrest) contains 6.8mmol (millimoles) of calcium. This is a complex measurement of the amount of a substance based on the relative atomic weights of its constituent atoms. You should not have to deal with millimoles in your everyday practice (except when recording a patient's blood sugar, which is also measured in mmol).

Once you are able to easily convert between the units, you can use various methods to work out the amount of medication you need to provide. If you are asked to give 500mg of paracetamol, and you have 500mg tablets, then no calculation is required! Where your medication strength does not exactly match what you have, or where the strength of medication contained in a liquid is required, you will find it helpful to use one of the methods below.

Calculating the number of tablets

If you divide the dose that has been prescribed (what you want) by the strength of the tablet that you have (what you have), this will provide you with the number of tablets you need. Ensure that the units you are using are the same, so dividing 500(mg) by 500(mg) is fine, but dividing 500(mg) by 0.5(g) will give you a quite different answer!

For example – you have 25mg tablets of diclofenac, and you have been asked to give 75mg. Dividing what you want (the prescribed dose of 75mg) by what you have (25mg tablets) tells you 3 tablets to administer:

$$\frac{\text{(What you want) 75mg}}{\text{(What you have) 25mg}} = 3$$

Calculating solutions/mixtures/injection volumes

This is slightly more complex. A tablet contains a specific amount of medication in each unit – e.g. paracetamol has 500mg in each tablet. Solutions are the same, but the ratio varies – e.g. amoxicillin comes as 125mg in 5mL and 250mg in 5mL strengths. This adds an additional step to your calculations.

You start by dividing your prescribed dose (what you want) by the stock strength (let us use amoxicillin 125mg/5mL, so our stock strength in this case is 125mg).

You then need to multiply the resulting figure by the stock volume (in this case 5mL) to give the amount of solution in mL. In this example, if we wanted to give 250mg, using the 125mg/5mL solution, we have the calculation:

$$\frac{\text{(What you want) 250mg}}{\text{(Stock strength) 125mg}} (2) \times \text{(stock volume) 5mL} = 10ml$$

If we still wanted 250mg, but were using the 250mg/5mL solution, our calculation would read:

$$\frac{\text{(What you want) 250mg}}{\text{(Stock strength) 250mg}} (1) \times \text{(stock volume) 5mL} = 5ml$$

A number of drugs are prescribed based on the patient's body weight. This simply involves an additional step prior to the drug calculation – e.g. the patient is prescribed a drug at 30 micrograms per kilogram body weight. To derive the dose required, a simple multiplication of the patient's weight in kg (e.g. 75kg) by the amount per kg (in this case 30 micrograms) gives a dose of 30 x 75 = 2250 micrograms. The dose calculation can then be processed in the normal fashion.

In addition to dosage calculations, you may be required to calculate the rate of an infusion. Infusion pumps provide a continuous infusion at a given rate, so it is important to be able to programme them to ensure an accurate hourly dose is delivered.

To calculate the flow rate, the prescribed volume (in mL) is divided by the duration of the infusion (in hours) – e.g. 1000 mL over 4 hours requires a flow rate of 1000/4 = 250 mL per hour.

Calculating the rate of an infusion which contains a medication requires a further step – first, the stock concentration must be calculated – this is the medication strength (generally in mg) divided by the volume of infu-

sion fluid in which it is contained – e.g. if we add 900mg of amiodarone to 500mL of dextrose, we have a stock concentration of 900/500 = 1.8mg/mL. Working out the required infusion rate (in mL/hour) then involves dividing the dose required (in mg/hour) by the stock concentration – e.g. if we want a rate of 60mg hour, the calculation will be 60/1.8, which gives an infusion rate of 33.3 mL/hour.

If you are asked for a minute rate (e.g. 1mg/min), then deriving an hourly rate simply involves multiplying the minute rate by 60 to give the hourly rate.

It is rare that you will have to prepare medications on your own. If you are in any way unsure, get someone to check your calculations. A few seconds spent checking a dosage or unfamiliar medicine may save you many weeks of anguish, and perhaps the life of your patient.

Applying Theory to Practice: Box 16.1 Answers to Exercise 16.15

A) 66mg (1000 x 0.066 – decimal point moves 3 places to the right)
B) 1350 micrograms (1000 x 1.35 – decimal point moves 3 places to the right)
C) 4400 mL (4.4 x 1000 – decimal point moves 3 places to the right)
D) 60000 micrograms (0.06 x 1,000,000 – decimal point moves 6 places to the right)
E) 1.6 milligrams (1600/1000 – decimal point moves 3 places to the left)
F) 0.0022 kilograms (2200/1,000,000 – decimal point moves 6 places to the left)

Conclusion

Accurate and competent drug calculations are part of every qualified nurse's clinical armament. You should ensure that you feel competent and confident to undertake the calculations discussed in this chapter before venturing to prepare infusions or undertake a drug round. The most important attribute is not a mathematical turn of mind, however, but rather a commitment to safety and accuracy in the patient's best interest. This is the cornerstone of all excellent nursing care. By demonstrating to your mentors or preceptors in clinical practice that you have some insight into medications and how to calculate the dose, you are far more likely to receive beneficial input from them. If at the start of your placements they identify you know little about commonly used medications they potentially will not trust you to administer drugs. When asked by mentors about drugs, never lie, be honest, no-one expects you to know every drug in the BNF! Both pharmacology and drug calculations play a major role in your future chosen career; remember practice may not make you perfect but it certainly helps.

Chapter 16 Summary Quiz

1. Drug metabolism is affected by relative:

A. Hormone secretion
B. Kidney function
C. Liver function
D. Clotting factors

2. Drug excretion is affected by relative:

A. Blood volume
B. Plasma concentration
C. Kidney function
D. Liver function

3. Which of the following is not one of the 'five rights' of medication administration?

A. The right patient
B. At the right time
C. Administered by the right person
D. Via the right route

4. Medication may be given by a variety of routes, which of the following is not one?

A. Oral
B. Rectal
C. Nasal
D. Mural

5. Subcutaneous injections are administered into the subcutis, the layer of skin below the dermis, composed primarily of:

A. Adipose tissue
B. Connective tissue
C. Elastic tissue
D. Muscle tissue

6. Into which of the following areas is a intramuscular injection not given?

A. The deltoid

B. The vastus lateralis

C. The pectoral muscle

D. The gluteus medius

7. Which of the following is not a class of antibiotic?

A. Penicillin

B. Cephalosporins

C. Macrolides

D. Aminoglycosides

8. What is the antagonist for opioids?

A. Naloxone

B. Protamine sulphate

C. Vitamin K

D. Charcoal

9. Which of the following is a side-effect of morphine?

A. Constipation

B. Respiratory arrest

C. Sedation

D. All of the above

10. Which of the following does not lower blood pressure?

A. ACE Inhibitors

B. Beta blockers

C. Calcium channel blockers

D. Histamine antagonists

Further reading

Department of Health (1988) *Guidelines for the Safe and Secure Handling of Medicines* (Duthie Report). DH: London. (This document is currently under review by the Royal Pharmaceutical Society.)

Department of Health (1999) *Review of Prescribing Supply and Administration of Medicines, Final Report.* DH: London.

Department of Health (2004) *Building a Safer NHS for Patients. Improving Medication Safety.* DH: London.

Green, B. & Gould, D. (2004) *Trounce's Clinical Pharmacology for Nurses*, 17th edn. Churchill Livingstone: London.

National Coordinating Council for Medication Error Reporting and Prevention (2007) *About Medication Errors: Definition.* http://www.nccmerp.org/aboutMedErrors.html (accessed 10 Feb. 2007).

Nursing and Midwifery Council (NMC) (2004). *Guidelines for the Administration of Medicines.* NMC: London.

The Medicines Act 1968. http://www.aroma-science.com/new/legislation/medicines_act_1968.htm (accessed 04/07/06).

http://www.testandcalc.com/quiz/index.asp

References

British Thoracic Society (BTS) and Scottish Intercollegiate Guidelines Network (SIGN) (2005) *British Guidelines on the Management of Asthma: A National Clinical Guideline*, revised edn. BTS & SIGN: London.

Department of Health (2004) *Building a Safer NHS for Patients. Improving Medication Safety.* DH: London.

McGavock, H. (2005) *How Drugs Work*, 2nd edn. Radcliffe: Oxford.

National Coordinating Council for Medication Error Reporting

and Prevention (2007) *About Medication Errors: Definition.* http://www.nccmerp.org/aboutMedErrors.html (accessed 10 Feb. 2007).

Nursing and Midwifery Council (NMC) (2002) *Code of Professional Conduct.* NMC: London.

Ryan, AA. & Chambers, M. (2000) Medication management and older patients: an individualised and systematic approach. *Journal of Clinical Nursing* 9: 732–41.

Glossary

A

Abrasions: (graze) superficial area of skin loss normally caused by friction.

Absorption the taking up of substances by the mucous membranes of the digestive tract.

Acetylcholine: Acetylcholine is one of many neurotransmitters in the autonomic nervous system (ANS) and the only neurotransmitter used in the somatic nervous system (SNS).

Acid base balance: the equilibrium between acid and alkaline necessary to maintain homeostasis. For the blood to function at an optimum level the serum pH must remain between 7.35 and 7.45.

Acidosis: is an increased acidity of the blood plasma, acidosis is said to occur when arterial pH falls below 7.35.

Action potentials: describes the cycle of events leading to a cell becoming electrically positive on the inside.

Acute coronary syndromes (ACS): is a set of signs and symptoms, usually a combination of chest pain and other features, interpreted as being the result of abruptly decreased blood flow to the heart.

Acute myocardial infarction (AMI): occurs when the blood supply to a part of the heart is interrupted. The resulting ischemia causes damage and potential death of heart tissue.

Adrenal insufficiency crisis: failure of the adrenal glands to secrete essential hormones i.e. mineralocorticoid and Glucocorticoids, if untreated will become life threatening.

Aetiology: the study of the causation of disease and how illness is introduced to the host.

Afferent: carrying towards - an afferent nerve carries impulses from the body to the brain.

Agonist: In pharmacology pertains to an excitory effect.

Allergens: a substance capable of inducing an allergic reaction, includes animal hairs, proteins and dust.

Allergic Reaction: being affected by an allergen, can result in various symptoms including a running nose, itchy skin and urticaria. Severe reactions can result in an anaphylactic reaction.

Alzheimer's Disease: a progressive form of **dementia**. Characterised by personality changes, disorientation and memory loss.

Amputations: can occur when a body part such as a toe or finger are partially or completely cut off.

Anaemia: collective term used to describe the end result of many disease processes in which the blood cannot carry enough oxygen.

Analgesics: pain killers; can be split into two main groups: Narcotics and non-Narcotics.

Anaphylaxis: A severe allergic reaction resulting in shock development.

Aneurisms: a localized, blood-filled dilation of a blood vessel caused by disease or weakening of the vessel wall.

Angioplasty/Percutaneous coronary interventions: the mechanical widening of a narrowed or totally obstructed blood vessel.

Antagonist pertains to an inhibitory effect.

Antibodies: cells that destroy or render foreign substances inactive.

Anti-Diuretic Hormone: a hormone found in most mammals, including humans. One of its most important roles is to regulate the body's retention of water, being released when the body is dehydrated; it causes the kidneys to conserve water, but not salt, by concentrating the urine and reducing urine volume.

Anti-platelet agents: drugs that reduce platelet activity, including aspirin and clopidogrel.

Antipyrexials: Medications such as Paracetamol used to reduce a patient's temperature.

Apex: anatomical term used to describe the top or tip (pointed end) of an organ or body.

Aphasia: deficient in use of language, usually due to damage to the cerebral hemisphere.

Apnoea: suspension of external breathing.

Appendicitis: inflammation of the appendix, can be life-threatening.

Apraxia: inability to maintain posture or perform learned movements.

Arachnoid membrane: a thin, delicate layer loosely covering the brain.

Arachnoid villi: point where most of the CSF is reabsorbed.

Arteriosclerosis: a disease affecting arterial blood vessels. It is a chronic inflammatory response in the walls of arteries, in large part due to the deposition of lipoproteins.

Articular cartilage: surface material of a joint.

Ascites: is an accumulation of fluid in the peritoneal cavity, attributed to cirrhosis in 75% of cases.

Aseptic: without disease, free from pathogens.

Asphyxia: a condition of severely deficient supply of oxygen to the body that arises from being unable to breathe normally.

Asthma: a disease synomimous with bronchial constriction and over production of mucous. Can be seasonal or brittle. A hypersensitivity reaction.

Asymptomatic: without symptoms.

Asystole: an absence of electromechanical activity throughout the heart traditionally referred to as a 'flat line'.

Atheromatous deposits: disposition of hard plaques of fat within the arteries.

Atherosclerosis: Fatty deposits that adhere to the inner lumen of arteries.

Atrial fibrillation: is a cardiac arrhythmia that involves the two upper chambers (atria) of the heart fibrillating rather than pumping in unison. It is defined as being irregularly irregular, and can often be identified as such when taking a pulse.

Atrioventricular (AV) node: an area of specialised tissue between the atria and the ventricles of the heart, which conducts the normal electrical impulse from the atria to the ventricles.

Auscultation: the technical term for listening to the internal sounds of the body, usually using a stethoscope.

Autonomic nervous system (ANS) regulating activity of smooth muscles, cardiac muscles and glands. Its activity is involuntary, outside of our control. The ANS is functionally divided into the parasympathetic and the sympathetic branches.

Autosomal recessive gene disorder: both parents need to carry the same altered gene, resulting in a 1:4 risk of having a child affected by the condition.

Avascular necrosis: reduction or cessation of blood flood to an area eventually causing death, the scaphoid bone provides an example.

Avulsions: forcing and tearing away of a body part or internal structure such as a small fragment of bone from a ligament.

Axons: the conducting area of a nerve cell. Electric impulses are conducted away from the cell body.

Azotaemia: The pathological presence of nitrogenous wastes, principally urea within the blood, commonly seen in renal failure, gastrointestinal haemorrhage and dehydration.

B

Bacteria: unicellular microorganisms, some of which can cause bacterial disease.

Bacteriocidal: destroy bacteria.

Bacteriostatic: inhibiting reproduction process of a bacteria.

Baroreceptors: detect the pressure of blood flowing through them, and can send messages to the central nervous system to increase or decrease total peripheral resistance and cardiac output.

Basal ganglia: area of the brain concerned with modifying and coordinating voluntary muscle movement.

Basal metabolic rate (BMR): the amount of energy, which is needed to maintain physiological equilibrium whilst at rest in a fasted state (kcal/day).

Beta-blockers: a class of drugs used for various indications, but particularly for the management of cardiac arrhythmias and cardioprotection after myocardial infarction.

Beta 2 agonists: drugs such as Salbutamol that cause relaxation of bronchial muscles, elevate blood pressure and increase the heart rate.

Bile: alkaline green/yellow fluid secreted by the liver and stored in the gallbladder. Aids digestion by emulsifying fats within the duodenum.

Bioavailability: how much and how quickly a drug reaches its intended target.

BIPAP: Bi-level Positive Airway Pressure; a breathing assisting device that is worn over the mouth or nose.

Bi-polar disorder: affects mood, thinking and behaviour and is characterised by mood swings. When in a high phase the person can display grandiose behaviour and express delusions but when low they become deeply depressed and due to the impulsive and emotion driven nature of the condition there is a high risk of suicide.

Bisphosphates: drugs that bind directly to bone

minerals because of their specific chemical structure. Once bound to the bone, these drugs inhibit bone loss by reducing the action of bone cells that normally degrade bone during the remodeling process.

Bladder: a hollow, muscular, and distensible organ that sits on the pelvic floor. It is the organ that collects urine excreted by the kidneys prior to disposal by urination.

Blood pressure: the force exerted by circulating blood on the walls of blood vessels, one of the principal vital signs.

Body Mass Index (BMI) chart: a scale designed to identify extremes of weight. Has been controversial due to its inability to be consistent with varying client demographics.

Bradyarrhythmias: abnormal and slow heart rates. Can result in haemodynamic collapse and cardiac arrest.

Bradykinesia is difficulty initiating movement and maintaining it. A patient will have a stooped posture and will move with a shuffling gait, they may loose their balance easily and fall. They can also have an expressionless face and blink infrequently

Brain stem: area of the brain containing the pons varolli, medulla oblongata and midbrain.

Broad complex tachycardia: a rate exceeding 100 per minute that may be of ventricular origin i.e. delayed.

Broad-spectrum antibiotic: an antibiotic with activity against a wide range of disease-causing bacteria.

Broca's area: motor control or area of speech within the cerebrum.

Bundle of His: a collection of heart muscle cells specialized for electrical conduction that transmits the electrical impulses from the AV node (located between the atria and the ventricles) to the point of the apex of the fascicular branches.

C

Calcification: hardening of an anatomical region caused by calcium salt deposits.

Calorigenic effect: heat and energy producing effect.

Cannula: indwelling device such as a venous cannula.

Capillary refill time: the rate at which blood refills empty capillaries. It can be measured by pressing a fingernail until it turns white, and taking note of the time needed for color to return once the nail is released. Normal refill time is less than 2 seconds. The capillary refill time (**CRT**) is a common measure of peripheral perfusion.

Cardiac Arrest: the sudden cessation of cardiac function, resulting in the loss of effective circulation

Cardiac cycle: is the term referring to all or any of the events related to the flow of blood that occur from the beginning of one heartbeat to the beginning of the next.

Cardiac output: is the product of the heart rate multiplied by the stroke volume (HRxSV=CO)

Cardiogenic Shock: is based upon an inadequate circulation of blood due to primary failure of the ventricles of the heart to function effectively.

Cardiovascular disease (CVD): is the collective name given to diseases affecting the heart and circulatory system

Cataracts: progressively developing clouding of the lens of the eye. Can be surgically removed.

Catecholamines: chemical compounds derived from the amino acid tyrosine containing catechol and amine groups i.e adrenaline/noradrenaline.

Central line: an indwelling venous or arterial cannula.

Central nervous system (CNS): the brain, spinal cord and nerves.

Cerebellum: the small area at the back of the brain, responsible for coordination of fine voluntary movements.

Cerebral Cortex: the outermost cellular layer of grey matter covering the cerebrum; controls higher mental activities.

Cerebral dominance: the dominance of activity between left and right sides of the brain.

Cerebral hemispheres are made up of four pairs of lobes: frontal, parietal, temporal and occipital.

Cerebrospinal fluid (CSF): a clear, colourless, odourless liquid that surrounds the brain and the spinal cord. It acts as a shock absorber, floating and cushioning the brain and spinal cord from trauma.

Cerebrovascular accident (CVA): is defined as a sudden loss of brain function leading to a neurological deficit that lasts for 24 hours or more.

Cerebrum: main part of the brain identified in pictures i.e. the largest part.

Chain of survival: Several key actions have been identified that improve the management of patient's potentially or actively experiencing cardiac arrest.

Chlamydia: a parasitic organism, commonly implicated in sexually transmitted infections.

Chloramphenicol: a bacteriostatic antibiotic, commonly used for eye infections.

Cholecystitis: (inflammation of the gallbladder) occurs when stones block the outflow of bile. The bile becomes concentrated and infected leading to a swollen and oedematous gallbladder. The patient presents with severe

right upper quadrant pain, fever, and occasionally jaundice. Cholecystitis can be acute or chronic and is treated by surgical removal of the gallbladder (**cholecystectomy**).

Choroid plexuses: projections of blood vessels from the pia mater into each of the ventricles of the brain.

Chronic obstructive pulmonary disease: a chronic and debilitating disease continuum in which localised irritation of the bronchioles and lungs results in increasing airflow obstruction which is usually progressive.

Chyme: partially digested food passing from the stomach into the small intestine.

Ciliated tissue: cells or tissue containing hair like projections, found in the airway tracts.

Circle of Willis: the anterior (carotid) circulation and the posterior (vertebrobasilar) circulation unite to become the arterial anastamosis.

Cirrhosis: Irreversible fibrosis (scarring) and the development of nodules severely affect liver function.

Clotting factors: Specific components of blood that combine to stop bleeding.

Coeliac disease: an autoimmune disorder of the small bowel that occurs in genetically predisposed people of all ages from middle infancy.

Colloids: thick fluids such as gelofusion which remain in the blood stream, referred to as plasma expanders.

Congenital: from birth.

CPAP: a device that delivers 'continuous positive airway pressure', regardless of inspiration or expiration making the effort to breathe easier. Can be delivered via mouth, nose or via breathing tubes.

C reactive protein (CRP): A globulin that appears in the blood in certain acute inflammatory conditions, such as infections.

Crepitus: cracking sound commonly found in arthritic joints and fractures.

Creutzfeldt-Jakob disease (CJD): a form of encephalopathy of viral origin.

Crystalloids: a fluid containing a true solution i.e. physiological saline.

Cyclizine: an anti-emetic.

Cystic fibrosis: a hereditary disease that mainly affects the lungs and digestive system, causing progressive disability and for some, early death.

Cystitis: inflammation of the bladder.

Cytology: study of the function and pathology of body cells.

D

Dalton's law: states that the pressure exerted by a mixture of gases are equal to the sum of the partial pressures of the gases in mixture.

Decussate: (decussation) the crossing of symmetrical structures in the form of an X.

Defibrillation: the application of an electrical current to the heart muscle may result in the chaotic rhythm and fibrillating muscle mass becoming organised again, thereby returning a cardiac output.

Delusions: abnormal beliefs that are not real.

Dementia: is not a disease but a group of symptoms which occur as a result of a number of different illnesses but which all cause degenerative changes in brain tissue leading to a progressive decline in cognitive functioning.

Dendrites: associated with each cell body creating a vast surface area to receive nerve impulses.

Depolarisation: discharging of an electrical current.

Depression: Although common, clinical depression is associated to the individual's ability to cope with everyday life.

Dermis: the true skin lying beneath the epidermis.

Diabetes mellitus: is a disease characterized by disordered metabolism and inappropriately high blood sugar (hyperglycemia) resulting from either low levels of the hormone insulin or from abnormal resistance to insulin's effects coupled with inadequate levels of insulin secretion to compensate.

Diaphragm: a sheet of muscle separating the thorax and abdomen.

Diarrhoea is defined as the abnormal passage of loose or liquid stools more than three times per day.

Diastole: the relaxation phase (filling) phase.

Diencephalon: part of the cerebrum containing the thalamus, hypothalamus and most of the third ventricle.

Diffusion: the net movement of particles from an area of high concentration to an area of low concentration.

Dimorphic: meaning it is both functionally and structurally different in males and females.

Diplegia: either arms or legs are affected.

Distribution: the passing or delivery of a substance within or throughout the body.

Distributive shock: as in hypovolemic shock, caused by an insufficient intravascular volume of blood. This form of relative hypovolemia is the result of blood vessel dilation, i.e septic shock and anaphlaxis.

Diverticular disease: inflammation of the diverticula, can lead to bleeding and ulceration.

Domperidone: anti-emetic.

Do Not Attempt Resuscitation Orders (DNAR): relates to the act of administering CPR. All UK hospitals should have an agreed DNAR policy, based on national guidelines.

Dopamine: Found mainly in the substantia nigra in the mid brain and in the basal ganglia. Its effect is the coordination of movement and control of behaviour.

Down's syndrome: a congenital anomaly affecting chromosome 21. Those affected experience mental and physical compromise.

Doxycycline: antibiotic.

Duodenum: 25cm long and containing the sphincter of Oddi where the common bile duct joins the small intestine

Dura mater: is the outermost layer of the meninges. It is a tough double-layered membrane attached to the bones of the cranium, housing the veins and arteries supplying the skull.

Dysarthria: difficulty in articulating words.

Dyspepsia: characterised by heartburn and a feeling of fullness.

Dysphagia: is the name for difficulty in swallowing and is common.

Dysuria: difficulty passing urine.

E

ECG -12 lead (electrocardiogram): uses 10 actual positions, but through combining some of these reveals 12 actual views of heart activity.

Effusion: the escape of fluid into a tissue or cavity.

Electrolytes: a liquid or fluid capable of conducting electricity.

Embolus: a clot originating from another area (clot on the trot).

Empyema: a collection of pus within the pleural cavity.

Epidemiology: studying the causes, incidence, distribution and control of disease in a population.

Epidermis: the external, non-vascular layer of the skin.

Epididymis: surrounds the testis conveying the spermatozoa from the testis to the vas deferens.

Epilepsy: a condition associated with convulsions, caused by an abnormal discharge of nerve impulses in the brain.

Epinephrine: a hormone when carried in the blood and a neurotransmitter when it is released across a neuronal synapse. It is a catecholamine, a sympathomimetic monoamine derived from the amino acids phenylalanine and tyrosine.

Epithelium: a tissue composed of a layer of cells, Epithelium lines both the outside (skin) and the inside cavities and lumen of bodies.

Epstein-Barr virus: a virus of the herpes family (which includes *Herpes simplex virus* and *Cytomegalovirus*), and is one of the most common viruses in humans.

Equinus position: people with equinus develop ways to "compensate" for their limited ankle movement, often leading to long term foot, leg and back problems. The most common methods of compensation are flattening of the arch or picking up the heel early when walking, placing increased pressure on the ball of the foot. Patients compensate by "toe walking", whilst others take steps by bending abnormally at the hip or knee.

Erythrocytes: red blood cells.

Erythropoietin: the production of red blood cells.

Euthanasia: the act of terminating the life of another who is experiencing irreversible illness or pain.

External respiration: the exchange of gases between the atmosphere and the pulmonary loop of circulation including the lungs.

Exudate: fluid that passes through a vessel or membrane into surrounding space or tissues.

F

Fallopian tubes: ducts that open out of the upper part of the uterus.

Fascia: the soft tissue component of the connective tissue system that permeates the human body. It interpenetrates and surrounds muscles, bones, organs, nerves, blood vessels and other structures.

Fascicles of the bundle of His/Purkinje fibres: a small group of nerve or muscle fibres.

Fasciotomy: incision of a fascia.

Filtrate: the liquid produced after filtering a suspension of a solid in a liquid.

Foetus: an unborn child.

Follicle-stimulating hormone (FSH): stimulates the graafian follicles of the ovary, in men stimulates the production of spermatozoa.

Fovea: a area of the retina, which is densely populated by cone, cells and limited numbers of cone cells.

Frank haematuria: presence of fresh blood in the urine.

Frank-Starling law/principle: The greater the stretch of the myocardium the greater the force of contraction.

Frazer Competence: Children are not deemed to be automatically legally competent to give consent. The

courts have determined that children can be legally competent if they have "sufficient understanding and intelligence to enable him or her to understand fully what is proposed". This concept is known as Gillick competency. The term Fraser competency is also used in this respect as Lord Fraser was the judge who sat on the case.

G

Gamma-amino butyric acid (GABA): Located in the hypothalamus, cerebellum, basal ganglia and spinal cord. It is the main inhibitory neurotransmitter.

Gametes: mature reproductive cell.

Gestation: the development process between conception to birth.

Glandular fever: *Infectious mononucleosis*, (also known as the kissing disease) is seen most commonly in adolescents and young adults, characterized in teenagers by fever, sore throat, muscle soreness, and fatigue.

Glaucoma: collective term used to describe diseases that damage the optic nerve caused be the effects of a raised ocular pressure.

Glial cells: supportive cells in the central nervous system. Glial cells do not conduct electrical impulses, they surround neurons and provide support and insulation between them.

Glomerular filtration rate (GFR) the rate at which plasma is passed through the gromeruli.

Glomerulus: minute section of the kidney containing arterial capillaries and connective tissue.

Glutamate: Widespread in the CNS where it has an excitatory effect. It is important in learning and memory.

Gonads: essential sex glands.

Glomerular filtration rate: the volume of fluid filtered from the renal (kidney) glomerular capillaries into the Bowman's capsule per unit time. Clinically, this is often measured to determine renal function.

Gluconeogenesis: manufactures new glucose from amino acids and glycerol when blood levels are low and glycogen stores are exhausted.

Glycogenesis: converts glucose to glycogen for storage.

Glycogenolysis: converts glycogen back to glucose for release into blood following secretion of glucagon by the pancreas.

Glucometer: a small medical device that tests the amount of sugar in the blood, taken from a finger prick.

Granulocytes: a category of white blood cells characterised by the presence of granules in their cytoplasm.

Grey matter: nervous system tissue consisting of cell bodies.

Guedel Airway: orophangeal airway device.

Guillan Barre Syndrome: the patient may complain of muscle weakness in the distal limbs and often numbness in the same region too. Gradually this weakness and numbness progresses and ascends, it can occur over several days or take up to several weeks to progress.

H

Haematemesis: vomiting blood associated with an upper GI bleed. Fresh blood is bright red and old brown blood is termed 'coffee grounds'.

Haematuria: Presence of blood in the urine; can be microscopic.

Haemoarthrosis: blood within a joint space, definition may also include synovial fluid or pus.

Haemodynamic collapse: loss of circulating volume or severe dilation of vessels resulting in a massive drop in blood pressure.

Haemoglobin: the iron-containing oxygen-transport metalloprotein in the red blood cells of the blood.

Haemolysis: the breaking open of red blood cells and the release of haemoglobin into the surrounding fluid.

Haemoptysis: describes the coughing-up of blood

Hallucinations: the feeling of having an experience, which is not real.

Haversian canals: These run longitudinally through compact bone and contain blood, containing lymph capillaries and nerves.

Head Tilt chin lift: manouvere opening the airway in an unconscious or arrested patient.

Heart attack: see acute myocardial infarction.

Heart blocks: a disease in the electrical system of the heart.

Heart rate: a term used to describe the frequency of the cardiac cycle. Usually it is calculated as the number of contractions (heart beats) of the heart in one minute and expressed as beats per minute (bpm).

Hemiparesis: (weakness) or paralysis affecting one side of the body.

Hemiplegia: paralysis affecting the arm and leg on one side of the body.

Heparin: naturally occurring anticoagulant, commonly used in immobile patients to prevent thrombosis.

Hepatic Encephalopathy is a reversible state of impaired cognitive function due to advanced liver disease.

Hepatitis (Alcoholic): (inflammation of the liver) occurs

in 20-30% of patients with a fatty liver who continue to drink, and may be mild, severe and life threatening. LFTs are raised and the patient may be jaundiced with right upper quadrant pain and nausea.

Hereditary: genetic factors responsible for the presence of particular characteristics in successive generations.

Herpes: a sexually transmitted, double-stranded DNA virus, called *herpes simplex virus* (HSV) type 2. This virus is closely related to herpes simplex virus type 1, which is the cause of common non-sexually-transmitted cold sores.

Hilum: concave in shape. This is where the nerves, blood and lymphatic vessels enter the kidney.

Homunculus: a small model of the human body.

Human chorionic Gonadotrophin (HCG): produced in the placenta during the first trimester of pregnancy, its presence in blood or urine confirms pregnancy.

Human Immunodeficiency Virus (HIV): virus that causes **AIDS**.

Humidified oxygen: adding moisture to supplementary oxygen to prevent the drying out of membranes and components of the respiratory tract.

Hydrocephalus: an excess of cerebral spinal fluid within the brain or the membranes. May be caused by infection, tumour or developmental anomalies.

Hydrostatic pressure: the pressure exerted by blood or other body fluids.

Hypercapnia: a condition where there is too much carbon dioxide (CO_2) in the blood.

Hypercholesterolaemia: is the presence of high levels of cholesterol in the blood.

Hyperglycaemia: results when there is a lack of the hormone **insulin.**

Hypersensitivity reaction: an exaggerated internal response to an allergen.

Hypertension: commonly referred to as high blood pressure, is a medical condition in which the blood pressure is chronically elevated.

Hypertrophy: the increase of the size of an organ or in a select area of the tissue.

Hypothalamus: links the nervous system to the endocrine system via the pituitary gland. The hypothalamus is located below the thalamus, just above the brain stem.

Hypoxaemia: is a pathological condition in which the body as a whole (generalised hypoxia) or region of the body (tissue hypoxia) is deprived of adequate oxygen supply

Hypoxia: see hypoxaemia.

Hypovolaemic Shock: a state of decreased blood volume; more specifically, decrease in volume of blood plasma.

I

Iatrogenic: ill health or adverse effect or complication caused by or resulting from medical treatment.

Idiopathic: no known cause.

Immunodeficiency: the inability or inadequacy of the immune system to respond effectively, leaving the body's defence system depleted and the individual vulnerable and susceptible to infections, diseases and malignancies.

Inferior: lower aspect or beneath.

Infertility: inability to reproduce.

Inflammatory response: a protective immune response characterised by localised heat, swelling and pain.

Insomnia: inability to sleep.

Insulin: hormone produced by the pancreas that enables the body to utilise glucose. Excess causes hypoglycaemia, deficit causes hyperglycaemia.

Interferons: When a virus infects a cell, the cell produces a protein called Interferon.

Internal respiration: describes the process whereby gases diffuse between the blood capillaries and the cells of the body.

Intracerebral haemorrhage (ICH): bleed within the brain.

Intubation: Tracheal intubation is the placement of a flexible plastic tube into the trachea to protect the patient's airway and provide a means of mechanical ventilation.

Inversion injury: where the ankle is twisted inwards.

Ischaemia: reduction of blood to an area, can result in pain and a reduced distal pulse if a limb is involved.

J

Jaw Thrust: a manoeuvre to open the airway whilst stabilising the C-spine.

Jejunum: second part of the small intestine.

K

Kidneys: organs that filter wastes (such as urea) from the blood and excrete them, along with water, as urine.

Korotkoff's sounds: the five phases of sounds heard when a stephoscope is placed over brachial artery to measure blood pressure with a sphymomanometer.

Korsakoff syndrome/psychosis: chronic condition following delirium and toxic states. Often involves hallucinations.

L

Lateral: meaning side, away from the midline.

Lateral horns: When looking at the core of grey matter, it appears to create the letter H. these Horns, which are paired projections of grey matter throughout the spinal cord, are appropriately determined by the direction of their projection. Therefore, the paired horns, which extend posteriorly, are known as the posterior horns, and the anterior horns are those, which project anteriorly. The shorter pair of lateral horns extend to the sides.

Leucocytes: White blood cells or leukocytes are cells of the immune system, which defend the body against both infectious disease and foreign materials.

Leydig cells: cells of the testis that produce the male sex hormone.

Limbic centre: area of the brain involving the senses such as emotions and feelings.

Lipogenesis: the production of fat.

Low molecular weight heparin: a type of heparin given via subcutaneous injection, which requires little monitoring.

Lymphodema: accumulation of lymph within subcutaneous tissue normally due to faulty lymph drainage.

Lymphoid: The lymphatic system is a complex network of lymphoid organs, lymph nodes, lymph ducts, lymphatic tissues, lymph capillaries and lymph vessels that produce and transport lymph fluid from tissues to the circulatory system. The lymphatic system is a major component of the immune system.

M

Malleolus: part of a bone shaped like a hammer i.e. the lower end of the fibula.

Malnutrition: (or under nutrition) occurs when the body's energy intake is less than the energy expenditure

Mannitol: osmotic diuretic often given in severe head injuries.

Mastectomy: removal of a breast.

Mean arterial pressure: a term used in medicine to describe a notional average blood pressure in an individual. It is defined as the average arterial pressure during a single cardiac cycle.

Medial: towards the middle.

Medulla oblongata: upper part of the spinal cord containing the autonomic control centres.

Meiosis: the division of sex cells, constriction of the pupil.

Menopause: the cessation of menstruation.

Menstruation: (period) the physiological shedding of tissue and blood from the non-pregnant uterus.

Metabolism: the end result of physical and chemical changes within the body affecting nutrition and substances such as drugs.

Metaclopramide: an anti-emetic.

Midbrain: part of the brain stem connecting the cerebrum with the pons and the cerebellum. Involved in motor coordination.

Miotics: drugs that constrict the pupil.

Multi-organ dysfunction syndrome: previously known as **multiple organ failure (MOF)**; altered organ function in an acutely ill patient requiring medical intervention to maintain homeostasis.

Mydriatics: drugs that dilate pupils.

Myelin sheath: a fatty white sheath surrounding nerve fibres.

Myofibrils: long fibrils that combine to make up a muscle fibre.

N

Narrow complex tachyarrhythmia: a heart rate above one hundred that conducts quickly i.e. originates above the ventricles.

Nasopharyngeal airway: a tube inserted into the nose, directed towards the throat with the intension of opening the airway.

Negative feedback system: Many biological process use negative feedback. Examples include the regulating of body temperature and blood glucose levels. The disruption of negative feedback can lead to severe results. In the case of blood glucose levels, if negative feedback fails, the glucose levels in the blood may begin to rise dramatically causing diabetes.

Nephron: is the basic structural and functional unit of the kidney. Its chief function is to regulate the concentration of water and soluble substances like sodium salts by filtering the blood, reabsorbing what is needed and excreting the rest as urine. Components consist of

- The Bowman's capsule and glomerulus
- The Proximal convoluted tubule
- The loop of Henle
- The distal convoluted tubule
- The collecting duct

Neuchal Transluceny: a measurement of the size of the translucent space behind the neck of the fetus using

ultrasound at between 10 and 14 weeks of pregnancy. Nuchal translucency tends to be increased in chromosome disorders such as Turner syndrome and Down syndrome,

Neuroglia: tissue that supports the central nervous system.

Neuropathy: umbrella term for disease of the nerves can cause a sensation of burning, severe pain tingling and numbness.

Neurotransmitters: a chemical substance that facilitates the transmission of nerve impulses within the brain and central nervous system.

Neutrophils: the most abundant type of white blood cells and form an integral part of the immune system.

NICE: National Institute for Health and Clinical Excellence.

Nitrates: a salt of nitric acid with an ion composed of one nitrogen and three oxygen atoms.

Non-granular leucocytes: pertaining to lymphocytes and monocytes.

Non-invasive ventilation therapy (NIPPV)**:** is the accepted initial mode of treatment in subsets of patients with acute respiratory failure, the foremost being exacerbation of chronic obstructive pulmonary disease.

Non-specific defence mechanisms: the non-specific defence mechanisms are very diverse. They include

- mechanical barriers to invasion i.e. the skin and mucous membranes
- mechanical reflexes such as coughing, sneezing and the watering of the eyes
- effects of body temperature
- effects of chemical substances such as sebum and gastric acid
- the activity of phagocytic cells such as neutrophils and macrophages

Norepinephrine/Noradrenaline: a catecholamine and a phenethylamine. It is released from the adrenal medulla of the adrenal glands as a hormone into the blood, but it is also a neurotransmitter in the central nervous system and sympathetic nervous system.

NSAIDs: Non-steroidal anti-inflammatory drugs. Drugs that inhibit prostaglandins reducing inflammation thereby stopping pain.

O

Obsessive compulsive disorder: occurs where the person experiences persistent obtrusive negative thoughts and carries out specific tasks or actions to prevent feared outcomes from occurring; examples include hand washing, checking, collecting, hoarding, touching and counting rituals.

Obstructive Shock: shock caused by obstruction of blood flow

Oesophageal Varices: increased portal pressure causes development of collateral circulation where blood supply bypasses the liver and is shunted mainly to veins of the lower oesophagus and stomach.

Oestrogens: promotes development of reproductive structures, in particular the changes in the endometrium with each cycle. Development of the secondary sex characteristics, including development of breasts, voice pitch, hair pattern and the depositing of fat at the hips and abdomen. They also help maintain fluid and electrolyte balance.

Ondansetron: an anti-emetic.

Opiates: the narcotic alkaloids found in opium, the main opiates derived from opium are morphine, codeine.

Orchiectomy: removal of testicle.

Oropharynx: the mouth to the pharynx.

Orthopaedic ward: also referred to as trauma ward; caring for those with injuries related to bone.

Orthopnoea: Inability to breathe when lying flat or tilted, usually due to heart failure and the accumulation of fluid in the lungs.

Osmosis: the movement of a substance such as water through a semi permeable membrane from a solution of a low pressure to one of a higher solute concentration. Continues until concentrations are equalised.

Osteoblasts: a bone-forming cell.

Osteoclasts: cells that remove/destroy unwanted bone.

Osteomalacia: bones are weakened by the loss of calcium and phosphorus. The bone calcification fails; as a consequence the bones become soft and rubbery and are easily deformed. In children this is called rickets.

Osteomyelitis: inflammation of bone caused by infection. Can be limb and life threatening.

Osteoporosis: loss of the density of bone with increasing bone space. Leads to bone weakness and pathological fractures.

Ovaries: sex glands of the female.

Ovulation: part of the menstrual cycle where the ovum is discharged after the rupture of the graafian follicle.

P

Palmer: palm of the hand.

Pancreatitis: (inflammation of the pancreas) occurs when pancreatic enzymes become prematurely activated. Autodigestion of pancreatic tissue causes local inflammation and oedema

Panic attacks: where physical symptoms are experienced associated with the body being highly responsive. These include palpitations, chills, hyperventilation, dizziness, chest pain, choking, nausea and stomach churning.

Paracetamol: is the active metabolite of phenacetin, it is effective for its analgesic and antipyretic properties.

Pathogenesis: the mechanism by which a certain etiological factor causes disease. The term can also be used to describe the development of the disease, whether it is acute, chronic or recurrent.

Patient at Risk Scores (PAR/MEWS). Early warning scores aimed to assist nurses in recognising physiological deterioration.

Patient group direction (PGD), meaning the nurse can dispense drugs without waiting for a written prescription.

PEEP: positive end-expiratory pressure.

Pelvic inflammatory disease (PID): Gynaecological condition caused by an infection, can be sexually transmitted spreading from the vagina to the upper parts of a woman's reproductive tract in the pelvic cavity.

Penumbra: literally meaning, "dim light"; the shadow that results when only part of the bright object is occluded.

Peripheral nervous system (PNS): Consists of neurons connecting the central nervous system (the brain and the spinal cord) to the rest of the body. Sensory neurons bring information to the central nervous system from sensory receptors of the body

Peritoneum: has two layers. The visceral peritoneum covers the abdominal organs and is continuous with the parietal peritoneum, which lines the abdominal wall. Between these layers is a potential space called the **peritoneal cavity** containing serous fluid, which lubricates the organs.

Phagocytosis: (eating cells) aimed at destroying foreign invaders (chemical or non-chemical), and dead or damaged cells.

Pharmacokinetics: the effects of the body on the drug

Pharmacodynamics: of the effects of the drug on the body

Phenylketonuria (PKU) is a very rare **autosomal recessive gene disorder.** This means that both parents need to carry the same altered gene, resulting in a 1:4 risk of having a child affected by the condition.

Phobias: focused aversions or highly reactive fears to specific phenomena, for example fear of spiders or heights

Photopic vision: the scientific term for human colour vision under normal lighting conditions during the day.

Pia mater: innermost layer of the meninges.

Pineal body: A tiny organ in the cerebrum that produces melatonin. Also called pineal gland or pineal organ

Pituitary gland: An endocrine gland located at the base of the brain that produces hormones, such as growth hormone, luteinizing hormone, follicle stimulating hormone and thyroid stimulating hormone.

Plasma: the yellow-colored liquid component of blood, in which blood cells are suspended.

Pneumonia: Pneumonia is an illness, which can result from a variety of causes, including infection with bacteria, viruses, fungi, or parasites.

Poly: used at the beginning of many words to mean many, multiple or excessive.

Pons: (Latin for bridge) lies between the medulla and cerebellum and appears as a broad band of transverse fibres.

Portal hypertension: A condition caused by cirrhosis of the liver. It is characterised by impaired or reversed blood flow from the portal vein to the liver, an enlarged spleen, and dilated veins in the oesophagus and stomach.

Positive inotropic effect: results in both an increase to the heart rate and force of contraction.

Postcentral gyrus: a prominent structure in the parietal lobe of the human brain and an important landmark.

Posterior: behind, back side.

Posterior (dorsal) horns: see **lateral horns**

Postictal: pertaining to the period following a seizure or convulsion; postictal drowsiness.

Postural blood pressure: recording the pressure changes in a patient from a lying to sitting position with their legs hanging over the bed. Can reveal a drop in the face of compensatory shock or reveal evidence of over active changes associated with anti-hypotensive medications.

Postural hypotension: also known as orthostatic hypotension results in dizziness caused by poor regulation of blood pressure after suddenly standing up. See **Postural blood pressure**.

Precentral gyrus: the convolution of the frontal lobe, contains the motor area.

Primary care: the first contact a patient has with the health care system, before being referred elsewhere. "Family doctors" and emergency departments are common sites for primary care.

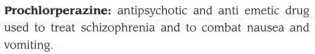

Prochlorperazine: antipsychotic and anti emetic drug used to treat schizophrenia and to combat nausea and vomiting.

Progesterone: works with oestrogen to prepare the endometrium for fertilised ovum and also prepares the mammary glands for milk secretion.

Prophylactic: is any medical or public health procedure whose purpose is to prevent, rather than treat or cure, disease.

Proprioception: sensory system that allows us to know the position of body parts and the motions of muscles and joints.

Proximal: used to describe the area of the limb closest to the body.

Puberty: A complex biological and psychological process involving sexual development and accelerated growth.

Pulmonary oedema: is swelling and/or fluid accumulation in the lungs. It leads to impaired gas exchange and may cause respiratory failure.

Pulseless electrical activity (PEA) organised electrical rhythm without a cardiac output/pulse, i.e. the patient is pulseless despite a potentially normal electrical rhythm.

Pulseless ventricular tachycardia (PVT): one of the cardiac arrests rhythms.

Pulse pressure: the change in blood pressure seen during a contraction of the heart, i.e. the difference between diasystolic and sytolic; roughly 40mmHg.

Pus: (pyarthrosis) collection of white blood cells in tissue fluid, it may be either a sign of infection or inflammation.

Pyelitis: inflammation of the renal pelvis.

Pyelonephritis: infection spreading from the renal pelvis to the cortex of the kidney. Commonly linked to infections below the ureters or within the bloodstream

Pyuria: Pus in the urine

R

Ranvier (nodes of): also known as neurofibril nodes, are regularly spaced gaps in the myelin sheath around an axon or nerve fibre.

Recombinant tissue plasminogen activator (rTPA): type of thrombolytic/fibrinolytics agent.

Renin angiotensin aldosterone axis (RAAA): a complex cascade of regulatory events leading to an increase in blood pressure and sodium retention.

Renal cortex: the outer portion of the kidney between the renal capsule and the renal medulla.

Renal medulla: the innermost part of the kidney. The renal medulla is split up into a number of sections, known as the renal pyramids.

Renal pelvis: the funnel-like dilated proximal part of the ureter in the kidney.

Repolarisation: recharging.

Respiratory effort: the amount of physical work a patient uses to maintain oxygenation whilst at rest.

Retroperitoneal: located behind the peritoneum and outside the peritoneal cavity.

Rhabdomyolysis: the rapid breakdown of skeletal muscle tissue due to traumatic injury, either mechanical, physical or chemical.

Rheumatoid Arthritis: This is a form of arthritis that affects the auto immune system. The immune system attacks the body tissues, which is usually triggered by an antigen in a genetically predisposed person, the synovial membranes and attacked and they go on to degrade and malform the articular surfaces of the bones.

S

Schizophrenia: a collective term for several mental illnesses characterised by disorganisation of the personality, progressive withdrawal from society and perceived abnormal behaviour.

Scotopic vision: is the primary source of vision.

Secondary Care: Services provided by specialists who generally do not have first contact with patients.

Section 2: a compulsory admission for assessment, which lasts up to 28 days.

Section 136: Is the police power to remove a person to a place of safety, preferably a hospital for assessment by a doctor and approved social worker. The section lasts for up to 72 hours.

Seizures: Simple partial seizures: do not affect consciousness. Symptoms may include rhythmic movements of the contralateral face. **Generalised seizures;** affect the whole cortex with the patient's level of consciousness usually being impaired, there is often no aura or warning. **Myoclonic seizures;** are classified by sudden muscle contractions of specific muscle groups with no loss of consciousness. **Typical absence seizures;** are distinguished by a transient loss of consciousness and awareness of the environment with a vacant appearance, which lasts just a few seconds. **Complex partial seizures;** are the most common type of seizure in adults, commonly lasting less than three minutes. **Tonic-clonic seizures;** involve bilateral extension of limbs followed by synchronous jerking movements. There is often a cry

before the seizure, a fall to the ground followed by incontinence, tongue biting, foaming at the mouth and loss of consciousness. There is a postictal phase and when patients wake they have muscle tenderness, transient confusion and exhaustion.

Self-harm: frequently occurs as a method of relieving pent up feelings of emotion or anger and is caused by low mood, depression, and feelings of self loathing or worthlessness.

Seminiferous tubules: this is where sperm are produced.

Septicaemia: blood poisoning. Rapid multiplication of bacteria and toxin production within the blood.

Serotonin: located mainly in the brain stem, where it controls mood, sleep, body heat and appetite.

Shock: a serious, often life-threatening medical condition where insufficient blood flow reaches the body tissues. As blood is the body's carrier of oxygen and nutrients, this leads to a deficiency of these essential inputs to life and an accumulation of waste products.

Sickle cell anaemia/disease: is a group of genetic disorders caused by sickle haemoglobin.

Sinoatrial (SA) node: is the impulse generating (pacemaker) tissue located in the right atrium of the heart, and thus the generator of sinus rhythm.

Skull: also the cranium; the bone encasing and protecting the brain.

Snellen Test: a visual acuity test easily performed via a chart.

Social constructionism: this philosophy challenges pre-conceived notions about how the world is understood by asking us to think about the way we all invent our own version of reality.

Solute: is a substance dissolved in another substance, known as a solvent.

Somatic (voluntary) nervous system: conducting impulses to skeletal muscles only.

Spastic cerebral palsy (spasticity): characterised by rigidity in muscles, which cause stiffness and restricted movement.

Specific defence mechanisms: certain types of cell designed to halt or terminate foreign invaders.

Spina Bifida: This is a congenital defect of the vertebral column, in which the laminae fail to unite at the midline.

Spirometry: measures lung function, specifically the measurement of the amount (volume) and/or speed (flow) of air that can be inhaled and exhaled.

Splenomegly: enlarged spleen.

Sterile: refers to anything that has been through a sterilisation process that effectively kills or eliminates transmissible agents (such as fungi, bacteria, viruses, prions and spore forms etc.) from a surface, equipment, foods, medications, or biological culture medium.

Stomach: an expandable storage sac between the oesophagus and the small intestine.

Stroke: the clinical designation for a rapidly developing loss of brain function due to an interruption in the blood supply to all or part of the brain, can be caused by thrombosis, embolism, or hemorrhage.

Stroke volume: The stroke volume can be defined as the amount of blood in the ventricles immediately before they contract (preload).

Subarachnoid haemorrhage (SAH): a bleed below the arachnoid space, associated with a high mortality and morbidity rate.

Subluxation: a partial dislocation of a joint in which the bones become out of alignment, but the joint itself is still intact.

Substantia nigra: part of the brain that produces dopamine.

Superior: towards the top or upper portion of the structure.

Synaptic cleft: small gap at a synapse, between neurons, where neurotransmitters are released.

Synovial joints: the most common and most moveable type of joints in the body.

Systole: the contraction phase.

T

Tachyarrhythmias: heart rate exceeding 100bpm can be of various causes including: atrial fibrillation and ventricular tachycardia.

Tachycardia: a heart rate of above 100 beats per minute.

Tachypnoea: increased rate of breathing.

Testosterone: male sex hormone (androgen).

Tetraplegia/quadriplegia: all four limbs equally affected.

Thalamus: located within the diencephalon, acts as a relay station for sensory inputs

Thermoregulatory Centre: the body temperature is monitored and controlled by the thermoregulatory centre in the brain. This centre has special cells sensitive to the temperature of blood flowing through the brain. Temperature receptors in the skin also send nerve impulses to this centre giving information about skin temperature.

Thrombocytes: cell fragments circulating in the blood

that are involved in the cellular mechanisms of primary homeostasis leading to the formation of blood clots.

Thrombolysis: aims to dissolve a thrombus occluding an artery and restore circulation in the acute phase of ischaemia.

Thrombus: where a clot or atherosclerotic plaque dislodges occluding a vessel causing ischaemia.

Thyroxine: is the major hormone secreted by the follicular cells of the thyroid gland.

Torsion: twisting; commonly affects the testicles or ovaries.

Trabecula: fibrous bands of connective tissues that extend into the interior of an organ from its surrounding to stabilise the functioning cells.

Transient ischaemic attacks (TIA): ischaemic episode affecting the brain, initially the patient may appear to have suffered a stroke but signs and symptoms will resolve within 24 hours.

Tremors: involuntary, purposeless movements with various causes including: Parkinson's disease, alcohol withdrawal, anxiety states and old age.

Troponin: a complex of three proteins that is integral to muscle contraction in skeletal and cardiac muscle, but not smooth muscle.

Tuberculosis: a common infectious disease caused by mycobacteria, mainly *Mycobacterium tuberculosis*. Tuberculosis most commonly attacks the lungs (as pulmonary TB) but can also affect the central nervous system, the lymphatic system, the circulatory system, the genitourinary system, bones, joints and even the skin.

Tympanic: meaning the tympanum, a thin semi-transparent membrane in the middle ear that transmits sound vibrations to the internal ear.

U

Ulna: the bone on the inner side of the forearm.

Ultrasound: a device that converts high frequency sound waves into heat which is reflected in differing degrees of various tissues.

Uraemia: A clinical syndrome synonymous with failing kidneys whereby excessive amounts of urea are found within the blood.

Urea: the waste product of protein metabolism. Can accumulate in the blood in the presence of renal failure or excessive production.

Ureters: the ducts that carry urine from the kidneys to the urinary bladder.

Urethra: a tube, which connects the urinary bladder to the outside of the body.

Urethritis: inflammation of the urethra; characterised by pain on urination (can be caused by localised inflammation/infection or linked to gonococcal infection)

Uric acid: an acid formed via the metabolism of proteins, can cause stone formations.

Urine: a liquid produced through the kidney, collected in the bladder and excreted through the urethra.

Urinalysis: a test performed on urine and one of the most common methods of medical diagnosis. A part of a urinalysis can be performed by using urine dipsticks, in which the test results can be read as color changes.

V

Vaccine: an antigenic preparation used to establish immunity to a disease.

Vagina: musculomembranous genital canal lying inbetween the urinary bladder and the rectum.

Venous return: the rate of blood flow back to the heart is the venous return, it normally limits cardiac output.

Ventricular fibrillation (VF): a condition in which there is uncoordinated contraction of the cardiac muscle of the ventricles in the heart. As a result the heart fails to adequately pump blood and hypoxia will occur followed by cardiac arrest.

Ventricular tachycardia: a rapid heart beat initiated within the ventricles, characterised by 3 or more consecutive premature ventricular beats, can be pulseless and lead to ventricular fibrillation.

VIP Score: visual infusion phlebitis score, a tool for assessing a cannula site for signs of infection/damage.

Viruses: a large group of disease producing agents only visible under microscope. Responsible for chickenpox, measles, herpes zoster and the common cold.

W

Warfarin: an oral anticoagulant, used to prolong the clotting time in patients at risk of clot formation.

Waterlow score: a structural tool that provides an estimate of the risk of a patient developing a pressure sore whilst hospitalised.

X

Xiphisternum: the end section of the sternum.

Y

Yankauer suction catheter: a wide bore tube facilitating the removal of fluids from the oropharynx.

Z

Zygote: A single diploid cell resulting from the fusion of male and female gametes at fertilisation.

Appendix: Answers to end of chapter quizzes

Chapter 2
1. B
2. A
3. B
4. D
5. C
6. D
7. A
8. A
9. D
10. A

Chapter 3
1. A
2. B
3. C
4. C
5. A
6. B
7. C
8. A
9. D
10. C

Chapter 4
1. B
2. D
3. C
4. D
5. C
6. C
7. A
8. B
9. D
10. C

Chapter 5
1. C
2. A
3. D

4. C
5. A
6. B
7. D
8. D
9. D
10. A

Chapter 6
1. C
2. B
3. B
4. A
5. C
6. D
7. A
8. C
9. A
10. B

Chapter 7
1. B
2. B
3. D
4. A
5. C
6. D
7. C
8. A
9. B
10. D

Chapter 8
1. A
2. C
3. C
4. D
5. C
6. A
7. A

8. B
9. D
10. C

Chapter 9
1. C
2. B
3. A
4. B
5. B
6. A
7. A
8. D
9. A
10. D

Chapter 10
1. A
2. C
3. A
4. D
5. A
6. B
7. B
8. A
9. D
10. A

Chapter 11
1. A
2. A
3. C
4. A
5. D
6. D
7. B
8. B
9. C
10. C

Chapter 15
1. C
2. B
3. ABC
4. C
5. The individual clutching at their throat
6. C
7. D
8. A
9. B
10. D

Chapter 16
1. C
2. C
3. C
4. D
5. A
6. C
7. C
8. A
9. D
10. D

Index

Locators shown in *italics* refer to boxes, figures and tables.

THE ENCYCLOPEDIA OF
MUSIC

INSTRUMENTS OF THE ORCHESTRA AND
THE GREAT COMPOSERS

THE ENCYCLOPEDIA OF
MUSIC

INSTRUMENTS OF THE ORCHESTRA AND
THE GREAT COMPOSERS

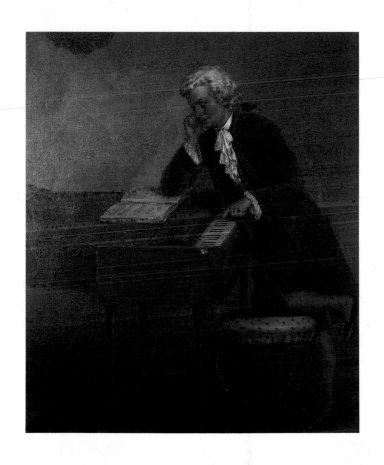

Max Wade-Matthews &
Wendy Thompson

HERMES HOUSE

This edition is published by Hermes House,
an imprint of Anness Publishing Ltd, Hermes House,
88–89 Blackfriars Road, London SE1 8HA;
tel. 020 7401 2077; fax 020 7633 9499

www.hermeshouse.com; www.annesspublishing.com

Anness Publishing has a new picture agency outlet
for images for publishing, promotions or advertising.
Please visit our website www.practicalpictures.com
for more information.

Publisher: Joanna Lorenz
Managing Editor: Judith Simons
Project Editor: Felicity Forster
Editor: Beverley Jollands
Photographer: John Freeman
Designers: Ian Hunt and Michael Morey
Jacket Design: Paul Vater at Sugar Free
Picture Researchers: Cathy Stastny and
 Daniela Marceddu
Production Controller: Claire Rae

Jacket Picture Credits: AKG, London (Bach,
 Mozart, Beethoven, Schubert); Lebrecht
 Collection, London (Brahms)

Previously published as separate volumes, *The World
Encyclopedia of Musical Instruments* and *The Great Composers*

Contents

Preface

If music be the food of love, play on!
WILLIAM SHAKESPEARE (1564—1616), "TWELFTH NIGHT"

People have been making music for a very long time, probably beginning with the voice and proceeding to simple rhythmic drumming – hitting a log with a stick or banging a rock with a club – and blowing a blade of grass or a conch shell. Since these humble beginnings there has been an explosion in instrument-making, accompanied by the rise of the composer particularly over the past six centuries.

Musical instruments

The very earliest evidence of music is provided by the remains of instruments. Clappers, flutes and drums have survived from before the last Ice Age, and these are the ancient ancestors of the thousands of musical instruments used in the world today.

The book begins with an exploration of the *History of Music-making and the*

ABOVE: *"Buffalo Dance" from George Catlin's* North American Indian Portfolio *of 1844. One of the dancers is keeping the rhythm with a shallow frame drum.*

Orchestra, presenting a general history of musical instruments, how they sounded and the kinds of music they were used for. The musical instruments of previous ages and different cultures have much to say, not only about music, but about social patterns, technology and skills, ritual and religion.

Even when they are not being played, musical instruments have a strong aesthetic appeal, which stems from their perfect blend of form and function. They are often lovingly made and beautifully decorated, with satisfying, rounded shapes and smooth surfaces that demand to be touched. Those who play them become deeply attached to them as the emotions expressed in music flow through them.

The *Encyclopedia of Musical Instruments* describes each family of instruments in detail: strings, woodwind and brass, percussion and

keyboards, ending with a section on the voice. As well as the standard orchestral instruments, folk instruments, traditional instruments from around the world, the precursors of modern instruments and those that have fallen into disuse are featured.

ABOVE: *A 16th-century trio of musicians playing together from a manuscript.*

ABOVE: *This Italian mosaic from the 2nd century BC shows strolling masked musicians.*

ABOVE: *A chamber group performing at an outdoor reception.*

There are plenty of folk tales and myths that tell of instruments with supernatural powers: warning drums, magic flutes, diabolical violins and pianos that play themselves. There is no doubting the magic of music, and musical instruments have a share of it.

The great composers

Owing to the invention of systems for writing down music in medieval times, scholars have added to their study of musical instruments a knowledge of composition methods and styles, and how these developed over the centuries.

ABOVE: *Musical instruments such as this double bass and bow have a strong aesthetic appeal.*

Beginning with a discussion of the first written musical notation dating from the 9th century AD, *Composition through the Ages* provides a survey of the principal milestones in the history of musical invention, culminating in the new and sometimes unusual sounds of the 21st century.

Within such a long period of development and innovation, some composers have stood out as having defined or developed particular styles of composition, or have created for themselves a significant place in music history. *Lives and Works of the Great Composers* covers the lives and times of the individuals who are seen as the most pre-eminent in Western music: Bach, Haydn, Mozart, Beethoven, Tchaikovsky, Wagner and Stravinsky, to name but a few. The book ends with a look at contemporary composers, such as Philip Glass, Arvo Pärt and Thomas Adès, with the promise of many exciting new developments extending well into the future.

ABOVE: *A painting from the mid 17th century by Jan Havicksz, entitled* The Harpsichord Lesson. *Baroque composers such as Pachelbel and Bach wrote major works for this instrument.*

ABOVE: *The symphony orchestra holds a central place in Western musical life.*

History of Music-making

and the

Orchestra

This anonymous 16th-century Italian painting entitled Concert Champêtre *("Concert in the Fields") depicts a virginalist playing* continuo *in company with a viola da gamba, lute and recorder.*

Introduction

Music is the universal language of mankind.

HENRY WADSWORTH LONGFELLOW (1807–82), "OUTRE-MER"

There are few people who do not react to music to some degree. The power of music is diverse and people respond in different ways. To some it is mainly an instinctive, exciting sound to which they dance or move their bodies. Other people listen for its message, or take an intellectual approach to its form and construction, appreciating its formal patterns or originality. Above all, however, there can be hardly anyone who is not moved by some kind of music. Music covers the whole gamut of emotions: it can make us feel happy or sad, nostalgic or energetic, and some music is capable of overtaking the mind until it is oblivious to all else. It works on the subconscious, creating or enhancing mood and unlocking deep memories.

ABOVE: *The Amati Quartet led by Attila Balogh was one of the foremost chamber ensembles of the 1980s and early '90s. This picture, taken in 1988, shows the quartet giving one of their recitals.*

Music is intimately bound up with important events in all our lives. There is hardly a ceremony, whether personal or national, that is not accompanied by music. It may be as simple as the nightly ritual of a mother singing her baby to sleep or as formal as the playing of a national anthem. It may be a spontaneous outpouring of mass emotion, such as the spectators singing before a football game, or it may be a highly wrought and carefully rehearsed performance of massed bands or choirs at a great state wedding or funeral.

The history of music is a part of the history of humanity. Ethnographic studies of ritual among primitive societies have provided plenty of evidence to show that music-making is a basic and universal instinct. Because it is not a concrete art form, we can have no knowledge of what music sounded like in the centuries before

ABOVE: *Instruments that were in use in the Iberian peninsula during the 13th century included a portative organ, cornetts, double bladder pipe, bagpipes, lutes and shawm.*

ABOVE: *A performance of* Carmen *at Blackpool Opera House in 1938. Bizet's most successful opera opened in Paris in 1875, during the last year of his short life.*

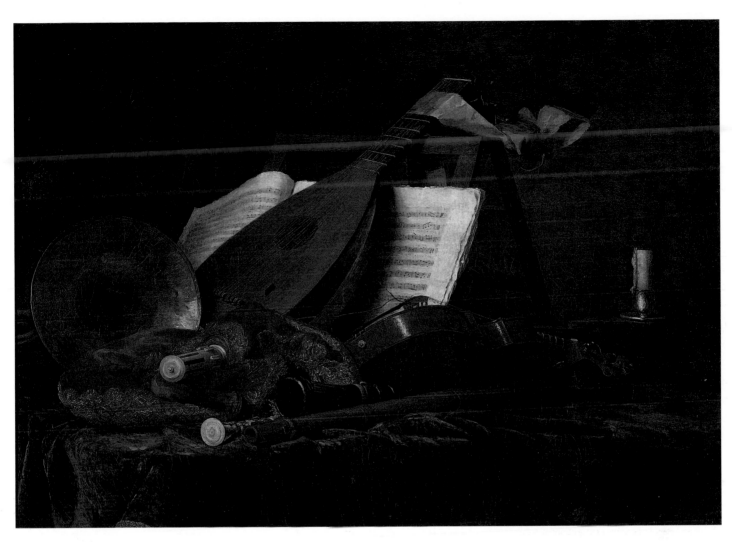

ABOVE: *This painting by Anne Vallayer-Coster, entitled* The Attributes of Music, *was completed in 1770, just before the French Revolution and the beginning of the Romantic period in music. The instruments (from left to right) are horn, cornemuse, lute, flute and violin.*

it began to be written down or, much later, recorded. But very early written accounts remain, as well as ancient instruments and pictures or carvings showing them in use, to convey some idea of the importance of music to ancient civilizations.

In the 20th century, there has been an unprecedented interest not only in the written remains of the music of previous generations, but in establishing how such music really sounded. As recently as the 18th century, musicians were expected to provide only new works for concert audiences, whereas modern music-lovers are avid for music from all historical periods, often performed on instruments and in styles that attempt to recreate the

effect intended by the composer. There are many ways in which we try to understand the lives of previous generations in order to set our own lives in a secure context, and music is a powerful way of evoking the past.

At the same time, musicians are constantly seeking new forms of expression. As in every other contemporary art form, originality is highly prized in music, and every new development in technology is explored by both composers and players. Recording techniques have made all forms of music instantly available to a universal audience, but have not diminished the demand for live performance, on a wider range of instruments than ever before.

ABOVE: *At the far left of this 15th-century Spanish painting are three singers reading from sheet music, accompanied by a band of six musicians on the right.*

What is Music?

Musick is a tonick to the saddened soul.
ROBERT BURTON (1577–1640), "ANATOMY OF MELANCHOLY"

When asked "What is music?" people will give various replies. Some will try to be scientific and say that music is a succession of sound waves. But that is also the result of scratching a blackboard with the fingernails, which most people would not describe as music.

The making of music is not restricted to human beings. Many animals, such as whales and birds, appear to use music as a means of communication. Natural music was utilized by the French composer, Olivier Messiaen, who used to go out into the countryside to transcribe birdsong, which he incorporated almost note-for-note into his orchestral and piano music. The American composer John Cage believed that the mechanical background sounds of everyday life could be described as music, and other composers have written works

ABOVE: Although birdsong is not created for a human audience, it is still music to human ears and one of the pleasures of life.

requiring all kinds of everyday objects to be used as "musical instruments".

Perhaps an easier question would be "What is not music?", though the answers would be just as varied. To some, the sounds made by a heavy metal rock band constitute music, while to others they are just highly amplified noise. Rock music of the 1950s and '60s, such as the songs of Buddy Holly, Jerry Lee Lewis, the Beatles or the Rolling Stones, was adored by its teenage fans but dismissed as unbearable noise by many of their parents. Many of Berlioz's contemporaries harked back to the "good old days" of Bach, while many early 20th-century music-lovers were none too impressed when confronted with the ground-breaking compositions of Stravinsky.

When André Previn was once asked the difference between popular and classical music, his reply was that there

was no such thing as popular or classical music, there was just good music and bad music. While there are many wonderful "classical" works, there are some that are not worth the manuscript paper upon which they were written. Conversely, as there are many popular songs that end up in the dustbin of history, there are many modern tunes that Mozart would have been proud to have written.

Beauty is in the ear, as well as the eye, of the beholder, and the

ABOVE: Drums are known to all cultures. This sculpture of a figure playing a small frame drum dates from AD 800, and is of the Peruvian Mochica culture.

ABOVE: The military drum was originally used as a means of signalling in battle, and was also beaten to set a rhythm that focused the minds of marching troops.

ABOVE: *Rattles made out of gourds are one of the oldest percussion instruments and have been found in every part of the world.*

Listening to music is a psychosomatic experience that, as well as promoting harmony and peace, holds a power for inner reassurance and satisfaction which stems from deep within the human spirit. Many people would count themselves the poorer without it. We do not have to go into the science and philosophy of music to find the answer to our question; we simply need to go into our own souls, for that is where music belongs.

appreciation of a piece of music depends to some extent on the listener's culture and upbringing. To someone born in the West, for example, the music of East Asia is mysterious and possibly difficult to listen to, because its idiom is unfamiliar. However, once its context is understood and Western preconceptions about musical conventions are set aside, it becomes more accessible. Even without understanding, all music has the power to exert an effect on the emotions.

ABOVE: *While the ringing of a single church bell might not be classified as music, a peal of three or more certainly is.*

LEFT: *The Portuguese* Quineto de Cristal *in 1882. Crystallophones were a 19th-century innovation and for a while were very popular in Europe and the United States. The glasses were arranged in five octaves and struck with small hammers. In time interest flagged, and crystallophones became historical curiosities.*

What is a Musical Instrument?

Music is the sound of universal laws promulgated.

HENRY THOREAU (1817–62)

Musical instruments and their story have always been part of human history, and the story of music begins with the story of humanity. Music, or sound, stood at the cradle of all religions. When primitive humans struck a piece of rock, stone or skin, or blew into an old bone or hollow branch, they perhaps concluded that what they heard was the voice of the object. They therefore assumed that by awakening the "voice" of the object, they could propitiate the unseen nature of which their life was a part.

The rhythmic articulation of time by means of an instrument of some kind is far older than the construction of a true musical instrument. Any objects that early humans happened to pick up when singing or dancing could become sound-producing "musical instruments". Implements created for use exclusively as musical instruments developed only very slowly and many, if not all, early instruments (such as the pot drum) were merely adaptations

LEFT: Very early in human history it was found that a very loud sound could be produced by blowing into a conch shell.

of artefacts already invented for some other purpose. Instruments are the working tools of music; they are the practical devices by which the acoustic properties of nature are managed for the artistic purposes of music that begin with the player. The musical instrument cannot be separated from the musician. In the hands of an incompetent amateur, the finest Stradivari may as well be a block of wood. However, in the hands of a virtuoso, even a crude violin can sound heavenly.

Obviously, we do not know the world's first "tunes". The development of music predates the invention of writing by thousands of years, and there is no way of knowing what

ABOVE: The conch shell is still used as a musical instrument in present-day China; at some temples the shell is blown to announce the beginning of prayers. This conch shell has been fitted with a bamboo mouthpiece.

ABOVE: Rhythm plays an important part in African music. These painted wooden rattles are from Nigeria.

The two elements – the body and the column or box of air – together form a coupled acoustic system.

Other very early instruments include hollow tubes such as reeds and bones, and conch shells, which are believed to have been used as signal instruments. It is possible that these were at first shouted into, until it was discovered that more pleasing sounds could be produced by blowing.

sounds the Neanderthals and early *Homo sapiens* enjoyed. The first "instrument" was certainly the human voice, and ritual chanting is likely to have been accompanied by rhythmic clapping or stamping. This in turn would have led to the striking of an object, such as a convenient log or stone, which could produce a different, and probably a louder, sound.

These early musical instruments, made of naturally sonorous materials, are termed "idiophones". Modern percussion instruments, such as gongs, wood blocks, cymbals and xylophones, are also examples of idiophones. Before long the early musician would have realized that the sound produced by hitting a solid log was different from that produced by a hollow log. The latter is an example of the coupled system of sound production, in which the vibrations are excited in one source with the collaboration of an associated structure – such as the air in the log. This discovery is the foundation of the design of modern wind instruments, such as the horn or oboe, and of the body and soundbox of stringed instruments, such as the violin.

ABOVE: Scrapers are some of the earliest percussion instruments and are known virtually everywhere. These examples from Laos are made from bamboo.

RIGHT: Shakers or rattles come in various shapes and sizes, such as a plastic ball, metal box, wicker basket and natural pod.

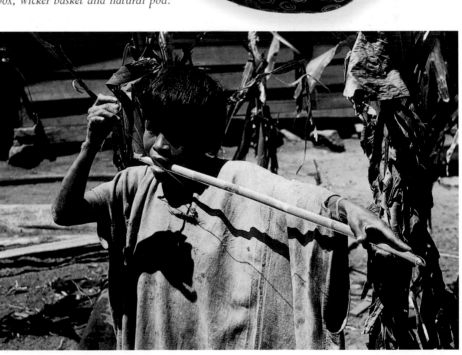

ABOVE: Musical bows are known almost all over the world. Often the mouth serves as a resonator while the string is set in vibration by either being tapped with a small stick, as in this example from Colombia, or plucked with a plectrum.

Music of Ancient Civilizations

*Provide me now a man that
can play well and bring him to me.*

1 SAMUEL 16:17

The earliest archaeological evidence of the use of musical instruments dates from about 3000 BC. By then, the Sumerians, an ancient society living in the fertile crescent of Mesopotamia, had assembled a range of musical instruments, including lyres, harps and reed-pipes, which may have been played as an ensemble. It is also known from written records that they practised antiphonal singing or chanting in their temples. There is no way of knowing what their music sounded like, but it is clear that it was a sophisticated part of Sumerian culture and that it had religious and ceremonial significance.

Egypt

The importance of music in ancient Egypt cannot be overestimated. Music was one of the concomitant joys of life; indeed, as a sign of this, the soundbox of the harp was sometimes fashioned to represent the sacred lotus flower in bloom.

ABOVE: This finely decorated 12th-century BC Egyptian harp is depicted on a tomb painting in Anhour Khaou's tomb in Thebes. In reality the left hand would have played the "back" of the instrument.

From the beginning of the New Kingdom in about 1550 BC, music, which was mainly performed by women, began to play a very prominent part in religious life. Many of the first musicians in the temples were the wives and daughters of priests, the more senior of whom enjoyed a high status second only to that of the king. The instrument of sacerdotal potency and ecclesiastical authority was the *sistrum*, a type of rattle with metal discs strung on a framework of wires, which symbolized divine power. Egyptian temple music was much more than just chanting and jingling. Harps, pandoras and pipes were also used to praise the gods, since it was part of the regular duties of the priest to extol the god in song, and dancing, accompanied by temple musicians, played an important part in many cults.

As time went on and the empire broadened, female slaves from captured nations were brought back to Egypt to serve as musicians. They attended academies of music where they were instructed in both singing and playing instruments. Music in Egypt was of such a high standard that even the Greeks commended it. Instrumental music was important in secular as well as religious life. Musicians played in homes as well as at feasts, in processions and at funeral ceremonies.

The earliest evidence of parallel pipes in Egypt is from about 2700 BC. Divergent pipes came into use – and in

ABOVE: A Theban tomb painting shows a musician playing double shawm pipes and another holding a lute-type instrument.

fact largely replaced the older instrument – in about 1500 BC. The divergent pipes were held with one pipe in each hand, with the proximal ends forming a V. Played exclusively by

ABOVE: This Egyptian wall painting dates from about the 15th century BC and shows a female musician playing an angular harp.

women, each pipe originally had four finger-holes, but later five or six became common. The right hand played the melody while the left pipe sounded a drone accompaniment.

The frame drum arrived in Egypt in about 1550 BC. Also played only by women, the drum accompanied many aspects of Egyptian life, ranging from the cult of Osiris to the dancing of the slaves in the Pharaonic court. Frame drums were similar in

ABOVE: A Hebrew coin dating from about AD 135 depicting a lyre.

appearance to the modern tambourine, complete with jingling metal rings, discs or pellet bells.

Israel

In ancient Israel, music had a place in almost every activity and at almost every event. The double-headed drum, in the form of the *tof*, is known to have been played in Biblical times, when women used it to accompany their songs and dances. Until about 1000 BC music was the spontaneous outpouring of the people. Later, however, with the establishment of a trained and official body of musicians to lead worship in the temple, it became more formal and more ritualized. Trumpets represented the power of God, and the cantillation of scripture was a potent reminder of the sanctity of God's word, setting it apart from the unsanctified conversation of daily life.

Pipes were also known in Biblical Israel where smaller pipes, called *halil*, were made of cane or metal. The Hebrew prophets plied their trade under the influence of music and were

often preceded by musicians playing drums, pipes and lyres. (The Latin word *praecinere*, which was used in translations of the scriptures to describe their activity, means both to prophesy and to play the pipes.)

By 200 BC the temple had an established choir of 12 men and a number of boys, who sang to the accompaniment of lyres, pipes and cymbals. Antiphonal singing, which had been a part of Sumerian religious practice and was known to the Egyptians, was adopted by the Jews for the singing of psalms.

ABOVE: This Egyptian tomb painting from Thebes, 1425 BC, depicts dancers performing to the music of a double shawm.

ABOVE: An impression of the Temple of Jerusalem, used as an illustration to a 1732 Bible, showing Solomon dedicating the Temple to the Lord. Music was a feature of the Temple life, and trained musicians were employed to lead the worship.

ABOVE: One of the oldest horns still used today is the Jewish shofar. They are made from a billy goat's horn or a ram's horn.

Classical Greece

That classical Greece was a musical Greece can be seen from the many modern musical words that owe their roots to Greek. Apart from "music" itself, they include "melody", "harmony", "symphony", "orchestra", "organ", "chorus" and "rhythm". The Greek work *mousike* embraced not only what is considered to be music today but also the text and accompanying dance. Greek poets did not just write the words, they also produced the work, trained the singers and dancers (who were mainly amateurs) and directed the accompaniment.

To the Greeks, music, singing and dancing were the main characteristics of a civilized society. They used music for many different purposes, ranging from celebration and the worship of gods to the boosting of morale. Musicians played to workers performing repetitive jobs, such as spinning and weaving, rope-making, grinding corn and treading grapes.

Music also played an important role in military exploits. An essential member of an Athenian trireme's crew was the aulete, or double-pipe player, who played to keep the rowers in time. Spartan armies marched to the sound of the aulos, which kept them at a steady pace without breaking rank. Aulos music also served as a morale booster to the troops, in much the same way as Scottish Highland regiments use the bagpipes today.

Greek contests

The notion of competition was dear to the hearts of the Greeks, and music was no exception. As a focus for competition, the art of *kitharodia* (singing to the self-accompanying of a kithara, or lyre) dates from about 670 BC. Choral contests were instituted about 50 years later, while in 580 BC the Spartans introduced aulos music into their public contests. These festivals were a magnet for performers, who came from great distances to take part.

Kithara versus aulos

During the 5th century BC, musical styles changed radically, as traditions were ousted by new ideas. Plato (c.428–347 BC), who was suspicious of change and denounced the new style as entertaining rather than edifying, complained about the "modern music" of his day, especially the use of the versatile aulos in preference to the kithara, which had also been adapted in an attempt to imitate the aulos and now had an expanded number of strings. Such was Plato's aversion to the aulos that he banned it from his ideal republic, believing that those who could not play the kithara were lacking in education.

Ancient Rome

Music was a rich and constant presence in Roman life. The everyday life of the Romans abounded in songs concerned with all subjects, ranging from reaping to weaving, from weddings to funerals and from love to satire. In the homes of the wealthy, music was often played during dinner, while in the theatre, plays and comedies often included the music of the *tibia* (the Roman version of the aulos) or the hydraulis, or water-pipe. The hydraulis also had a place in the arena, where it was often played with brass instruments, such as the *cornu* and *tuba*, to accompany chariot fights and gladiatorial contests

ABOVE: That music played an important part in Greek cultural life can be seen from this 5th-century BC vase painting depicting a young man learning to play the lyre.

ABOVE: *This Etruscan wall painting of the early 5th century BC shows an ambulatory musician playing an aulos, or double pipe. The player was known as an aulete.*

ABOVE: *The Roman Colosseum, seen here as it was in 1835, was a centre of Roman entertainment, much of which was to the accompaniment of music.*

in the arena. Pantomimes, another popular Roman entertainment, regularly incorporated choral singing, instrumental music and dancing.

Cult music in Roman life ranged from elaborate festival performances to accompaniments for the ritual slaughtering of an animal, when the playing of the *tibia* drowned out the cries of the doomed creature. Roman professional musicians had their own associations, which furnished

performers for both public and private entertainments: extravagant fees were not unknown for the more popular musicians. Because of their connection with the state cult, these musicians benefited from certain privileges, such as being allowed to roam the streets unhindered, even though they were masked and frequently drunk.

ABOVE: *Second-century Roman mosaic of a hydraulis, the ancestor of the modern organ. Under the pipes was a keyboard that operated perforated sliders. When a key was pressed, a slider was pushed into position to release pressurized air from the wind canal and thereby sound the note. The scene also shows a cornicin, a large and powerful circular horn.*

ABOVE: *First-century BC relief from Denmark depicting Celtic carnyx players. These instruments have a warlike appearance with their bells shaped like grotesque boars' heads.*

India

The origin of the classical music of northern India is shrouded in obscurity. It is a mixture of many ancient cultural influences and the result of a long process of integration of various types of music that makes it one of the world's greatest art forms. The Sanskrit hymns of the *Rig Veda*, composed between the 14th and 10th centuries BC, were – and still are – intoned, and it is possible that the style that is used today has survived virtually unchanged from the time of their composition.

Hindus believe in the power of *samgita*, which encompasses vocal music, instrumental music and dance, to influence the universe and to play a part in freeing the individual from the cycle of birth, death and rebirth.

Raga

The *raag* is the mainstay of northern Indian classical music. There are some 200 main *raga*, each with its own scale pattern and specific rules. Some are linked with specific seasons and times of day, while some are feminine and others masculine.

The performance of a *raag* always follows a set pattern. It begins with the

ABOVE: This 17th-century painting from India depicts lotus-flower dancers performing to the music of a dhola *drum and sitar.*

ABOVE: This painting of Indian marriage celebrations in 1561 shows guests dancing to the rhythm of tambourines, tabla drums, trumpets and cymbals.

alapa, a slow, meditative mood-setter that introduces the notes of the scale in free time and is unaccompanied by drums. This can last several hours, although more usually it is a matter of minutes. The next two sections are the *jorh* and the *jhala*, in which the soloist begins to introduce a rhythmic element and explore complex variations.

The final section, the *gath*, introduces the tabla, a set of two drums played with fingertips and palms. The right-hand drum is the *tabla* and the left-hand one the *bayan*.

Both drum heads are made of skin with a paste of flour and iron filings in the centre. The *tabla* body is made of wood and that of the *bayan* of metal.

Qawwali

Another type of music associated with northern India (and Pakistan) is *qawwali*, a spiritual song that is intended to transport the mystic towards union with the creator. *Qawwali* music can be traced back at least as far as the 9th century, and in its present form to the late 13th century.

A feature of modern *qawwali* is the harmonium, an instrument introduced to India by Christian missionaries around AD 1900. Although the harmonium has the advantage that it does not need constant retuning, it does not meet with universal approval and is banned from All Indian Radio because it does not conform to the traditional flexible intonation of *sruti* music, in which the "same" note can acquire different, but recognizable, pitches in ascent and descent. Neither can the glides and swings of *gamaka*

ABOVE: *This Indian scene depicts the celebrations during the birth of Timur. The musicians are playing instruments such as cymbals, tabla drums and trumpets.*

music be achieved on the harmonium. The celebrated musician Rabindranath Tagore once went as far as to call the harmonium "the bane of Indian music".

Indonesia

The most famous music of South-east Asia is the vibrant, thunderous gamelan, the percussion orchestra, consisting of gong-chimes, metallophones and gongs, which is played in Java and Bali. The tradition goes back well over a thousand years and is believed to predate the Hindu-Buddhist kingdom that was founded in Bali in the 7th century, when the Balinese arrived from Java, having been ousted by the arrival of Islam.

In no other country is music such an integral part of the daily life of the community. There is a greater concentration of orchestras in Bali than

anywhere else in the world. Here, however, as in the rest of the Indonesian archipelago, music does not have a particular religious significance, as it does for Hindus in India.

Spanning over five octaves, gamelan music is like a tree, with some instruments representing the trunk, some the branches and some the flowers. The various instruments of the gamelan include drums, bamboo flutes, cymbals, the *rebab* (an upright fiddle), the great gong, which can be up to 1m/3ft in diameter, and the *trompong* (a row of ten gong chimes set in a wooden frame). One group plays the core melody, while another group stresses this at regular intervals, generally one note in four. A third group expands the core melody with a range of up to three octaves, while a fourth doubles the melody an octave above. As well as these groups, various gongs provide punctuation and drums conduct the rhythmic undercurrent.

Javanese gamelan music is courtly and gentle; the players use padded mallets and the tempo is slow and serene. In Bali, the style is much brighter, louder and more exuberant, using wood or horn hammers and employing a greater dynamic range.

ABOVE: *The young Indian prince Shri Raga listens to the music of the vina, an instrument characterized by a long string carrier and gourd resonator.*

ABOVE: *Balinese gamelan percussion orchestras go back well over a thousand years. Trompong players are shown here, with tuned gongs in the background.*

ABOVE: This 18th-century Chinese illustration depicts a man playing a kuchin, *a form of long zither. Traditionally, all dimensions of the* kuchin *have a cosmological meaning.*

China

Chinese music dates back millennia and is one of the oldest and most highly developed of all musical systems. The Chinese concept of music theory is different from that of the West in that the emphasis is placed on the philosophical, cosmological and educational values of music.

Music played an important part in the lives of the ancient Chinese and was closely associated with matters of state and government. To the Chinese, music is part of nature and is organically integrated with the cosmological universe. The earliest Chinese musical notation dates from the 4th century BC, while two centuries earlier Confucius had compiled a book of songs.

Chinese instruments

Since ancient times, Chinese musical instruments have been classified according to their major acoustical material – metal, stone, clay, leather, silk, wood, gourd or bamboo – and how they are played.

The *ch'in*, or classical long zither of China, can be dated back to the T'ang dynasty (AD 618–907). Played with a curved horsehair bow, the modern instrument has no bridges and the stopping places for the ten pairs of silk strings are indicated by ivory discs inlaid into the soundboard. The Thai *chakay*, on the other hand, is played with a single plectrum, usually made of ivory, metal or tortoiseshell.

Another typical traditional Chinese instrument is the *qin*, a seven-stringed

ABOVE: The Chinese yün-luo *gong chimes are of Mongolian origin and consist of between 10 and 24 small bronze bowls suspended vertically in an upright frame.*

zither that has been a favourite subject of poets and painters for over a thousand years. The most delicate instrument in the Chinese repertoire, the *qin*'s ethereal harmonics are a joy to hear.

By the 8th century, the *sheng*, or reed-pipe mouth organ, had 17 pipes. This number became the norm, and today it is tuned chromatically and played polyphonically in triads. Although historically the *sheng* was played at funerals and at court, the *lu-sheng*, traditionally a dance instrument, is now a regular feature of the Chinese orchestra.

The Chinese bronze *bo* cymbal of the Hai Province differs from the Turkish cymbal in that the rim turns out slightly. Used in the Peking opera, these cymbals are about 20cm/8in wide. In the south of the country, in Canton, the cymbal of choice is the *dabo*, held by a small central knob.

Chinese temple and court

The ritual temple music of southern China lives on in the Temple of

ABOVE: Dancers from the traditional Chinese opera in Canton. In spite of the political upheavals in China, Cantonese opera has survived.

ABOVE: Three female musicians playing Chinese drums and a flute painted on a vase of about 1640.

Sublime Mysteries in Suzhou. Here the monks play a wide range of music, including pieces for silk and bamboo instruments, flutes and oboes, long trumpets and a whole battery of percussion. In orchestral, ensemble and solo instrumental court music, multipart form dominates. Four stages of court music development are most commonly heard: the introduction, the elucidation of the theme, the transition and the summing-up.

Chinese opera

Kunqu opera, which evolved in the 16th century in Kiangsa province, is a sophisticated opera based on an earlier form of literary drama. Based on written librettos, its tunes are slow-

ABOVE: A row of Chinese Miao people playing lu-sheng *mouth organs and long bamboo trumpets.*

moving, with a regular 4:4 rhythm. The principal instruments used in *kunqu* are the *titzu* and *hsiao* (the transverse and end-blown flutes).

In 1790 the visits of various acting companies to Peking, for the 80th birthday celebrations of Emperor Ch'ien-lung, introduced to the capital the operatic styles that were to go on to form the core of "Peking opera". Performed in teahouses, its characters, unlike those of Western opera, are categorized by the kind of person they represent rather than by vocal range. The four main types are: *sheng* (male), *tan* (female), *ching* (warriors and gods) and *ch'ou* (clowns).

ABOVE: This quintet of Chinese musicans are playing (from left to right) a two-stringed dutar, paipan *(clapper),* chettö *(flute),* sheng *(mouth organ), and* pipa *(lute).*

ABOVE: Top row — three trumpets, drum, two erh-hu *(fiddles),* kuchin *(zither). Middle row —* yün-luo *(gong chimes),* lo *(gongs), two* chettö *(flutes), drum. Bottom row — drum, three* pipa *(lutes),* sheng *(mouth organ).*

Japan

Japanese musical history can be divided into several stages of development. The first stage is the period up to the 6th century when the country, which had previously been ruled by a number of clans, was developing into an imperial state. Shinto became the state religion, and the music and dance associated with it became the main body of court music. The second stage, which lasted for the next three centuries, saw the introduction of continental Asian music and dance, as well as Buddhism. It was during this time that *gagaku* came into being.

Gagaku court music is the oldest surviving music in Japan and has been preserved at the imperial court and at a few temples. Nearly 20 different types of instrument are used in *gagaku*, including the *sho* (a reed-pipe mouth organ), flute, drums, gongs and chimes. The various types of *gagaku* include *kangan* (instrumental ensembles), *bagaku* (dance music) and the ritual music for Shinto ceremonies.

ABOVE: Japanese girls playing a samisen *(a guitar-like instrument with three strings) and a* koto *(a 13-stringed zither).*

ABOVE: The shakuhachi, *a bamboo end-blown flute with five finger-holes. The instrument originated in China and was taken to Japan by Buddhist priests in AD 935.*

The third stage in the development of Japanese music came in the period between 900 and 1573. It was then that the theatrical form called *noh* was developed. A marriage of drama, theatre, music and dance, the beauty of *noh* lies in its refined symbolism and sophistication.

The last period saw the Japanese version of the zither, the *koto*, come into fashion. The *koto*, which has 13 silk strings that pass over movable bridges, is played mainly by women, who wear three long ivory plectra on the right hand: one on the thumb, one on the index finger and the third on the middle finger. The left hand is used to dampen the strings and change the pitch. Other Japanese classical instruments of the period include the *shakuhachi* (bamboo flute) and the *biwa* (lute).

Korea

The music of Korea can be traced back over 5000 years and is based on two modes, the *p'yongjo* (common in court music, such as *aak*, and folk songs) and the more widely used *kyemyonjo*. The greatest period of musical development in Korea was during the reign of King Sejong (1418–50). Not only did Sejong reputedly devise the Korean alphabet,

ABOVE: A Korean musician playing the koto, *a kind of zither.*

ABOVE: *A Korean musician playing the* soduang, *a two-stringed instrument with a round resonating box covered with leather at one end and open at the other to admit the neck.*

but he also created an advanced system of musical notation.

Korea treasures its musical heritage, and classical Korean music is actively promoted at the Seoul National Classical Music Institute, where leading musicians are classed as national treasures.

The Korean tradition of *samulnori* drumming goes back at least a thousand years. Played by a quartet of musicians on drums and gongs, *samulnori* originated in the rural farmers' dances that are still performed by dancers wearing hats with long ribbons that swirl into spectacular shapes as the dancers move their heads.

Korea is also known for large orchestras of flutes, oboes and bronze and stone chimes that still play on the first Sunday in May at the ancestral shrine in Seoul. This is a very colourful sight: the massive frames of the chimes are richly decorated with dragons and birds, and contrast with the bold, bright costumes of the musicians.

The *kayagum*, a 12-stringed zither, provides the accompaniment to vocal music and is also played as a solo instrument accompanied by the *changgo* (an hourglass-shaped drum) and the *taegum* (a wooden flute). It has been said that the beauty of *kayagum* music is that when a melody makes a leap down it sounds like a waterfall, and when it reaches the bottom the note vibrates in the same way that water bubbles at the foot of a waterfall.

ABOVE: *A Korean* cholgo, *or temple drum, resting on a wooden stand shaped like a tortoise. In ancient mythology the world was deemed to rest on a tortoise.*

ABOVE: *A Korean* honga *orchestra playing Confucian ritual music. A feature of the orchestra is the* pyongyong *or stone chimes. Sixteen tuned stones are freely suspended in a wooden frame in two rows and are struck with a mallet made of cow horn; they continue to emit a clear sound for several minutes.*

European Music in the First Millennium

The chime of minstrel music, dulcimer, and harp with many strings,
a pleasant dinning makes to him who heareth not distinct the note.

DANTE ALIGHIERI (1265–1321)

During the first millennium there seems to have been little innovation in Western music, but an exception was the introduction of Gregorian chant in church services. This was a reshaping of the older Roman chant, in which melodies were sung to the accompaniment of a sustained note on, it is believed, a stringed instrument.

ABOVE: *Gregorian church chant from* De Harmonica Institutione *of Benedictine Abbot Regino von Prum, AD 915.*

Pope Gregory I (AD 590–604) is said to have ordered the collection and codifying of the plainsong used in the Roman church, and his name became associated with this form. The chants were written down by monks, using a form of letter notation above the lines of text. The appearance of "neumes" in the 9th century led to a more exact method of defining pitch.

The teaching of the chant was put on an official footing in the church by Pope Vitalian (AD 657–72), who was instrumental in founding the Scola Cantorum, based on the model of the Byzantine court. It was under Charlemagne (AD 742–814) that the Gregorian chant became widely used. With the associated antiphonal psalmody (a liturgical chant that was sung in association with a psalm), it was sung all over Europe.

The chant's system of eight tones was directly related to the eight church modes. It was for unaccompanied voice for, according to St Aloysius, any form of musical instrument was a tool of the devil, while St Augustine expressed concern over the seductive "peril of pleasure" created by beautiful singing. However, in the 9th century Benedictine culture began to include the advancement of music. The monastic revival of the late 10th century saw the gradual introduction of organs into churches, although these were not originally used as an accompaniment to the singing, but rather served for signalling purposes, both to call people to worship and to denote points of the service, like the bell at the elevation of the host.

ABOVE: *This 8th-century illumination shows King David playing the crwth, accompanied by four horns and two dancers. Scribes are writing down the words.*

ABOVE: *This drawing from the late 10th century shows Pope Gregory dictating to Deacon Peter.*

Secular music

Songs were, of course, also sung outside the church, especially on long journeys such as those to the various crusades and on pilgrimages. It is known that music played a role in the building of Notre-Dame (1163–1250), when the workers sang as they worked. Indeed, at this time Paris was the musical centre of the Western world, and its university was one of the first officially to teach music.

One of the leading French musicians of the time was Léonin, who was active in Paris between 1163 and 1190. Léonin played a part in the early development of polyphony, by composing *organum* (a medieval form of part-writing) for two voices taken from the solo portions of graduals and alleluias for all the principal feasts of the ecclesiastical year. The main significance of this work was the introduction of a rational system of rhythm into polyphonic music. After Léonin's death, his work was modified by his pupil Pérotin.

This was the age of the peripatetic musician. There were two main classes: the troubadour (a cultivated travelling musician, generally of noble birth) and the minstrel (a professional entertainer, of more lowly birth). In Germany, the 12th, 13th and 14th centuries saw the heyday of the *Minnesinger*, the German equivalent of the French troubadours. All these singers were both poets and composers of their own songs, for at this time very few sang other people's music.

ABOVE: *While peripatetic minstrels were a feature of the medieval landscape, some houses retained their own musicians. This trio is playing a tabor, pipe, small harp and lute.*

ABOVE: *A group of four early 14th-century German troubadours playing the unusual combination of two trumpets, drum and bagpipes.*

Structuring Music

Music is the reaching out towards the
utmost realities by means of ordered sound.

RALPH VAUGHAN WILLIAMS (1872–1958)

The Greek mathematician Pythagoras (c.570–500 BC) carried out the earliest known acoustical experiments. Knowing that the shorter the length of a string the higher the pitch will be, Pythagoras demonstrated that pleasing intervals were sounded when a string is divided into certain ratios. When the length is halved, an octave is formed; when it is reduced to two-thirds the pitch is raised by a perfect fifth; when reduced to three-quarters it gives the perfect fourth. The same applies to the length of a column of air in a wind instrument. Over the years the remaining intervals of the scale were filled in with tones and semitones and thus began the gradual progress that culminated in the recognition of

ABOVE: The number of lines in each staff varied. This music from the Furtmeyer Missal, *written for the Archbishop of Salzburg in 1481, is on a four-line staff.*

tonality, or key. This concept has since remained the basis of musical composition in the West, though smaller intervals, called "microtones", occur in other musical cultures, such as in Indian music, and have been used by some experimental composers of the 20th century.

Harmonic vibrations

It was not until the 17th century that the relationship between the frequency of vibration and the length, diameter, tension and density of the string was established. It was Galileo (1564–1642) who discovered that if either the string's thickness or length is doubled, the frequency of vibration, and consequently the pitch, is halved. For this reason, bass strings can be

made thicker than treble ones – if they were all of the same thickness the lowest string in a piano would have to be about 6.5m/7 yards long.

Notation

The staff originated in medieval Europe as a means of recording plainsong. At first it was a single line around which the neumes, like small ticks, were placed to show the approximate melodic and rhythmic shape. Additional lines were added in the 11th century and the spaces, as well as the lines, were used to position the notes. By the 16th century, today's exactitude of recording pitch was arrived at when a pair of five-line staves became the norm, arranged as a "grand staff" with the top five lines

ABOVE: The frontispiece of Franchino Gaffari's Theorica Musicæ *(1492) showing Pythagoras playing instruments such as tuned bells, musical glasses and pipes.*

ABOVE: This 12th-century plainchant from the Missale Romanum *shows the neumatic notation of the day. There is only one line of "notes" which rise and fall.*

ABOVE: *This manuscript, entitled* Sumer is Icumen In *(c.1240), uses a six-line staff.*

Novel notation

During the 20th century,
various avant-garde composers
have experimented with new
forms of notation, including
squiggles, blobs, graphs and
wiring diagrams. Only one
system made an impression,
albeit very minor, and that was
only because a very rich man,
Cornelius Pot, was behind it.
Pot, a Dutchman, invented
Klavarskribo in 1931.
Intending it as a new method
of piano notation, he even
founded the Klavarskribo
Institute to promote it. By
1950 he had produced some
10,000 works transcribed
into Klavarskribo notation
but, in spite of copies
regularly turning up in second-
hand music shops, no known
pianist can read it.

forming the treble clef and the bottom
five lines the bass clef.

The *flat* sign, which originally
applied only to the B line, originated as
a lower case *b*. The natural sign was a
square gothic *b* that was later modified
to give today's symbol. The *sharp* sign
originated as a cancelled *b* with a
stroke through it.

Tonic solfa

The tonic solfa had its roots in the
11th century when a monk named
Guido d'Arezzo devised a way to help
singers learn a new melody by relating
its notes to the pitches of certain
syllables associated with a well-known
tune. The tune he chose was a Latin
hymn in which the first syllables of the
first six lines were each set one note
higher than the previous one. Using
the first syllable of each line as his
model, he came up with Ut, Re, Mi,
Fa, So, La. Apart from the change of
Ut to Doh and the addition of Ti, these
syllables are still used today.

Strings

There's not a string attuned to mirth
but has its chord in melancholy.

THOMAS HOOD (1799–1845)

I f we believe Greek legend, it was the twang of a bowstring that first made the god Apollo aware of the musical properties of a vibrating string. The fundamental pitch at which a stretched string, held in tension between two points, is heard, depends upon its length, thickness, weight and tension, together with the properties of the soundbox or soundboard. The frequency at which a given string will vibrate is inversely proportional to its length, proportional to the square of its tension and inversely proportional to the square of its mass, while the amplitude varies with the energy imparted and transmitted.

Materials

A string for a musical instrument may be made of any material that can produce a musical sound when it is held under tension and plucked, bowed or struck. Although most early

ABOVE: These two putti, one playing a small harp and the other the portative organ, are from the frieze of musical angels in the Chapel of Isotta degli Atti in Rimini.

strings were made out of gut or silk, many other materials have also been used, such as gold wire strings found in Persia dating from the 5th century BC. More recently, nylon or steel strings have become common, and many strings are bound with fine wire.

Gut strings were made from the guts of lambs, from seven to eight months old. After cleansing and pickling in an alkaline solution, the guts were twisted together under tension before being polished with pads made of hair. The final diameter of the string was determined by the number of guts used, which ranged from two for the smallest mandolin string, up to 120 for a double bass.

Methods of string-playing

There are three ways to excite the string: plucking, bowing or striking. Although plucking excites an active range of high harmonics, they are short-lived. Plucking imparts energy by a single impulse and there is no means of maintaining the vibration. The optimum place to pluck a string is about one-seventh of its length from the end, as this will give the best selection of harmonics as well as amplitude. If the string is plucked either with the fingernails or with a plectrum, it is displaced at a sharp angle and a bright sound is produced, as opposed to the duller sound made when it is plucked with the pad of the finger or thumb.

ABOVE: A mid 13th-century fiddler playing with a large arched bow. The stick extends beyond the end of the hair, the projection serving as a handle.

ABOVE: This 13th-century illustration of King David shows him playing a harp whose arching neck terminates in an open-mouthed zoomorphic head.

A more solid sound is obtained by striking the string (as on a piano or a dulcimer). A struck string vibrates longer, giving a slower decay in the upper harmonics. However, in the stiffer and tenser lower strings of the piano the vibrations tend not to subdivide indefinitely into the shorter lengths, causing the upper harmonics to be weaker, with most of the energy going into the lower harmonics. Like the plucked string, the struck string has only a single impulse for each note sounded.

One of the more pleasing sounds achieved from a string is by using a bow, which maintains the supply of energy for vibration and thus permits the playing of sustained notes. The sound depends on the position of the bow and the width of the hair brought into operation. Different sounds can be produced by bowing slowly with the full width of the hair, bowing near the centre of the string, bowing swiftly with the edge of the hair, or bowing near the end of the string.

Types of string

TOP ROW, FROM LEFT TO RIGHT: Until the 1970s many violinists used gut strings exclusively, but as the high-tensioned E string had a tendency to break easily, it was replaced by wire.

Viola strings are usually made of gut. The lower two, or sometimes all, are wire-wound.

Harp strings are like piano strings, except that they are plucked.

Most classical guitar strings are made of nylon. They are usually sounded with the left side of the fingernails, but some players prefer to use the right side of their nails.

BOTTOM ROW, FROM LEFT TO RIGHT: Acoustic guitar strings can be made of gut or steel, played with fingers or plectrum.

Mandolin strings are laid in four courses of two. Tuned to the same pitch as the violin, the strings are played with a plectrum.

The strings of the sitar are carried over two bridges, first the "small" bridge and then the "main" bridge. Tuning is achieved by the pegs, and beads are used for fine tuning.

The strings of a piano range in thickness from very thin top strings to the thickly wound bass strings shown here.

Bows

The Devil rides upon a fiddlestick.
WILLIAM SHAKESPEARE (1564–1616), "HENRY IV PART 1"

The use of a bow as an instrumental accessory originated in the Byzantine Empire but, because of the weak tone of early bowed instruments compared with that of plucked ones, it was considered to be worthy only of the "common people". It was introduced into Europe in the 11th century by the Islamic conquerors of Spain, and within 100 years the bow had become known and was being used over most of western Europe.

Early bows

The form of the early bows, which were in the shape of fully drawn hunting bows, differed greatly from those in use today. As its name suggests, the bow originally had a convex shape, designed to hold a band of horsehair under tension so that it could be drawn across the strings of an instrument to set up a sustained vibration. In time the bowed shape became longer and more slender,

ABOVE: *Early bows, as the name implies, were similar in appearance to bows used in archery, with a high arched stick.*

though it was still convex. By the 12th century, bows with a curve at one end – a type still occasionally found in eastern Europe – had become popular.

The horsehair was tied directly to the stick at both ends, and the player varied the tension while using the bow, to facilitate the playing of single strings or multiple stopping (drawing the string over more than one string simultaneously). To allow for this, the bow was held in the fist and pressure was exerted on the hair with the fingers.

Early bows differed greatly in size; they could be as small as 20cm/8in. In the 16th century, the violin was becoming a popular instrument for dance music, and short bows of about 35cm/14in were adequate for this purpose. Concert bows were substantially longer, and some were more than twice the

size of the instrument being played. Some bows had sticks that extended well beyond the end of the hair, the projection serving as a handle.

Modern bow

In the second half of the 18th century the bow underwent a number of radical changes, principally to suit the development of the violin as a solo, virtuoso instrument. The new designs were the work of François Tourte (1747–1835) and Wilhelm Cramer (1745–99). Cramer designed a concave bow, which quickly led to the abandonment of the convex version. Tourte widened the ribbon of hair to about 1cm/⅓in, composed of 150–200 strands cut

ABOVE, FROM TOP TO BOTTOM: *The ribbon of the modern violin bow is made of horsehair. The viola bow is similar to the violin bow but is slightly larger.*

ABOVE: *The standard length of the cello bow is about 68cm/27in.*

ABOVE: *The double bass bow is shorter and heavier than the cello bow, and can be held either from above or underneath.*

ABOVE: *Detail from Bellini's* Maria with Child and Saints *(1505) showing an angel playing a large viol with a bow that shows the trend for the arch to become lower.*

ABOVE: The insipid tone of early bowed instruments was due to the bow stick being weak. The player could not tighten the hair and so the strings could not be firmly gripped.

from white horses' tails. He attached this to a strong, movable frog, so that the tension on the hair could be adjusted and set at the beginning of the performance. The bow could now be held lightly with the fingertips, instead of being grasped firmly in the whole hand. This allowed much greater flexibility and delicacy of playing style, which facilitated the rise of the great 18th and 19th-century violin virtuosi.

ABOVE: This illustration of 1830 shows the "old" and "new" styles of bowing the violin.

Bach bow

The Bach bow was created by Knud Vestergard of Viby, Denmark to play the Bach solo violin sonatas "precisely as written", and is associated with the violinist Telmányi. The bow has a very high arch, with as much as 10cm/4in separating the bow stick and the hair at the highest point. When playing on individual strings the bow hair can be tightened by a lever worked by the thumb. By loosening the hair the player is able to encompass all the strings, and thus sustain multiple stops continuously. The creation, however, succeeds in playing Bach's music only as imagined by the bow's 20th-century inventor – not as Bach intended or heard it.

Tourte also fixed the length of the violin bow at about 75cm/30in and the playing hair at about 65cm/25in. To make the stick he chose red Brazilian pernambuco wood for its combination of strength and lightness. These innovations in design established the form of the standard modern bow, which is sometimes referred to as the "Tourte bow".

ABOVE: Early 14th-century fiddler playing with a high arched bow. The player is gripping the bow where the stick extends beyond the end of the hair.

ABOVE: The modern bow, as used by American violinist Isaac Stern (born 1920). Stern's playing – particularly of the Barber and Bruch concertos – has thrilled audiences for over 50 years.

Reeds

There's music in the singing of a reed.

<small>LORD BYRON (1788–1824)</small>

The sound of a reed instrument is initiated by the vibration of the reed, which sets up the vibration of the air column in the tube of the instrument. Reed instruments fall into two main categories, according to the use of the reed: they are known as "bleating" and "free". The ancient Greek aulos was an early bleating reed-pipe and is known to date back to at least 2800 BC.

Reed preparation
In ancient Greece, cane for making aulos reeds was cut during early summer, when at its most elastic,

ABOVE: A selection of different types of single reeds (from top to bottom) — clarinet, alto saxophone, tenor saxophone and baritone saxophone.

and laid out to season in the open. It was scraped and cleaned during the following spring, and cut into segments at the nodes: each internode furnished two reeds. Segments closer to the root were suitable for the left-hand pipe of the aulos and those closer to the tip of the stem were used for right-hand pipes. This is an indication that the left-hand pipe was the lower pitched of the two.

Today, reeds are still cut from the stem of the large semi-tropical grass *Arundo donax* or *Arundo sativa*, commonly, but inaccurately, called cane. The plants are specially cultivated in parts of Spain and southern France. They are now factory-cut, but many players learn to cut their own, a very skilled art. Various attempts to find substitutes for *Arundo donax* have been made from time to time, and materials as diverse

ABOVE: A single reed.

as silver and whalebone have been tried, but have never been successful. A recent development has been the use of manmade fibres, although the general consensus is that artificial reeds sound coarser than those made from natural cane.

Bleating reeds
A reed that beats against a surface is known as a "bleating" reed, and instruments that work on this principle can also be subdivided according to whether they use single or double reeds. The single reed, typified by that

ABOVE: A selection of oboe double reeds — two baroque, classical, classical oboe d'amore, modern oboe, modern oboe d'amore, two cor anglais and bass oboe.

ABOVE: The idea for a reed instrument must have evolved from people finding that blowing on a blade of grass produced a sound. This engraving is from Bonanni's Gabinetto Armonico *(1723).*

ABOVE: The various stages in making a reed. Top — the cut cane, Middle — the cane is cut in half, split and the scrape is shaped. Bottom — the final stages in shaping, trademarking and packaging the reed.

of the clarinet, is a narrow slip cut to length, flattened on the inner side, and on the other side scraped down to a feather edge at one end. It is fastened to the mouthpiece of the instrument and vibrates against it.

The double bleating reed, typified by that of the bassoon, is made up of two slips of "cane", hollowed out on the inside until quite thin and again scooped to a feather edge on the outside. The two slips are then bound together and mounted in a short metal tube, known as the "staple".

Free reeds

The free reed is found mainly in certain organ pipes and bellows-blown instruments such as the harmonium and accordion. It is also used in the harmonica (mouth organ) as well as in the traditional Chinese *sheng*. The pitch

of the reeds, which are fastened over slots cut into the metal frame, can be lowered by filing near the fixed end, or raised by filing near the free end. A major development in the history of the accordion was the introduction by firms such as Höhner, founded in Trossingen in 1857, of high-tempered steel reeds, which helped to ensure the instrument's popularity.

LEFT: Although most professional oboe players make their own reeds, the process takes time and skill, and ready-made reeds are available.

Valves

*The irremediable vulgarity of the cornet's timbre
has kept it away from the symphonic orchestra.*

MICHAEL BRENET

In 1815 a notice appeared in the *Allgemeine Musikalische Zeitung* that was to change the evolution of the brass instrument forever. Heinrich Stölzel, a 38-year-old horn player in the orchestra of Prince von Pless in Upper Silesia, announced that he had produced a horn on which a scale of nearly three octaves could be achieved by means of two airtight valves that were pressed down by "piano keys" and returned by springs. Although Stölzel is often regarded as the sole inventor of the valve, it is believed that he was ably assisted by his fellow musician Friedrich Blühmel.

ABOVE: *An 1848 view inside Adolph Sax's factory showing brass instruments being produced.*

Function of the valve

The purpose of the valve is to admit vibrating air into, or exclude it from, auxiliary tubing of sufficient length to lower the basic pitch of an instrument by a certain musical interval. The length of this tubing must be in proportion to that of the main tubing; the length for a whole tone is about one-eighth of the whole and that for

ABOVE: *A trumpet has three piston valves and two finger grips.*

a semitone about one-fifteenth. On a three-valved instrument the depression of the first valve lowers the pitch of the instrument a whole tone; depression of the second lowers it a semitone; and the third a whole tone plus a semitone. This combination, with different harmonics obtainable by altering the pressure of the lips, allows a complete scale to be played.

Once the valve has been depressed and released it is instantly returned by a spring; the most common method is to have the spring push the valve back up from the bottom.

Although valves are traditionally made of brass, sometimes plated with silver or nickel, other materials have been used. The Boosey "Solbron" was made of bronze while, for its

tubas, the Swiss Hirstbrunner Company produces the "Trypen" valve, which is made from a combination of brass and plastic. The most efficient valves, however, are those made from "Monel", which is a copper-nickel alloy.

Piston valve

In the years between 1820 and 1840, various experiments resulted in the production of two different types of valve: piston and rotary. In 1835 Wilhelm Wieprecht produced his robust short-stroke Berliner Pumpen

LEFT: *The piston valve is returned to its open position by means of the spring, while the coquilles connect with and admit air into the additional tubes that change the pitch of the instrument.*

ABOVE: *Each piston valve has its own tuning slide; the further out the slide is pulled, the lower the note produced.*

ABOVE: *The flugelhorn uses piston valves to produce the different pitches required.*

valves. These had horizontal passageways and were used on all types of brass instruments. In 1839 this was improved upon by Etienne-François Périnet, who made a lighter and narrower valve, in which the coquilles were positioned obliquely in the piston. The main advantage of this valve was that it could be worked faster and the air column moved around a curve instead of, as with Wieprecht's valve, around a 90° bend.

ABOVE: *Tuba valves are, of necessity, bigger than trumpet valves and as such take longer to return to the open position after being depressed. This means that as a rule the tuba does not play fast music and is usually not expected to play notes shorter than semi-quavers.*

Today, many euphoniums and tubas have four valves. The extra valve not only helps to keep the instrument in tune, but also allows the musician to play lower harmonics. Most makers place the extra valve at the back of the instrument, where it is operated by the first finger of the left hand. However, the Yamaha Company of Japan positions its four valves together, parallel with the bell, and all are operated by the fingers of the right hand.

Rotary valve

Although several people experimented with rotary valves, Joseph Riedel of Vienna produced the design that is used in modern horns. Riedel's valve, which was patented in 1832, has two passageways that pass through the rotor, one on each side of a central spindle. When the valve is operated the cylinder rotates through 90°, directing the air into the valve tube much as water flows through a tap.

ABOVE: *Close-up view of the rotary valves on a French horn. Rotary valves were invented by Joseph Riedel in 1832.*

Drum Heads and Sticks

The noisy drum has nothing in it, but mere air.

THOMAS FULLER (1608–61)

When a drum is struck, the membrane vibrates in both a circular and a segmental pattern, producing a fundamental tone and various harmonic overtones, the number and strength of which affect the timbre of the instrument. The timbre and apparent pitch of the drum also vary according to the type of beater used, the degree of hardness or softness of the beater and its contact area on the drum head. Hard beaters produce high overtones while light ones have virtually none.

The sound of the drum is also influenced by the place where the membrane is struck. If this is at the edge, high overtones will be elicited, while if it is hit at or near the centre, deeper tones will predominate. Percussionists get to know their instruments and know the place on the membrane (the "beating spot") that is best to strike.

Drum heads
The first drum heads were made of hide, but animal skin reacts strongly to changes in atmospheric humidity,

ABOVE: *The Indian* dhol *has two indefinitely pitched heads, each with a loud, deep sound. The drum is used to herald public announcements and to lead processions.*

so today artificial materials such as plastic are used. Early side drum heads were tensioned with ropes drawn into V-shapes, with leather buffs at the point of each V which were drawn to tighten the ropes and thus increase the tension. Other methods were introduced later, the most usual being rods with screw nuts. Until World War II, most drums were single-tensioned, with one screw working on both heads. However, as most players prefer to have one head tighter than the other, double-tensioning was introduced, whereby each head is separately controlled by rods that screw into blocks halfway down the shell.

RIGHT: *One of 12 musical angels painted by the Italian painter Fra Angelico in 1433. This one is playing a drum with a parchment head.*

Drum sticks
There are three main types of beater head: hard, medium and soft. The choice of suitable sticks or beaters depends on the tonal effects required, as different types of stick or beater will influence the sound of the drum in three ways: volume, tone and attack. The harder the head of the beater, the louder the sound will be.

All drums have a sound-spectrum: they will produce a wide range of different sounds. A thin, hard-headed stick will bring out the higher sounds, causing the drum to sound bright and clear. A soft-headed beater, on the other hand, will elicit the low tones, producing a mellow, muffled sound. Hard beaters will produce a crisp,

ABOVE: *The military side drum is covered with a head of either calfskin or plastic.*

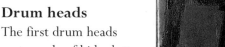

Timpano, timbale and bass drum heads

ABOVE: A timpano with a plastic head. The timpanist tunes the head to the required pitch by means of a foot pedal, a device that was invented in 1881 by Carl Pittrich.

ABOVE: The screw-tensioned heads of timbales are made of plastic and usually tuned a certain distance apart. They are usually played in pairs with wooden sticks.

ABOVE: This military bass drum has a plastic head. Plastic, unlike organic hide, is not affected by moisture and is therefore suitable for use in military parades in wet weather.

well-defined attack, while soft beaters, which tend to have larger contact areas, will give a less distinct delivery, the sound being smothered by the spread of the beater head at each contact with the drum.

In general, hard wooden sticks are used for snare drums, while sticks with hard to medium rounded heads (of wood, woven yarn, plastic or hard rubber) are used for playing xylophones and vibraphones. Instruments such as the marimba are played with soft-headed beaters, while timpani can be played with sticks in three degrees of hardness, according to whether the core is covered with soft, medium or hard felt. Some timpani sticks are double-ended, with felt heads on one end and wooden ball-shaped heads on the other, so that the sticks can be quickly reversed as required by the music.

BELOW, FROM LEFT TO RIGHT: Sticks for the bass drum, glockenspiel, vibraphone, rototom, timpani and xylophone.

ABOVE: A percussionist may need a number of different sticks and beaters for a given performance. A selection of sticks is shown here in a container suitable for travelling.

Keyboard Keys and Hammers

Seated one day at the organ I was weary and ill at ease,
And my fingers wandered idly, Over the noisy keys.

ADELAIDE A. PROCTER (1825–64), "A LOST CHORD"

Early European keyboards were simple devices with heavy levers operated with the hands rather than the fingers. The spacing between the keys on early organs, the oldest keyboard instruments, was the same as that for the pipes, sometimes as much as 10cm/4in. Up to the 13th century keyboards were diatonic, with C as the first key. When the B flat was added, this was not intended only for the playing of melodies but also as an aid to transposition. Used solely to accompany plainsong, early keyboards had a range not exceeding two octaves – matching that of the voices of the monks. In the 14th century, with the development of polyphony, the keyboard compass began to widen, and

ABOVE: Detail from Court Concert at Prince Bishop's of Lüttich in Seraing Palace *by Paul Delcloche (1753). This finely decorated piano still lacks a pedal.*

ABOVE: The piano keyboard consists of white and black keys. The white keys are the natural notes while the black ones cover the sharps and flats.

by 1330 most of the chromatic keys that we know today had been added.

Closed-case keyboard instruments, in which the tuned strings are held taut above a sounding board, include those in which the strings are plucked, such as the harpsichord and spinet, and pianos, in which they are hammered. Since the harpsichord player cannot control the force with which the strings are plucked, larger instruments frequently have a second keyboard that can be used to add variety in weight and sound quality. Both piano and harpsichord keyboards have the keys for the diatonic notes at the front, with the keys for the other five notes of the chromatic scale (the black keys) arranged between and a little behind them. The modern full-size piano keyboard has 88 notes.

ABOVE: Detail of the strings of a grand piano made by the Berlin firm of Bechstein.

ABOVE: *The piano hammers hit the strings from underneath. Over the strings is the row of dampers that stop the sound.*

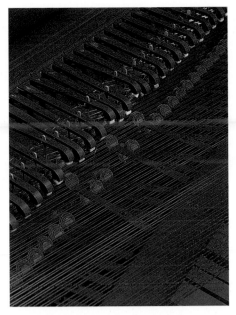

ABOVE: *The hammers of a square piano, in which the strings are arranged horizontally in a rectangular box-like case.*

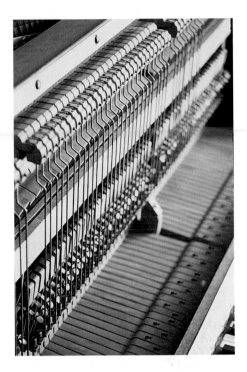

ABOVE: *Interior view of an upright piano.*

Hammerheads

Several materials have been used for covering piano hammerheads. Early German pianos used buckskin, but this suffered from variations in thickness and elasticity. Early 19th-century leather-covered hammers were light, but as the mass and tension of the strings increased, makers tried to increase the weight of the hammers by loading them with lead. This, however, also increased the effort required to play the instrument and the method was quickly abandoned. In England, a coarse woollen cloth was tried, but it was clear that a softer, more durable

material was needed and in 1826 Jean-Henri Pape patented felt hammers that were a blend of sheep's wool and rabbit fur. This material remained in contact with the string for longer before rebounding, thereby producing a fuller, rounder tone than that achieved by leather.

Bass hammerheads, which are much thicker and heavier than those that strike the treble strings, are pricked with holes to give them a softer texture. The softer the felt the more slowly it rebounds from the string, thus preventing unwanted high overtones. If the felt is untoned it produces an uneven tone, many of the notes sounding duller or brighter than their neighbours.

Piano action

In a grand piano the hammers strike the strings from underneath and fall back by gravity, the action being, therefore, more responsive than in the upright piano, which has to rely on springs to return the hammers. For this reason the quick repetition of notes on the grand piano is generally

more efficient than on the upright. Quick repetition is also facilitated by the escapement, which allows the hammer to rebound from the string and be ready for the same note to be struck again. By catching the hammer before it reaches its original position, the note can be repeated more quickly than would be possible if the hammer travelled the full distance.

ABOVE: *Clavichord hammers are responsive to the force of the player's finger movements.*

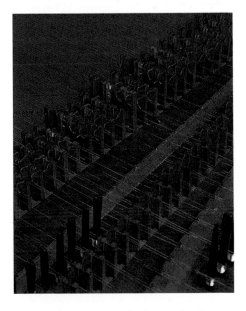

ABOVE: *Interior view of a harpsichord, showing the jacks under the strings.*

Evolution of the Orchestra

Musicke is said to be the rejoycing of the heart:
Musicke comforteth the mynde and feareth the enimie.

JOHN FLORIO (1553–1625), "FIRST FRUTES"

The word "orchestra" comes from the Greek, and originally meant the place where the Greek chorus sang and danced. In the Roman theatre, this space was reserved for the seats of senators. Later it was applied to the stage itself. The term was revived in the late 17th century, and by the early 18th century it had been applied in France to the players themselves.

The roots of the modern orchestra go back to the 16th-century consorts employed in noble households, and to the groups of instrumentalists

ABOVE: Five musical angels from a triptych by Hans Memling painted in about 1480. The instruments depicted are the psaltery, tromba marine, lute, sackbut and tenor shawm.

ABOVE: Fifteenth-century Italian fresco of an angel playing a sackbut – a standard instrument in civic bands at this time.

especially assembled for important occasions such as royal weddings and funerals. During the 17th century the composition of orchestras varied from place to place: strings were preferred in Italy, France and England, whereas the German courts preferred brass ensembles.

Municipal consorts

Musicians were employed by European civic authorities from as early as the 13th century. The first town known to have availed itself of a regular musician was Brunswick, Germany, in 1227. Florence in Italy and Ypres in Belgium had civic musicians by 1291 and 1297 respectively. In Germany, town musicians were known as *Stadtpfeifer* (town pipers) and in England as waits.

The duties of these official musicians were many and varied, ranging from civic functions to church festivals and celebrations.

English waits

The word "wait" derives from either Anglo-Saxon *wacian* or Old High German *Wahta*, both meaning "watch" or "guard". In time the word began to be used for the shawm, the instrument played by the watch, which was generally dubbed the "wait pipe". Many English towns possessed waits at an early date, York (1272) and Norwich (1288) being among the first recorded. The musical part of the waits' duties grew and by the mid 14th century three waits were included in the Royal Band of Edward III. By the

15th century most towns employed waits, whose main function it was to attend the mayor on ceremonial occasions and, in some towns, to play in the streets at night.

Most bands of waits performed only in their local area, but some travelled farther afield. In 1589 Sir Francis Drake employed five Norwich waits, equipped with their shawms, trombone and recorder, to provide shipboard entertainment for his expedition to Lisbon – forming what must have been the first ship's band.

German Turmmusik

Although Germany had had *Stadtpfeifer* since the 13th century, in the 16th century a phenomenon known as *Turmmusik* (tower music) became common. This was music played from the church or town-hall tower. The repertory of these bands consisted in the main of harmonized chorales but also included occasional *Turmsonaten*, which were played by instruments such as cornetts, trombones and trumpets, in four or five-part harmony.

ABOVE: Detail from a mural The Nuremberg Town Band, *painted in about 1500 by Albrecht Dürer. Pictured are two trombones, two cornetts, two shawms and a drum. Later that century a greater variety of instruments was in use, including recorder, viol, fiddle, cornett, guitar, lute, bandora and bagpipes.*

ABOVE: A 15th-century consort consisting of musicians playing small kettledrums, fiddle, horn, triangle, lute and bagpipes.

Sixteenth-century consort

The main instrument of a medieval consort was the shawm, a double-reed woodwind instrument that was first used in western Asia for dance and ceremonial music, and was brought to Europe by returning crusaders in the 12th century. The forerunner of the oboe, it had a piercing, brilliant tone, which made it especially suited for playing outdoors. It was initially used in folk music, and much later in opera.

Like its eastern prototype, the eight-holed European shawm was made from a single, conically bored piece of hardwood, terminating in a bell.

By the beginning of the 16th century shawms were being used in consort, and several sizes were made. The type instrument was the seven-holed treble, which was about 66cm/26in long. The shrill-toned soprano shawm was tuned a fifth above the treble and was about 48cm/19in long. The alto shawm, tuned a fifth below the treble, was about 76cm/30in long. The tenor shawm, which was tuned a fifth below the alto, was 112cm/4ft long and had a long S-shaped staple on which the reed and pirouette were mounted.

The bass instrument, which was known as the "bombarde" due to its resemblance to the newly invented artillery piece, was tuned an octave below the tenor and was 1.8m/6ft long. It had two keys at the front and two at the rear. There was also a giant bass shawm of about 3m/10ft in length which when played was passed under the musician's arm with the bell resting on the floor behind him.

Baroque Orchestra (1600–1750)

Handel's entertainments are calculated for the Quality only,
people of moderate fortunes cannot pretend to them.

In the 17th century, instrumental music was still the privilege of the great aristocratic and royal households that had the means to employ full-time orchestras and composers. Indeed, the only way that a composer could earn a living was to be employed as a servant by some wealthy patron, either a leading church dignitary or a member of the aristocracy.

A feature of Baroque music was the *basso continuo*, or figured bass, and most music was written for strings and a harpsichord. The harpsichord shared the bass line with the cello, but also added chords that helped to thicken the harmonic texture.

Italy

One of the first orchestras resembling those of today was formed in 1607 by Claudio Monteverdi (1567–1643).

ABOVE: Jean-Baptiste Lully (1639–87) is seen here with the score of Armide et Renaud, *which he composed in 1686.*

Language

By the early 17th century Italian composers had begun to write expression marks into their music, which is why today Italian is still, by convention, the language of Western music. Indeed such was the influence of Italy that some 19th-century English musicians adopted Italian versions of their plain English names, believing – not without good reason – that this would impress their public. The composer John Cooper (c.1570–1627) became Giovanni Coprario, and the Irish tenor and friend of Mozart, Michael Kelly (1762–1826) called himself "Ochelli". Charles Dickens satirized this curious affectation in his story *The Dancing Academy*, in which the dancing master is a certain Signor Billsmethi.

Employed by the Duke of Mantua at one of the richest courts in Italy, Monteverdi was able to use a 40-strong band of strings, flutes, cornetts and trombones for his opera *Orfeo*. The fusion of brass and strings – as opposed to the earlier orchestration of strings and woodwind only – had been adopted by many bands in northern

Italy, particularly that of St Mark's, Venice, where Monteverdi ended his career.

This was a period when opera flourished in Naples in the hands of Alessandro Scarlatti (1660–1725). However, in Italy instrumental music also began to be played in its own right, independently of opera, and the concerto came into being. Two of the foremost Italian composers of this form were Arcangelo Corelli (1653–1713) and Antonio Vivaldi (1675–1741). Both wrote *concerti grossi*, characterized by the interplay between a large and a small group of instruments.

France

The *Vingt-quatre Violons du Roi*, which confusingly sometimes numbered 25, was set up to provide music at the court of Louis XIII (1601–43). It served as a training ground for the most brilliant players in France, as well as establishing a stylized method of playing dance music. The band, which had the reputation of decorating and embellishing everything it played, played from memory and as a result some of its performances were nothing short of disastrous. However, when Jean-Baptiste Lully became Louis XIV's *Compositeur de la Musique Instrumentale* he set up his own band, the *Petits Violons*. This band, whose members were the first to wear a uniform and to use their bows in the same direction, was greatly admired and soon became a model for the rest of Europe.

Public concerts

Although music had been banned in England during the Commonwealth (1648–60), on his return from exile in France it was not surprising that Charles II was quick to introduce French music and customs to the English court. One of the Royal violinists was John Banister who, in 1672, started organizing musical performances at his home, which an invited audience would pay to hear.

At the beginning of the 18th century, public concerts as we know them today were still unknown, and musical performances were restricted to the homes of the nobility. However, as the standard of living gradually rose, so did the mercantile class, whose new opulence stimulated a desire for novelty in all forms of artistic expression, including music. It was, however, still music by the upper classes for the upper classes.

Some of the earliest public paid-entry concerts in France were the *Concerts Spirituels*, which began in 1725 in a hall in the Tuileries, Paris.

ABOVE: The Concert *(1690) by A. D. Gabbiani shows seven Modena court musicians playing violins, cello and harpsichord.*

These were primarily performances of sacred music, sung in Latin, which took place on holy days in the church calendar (when the opera was closed). The difference between these events and those organized by Banister in England was that whereas Banister's audience consisted solely of invited guests, there were no restrictions on admission to the Paris concerts.

ABOVE: In the middle of the 18th century the rich still employed musicians to perform in their homes. This painting shows a group of patrons listening to a singer accompanied by a chamber band consisting of a harpsichord, two violins, viola and cello.

ABOVE: Johann Sebastian Bach performing on a piano before his patron Frederick the Great in May 1747.

Classical Orchestra (1750–1830)

Orchestral music is one of the glories of the world.

GEORG SOLTI (1912–97)

The love of orchestral music had become so widespread by the year 1775 that it was said that even "common servants" could be met who pretended "as much judgement of an opera tune as my Lady Duchess". It was also a period when professional performers began to make large fortunes and composers were able to make an independent living, without having to tie themselves to any one court or church. Two of the first truly independent composers were Wolfgang Amadeus Mozart (1756–91) and Ludwig van Beethoven (1770–1827).

ABOVE: London's 18th-century Vauxhall Gardens were the centre of social intercourse for the upper classes. Anybody who was anybody spent time there chatting to the background music of the house band.

Instrumentation

Mozart wrote his early symphonies for the forces he had available, namely strings, two oboes and two horns. By 1782, however, he was independent and began writing for his ideal orchestra, which included flutes, clarinets, bassoons, trumpets and kettledrums. It was, however, Joseph Haydn (1732–1809) and Beethoven who established the nucleus of the modern symphony orchestra; by 1800 the average size of the orchestra was about 40.

Mannheim

One of the first "modern" symphony orchestras was founded by Johann Stamitz (1717–57) at the court of Duke Karl Theodor at Mannheim, Germany, in 1742. The Mannheim orchestra consisted of 50 virtuoso players, making it the largest regular ensemble in Europe at that time. "Its *forte* was like thunder, its *crescendos* like mighty waterfalls, its *diminuendos* like a gentle river disappearing into the distance, its *pianos* like a breath of spring." When a long *crescendo* began it was not unknown for the audience gradually to rise from their seats. This *crescendo* became known as the "Mannheim Steamroller", while an expressive falling phrase was the

ABOVE: Mozart was one of the few musical child prodigies whose genius developed with maturity. By the age of two he was already discovering chords on the keyboard and, by the time he was five, was performing on and composing pieces for the instrument. As well as 18 masses, 21 concertos and 41 symphonies, Mozart also wrote 12 operas, two of the most popular being The Marriage of Figaro *and* The Magic Flute.

"Mannheim Sigh", and various interpolated woodwind trills and turns were "Mannheim Birdies".

Subscription concerts

By the end of the 18th century concerts were being held frequently. Although they were now public events rather than private parties held in the homes of the nobility, they remained an exclusive form of entertainment due to the high price of subscriptions, which had become established by 1760. By charging in advance in this way, promoters of concerts knew just what money was available and thus were able to hire the finest performers they could afford. It was not until the middle of the 19th century that there was a change from subscriptions to the selling of tickets at reasonable prices.

In the days of Mozart and Haydn the audience did not sit quietly as (in theory) they do today, but engaged

in many activities, including eating, drinking, chattering to their friends and falling asleep. It is said that Haydn wrote his Symphony No. 94, nicknamed the "Surprise", to wake them up.

Music festivals

A phenomenon unique to British society during the Classical period was the music festival. Lasting two or three days, these were held in many provincial towns in aid of local charities, drawing in the famous musical names of the day to give local people a chance to hear what London audiences were able to enjoy on a regular basis. The annual *Three Choirs* festival, held in Gloucester, Worcester and Hereford, was one of the first to be founded, in 1724. Leicester held two such festivals in 1771 and 1774 and, in July 1803, just over the border in Warwickshire, Nuneaton held a two-day event. In 1823 and 1825 York held two very successful festivals and, in 1826, under royal patronage, over £2400 (US$1485) was raised in Birmingham, a town that had been holding triennial festivals since the 1790s. The forward march of

ABOVE: The band of strings and horns at the San Beneto Teatro. The musicians are placed in two serried ranks at the side of the hall in Venice.

ABOVE: Beethoven, who had received his early musical education from his father, became a professional musician at the age of 11. Over the next few years he took lessons from Mozart and Haydn. Soon his aristocratic patrons recognized the worth of his work and gave him financial support for the rest of his life.

ABOVE: By the early 19th century renowned opera singers such as Giuseppe de Begnis were performing virtuoso parts full of technically difficult vocal pyrotechnics.

19th-century musical life in Britain continued in 1813 with the founding of the London Philharmonic Society, whose main aim was to perform the great orchestral works of the day.

Romantic Orchestra (1830–1910)

*It is scarcely credible that a distinct Romantic school
could be formed in music, which is in itself romantic.*

Robert Schumann (1810–56)

By the 1850s the orchestra was increasing in size, and by 1880 it was not unusual to see an ensemble of 100 or more instrumentalists. Composers were beginning to treat the orchestra as a homogeneous whole rather than as diverse sections, with an increasing awareness of the importance of internal balance.

One of the greatest Romantic composers was Richard Wagner (1813–83) who, unlike earlier composers, was not content simply to write for the instrumental forces already present in the orchestra. As well as introducing existing instruments to the orchestra, he even specified the making of new ones, such as the bass trumpet and the Wagner tubas for *The Ring*. Hector Berlioz (1803–69) was also an

ABOVE: A scene from the première of Wagner's Rienzi, *performed at the Dresden Hoftheater on October 20, 1842.*

ambitious composer, and in his *Requiem* he called for a chime of 16 timpani. Gustav Mahler (1860–1911) wrote on an equally grand scale, and his Eighth Symphony was written for a chorus of 500, as well as 350 children's voices, seven soloists and an augmented

orchestra – not for nothing was this work nicknamed the "Symphony of a Thousand".

On June 17, 1872 the largest orchestra ever formed took part in a concert at the World Peace Jubilee in Boston, Massachusetts. The orchestra of 1000 instrumentalists and choir of 20,000 voices were conducted by Johann Strauss the younger, who was on a tour of the United States. Armed with a long illuminated baton and 100 assistant conductors, he led the band (as Strauss later recalled) in an "unholy racket" such as he had never before or since heard.

Larger orchestras meant higher overheads and, as many orchestras no longer had royal patronage, it was only through the efforts of the rich music-lovers who sponsored events that most orchestras survived. Bigger concert halls were built to accommodate the large paying audiences that were needed at concerts to make the orchestras viable.

Promenade concerts

The concept of the promenade concert originated in France, where successful concerts were mounted in Paris by Philippe Musard and Louis Antoine Jullien. The format was brought to Britain, and the first London promenade concert was held in December 1838. Unlike promenade concerts today, where the audience is static, those attending these early events literally did promenade, chatting to their friends as the concert progressed. Music was a secondary

ABOVE: Richard Wagner, one of Europe's finest Romantic composers, is seen here conducting the Siegfried Idyll *on the steps of his house as a surprise for his wife Cosima on the morning of her birthday in 1870.*

ABOVE: *The cover of the sheet music for the* Promenade Quadrille *showing the Covent Garden Orchestra in London, 1870.*

concern, as the audience used the opportunity to show off their fashions.

Orchestral tours

By the 1840s, large musical groups were beginning to tour, both nationally and internationally. This was mainly due to the advent of the railways, which were able to transport large numbers of people (and baggage) much faster than horse-drawn coaches. At last people in the provinces were able to see and hear what those in the capital cities had been enjoying for many years. This led to a resurgence of interest in music, and many towns throughout Europe formed their own amateur bands and choirs.

The music of preceding generations began to be revived. In contrast to the 18th century, when most of the music played was contemporary, during the 19th century the works of

RIGHT: *An illustration of an English orchestra from the early 19th century.*

dead composers, such as Beethoven, Mozart and Handel, found a place in almost every concert.

It was not only bands that were taking advantage of the better transportation; composers and soloists such as Franz Liszt (1811–86), Niccolò Paganini (1782–1840) and Felix Mendelssohn (1809–47) also began to make provincial tours, to the delight of those who were unable to travel to hear them play in the big cities.

ABOVE: *A scene from a performance of Wagner's* Tannhäuser *at the Bayreuth Festival of 1972.*

ABOVE: *An early 19th-century performance in London's Vauxhall Gardens. A feature of the band are the two black musicians – one with a tambourine and the other with a Turkish crescent. An important development during the 18th century was the adoption by European bands of "Turkish" or "Janissary" music. The instrumentation depended heavily on percussion, and a feature of these bands was that percussion instruments were usually played by young black men. Dressed in the most exotic manner, they performed incredible acrobatics as they played.*

Modern Symphony Orchestra

There are two golden rules for an orchestra:
start together and finish together.

THOMAS BEECHAM (1879–1961)

After World War I the cost of mounting such colossal works as Mahler's Eighth Symphony became prohibitive and composers turned their pens to smaller combinations. One such composer was William Walton (1902–83) whose *Façade* was greatly influenced by jazz, as was *The Rio Grande* by Constant Lambert (1905–51). The divide between "serious" music and jazz narrowed, with jazz idioms also coming to the fore in Walton's *Belshazzar's Feast*, in which the squeaking flute sounds like a slate pencil scraping on a hard stone wall. Another composer who used both new and old musical forms was Michael Tippett (1905–98), who

ABOVE: The modern symphony orchestra usually consists of over 90 players, requiring a large concert hall for its performances. The Philharmonia Orchestra is shown here performing at the Royal Festival Hall in London.

ABOVE: For maximum volume, modern composers may include a large choir and percussion section in their compositions. The Bournemouth Symphony Orchestra and Choir are seen here under the direction of Kees Bakels. Founded in 1893, this orchestra has become one of Britain's foremost provincial orchestras and has been conducted by many great maestros.

incorporated motifs from spirituals in *A Child of Our Time* and blues and boogie-woogie in *Songs for Dov*.

In the 1950s the idea developed among composers that each separate instrument should be distinctly audible playing its individual part, rather than hearing the orchestra as an entity, a single giant instrument. Players now had to work much harder than before to give richness or beauty of tone-colour to the music.

Conductorless orchestra

The post-revolutionary Pervyi Simfonicheskii Ansambl (First Symphonic Ensemble) was formed in the USSR in 1922. The unusual aspect of the orchestra was that, believing that in the ideal Marxist state all men are equal, its members felt that there was no need to be led by the dictatorial

baton of a conductor; instead they were led by a committee. Although it was a partial success, the principal difficulty with the concept was in changing tempo. The orchestra survived for ten years and had to be disbanded only when the individual talents began to rebel against the rigid control under which they were expected to play.

New instrumental techniques

Twentieth-century orchestral practice provided composers with a vast range of techniques. One composer who developed a remarkable effect was the Spanish composer Roberto Gerhard (1896–1970), who devised the ethereal ringing tone produced by stroking the edge of a cymbal with a double bass bow. Another novel use of the orchestra was that produced by Pierre Boulez (born 1925) in *Don* from *Pli selon Pli*, where he used the orchestra not as families of woodwind, brass and strings, but as three groups of high, medium and low-voiced instruments, irrespective of their colour.

ABOVE: A modern symphony orchestra stands to acknowledge the audience's applause.

Some composers, although writing music for the instruments of a conventional orchestra, arranged the instruments in unusual combinations. In his *Music for Strings, Percussion and Celeste*, Béla Bartók (1881–1945) divided the strings into two chamber groups placed on either side of a piano, harp, celeste and percussion section.

Another composer who experimented with new effects was Claude Debussy (1862–1918). His symphonic sketch *La Mer*, composed in 1905, was finished while he was staying at the Grand Hotel at Eastbourne in England, overlooking the sea, and is a well-known example of his impressionistic approach to composition. Although Debussy used large forces for his orchestral works, it was less to enhance volume than to create colour in his music.

Other new orchestral effects have been created by the woodwind deliberately overblowing, brass players being instructed to whisper, shout or yell into their mouthpieces, and string players being asked to produce harsh, grating sounds by bowing between the bridge and the tailpiece of their instruments. Compositions like these are set to continue breaking all the rules well into the 21st century.

ABOVE: A large symphony orchestra accompanying a group of jazz soloists.

Authentic Music

The tragedy in the interpetation of music of the past lies in the fact that it is confined to concert halls, congresses of musicology, or conservatory classes. Music needs air, sunlight and liberty to be alive.

WANDA LANDOWSKA (1877–1959)

It has recently become fashionable to perform music with an authentic orchestra, using the number and type of instruments that the composer would originally have intended. Players and scholars alike have investigated early music and instruments in an attempt to discover just what was played and on what instruments, how it sounded and how it was performed. Indeed, such is the current situation that a concert of early music is likely to attract a larger audience than one of modern music.

There are special problems confronting the performer of authentic music, and each of these must be considered before calling a performance truly "authentic". Design and colour cannot be separated. In the same way that an outline drawn by Raphael could not be coloured in with Cézanne's palette, a modern violinist will not play in the same manner as Corelli. Even if he is playing on a 300-year-old instrument, he still has to know how the music was intended to be played.

Although modern composers use instruments which, by name at least,

ABOVE: *Authentic music performances can be a living history experience. In this case a Salzburg violinist is dressed in 18th-century costume to enhance the period effect.*

would have been familiar to Haydn and Beethoven, the style of playing and the sounds produced are totally different. Orchestral sounds changed completely with the introduction of Boehm flutes, Triébert oboes, Klosé clarinets and Heckel bassoons, not to mention valved horns and electronic instruments.

Another factor to bear in mind is the size of the orchestra's string section in relation to the wind section. In the 18th century it was unusual for an orchestra to have more than eight violins, 12 being rare. By the time of Beethoven's death a violin section of 32 had become common. However, there was no relative increase in the woodwind section. It follows therefore

RIGHT: *A modern group of musicians dressed in late 18th-century costume recreating an orchestra playing Mozart's* Te Deum.

LEFT: A chamber group of musicians performing in the style of the early 19th century.

Johann Stein to tune Mozart's piano had a frequency of 422Hz – half a tone lower than modern pitch. From 1800–50 the pitch in France rose from 423 to 446Hz. In 1880 Steinways were tuning their pianos to 457Hz – a quarter-tone above the present pitch.

The first attempt to fix a standard was made in 1834, but had no success. In 1889 it was decided to stabilize the pitch at 435Hz and by international agreement in 1939 "concert pitch" was fixed at a frequency of 440Hz.

that a work by Mozart played by a modern orchestra will not sound like the sonorities Mozart heard – the wind being lost under a mountain of strings. Unless the orchestra plays with the correct numerical relationship between the strings and wind, as the composer understood It, the sound will never be "authentic".

Any instrument that is used over a period of time undergoes changes. These changes invariably alter the sound produced and, as composers score for instruments according to how they perceive the sound they make, so does the way they write for them. Elgar did not write for the horn in the same way that Beethoven or Purcell did.

Pitch

It is not only the instruments, but also the pitch that has altered. From 1762–89 the tuning-note (A) varied between frequencies of 377 and 428 cycles per second, or Hertz (from a minor third to half a tone below the modern standard). Apart from this variation, musicians in different regions tuned to different pitches at the same time. France preferred a low, Germany a middle and England a high pitch. The tuning fork used in 1780 by

LEFT: Performers of early brass instruments playing Turmmusik *(tower music). The narrow bore of the two trombones indicates that these instruments are related to sackbuts.*

ABOVE: The Academy of Ancient Music was founded in 1973, and its ensemble is dedicated to giving authentic performances on period instruments of a mainly 18th-century repertoire.

Chamber Music

*Chamber music concerns itself as a world of sound
that has external boundaries but no internal ones.*

HANS WERNER HENZE (BORN 1926)

Originally, the term "chamber music" described intimate music for small groups of solo instruments performing in a drawing room before either a small audience or with no listeners at all. Chamber music differs from other orchestral music in that generally only a single instrument performs each part, whereas in an orchestra the parts are played by groups of instruments.

Although there had been a lot of small-scale ensemble music in the Middle Ages, the medieval court was a place of public exhibition, with very little opportunity for domestic music-making. However, with the rise of instrumental music and an increasing interest in amateur vocal and instrumental music-making in the 16th century, music began to play an important part in the homes of the well-to-do.

Many great houses maintained one or more professional musicians and in 17th-century Italy some princely establishments appointed musicians who had special responsibility for the performance and composition of chamber music. Monteverdi held such a post in the household of the Duke of Mantua, and his contemporaries in similar posts included Enrico di Foggia and Sigismondo d'India.

ABOVE: A painting by Max Buri (1868–1915) showing a group of German village musicians in about 1910.

Another development of the period was the tendency to arrange vocal music for instruments. From the mid 16th century consort music for viols flourished, with compositions being circulated in manuscript copies. Some were published by composers such as Michael East (c.1580–1648) and William Byrd (1543–1623), who issued their collections in 1610 and 1611 respectively. During the 16th and 17th centuries many consorts were formed, the music of which led to the invention of new dances such as the slow, stately pavan and the quicker galliard, as well as the musical forms of *ricercare* and *canzona*, which in turn led to the development of the 17th-century sonata and fugue.

In the 17th and 18th centuries chamber music was encouraged in Germany by the flourishing *collegium musicum*, in Italy by the spread of music academies and in England by the formation of music clubs.

Eighteenth-century chamber music began to include wind instruments, especially in France where music for

ABOVE: A Musical Evening by Michel Ange (1680–1730). The painting shows a chamber ensemble (harpsichord, cello, violin and flute) performing to a group of friends.

ABOVE: One of the finest musicians of the 20th century, Yehudi Menuhin, with his sister Hephzibah and the French cellist Maurice Gendron.

ABOVE: This painting by Pieter Fabris shows a group of mid 18th-century chamber musicians playing in Lord Fortrose's apartment in Naples, Italy.

various combinations of violin, flute, oboe, bassoon and harpsichord was first published. This flexible instrumentation, much of which included a fully written-out harpsichord part, as opposed to the *continuo* required hitherto, seems to have been a development prompted by publishers rather than composers.

In the homes of the nobility regular music evenings were held, at which small groups of musicians played for the family and their guests. Some of these groups were professional musicians who were sponsored by the family. One such ensemble was the Rasumovsky Quartet in Vienna, which was founded and paid for by Count Rasumovsky, the Russian ambassador to Vienna, who played second violin in the group. It was considered one of the best in Europe and even Beethoven wrote pieces especially for it.

New instrumentation

In early 20th-century France there was a proliferation of works for combinations unknown before 1900.

There was a concentration on the flute and the harp – uncommitted instruments that suited the impressionistic age. Examples include the enchanting *Introduction and Allegro* by Maurice Ravel (1875–1937) and Debussy's trio, Sonata for Flute, Viola and Harp.

Another French chamber composer who went in for unconventional instrumentation was Pierre Boulez, who scored *Le Marteau sans maître* for flute, viola, guitar, vibraphone or xylophone and percussion. Igor Stravinsky (1882–1971) was also an innovator and his *L'Histoire d'un soldat* (1918) was scored for clarinet, bassoon, cornet, trombone, violin, double bass, three actors and a dancer.

However, it will take a lot to beat Schoenberg's scoring of *Pierrot Lunaire*

ABOVE: Florilegium was founded in 1991 to play the music of the 17th and 18th centuries. The group is one of the most exuberant chamber ensembles in Europe.

ABOVE: *An 18th-century string quartet playing at double music desks that are reminiscent of the double prayer desks of two centuries earlier.*

specialized individuals, and might offer little to the amateur performer, who instead takes refuge in more accessible works from earlier eras.

String quartet

This chamber group was evolved by Joseph Haydn while he was employed by the Esterházy family at Eisenstadt near Vienna in the late 1750s. For the first time, chamber music abandoned the harpsichord and the new ensemble may have been used for outdoor serenades, for which it was too much trouble to carry the harpsichord outside. Altogether, Haydn wrote over 70 quartets, most of them in sets of six.

One of the novel features of the string quartet was that all the instruments had an equal share of the tunes, and for this reason the music was fun to play.

ABOVE: *The San Francisco-based Kronos Quartet was founded in 1973 and exclusively devotes itself to playing music of the 20th century and beyond.*

in 1912. This extraordinary work was written for flute, clarinet, bass clarinet, violin, viola, cello, piano and a narrator. The inflexions of the latter's voice are included in the score.

Modern chamber music

In the 20th century a reaction against the large Romantic orchestrations of the 19th century led to a renewed interest in chamber music. This was not the chamber music of the past, such as piano trios, string quartets and quintets, but small groups with new sounds and unusual combinations of instruments, with an emphasis on mixed ensembles of wind and strings and often also with vocal as well as percussion elements.

Modern chamber music has moved from the private house to the concert hall, and organizations such as the Library of Congress and the Dutch Donemus Foundation, or wealthy

individuals such as Walter Cobbett have been, and still are, active in promoting it.

The original social function and context of chamber music has now wholly disappeared. Much modern chamber music can be both difficult to play and demanding to listen to. It is often written for highly skilled and

ABOVE: *Although piano duets using one or two pianos are common, it is most unusual for more than two to be played together. This photograph from a 1920s advertisement shows four musicians, each playing a Bechstein grand piano.*

ABOVE: An early 19th-century quartet playing at a quadruple music desk especially designed for quartets.

This is still the case today: the sign of a good string quartet is a sense of equality.

The string quartet (like the brass band) suffers from a lack of colour contrasts – but this can be overcome not only by the differences in tone between the instruments, but by the way they are played. For instance, the instruments can be either played with the bow (*coll'arco*) or plucked with the fingers (*pizzicato*). The violin player may play notes on the G string that would normally be played on other strings. This gives a warmer quality to the sound.

Another trick to thicken the sound is the use of double-stopping, in which more than one string is played on an instrument at the same time. Two composers who used double-stopping to great effect were Debussy and Grieg. Contrasts can also be achieved by resting instruments before bringing them all in together for a climax. Haydn, Mozart and Beethoven were all masters of the string quartet and often doubled instruments for special effects.

In the 18th century it was taken for granted that music should be composed with amateur capabilities in mind. However, if a composer writes simple music today it is sometimes frowned upon and regarded as fit only for learner musicians. Although Mozart, Beethoven and Schubert all enjoyed writing string quartets, the form died out in the 19th century, but was revived in the 20th century, notably by Bartók and Shostakovich. Other 20th-century composers who are noted for their string quartets are Schoenberg, Hindemith, Walton and Tippett, whose five quartets included influences from the 16th-century madrigal.

Chamber orchestras

After World War I, economic factors saw an end to some of the large orchestras that had been dominant at the beginning of the 20th century, and composers increasingly wrote for smaller combinations of instruments. In the decades between the two World Wars a number of chamber orchestras were founded, the best known of which was the Basle Chamber Orchestra, which was set up in 1926 and was conducted by Paul Sacher.

In London, the Boyd Neel String Orchestra was founded in 1933. In an attempt to get the best of both worlds, it adopted an 18th-century repertoire and instrumentation while at the same time encouraging contemporary composers to write new works for it. In an attempt to stimulate interest in chamber music, similar orchestras, such as the Swiss Melos Ensemble, were founded all over Europe.

ABOVE: The English Chamber Orchestra was founded by Arnold Goldsbrough in 1948. One of its prime engagements was under Benjamin Britten at the Aldeburgh Festival.

ABOVE: The Austrian Alban Berg String Quartet was founded in 1971 and has won international distinction with its recordings of the complete Bach, Brahms, Berg and Webern quartets. They are seen here playing at the Royal Festival Hall, London, in 1998.

European National Music

Tell me where you live,
and I will tell you how you compose.

ROBERT SCHUMANN (1810–1856)

The 19th century was a period of European nationalism, not just in military matters but also in the arts, including music. For two centuries, the dominant musical figures in Europe had been German – from Bach to Beethoven – but the Romantic movement, which stressed personal feelings, led to composers striving to express their own traditions, and drawing on the musical influences of their own countries.

United Kingdom
Since the death of Henry Purcell in 1695, the United Kingdom had not produced a major composer, but the successful career of Arthur Sullivan (1842–1900), composer of the Savoy Operas, revived British music and paved the way for a generation of recognizably "English" voices, notably Edward Elgar (1857–1934) in whose music a mixture of nobility and nostalgia defined the British spirit at the end of the Victorian era. Frederick Delius (1862–1934) wrote works full of pastoral lyricism, and Ralph Vaughan Williams (1872–1958) rediscovered and reworked the rich vein of English folk music.

Czechoslovakia
One of the first orchestral composers to compose works with a definite national character was Bedřich Smetana (1824–84). Although he seldom used actual folk songs in his music, unlike his close friend Antonin Dvořák

(1841–1904), Smetana's work was unmistakably Czech. Absorbing the traditions of Berlioz and Liszt, Smetana was also an excellent pianist in the style of Clara Schumann. In 1861 he was appointed head of the Department of Music in the newly formed Prague

ABOVE: Scandinavian scenery inspired composers such as Sibelius and Grieg.

Society of Arts and it was during the tenure of this office that he wrote his most famous opera, *The Bartered Bride*. After suffering for some time from a whistling in his ears, in 1874 Smetana suddenly became stone deaf, but, like Beethoven before him, went on composing, including arguably his best work, *Má Vlast* ("My Country"), a set of six musical landscapes.

Finland
Another 19th-century composer whose music is evocative of his country is the Scandinavian Jean Sibelius (1865–1957), who was born in the

ABOVE: Sir Edward Elgar was England's greatest national composer of the 20th century. His work includes such typically English compositions as the four Pomp and Circumstance *marches and the* Enigma Variations. *A great friend of Adrian Boult, Elgar fixed a sign on his cottage gate, "Please Boult the Gate".*

Finnish town of Hämeenlinna. Although intended for a legal career, he soon abandoned his law studies to devote himself entirely to music. In 1892 a performance of his first large-scale orchestral work, the *Kullervo* Symphony, created such a sensation that he soon became established as Finland's leading composer. One of his most popular works is the tone poem *Finlandia*, which he composed in 1899 and which was banned by the Tsar because it roused such nationalistic fervour. Although his inspiration was intimately connected with Finnish landscape and literature (such as *Kalevala*, the national folk epic), Sibelius's achievements lie principally in his remarkable mastery of form.

Norway

Edvard Grieg (1843–1907) turned to his native folk music for inspiration, having learnt the folk songs of Norway from his mother. One of his most popular works is his incidental music to Ibsen's play *Peer Gynt*, in which he evokes trolls, mists and mountains in a work that is unmistakably Scandinavian.

Germany

One of the most obvious examples of overt nationalism in 19th-century orchestral music must be the work of Richard Wagner (1813–83), whose love of everything Aryan was to make him the darling of the Nazis, who conveniently forgot his Semitic ancestry. Wagner drew inspiration from

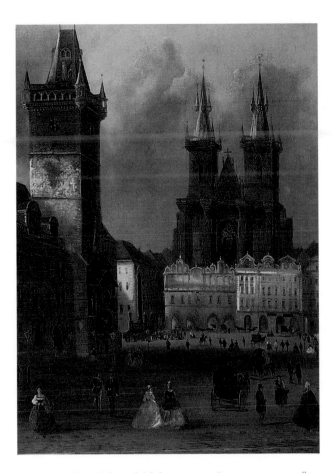

ABOVE: In the 18th and 19th centuries Prague was one of the main musical capitals of Europe. This scene of the Old Square is as it was in the days when Mozart walked its streets, and would have been familiar to Czechoslovakia's two great national composers, Dvořák and Smetana.

ABOVE: The Battle of Polotsk, 18 August, 1812. One of the compositions that most brings to mind "Mother Russia" is Tchaikovsky's 1812 Overture, which describes in music the day when Napoleon's army was finally defeated. The work has many musical effects, from the roar of cannon to church bells ringing out the news of victory.

the legends and myths of Germanic folklore, producing epic operas such as *Tristan und Isolde* and *Tannhäuser,* as well as the renowned *Der Ring des Nibelungen.*

France

Camille Saint-Saëns (1835–1921), as president of the Société Nationale de Musique, declared himself in favour of the "essential French qualities of logic, reason and clarity", and imparted these qualities to his huge musical output, including operas, choral and orchestral works, organ and chamber music. Gabriel Fauré (1845–1924) was a pupil of Saint-Saëns, and composed ravishing songs and choral works of great delicacy and elegance.

Russia

Russian music is full of the sounds of "Mother Russia", from Tchaikovsky's patriotic *1812 Overture* to the folk-based compositions of musicians such as Mikhail Glinka (1804–57). Glinka was regarded as the "father" of Russian music, and inspired a group of composers, known as "The Five", who set out to develop a pure Russian style. They included Alexander Borodin (1833–87), whose opera *Prince Igor* relates the story of the 12th-century struggles of the Russians against the Polovtsy invaders, and Modest Mussorgsky (1839–81) whose masterpiece is the opera *Boris Godunov,* based on Pushkin's drama about the 16th-century Tsar.

Folk Music

*The best way to get to knowing any bunch of people
is to go and listen to their music.*

Woody Guthrie (1912–67)

While most music tends to cross boundaries, folk music differs from area to area. The folk music of Northumberland is different from that of southern England; the music of Hamburg is different from that of Munich or the Tyrol; in Russia, the folk tunes in the west are different from those in the east. The workers on the American cotton plantations sang songs that were unknown in the industrial cities of Boston and New York. The words and tunes of folk songs were transmitted aurally, and might have existed in several versions in different places, as they were subtly altered over the years.

In Britain, most songs were traditionally sung only by men. Women exercised their vocal chords only while working or in the home, and were very rarely heard in public.

ABOVE: This print from the 1830s shows a party of villagers folk-dancing outside an inn in Süd Tirol, Austria, now part of northern Italy.

Work songs

Many traditional songs were about work, especially the hard conditions associated with occupations such as working in the fields, down the mines or on ships. Singing made hard work easier and many songs were of the call and response type, in which the leader or shantyman would sing out the story and the rest of the workers would join in the chorus. Another type of work song was the street cry, with which street vendors advertised their wares.

Ballads

The ballad was a song that told a story, and might be based on contemporary news events of the day, such as a battle or a mining disaster, or on legends or fictional tales. In the days before radio or television, when few working people were able to read newspapers, singing or listening to these ballads was one way to escape briefly from the

ABOVE: The composer Béla Bartók travelled extensively all over Hungary and neighbouring states, making recordings of folk songs.

daily grind. There were also many shorter songs, which might be pithy and humorous or lyrical and romantic.

Instrumental accompaniment

At work in the fields, or in the home, most folk music was sung unaccompanied. In Biblical Israel songs were sung to the accompaniment of the harp, while in classical Greece the singer was accompanied on the kithara. In medieval Europe folk songs were sung to pipe and tabor and later to the hurdy-gurdy or bagpipes. Bagpipes were purely a folk instrument, being thought to be crude and fit only for the tavern, in contrast to the viol, favoured by the more well-to-do.

Dancing

Feast days and their associated rituals have invariably included both music and dancing, such as the May Day Morris dancing of southern England and the sword dances of the north. These two very different traditions of folk-dancing reflect the Viking occupation of the north-east of Britain.

Originally, dances like these were performed only on certain occasions, and were part of religious ceremonies to celebrate the passing of the seasons and to bring good luck to the harvest. Though the original significance of these dances has been lost, they are

ABOVE: Before radio and television people made their own amusements, and one of the few pastimes available for the "labouring poor" was dancing. This print of 1804 shows a Polish man dancing before his friends.

ABOVE: One of the joys of life in the southern states of America is when the family play their instruments on the porch.

ABOVE: Morris dancing is thought to be associated with fertility. There are many groups who try to recreate England's past.

still performed on festive occasions, such as village fête days.

Some folk dances have become popularized far beyond their point of origin. The waltz originated as a peasant dance in southern Germany, but has become known – in its more refined state – all over the world. Another genre that has become popular way beyond its native shores, due both to migration and, latterly, to a film and stage show, is Irish dancing.

As with folk songs, the instruments that provided the music for these dances were small and portable, such as the fiddle. The accordion, invented in the early 19th century, became popular as an accompaniment for open-air dancing, and a 20th-century innovation in Morris sides is the inclusion of the concertina.

Contemporary folk music

In the 1960s, with the growth of the American civil rights movement and the increasing aversion of young people to America's involvement in the war in Vietnam, folk songs experienced a

revival of interest as a means of political protest, sung by professional folk singers such as Joan Baez (born 1941), Pete Seeger (born 1919) and Bob Dylan (born 1941). Many of Bob Dylan's "protest" songs of the mid '60s have become folk classics, such as *Masters of War*, *The Times They are A-changin'* and *With God on our Side*. Country Joe McDonald's chorus, "And it's one, two, three, what are we fighting for?" has become the universal anti-war anthem.

ABOVE: One of the new-style folk singers of the 1960s was Bob Dylan, whose songs relate to the protest movement of that time.

Revolutionary Music of the 20th Century

Think nothing. Wait until it is absolutely still within you.
When you have attained this begin to play.

<small>KARLHEINZ STOCKHAUSEN, INSTRUCTIONS TO PERFORMERS OF "ES"</small>

As the 20th century dawned, some composers turned away from the hitherto accepted rules of harmony and composition and ventured out into the realms of polytonality, atonality and microtones.

Atonal music

In 1908 the Austrian composer Arnold Schoenberg (1874–1951) changed the whole basis of harmony. He abandoned

By numbers

A composer who drew inspiration from unusual sources was the Russian Joseph Schillinger, who emigrated to the United States in 1930. At one concert he asked his audience which composer the new work he had just played reminded them of. Suggestions included Mozart, Bach and Beethoven; however, nobody could guess Schillinger's actual source, which had been the stock-market quotations. Schillinger had plotted the figures on a sheet of graph paper and given each a proportional musical value. Schillinger also taught music, and amongst his pupils was Glenn Miller, whose *Moonlight Serenade* was written as an exercise set by Schillinger.

ABOVE: Arnold Schoenberg decided to abandon tonality in 1907 when he wrote his Second String Quartet, a work in which the keys are not stated but "sensed".

the idea of the central keynote and regarded every semitone of a chromatic scale as being of equal importance. One of his early atonal compositions was the opera *Expectation*, a work for soprano and orchestra. Although some listeners admired Schoenberg's work, many more found it unintelligible, preferring tonal music that was more pleasing to the ear.

Microtones

Another innovation of the 20th century was the use of microtones. Although microtones were, and still are, common in eastern music, and are found in some eastern European folk music, the smallest interval generally

used in European music was the semitone. The main promoter of microtones in Europe was the Czech composer Alois Hába (born 1893), who divided the notes of the scale into intervals of one-third, one-quarter and one-sixth of a tone. Due to the construction of European wind instruments, such music is only easily playable on strings and trombones.

Polytonal music

Polytonality is the use of two keys simultaneously. Again, to most listeners this is very grating on the ear, but the genre did find some early supporters. One of these was Charles Ives (1874–1954), an insurance salesman who wrote music in his spare time. Some of his music is very complex to perform: in its original form, his Fourth Symphony, for instance, needs four conductors to

ABOVE: Charles Ives was the first American composer to break away from the German style that had influenced most American music during the late 19th century.

ABOVE: *Dimitri Shostakovich was greatly influenced by his compatriots Rimsky-Korsakov, Tchaikovsky and Prokofiev.*

keep the players together. Another exponent of polytonality was Igor Stravinsky. His music for the ballet *The Rite of Spring* begins with a bassoon solo that is scored deliberately at the top of the instrument's range because he wanted the player to strive to reach the note to give the sound the quality of struggle. At its first performance in Paris in May 1913 the audience almost caused a riot. At one point the manager of the theatre, in an attempt to restore calm, was heard to say "Listen before you boo." When the composer Camille Saint-Saëns heard the work, he just kept repeating *"Il est fou."* Yet the work has since become an established and popular part of the orchestral repertoire.

Aleatoric music

Some of the music of Karlheinz Stockhausen (born 1928) never sounds the same twice over because it is aleatoric: it includes the improvisatory elements of chance and free choice. Stockhausen has abandoned conventional notation altogether and writes "text scores" in which he explains in words how the music should be played. In *Gold Dust*, for instance, he even suggests that the musicians should starve themselves for four days and nights before the performance.

Another composer who explored the operation of chance was John Cage (1912–92), whose *4' 33"* consists of

four minutes and 33 seconds of silence, the idea being that the music is created by the sounds provided by the natural environment at the time. This work was satirized by the musician and humorist Gerard Hoffnung, who in the mid 1950s announced that he had written a work that included three bars of silence. The first and third bars, so Hoffnung explained, were in 5:4 time, but the second bar was in 3:4 time, "thereby giving the whole work a quasi-Viennese flavour".

ABOVE: *Karlheinz Stockhausen abandoned both conventional musical notation and instrumentation, utilizing "instruments" such as iron chains and shortwave radios.*

ABOVE: *Igor Stravinsky had a rich and diverse musical output. Here he is shown conducting a 1951 rehearsal of his opera* The Rake's Progress *in Venice, Italy.*

Many of Cage's works for dance companies and concert performances exploited his invention of the "prepared piano", in which he created percussive effects by placing objects such as rubber bands and paperclips between the strings. He also wrote *HPSCHD*, a piece for seven harpsichords and 51 tape machines, and *0'00"* which was for any musician playing any instrument in any way.

ABOVE: *The composer and pianist John Cage was a pupil of Schoenberg. His music exploits a variety of percussive and novel sound effects produced by orthodox instruments, modified instruments such as the "prepared" piano, and objects such as radio receivers, chairs and even dead fish.*

Brass Bands

Brass bands came into existence in England and Wales in the 1830s as a result of the philanthropic efforts of factory owners to enrich the lives of their work forces. They saw brass bands as valuable adjuncts to their works, and in an era of increasing leisure, the bands became a popular pastime.

Improvement in the manufacture of brass instruments at around this time made both fingering and blowing easier, and the advent of the railways made travel feasible for working people. It was not long before bands began to compete with one another in friendly rivalry.

Contests

The first known brass band contest, at which five bands took part, was held at Burton Constable, near Hull, in 1845. In those early days the participating bands were restricted

ABOVE: Brass baritones from an Austrian town band giving an outdoor performance in Salzburg, Austria.

to 12 players (as opposed to 25 today) and played arrangements of works by composers such as Weber, Rossini and Mozart.

The most distinguished of these early bandsmen was Enderby Jackson, a conductor and arranger who, in 1854, established the principle that all participating bands in a contest should play the same test piece.

Today the British National Brass Band Contest, held in London at the Royal Albert Hall, is the highlight of the British bandsman's year. Since 1978 the more ambitious British bands have also been able to compete with their European counterparts at the European Brass Band Championships.

United States and beyond

Brass bands became popular in the United States almost as early as they did in Britain. One of the first bands to be formed in the United States was the Brass Band of New York, established by Alan Dodworth in 1834. Brass band

ABOVE: The "Besses o' th' Barn" band from Whitefield, Lancashire, was one of England's foremost brass bands. It was founded in 1818 and is seen here during its successful tour of France in 1905.

concerts soon became a part of the American way of life. It was truly music for the people, with bandstand gazebos in almost every park. Some of these, such as that in New York's Central Park, were paid for by the railway company as a way of increasing fare income by transporting out-of-town concertgoers into the city. On Boston Common, concerts were so well attended that some are said to have attracted crowds of up to 10,000 people.

By 1900 the brass band movement had reached its zenith in England and Wales, with some 20,000 brass bands. Although their number declined after World War II, there was a revival of interest from the 1960s. This resurgence occurred not only in Britain, Australia, New Zealand and the United States but also in Europe, where British-style brass bands were formed in the Netherlands, Sweden, Switzerland, Norway and Belgium.

Repertoire

Brass bands play a mixture of transcriptions of orchestral works and original compositions. Notable early

ABOVE: The Durham Miners' Gala is one of the most eagerly anticipated events in the British brass bandsman's diary. Many bands take part in the event, both marching through the town and giving static concerts.

arrangers of music for bands include J. Ord Hume, Samuel Cope and William Rimmer. As well as orchestral composers such as Arthur Bliss, Gustav Holst and Sir Edward Elgar, all of whom wrote for brass band, the brass band's repertoire has been greatly enhanced by men such as Eric

Ball, Geoffrey Brand and Granville Bantock. At first, some of this new music was treated with suspicion, and it was not unknown for band conductors, unaccustomed to anything but the harmonies of marches and hymn tunes, to change "wrong notes" to their own satisfaction. It is reported that one conductor with a limited knowledge of Italian went into a music shop after receiving a new score with the intention of buying "some of those new-fangled *senza mutes*".

These days, band concerts in the park are still enjoyed by thousands of people who like nothing better than relaxing in the sunshine listening to a "good drop of music".

LEFT: The continued survival of brass bands in Britain depends on young people taking up brass instruments to fill the ranks of older musicians. The presence of so many youth bands in the country assures the future of the brass band movement.

Military Bands

Explain it as we may, a martial strain
will urge a man into the front rank of battle.

Henry Theodore Tuckerman (1813–71)

Soldiers of the world have always marched to music, even if it was only the rhythmic tread of their own feet. By 1600 BC Egyptians were marching to trumpet and drum, and a thousand years later Roman trumpeters played on the march. Trumpets were an integral part of Caesar's army and on that fateful day, while standing by the bridge crossing the Rubicon, the trumpets blew a thunderous blast. In 6th-century Persia the regiments marched to bands of drums, pipes and trumpets. Four hundred years later their descendants were still enjoying the stirring music of large bands of drums, cymbals, trumpets and other wind instruments.

European military bands

Military bands came to the attention of western Europeans during the Crusades from the 11th to 13th centuries, when they encountered Saracen bands consisting of *surnay*

LEFT: A Prussian military band shown on the sheet music for Preussicher Zapfenstreich *by H. Saro, published in 1885. A feature of the band is the Turkish crescent surmounted by the Prussian Eagle.*

(oboes), *nafir* (trumpets), *buq* (horns) and *naqqara* (kettledrums). During the late Middle Ages European armies began to copy these bands loosely, employing combinations of shawms, bagpipes, trumpets and drums. The duties of the musicians were mainly to play at tournaments and to accompany the soldiers on campaign.

Janissary bands

An important development during the 18th century was the adoption by European military bands of "Turkish" or "Janissary" music. The instrumentation of these bands included oboes, fifes, side drums, kettledrums, cymbals, triangles, Turkish crescent and bass drum. Such was the fad for this type of music that some regiments in Poland, Russia and Prussia even imported whole bands, complete with musicians, from Turkey. Today, remnants of the Janissary era live on in the leopardskin apron worn by bass drummers and the shape of the lyre glockenspiel.

The trend was reversed in the early 19th century when, in 1826, the Sultan of Turkey disbanded his corps of Janissaries and invited Giuseppe Donizetti (brother of the composer) to reorganize Turkish bands on the lines

ABOVE: Russian horn bands were a feature of the late 18th and early 19th centuries. Such was the popularity of these combinations with the Russian nobility that they often sold them to one another — players as well as horns.

ABOVE: *For centuries, armies have used drums to keep their marching troops in step. Here an 18th-century side drummer leads a platoon of troops past the National Theatre in Prague.*

ABOVE: *Brightly dressed army side drummers playing at the Battle of Fontenoy in 1745.*

of European ones. Persian bands followed suit and adopted Western instrumentation in about 1840.

New instruments

By the end of the 18th century military bands were increasing in size, mainly as a result of adding extra percussion instruments, which in turn made it necessary – for purposes of audibility – to increase the wind section. Clarinets, both B flat and E flat, were introduced into military bands and soon outnumbered any other instrument. Performing the same role as the violins in the symphony orchestra, there were two main reasons for the clarinet replacing the oboe in military bands. First, it is much easier for a marching musician to play the single reed clarinet than the double reed oboe and

second, the softer sound of the oboe tends to become lost when playing with modern brass instruments.

American Civil War bands

During the American Civil War military bands proliferated on both sides of the conflict and were heard on all occasions, from ceremonial parades to battle marches. A good band was a source of tremendous pride and was long remembered by those fortunate enough to witness the "dawn of peace".

Sometimes Union bands played in competition with their southern counterparts. One such impromptu concert happened during a lull in the Battle of Spotsylvania in 1864. Each side brought their band to the front line where, for an hour or so, the bands played alternate tunes. The concert ended with the Confederate band bringing tears to the eyes of the battle-hardened men of both sides with their heart-rending rendition of *Home Sweet Home*.

ABOVE: *Members of military bands often "double" on stringed instruments. The bands of the Austrian Empire were no exception and here Johann Strauss the Younger is seen conducting a military orchestra at a royal ball in Vienna.*

Military schools of music

A major event in the evolution of European military bands was the celebration of peace at the end of the Crimean War in 1856. Military bands of all the allied nations took part, giving the bandsmen an opportunity to hear each other play and compare standards. In the wake of the British bands' poor showing (particularly embarrassing when they played the national anthem in different keys), the Royal Military School of Music was founded at Kneller Hall in Twickenham, near London.

At this time British military bandmasters were still mainly civilian musicians and – more surprisingly – were in many cases foreign. Three examples were Francis Ptacek, a member of the Prague Conservatoire who was director of the band of the Leicestershire Militia; Herr Sawerthal,

ABOVE: *Marching bands are popular in the United States, Australia and, to a lesser degree, Britain. This Sydney annual marching band festival takes place in Australia every August.*

the bandmaster of the Royal Engineers; and Karl Tieke, the composer of the evergreen march *Alte Kameraden*, who was the director of the band of the Royal Irish Dragoon Guards.

It was not until 1887 that an army bandmaster, Dan Godfrey, the director of the band of the Grenadier Guards, received a commission. Today all directors of full-time military bands are of officer rank.

Civilian "military" bands

During the 19th century the term "military band" became something of a misnomer as it began to be used more loosely, referring also to civilian bands using military band instrumentation for public concerts. One of the most popular of these civilian bands was the renowned Jullien Band.

Jullien

Louis Antoine Jullien (1812–60) was the son of a military bandsman. After a period of study at the Paris Conservatoire, he began promoting concerts of dance music at the Jardin Ture, where he became known as the "Napoleon of Music".

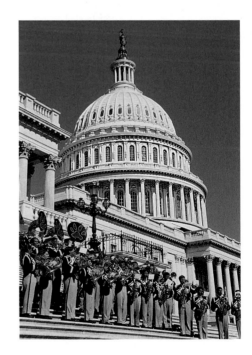

ABOVE: *Almost every school in the United States has its own band. This one is proudly playing on the steps of the Capitol building in Washington DC.*

ABOVE: *The drum corps of the Grenadier Guards playing at the annual "Trooping of the Colour" in London.*

ABOVE: One of the best-known annual events in Germany is the Oktoberfest. *Held in Munich, this beer festival is enlivened by the many bands that perform.*

In 1840 he moved to England, and made his debut in Drury Lane in June.

Thanks to a spotless white waistcoat, as well as his ambrosial curls, superb moustache and the magnificent air with which he wielded his baton, Jullien was the object of unsparing ridicule.

ABOVE: Jullien's concerts were always sold out well in advance. Despite this, he was never able to pay off the debts he had amassed in Paris, and he died bankrupt.

He was a devotee of Beethoven, and whenever he conducted works by that composer he would have a new pair of white gloves presented to him which he would wear while he conducted.

Each year Jullien tried to bring some novelty into his concerts. In 1849 he introduced the *monstre* ophicleide (a brass instrument later superseded by the tuba) which at that time was the largest wind instrument ever made. In 1851 he toured with a French drum corps, which appeared in full military uniform by permission of Prince Louis Napoleon. In the same year, appreciating the discomforts, if not the dangers, of passive smoking, Jullien requested that his concerts be non-smoking events.

Sousa

Another famous civilian wind band was that formed by John Philip Sousa (1854–1932) in 1892. Sousa was born in Washington DC, and from the age of six he learnt to play the violin, as well as studying various band instruments, harmony and musical theory. In 1867 he followed in his father's footsteps and became a professional trombonist, but later turned to the violin and conducting. Between 1868 and 1892 he built up a promising reputation as bandmaster of the United States Marine Corps Band. In 1892 he left the service to form his own famous band, which toured Europe several times as well as making a two-year world tour in 1910–11. Sousa, who is justly called the "March King", composed 136 marches, including *The Washington Post*, *The Stars and Stripes Forever*, *Liberty Bell*, *High School Cadets* and *El Capitan*. Sousa is also remembered for the redesigned helicon first made for his band in 1899, now known as the sousaphone.

ABOVE: Sousa was justly known as the "March King" — he composed 136 marches. His band became famous worldwide and he made a two-year world tour in 1910–11.

Country Music

*You got to have smelt a lot of mule manure
before you can sing like a hillbilly.*

HANK WILLIAMS (1923–53)

For many, country music is summed up as songs about orphaned children, lost mothers, betrayed lovers, train wrecks and coal-mining disasters. However, there is actually a lot more to country music than sentimentality and sickly patriotism. It is not just "hillbilly music" but has a century of tradition, with many styles evolving and co-existing over the decades. It is a blending of the two distinct traditions of the American settlers: European ballads, story songs and dance music, and African-American blues and work songs.

ABOVE: *The fiddle is one of the most popular instruments with country musicians. It is used in many types of country music, from bluegrass to the sentimental tones accompanying the songs for which the genre is famous.*

ABOVE: *Hank Williams was America's greatest honky-tonk performer, whose early death ensured him a permanent place in country music's pantheon of stars. One of his best-known songs is* Cold, Cold Heart.

The commercialization of this blend came in the mid 19th century with the minstrel shows that were created by white performers parodying black manners. These shows gave birth to two distinct forms of entertainment. In the North they evolved into vaudeville, while in the South they nurtured home-grown banjo and fiddle players.

Another seedbed for country music was the southern rural church where singing was – and still is – a central part of the service. Although the white and black churches had different styles, they merged into a tightly harmonized music called "bluegrass". An early example of this type of music was that sung by the Carter Family from Virginia, whose songs were based on the ultimate embodiment of home and family values. Their unornamented, nasal, simple four-square harmonies were entirely white with no black influences whatsoever.

In marked contrast to the "home harmonizers", there were more progressive singers, such as Jimmie Rodgers (1897–1933), who sang a combination of jazz, blues and country. Although he recorded with many bands, his most moving performances were those in which he was accompanied only by his guitar – songs such as the autobiographical *T. B. Blues*, *T. for Texas* and *Waitin' for a Train*, which is one of the most popular train songs ever.

ABOVE: *This country fiddle player is being accompanied by an accordion player.*

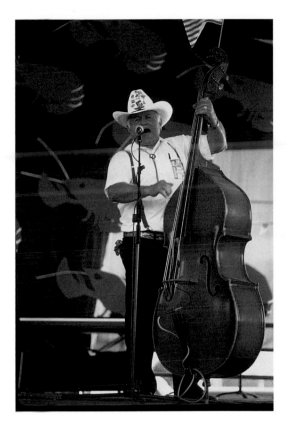

ABOVE: *Before the advent of the electric bass guitar, every country band had a string bass. Some bass players were very versatile and were able to produce remarkable effects on their instrument.*

Rodgers influenced many country singers, including the legendary Hank Williams (1923–53). Williams sang in the first person and dealt head-on with issues such as adultery and alcoholism. His many songs are still part of almost every country singer's repertoire and there is hardly ever a country music concert anywhere that does not include at least one Hank Williams song.

Grand Ole Opry

Country music spread into the homes of Americans via radio programmes, in particular Chicago's *National Barn Dance*, the *Louisiana Hayride* from Shreveport, and WSM Radio's *Grand Ole Opry* from Nashville, Tennessee. In the mid 1950s Nashville became the centre of country music and the "Nashville Sound", featuring tickling

pianos and a strong string section, became known throughout the world. Nashville remained the bastion of country music throughout the 1960s, but remained very conservative, both artistically and politically. In the '60s and early '70s there was, for example, an unhealthy number of songs supporting America's involvement in the Vietnam War, notably Merle Haggard's *Okie from Muskogee* and *The Fightin' Side of Me*, which cemented his stardom but enraged liberals everywhere. The slushy sounds of Nashville were rejected by singers such as Waylon Jennings (who had played with Buddy Holly) and Willie Nelson. They left Nashville and went to Texas where they established what has become known as "outlaw country". During the 1980s and '90s mainstream country music has become more and more like pop, so that in many cases it is hard to spot the difference.

ABOVE: *Willie Nelson (born 1933) is one of the most influential songwriters and singers country music has ever known. His laid-back style of singing once led one reviewer to announce that by the time Nelson had sung one line, Dolly Parton would have sung a complete song! One of Nelson's best-known albums is* Tougher than Leather, *which deals with the effects of fate on life.*

ABOVE: *Many solo country singers have teamed up with a colleague to produce duets. One of the most successful of such pairings is Dolly Parton and Kenny Rogers.*

Jazz

If you're in jazz and more than ten people like you,
you're labelled commercial.

HERBIE MANN (BORN 1930)

Jazz is a truly American music, being a combination of that country's two dominant cultures – African and European. As a genre it is almost unique in embodying both rural and urban sounds, as well as ranging from the raw sounds of New Orleans Dixieland bands to the sophistication of New York cool jazz groups.

New Orleans

Dixieland jazz evolved from the ragtime music of the late 19th century, which was epitomized by the work of Scott Joplin, composer of piano rags such as *The Entertainer*. Finding the steady ragtime 2:4 time monotonous, some musicians doubled the time to 4:4 and began to play the melody just a little ahead of or behind the beat, which gave an unevenness to the pulse.

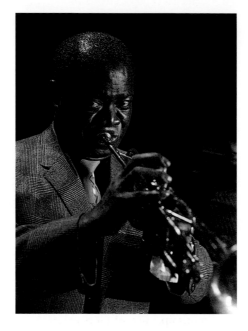

ABOVE: Louis Armstrong single-handedly transformed jazz from a collective art to one of solo expression. His clear, ringing trumpet-playing was impeccable.

These subtle rhythmic changes increased the swing of the music, producing the fast, happy, high-energy music now known as traditional jazz.

One of the earliest exponents of the genre was Buddy Bolden (1877–1931), who is remembered for his blues songs, such as *Careless Love*. Another of the early traditional players was Jelly Roll Morton (1885–1941), a brilliant pianist, arranger and composer, who is best remembered for his *Tiger Rag*.

Another early New Orleans bandleader was "King" Oliver (1885–1938), who moved to Chicago in 1918 and formed his own band, the Creole Jazz Band, in 1922. One of the musicians Oliver invited to join him was Louis Armstrong (1901–71), who had started his professional life playing trumpet in the red-light district of New Orleans for 15 cents a night. Armstrong, a master of improvisation, formed his own band in 1925 and revolutionized jazz for all time. He was the first to create solo improvised melodies that complemented the basic theme, and thus established the central role of the soloist in what had previously been an ensemble form. His technical virtuosity was breathtaking – he was, for instance, able to hold high notes effortlessly for three or four bars at a time.

Chicago "traditional" jazz

Influenced by what was happening in New Orleans, the Chicago of the early 1900s was also a centre of jazz. Led by Nick LaRocca, the Original Dixieland Jazz Band – which was composed

ABOVE: When one thinks of jazz, one automatically thinks of New Orleans, a city where almost every bar and club has its own house band.

ABOVE: *As well as being a comedian and film maker, Woody Allen is an enthusiastic jazz clarinettist, his favourite being New Orleans jazz. He is seen here guesting in a band show.*

melodic improvisation is very free in cool jazz and players often use counterpoint to play two improvised melodic lines at the same time. Two of the best-known exponents of cool jazz are Miles Davis (1926–91) and the Dave Brubeck Quartet.

ABOVE: *Thelonious Monk was one of the greatest jazz pianists. Born in New York City, he began playing at his local Baptist church. Although he had his own big band, he is better known for his jazz quartet.*

solely of white musicians – made the first ever jazz recordings in 1917. One man who was inspired by the band was the legendary Bix Beiderbecke (1903–31) who, after hearing a recording by LaRocca, persuaded his parents to give him a cornet. He formed his own band – the Wolverines – in 1923, but by 1925 he had gone solo and was performing with various touring bands. Although he died at only 28, Beiderbecke was the man chiefly responsible for introducing Dixieland jazz to a white audience, and without him the genre would never have become so popular.

Bebop and cool jazz

An offshoot of classical jazz is bebop, which developed in Harlem in the early 1940s. The onomatopoeic name was coined by young musicians including Dizzy Gillespie (1917–93), Charlie Parker (1920–55) and Thelonious Monk (1917–82) to describe the style that emerged during their jam sessions, characterized by upbeat rhythms, fast tempo and improvisation. Bebop later became accepted as the nickname for the

whole wave of new jazz that exploded after World War II.

Cool jazz ("modern jazz") musicians take a more intellectual approach to their music. Disdaining any kind of showmanship, they often play with their backs to the audience. The rhythm is muted, the drummer simply keeping the beat, on which the players stay rather than syncopating. The

ABOVE: *Dizzy Gillespie, trumpeter, composer and bandleader, was responsible for giving jazz a whole new style that included whole-tone scales and altered chords.*

Big Bands

To swing is to affirm.

FATHER G. V. KENNARD

In the mid 1920s the move began to form larger jazz bands, which were in fact small orchestras. Two of the early dance bands of the era were those led by Paul Whiteman (1890–1967) and Fletcher Henderson (1897–1952).

Whiteman, a classically trained violinist, formed his first (all-white) small band in 1919. In 1924 he organized the first ever concert of jazz music at New York's Aeolian Hall, at which the highlight was George Gershwin playing his *Rhapsody in Blue* for the first time. Whiteman's orchestra was so successful that at one time there were no less than 28 different "Whiteman" bands touring the United States.

Fletcher Henderson, whose band consisted of all black musicians,

ABOVE: *Glenn Miller formed his band in 1938, and within a year his trademark sound of soothing reeds – for example in* In The Mood *– had become world famous.*

played at New York's Roseland Ballroom. However in 1923, after Louis Armstrong had played for a short time with the band, Henderson changed his style from polite dance music to swing jazz. Henderson is remembered especially for his revolutionary "call and response" arrangements, which split the band's instruments into two groups, the first group stating a melody and the second responding to it.

Instrumentation

One of the important innovations of the big band was the introduction of the saxophone. One of the first jazz saxophonists was Coleman Hawkins (1904–69), who introduced the instrument to Henderson's band in

1923. Between the 1930s and '60s, saxophones were to feature strongly in the "big band" orchestras led by people such as Glenn Miller and Duke Ellington in the United States, Henry Hall in England and Bert Kaempfert and James Last in Germany.

Big band leaders

One of the most talented jazz musicians was Duke Ellington (1899–1974). His compositions are still standard works in most bands' repertoires and include classics such as *Satin Doll* and *Mood Indigo*. Ellington, whose band was at its peak during the 1930s, introduced the "jungle style", in which growling trumpets and wailing clarinets gave the music an unmistakable African feeling.

ABOVE: *George Gershwin was one of America's most versatile songwriters. With his brother Ira he wrote musical comedies, such as* Funny Face *and* Tiptoes.

ABOVE: *Duke Ellington: pianist, bandleader and composer.*

ABOVE: *Noted especially for his minimalist piano style, which he had perfected by the end of the 1930s, Count Basie was one of the finest jazz pianists of the 20th century.*

Another jazz man to hit the scene in the 1930s was the clarinettist Benny Goodman (1909–86). Goodman was well known for his sight-reading skills and was the first white jazz musician to break the colour barrier and work with black colleagues. Goodman's band, which was noted for being the best rehearsed and most precise, played the "pop" music of its day.

Kansas City swing

Count (William) Basie (1904–84), who became the leader of Kansas City swing, began his career as pianist in the Bennie Moten band, one of the first to feature the combination of five brass, four reed and four rhythm players. After Moten's death in 1935, Basie began to build his own ensemble from the remnants of his mentor's band. He soon became one of the most successful jazz bandleaders, and led his band until his death in 1984. The band was noted for its "head arranging", in which riffs were improvised during performances, the other musicians having hastily to adjust their parts.

Western swing

Western swing is a combination of string-band music with jazz styles that developed in the late 1920s. One of the first bands to feature the new type of music was the Light Crust Doughboys, which featured the fiddler Bob Wills (1905–75). Wills soon left to form his own band, the Texas Playboys, which became the epitome of western swing. Wills incorporated old-time country fiddling, jazz, blues, boogie-woogie and the Tex-Mex sounds that became so popular in the 1960s.

ABOVE: *Although the early days of Basie's band were exhilaratingly wild, under his leadership they became the most disciplined and sleek big band of the era.*

ABOVE: *Benny Goodman, the "King of Swing", was at home in jazz and classical music.*

ABOVE: *Duke Ellington was the master of swing and endured long after the period was history. He led arguably one of the greatest swing bands of all time.*

Rock and Pop

You have to blame Thomas Edison for today's rock 'n' roll.
He invented [sic] electricity.
STAN GETZ (1927–91)

Rock music evolved from the blues. After the end of World War II many African-Americans from the Deep South moved to northern cities such as Chicago, in search of work and to escape the racialism that was — and to some extent still is — rife in the former Confederate States. Here, musicians created an urbanized rhythm that served as a foundation for pioneer rock 'n' rollers such as Little Richard and Chuck Berry.

Electric guitar
Although the first solid-body electric guitar was built by Les Paul, it was first mass-produced by Leo Fender, and became a key element in rock 'n' roll. Fender, a California-based guitar and

ABOVE: The Beatles, who began their musical career in a nightclub in Liverpool, became the world's top pop group with hit records such as She Loves You *and* A Hard Day's Night.

amplifier manufacturer, had often been asked by musicians if he could give more volume and at the same time eliminate screech and feedback from the electrified instruments of the time. He came up with the solid-body guitar that he developed just after World War II. His first model, the Broadcaster, entered mass production in 1948, and its sharpness and attack made it an instant success, especially with country musicians. In 1950 its name was changed to the Telecaster, and it was this instrument that gave the rock of that decade its distinctive sound. In 1951 Fender introduced his solid-body bass guitar and, five years later, his futuristic Stratocaster.

One of the pioneers of electric guitar-playing was Muddy Waters (1915–83), who moved up to Chicago from Mississippi. In 1944 he bought his first electric guitar, one made by Fender, and within two years had formed his first electric combo.

African-American music
The importance of African-American music cannot be overestimated. From the Motown sound of the 1960s, through soul and disco to the rap of the 1990s, the exciting sounds of black music have dominated and led the way in many popular music trends. More than anything else, rock music has helped to integrate black and white America, breaking down the racial barrier that has plagued the country.

The 1950s
Many of the young white singers of the 1950s derived their inspiration from black music, including Elvis Presley (1935–77), who became one of the most influential rock 'n' roll singers of the 20th century. Born in Tupelo, Mississippi, as a boy Elvis was always in demand for singing at church services and revival meetings, and was greatly influenced by black blues singers. Indeed, when people who did not know him heard him singing, they could not believe that he was white. Presley's romantic, suggestive ballads, which were matched by his gyrations on stage, made him one of the first mass idols of American adolescent culture (as well as getting him banned from many television stations).

ABOVE: Elvis Presley was the foremost and most influential popular singer of the 1950s and '60s. His style ranged from country to rock and mainstream.

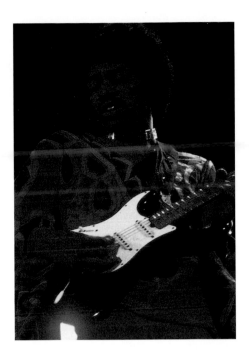

ABOVE: *The legendary rock guitarist Jimi Hendrix, born in Seattle, had his first hit in Britain with* Hey Joe *in 1967.*

Another pioneer was Buddy Holly (1936–59), whose short career was the inspiration for many singers of the 1960s, including Mick Jagger. Holly was a shy, bespectacled youth from Texas whose life was tragically cut short in a plane crash in 1959.

Rock 'n' roll was synonymous with rebellion and no one was more rebellious than Jerry Lee Lewis (born 1935), who shocked the morality of the age by marrying his 13-year-old cousin. It was not until the mid 1960s that Lewis once again gained public approval.

ABOVE: *Abba, whose name was taken from the initial letters of the members' names, were one of the few pop groups outside America or Britain to gain international stardom.*

Pop music

The 1960s have been rightly dubbed the "Swinging Sixties", and musically they were dominated by the Beatles and the Rolling Stones. Whereas the Beatles based their music on the rock of the 1950s, the Rolling Stones were rhythm-and-blues-based. Both bands had great success, and in one way or another have influenced almost every other rock band since.

While many bands were conventional, some performers mirrored the violence of the time (especially the United States' involvement in Vietnam). One of these was Jimi Hendrix (1942–70), who was one of the greatest guitarists of the '60s and had been a member of James Brown's backing band, the Famous Flames. His erotic stage actions, suggestive lyrics and guitar-smashing antics brought him much criticism — on one occasion he doused his guitar with lighter fuel and set it on fire. Other like-minded bands included The Who and the Sex Pistols.

ABOVE: *Frank Zappa (1940–1993) started writing music at high school, inspired by the rhythmic experimentation of the avant-garde composer Edgar Varèse.*

ABOVE: *Vanessa Mae (born 1976) became one of the youngest musicians to play with the London Philharmonic and took the music world by storm with her album* The Violin Player.

Another band of the 1960s and '70s, Frank Zappa's Mothers of Invention, was used as a vehicle for band-audience involvement. Music was only a part of the performance, which also included satire and comedy. Anything could happen, from a bag of vegetables being opened and examined to "dead air", when the band stopped and completely ignored the audience. On one occasion, when the audience had become unsettled and angry, Zappa approached the microphone saying, "It brings out the hostilities in you, doesn't it?" Zappa went on to become a film producer and classical composer, and died in 1993.

There was a respite from "heavy metal" when in 1974 a breath of fresh air entered the pop charts with Abba. This Swedish quartet, who depended more on television and radio than live concerts to build an image, achieved their breakthrough by winning that year's Eurovision Song Contest with *Waterloo*, a song that became a top-ten hit in many countries and many languages.

Famous String Players

*To play great music you must keep
your eyes on a distant star.*

YEHUDI MENUHIN (1916–99)

The idea of a stringed instrument being a virtuoso instrument emerged during the Baroque period, when composers such as Arcangelo Corelli, who was a violinist, began to exploit the strings' expressiveness in *concerti grossi* and solo sonatas. Eighteenth-century refinements in stringed instrument design allowed for increasing technical brilliance by a number of great Italian virtuosi, culminating in the talents of the violinist Niccolò Paganini (1782–1840), who confirmed the star status of the soloist. He was also an expert on the mandolin, guitar and viola.

Violin

The great violinists of the Romantic period included Rudolphe Kreutzer (1766–1831), for whom Beethoven wrote his *Kreutzer Sonata*, and Joseph Joachim (1831–1907), to whom Brahms's Violin Concerto was dedicated. Fritz Kreisler (1875–1962) showed an early talent for the violin and by the time he was 15 had

ABOVE: Yehudi Menuhin was one of the most respected musicians who has ever lived. His violin-playing inspired young players.

ABOVE: David Oistrakh coupled the technical brilliance of Heifetz with the warmth of Menuhin. He can truly be said to be one of the greatest violinists of all time.

achieved worldwide success. His playing epitomized Viennese lilt and warmth, while his almost constant vibrato made him one of the founders of the modern school of violin-playing.

As well as being the foremost composer of his generation, Paul Hindemith (1895–1963) was also an outstanding viola player, playing in the Rebner and Amar Quartets, and the Opera Orchestra in Germany from 1915–23. Also an accomplished violinist, it was said he could play every instrument in the orchestra.

Yehudi Menuhin (1916–99) began his career as a child prodigy, and was at home in all types of music, achieving a unique tone and mastery of rhythm. He will always be remembered for his playing of the Elgar Violin Concerto under the direction of the composer, and as a humanitarian for the schools he founded for musically gifted children in England and Switzerland.

David Oistrakh (1908–74) achieved national recognition in the former Soviet Union after performing Glazunov's Violin Concerto in 1927. The Soviet authorities prevented him from performing outside the USSR until the early 1950s, but from then on he took the international stage by storm. He remained a Soviet citizen all his life and was committed to contemporary Russian composers such as Prokofiev and Shostakovich.

The Israeli violinist Itzhak Perlman (born 1945), although a victim of poliomyelitis at the age of four, was giving public recitals when he was ten years old. In his subsequent career, Perlman's charismatic stage presence, combined with his instinctive directness of musical expression, brilliant technique and a concern for refinement of detail, has brought him international recognition.

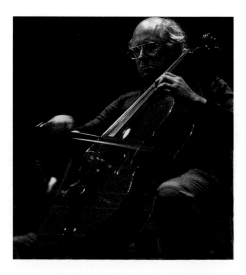

ABOVE: Mstislav Rostropovich was a close friend of Benjamin Britten, who wrote several cello works for him.

ABOVE: *The charismatic Jacqueline du Pré made her debut at the age of 16.*

Cello

As the cello took a more prominent role in chamber music during the 18th century, composers such as Liugi Boccherini (1743–1805) began to recognize its potential as a solo instrument. An early British virtuoso, Robert Lindley, began playing when he was five years old. His technique was said to be so brilliant that he was able to play first violin parts on his cello. In 1794, aged 18, Lindley played before the Prince Regent and, by 1826, had become lead cello with the Italian Opera in London.

Pablo Casals (1876–1973) probably did more for the cello than any other player. Although he is mainly remembered for his masterly playing of the Bach solo cello suites, Casals was also a conductor and a member of a chamber trio, and founded an annual festival of chamber music in France. Another influential cellist of the 20th century is Mstislav Rostropovich (born 1927), who has been immensely successful in playing the works of composers such as Shostakovich, Prokofiev and Britten.

The talent of Jacqueline du Pré (1945–87) was recognized at a very early age. She launched her professional career in 1961 with a concert at London's Wigmore Hall, at which she played a cello of 1672 by Antonio Stradivari. One of the great musical icons of the 20th century, she was admired by her audiences for the love she radiated in her playing, which was noted for its instinctive feeling for style as well as its technical proficiency. In 1973 her career was suddenly interrupted by the onset of multiple sclerosis, but she continued to teach.

Harp

Nicholas Bochsa (1789–1856), though a skilful player of almost every instrument, was best known for his expertise on the harp, an instrument on which he was constantly discovering new musical effects. Harpist to Louis XVIII, in 1817 he had to leave his native France hurriedly, due to his part-time business in forged documents. One of Bochsa's favourite pieces was his *Fantasia for Harp and Violin* which he often played with

ABOVE: *Since making her London debut in 1963, Marisa Robles has become a professor at the Royal College of Music.*

ABOVE: *John Williams is a very versatile guitarist, playing classical, jazz and pop music – he founded the pop group, Sky.*

Nicholas Mori, who was said to have handled his violin as tenderly as a mother her child, but as playfully as the child its toy.

The Spanish harpist Marisa Robles (born 1937) is one of the foremost players of the 20th century, noted for the quicksilver quality of her playing.

Lute and guitar

The eminent Spanish guitarist Andrés Segovia (1893–1987) was largely self-taught, but championed the guitar as a concert instrument, commissioning many new works. One of his pupils was Julian Bream (born 1933), who also took up the lute and quickly became a leading performer on it. In 1971, Bream began giving encouragement to guitar and lute makers by inaugurating the Semley Festival in Wiltshire to promote rare chamber music.

John Williams (born 1942) also studied guitar with Segovia. As a composer, he is particularly active in crossover projects, using tapes and electronics in his music and drawing on non-Western influences.

Famous Woodwind and Brass Players

*It takes perhaps a thousand poor musicians
to produce one virtuoso.*

RALPH VAUGHAN WILLIAMS (1872–1958)

As with other orchestral instruments, the expansion of the solo repertoire for woodwind and brass went hand in hand with technological advances that enabled the instruments to be played with far greater range and expressiveness.

Flute

Although Vivaldi and Mozart wrote for the solo flute, it was neglected during the 19th century, but found favour with French impressionists such as Debussy, and many modern composers have since written for it. The virtuoso James Galway (born 1939) is widely known as a popular soloist, but also spent many years as an orchestral player, including a period as principal flautist with the Berlin Philharmonic under Herbert von Karajan. A strong advocate of contemporary music, Galway's bright tone and twinkling vibrato has brought him thousands of fans all around the world.

Jean-Pierre Rampal (born 1922) was an all-round musician of astonishing versatility. His repertoire ranged from Baroque to contemporary, while his playing was noted for its pure tone, subtle dynamics and exquisite phrasing.

Oboe

The sweet tone and expressive playing of Leon Goossens (1897–1988) set new standards for the instrument. Principal oboe with Henry Wood by the time he was 16, Goossens's phrasing, superlative finger technique and breath control were to influence many composers to write concertos for the oboe.

Another leading 20th-century oboist is the legendary Heinz Holliger (born 1939), who is an eminent exponent of sounding chords, double trills and

ABOVE: Leon Goossens was one of the finest oboe players of the 20th century. A member of a very musical family, he was brother to the conductor Eugene and the harpists Sidonie and Marie.

glissandos. He is not shy of experimentation; his work with sounds produced by a microphone placed within the bore of his instrument encouraged composers such as Hans Werner Henze to write for the oboe.

Clarinet

One of the 20th century's finest clarinettists was Benny Goodman (1909–86), a musician who was equally at home in classical music and jazz. He formed a 12-piece jazz band in 1934, but did not forsake his classical roots, for he later recorded the Mozart Clarinet Quintet with the Budapest Quartet, as well as commissioning works from Aaron Copland and Paul Hindemith.

ABOVE: One of Ireland's most popular musicians, James Galway has entertained millions with his flute-playing, performing both classical music and popular songs.

ABOVE: Barry Tuckwell studied horn technique with the virtuoso Dennis Brain (1921–57) on his arrival in England in 1950. He was Professor of Horn at the Royal Academy of Music (1963–74), launching his solo career in 1968.

Horn

Barry Tuckwell (born 1931) began his musical career in Melbourne, Australia, at the age of 15 and played with the Sydney Symphony Orchestra. He was principal horn with the London Symphony Orchestra from 1955 to 1968, in which year he founded the Tuckwell Wind Quintet. The leading horn player of his generation, Tuckwell is famed for his outstanding ability to make light of extreme technical and musical difficulties, achieving his marvellous tone by playing a large-bore Holton double horn, rather than the lighter-toned instrument preferred by many of his contemporaries.

Trumpet

One of the finest trumpet players was Louis Armstrong (1901–71), a man who almost single-handedly transformed jazz from a collective art to one of solo expression, exemplified in a series of 1920s recordings known as the "Hot Fives" and "Hot Sevens". His clear ringing trumpet sound

influenced many modern trumpet players, both jazz and classical.

The innovative player Maurice André (born 1933) has brought the trumpet to a whole new audience. One of his main contributions to trumpet-playing has been his pioneering of the small, four-valved piccolo trumpet. He has transcribed for it many Baroque compositions originally written for other wind instruments.

Another champion of modern trumpet music is Håkan Hardenberger (born 1961). He has had various works written specially for him, including Harrison Birtwistle's trumpet concerto *Endless Parade*. A master of musical effects, Hardenberger's playing combines technical brilliance with a great beauty of sound.

Wynton Marsalis (born 1961) comes from New Orleans, and is chiefly known as one of the most famous jazz trumpeters of his generation. However, such is his catholic taste that he is as much at home with Haydn's trumpet concertos as he is with the

ABOVE: Håkan Hardenberger is one of the world's top trumpet players, famous for his flawless technical ability and the beautiful quality of his tone.

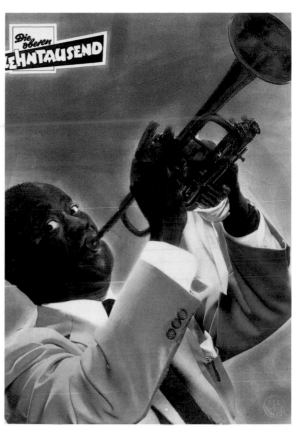

ABOVE: The great jazz trumpeter Louis Armstrong in a scene from High Society.

Lincoln Center Jazz Orchestra. He is also a composer, and in 1997 won a Pulitzer Prize for his operatic piece *Blood on the Fields*.

Trombone

Many technical developments of the 20th century have been due to the influence of jazz musicians. One of the foremost jazz trombonists of the second half of the century is the German virtuoso Albert Mangelsdorff (born 1928). He played with various German jazz groups before forming his own band in 1958. In 1964, influenced by his recent tour of Asia, he started introducing eastern elements into his playing. His main claim to fame, however, is that he was the first trombonist to succeed in playing three and four-note chords on his instrument, a feat that he achieved by a skilful combination of lip and vocal sounds.

Famous Concert Halls and Orchestras

...For we must have music, We must have music
To drive our fears away.

NOEL COWARD (1899–1973)

Until the 18th century, public concerts as they are known today did not exist. One of the first rooms to be devoted to formal concerts was that opened in London by Thomas Hickford in 1711. From then on other custom-built concert halls and opera houses gradually started to appear all over Europe.

German patrons of music built concert halls on a grand scale. At Schwetzingen, the Elector of Palatine built a new opera house capable of holding an audience of 5000, while Duke Karl Theodor of Württemberg bankrupted his entire principality to provide sensational opera productions at Mannheim.

The Berlin Opera House was built by Frederick the Great of Prussia (1740–86). A notable flautist and patron of music, Frederick was deeply immersed in French culture and maintained a French-speaking court. Opened in 1773, the Opera House, which employed singers from Italy and dancers from France, was equipped with parking space for 1000 carriages. The staircases were so wide that sedan

ABOVE: *The Amsterdam Concertgebouw Orchestra was founded in 1888. Its hall is renowned for its magnificent acoustics.*

chairs could be carried up to the fourth tier of the boxes, and three enormous chandeliers illuminated the whole auditorium.

In London, purpose-built concert halls included Carlisle House, Soho Square (1764); the Pantheon, Oxford Street (1772); and the Hanover Square Rooms (1775). Halls were also opened in some major provincial centres, such as Bath, which, thanks to its spa, was the centre of English fashionable society in the 18th century.

Throughout the 19th century the orchestras involved in London concerts contained so many of the same players that it would be difficult to describe each orchestra as different. Players had little or no

financial security and were engaged for each concert, not for the entire season. The custom of sending a deputy to the rehearsals, or even the concert, had become established, meaning that the composition of the orchestra was constantly changing.

One of the first conductors to recruit musicians for an entire season was Charles Hallé (1819–95). Hallé had made his reputation in Paris, but was driven to England by the revolution of 1848 and eventually settled in Manchester, which had an influential German community. He threw himself heartily into the town's musical life and in 1857 founded what was to become the celebrated Hallé

ABOVE: *This painting by Ludwig Edward Lutke shows the German State Opera House in Berlin, c.1845.*

ABOVE: *The New York Metropolitan Opera House was founded in 1883 but was rebuilt after a fire destroyed the original building.*

Orchestra. Its members were always present at both rehearsal and concert, making the orchestra the most disciplined and efficient band in the country. They never sounded, as did so many other orchestras, like a bunch of instrumentalists thrown together for a single event.

During the 20th century several great orchestras have been founded in London, including the London Philharmonic, which was founded in

ABOVE: Musical events held at the Royal Albert Hall in London range from brass band contests to rock concerts.

1932 by Thomas Beecham, and the BBC Symphony Orchestra, which was founded in 1930 and was the first orchestra to offer an annual salary and paid holidays.

As the 20th century progressed, orchestras faced the problem of financial support. The Boston Symphony Orchestra was founded in 1881 by the financier Henry Lee Higginson. He gave his conductors absolute artistic freedom and kept the orchestra at the highest level of achievement. Its financial future was assured by Higginson's creation of a body of 300 guarantors. Further south, the New York Philharmonic was founded in 1842. For the first 66 years of its existence it was run by an internal committee of musicians.

However, in 1908, due to financial difficulties, the orchestra was taken over by a syndicate.

The Berlin Philharmonic Orchestra, which acquired its high international reputation under the directorship of Herbert von Karajan, is funded by the city of Berlin, and has its home in an acoustically brilliant concert hall affectionately known as the "circus tent". Although it has a capacity of 2000, the seats virtually surround the orchestra, giving the hall a feeling of intimacy.

The audience at the Royal Albert Hall in London is seated in a vast ellipse, but had to suffer poor acoustics until they were remedied in the 1960s. The brick and glass building was built from 1867–71, and is universally known as the venue for the annual Henry Wood Promenade Concerts, which have been performed there since World War II when their former home, the Queen's Hall, was destroyed.

The Sydney Opera House on Bennelong Point is one of the city's most notable features. Designed by

ABOVE: Kurt Masur conducting the New York Philharmonic Orchestra in 1999. Masur made his United States debut in 1974.

Jørn Utsen, the building was largely financed by the Australian lottery and was opened in 1973. Its programme offers 16 different operas a year and there is a performance almost every night during the winter.

The world's largest opera house is the Metropolitan Opera House at the Lincoln Center in New York, completed in 1966 with an audience capacity of 4065.

ABOVE: Looking like something that has just emerged from the sea, the main features of the Sydney Opera House in Australia are its nine flying roofs, the highest point of which is 67m/220ft above sea level.

Encyclopedia
of
Musical
Instruments

The modern symphony orchestra consists of around 20 different musical instruments. These can be categorized into four main groups: strings, wind, percussion and keyboards.

Strings

How Stringed Instruments Work

What can be more strange, than that the rubbing of a little hair and
cat-gut together should make such a mighty alteration in a man.

JEREMY COLLIER (1650–1726)

Although the orchestral term "strings" is used only for the violin family, there are many other stringed instruments, played with or without a bow, that come under the general term "chordophone". In every case, the mechanics are the same.

One group of stringed instruments, which includes the harp and lyre, is played with open strings – each string producing only one note. The other group, into which most other stringed instruments fall, consists of those played with "stopped" strings: each string can be held down, effectively changing its length, so that it will produce a range of notes.

Sound production

There are two distinct types of construction of stopped-string instruments, each with its own acoustic implications. The lute is a perfect example of one type, with a flat soundboard and a bowl-shaped back, with no connecting ribs or soundpost. Instruments of the second

ABOVE: *Detail of two violins, showing the f-holes and parts of the bridges.*

type, by far the most common, have flat soundboards and flat or moderately arched backs, joined by side ribs. In both cases the sound is produced by the vibration of the strings being transmitted into the soundbox via the bridge.

The pitch produced by a string depends not only on its length but also on its thickness, weight and tension. In most instruments it is impractical to vary only the length of the strings, as the lower strings would have to be so long as to be unwieldy, so strings of different thicknesses are used: they may then all be of the same length. The tension of the string is also important. Too slack a tension sounds

ABOVE: *Unlike violins, violas and cellos, viols have frets on their fingerboards.*

ABOVE: *The string family (from left to right): two violins, a viola and a cello. The central motif of the stained-glass window is a lyre, a universal symbol of music.*

there was no clear demarcation between the body and the neck. Examples of such instruments are the mandora and the rebec.

The mandora evolved into the mandolin, while the rebec has survived in the form of the *lyra* of modern Greece and Crete and the Bulgarian *gadulka*. Used as a folk instrument to accompany songs and dances, the traditional *lyra* or *gadulka* has three gut strings that are played with a horsehair bow. It is held vertically while it is played, with the lower end tucked into the player's belt when standing, or held on the hip when seated.

feeble, while too thick a string is hard to get vibrating and restricts the higher harmonics. Low strings are usually wound with a fine wire on a moderate core to allow them to be held under sufficient tension without excessive mass or stiffness.

Shape of stringed instruments

Although stringed instruments come in various shapes and sizes, many have waisted bodies that allow both freedom for the bow and a more complex vibration. Stringed instruments were, however, waisted many centuries before the advent of the bow, and instruments so shaped appear in Babylonian sculptures. The shape may have been used not only for musical effect but perhaps because it had some symbolic or ritual association with the female form.

Early stringed instruments were usually carved from a solid block of wood that tapered in such a way that

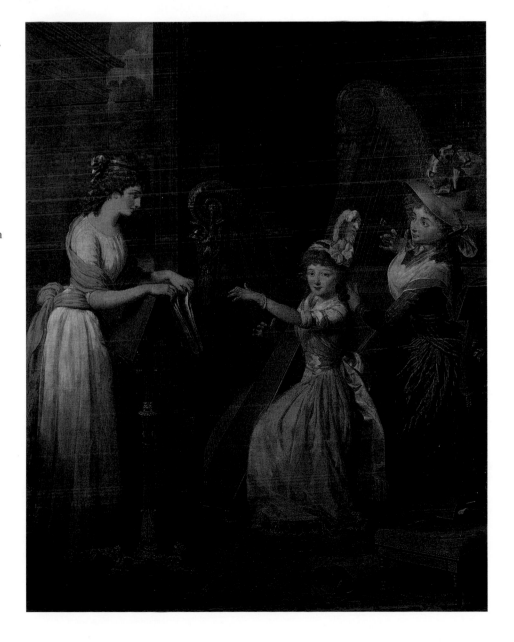

RIGHT: *This painting by Jean-Baptiste Mauzaisse (1784–1844) depicts the daughters of the Duke of Orleans being given a harp lesson by their tutor Mme de Genlis. The young musicians are playing pedal harps.*

Violin

The true mission of the violin is to imitate the accents of the human voice, a noble mission that has earned for the violin the glory of being called the king of instruments.

CHARLES-AUGUSTE DE BÉRIOT (1802–70)

The violin is the lead voice and most numerous instrument of the modern orchestra. The average orchestra has about 35 violins, which are divided into two sections – first and second. The violin's four strings give the instrument a range of over four octaves, including all the semitones and many microtones. Its extraordinary musical versatility, coupled with its emotional appeal and agility, makes possible – depending on the skill of the player – an expression of moods ranging from the tender lyrical music of Mozart to the dramatic tones of Wagner.

Origin

Although no one knows who invented the violin, some of the earliest instruments were made by Giovan Giacoba dalla Corna and Zanetto Montichiaro, both of whom are named in Giovanni Lanfranco's *Scintille di Musica* (1533). The first "famous" violin maker, however, was Andrea Amati (1525–1611), who was born in Cremona and became the founder of the Cremonese school of violin-making.

ABOVE: The scroll and pegs of a violin.

Although the violin family (violin, viola and cello) has been the mainstay of the symphony orchestra since its rise in the 17th century, the three-stringed violin had been in existence since the early 1500s. It was certainly known in 1508, for it appears in a wall painting of that date in the Sala del Tesoro at the Palazzo di Ludovico il Moro in Ferrara. Twenty or so years later, Gaudenzio

Ferrari depicted the instrument in *The Madonna of the Orange Trees*, painted for the church of San Cristoforo in Vercelli. The same artist included violins in his fresco in the cupola of Saronno Cathedral in 1535.

These early three-stringed violins were an amalgam of two other instruments that were well known at this time – the fiddle and the rebec. The new instrument combined the

LEFT: *The violin is the lead instrument in the orchestra. This one was made by Anton Kreutzinger in 20th-century Germany.*

sonority and playing potential of the former with the simplicity of the latter.

Construction

Although the violin appears to be of simple construction, it is in fact made of over 80 separate parts. The soundboard is generally made of European spruce and the back and the ribs are made of maple. Maple is also used for the neck, pegbox and scroll, while the fingerboard, which runs along the neck and extends over the soundboard towards the bridge, is generally made of ebony.

Originally, all four strings were made of gut. However, from about 1700, to improve the tone, the G string was wound with silver wire. Modern instruments still have the G, D and A strings made in this fashion, while the E string is generally constructed of steel.

The mid 18th century saw some major modifications in the construction of the violin. The emergence of purpose-built concert halls and the resultant larger audiences created a demand for instruments capable of producing greater volume and brilliance of tone. To achieve this, the neck and fingerboard were

ABOVE: This violin was made by the Italian craftsman Giuseppe Guarneri (1666–1739) in about 1695. Guarneri was the younger son of Andrea Guarneri, who had served as an apprentice to Nicola Amati and began the second great dynasty of Cremonese violin makers.

lengthened, the bridge was made higher, the soundpost was thickened and the soundboard was made thinner.

Another modification was that the number of nails attaching the neck was reduced from four to three. The neck had to be nailed, as glue would have adversely affected the tone. Modern violins have the neck mortised into the upper block so that nails are no longer needed.

RIGHT AND BELOW: A collection of modern violins. These instruments were made in the early 1990s by David Lipkin and Haim Algranati, London.

Key features

TYPE: stringed

TUNING: *g, d', a', e"*

NOTABLE PLAYERS OF THE VIOLIN: Niccolò Paganini, Joseph Joachim, Eugène Ysaÿe, Jascha Heifetz, David Oistrakh, Yehudi Menuhin, Isaac Stern, Itzhak Perlman, Kyung-Wha Chung, Nigel Kennedy, Anne-Sophie Mutter.

ABOVE: The Bavarian village of Mittenwald has been a centre of violin-making since 1684 when Matthias Klotz, who was born in the village, returned from Cremona. Johann Reiter, a craftsman of Mittenwald, is seen here working in his shop.

ABOVE: A depiction of a violinist on a Swedish-made carpet designed by Per Nilsson in 1781.

The violin outside Italy

By about 1550, four strings had become standard and schools of violin-making had been established in Venice, Cremona and Brescia. The makers not only catered for Italian musicians, but also exported instruments to England, France, the Low Countries and Germany. Charles IX of France bought 12 violins from Andrea Amati of Cremona, while the English were such avid customers that they were accused of "dispeopling" Italy of violins. Even in the 16th century, large sums were being paid for fine violins; one sold by Gasparo da Salo of Brescia in 1588 fetched over four times his housemaid's annual wage.

Music for the violin

At first, the violin was used only for doubling the voice and to accompany dancing. For the former purpose, the violinist used the vocal score, while dance musicians played from memory, so no music for the violin was published until the end of the 16th century. The first music known to have been published specifically for the violin was the *Balet Comique de la Royne*, which was devised for the French court by Balthazar de Beaujoyeulx in 1582. It included two dances that were scored for ten violins in four parts. This royal patronage was a breakthrough indeed, for up to this time the violin had been looked down upon, with "virtuous people" preferring the viol, which produced

ABOVE: *Known as the* Emile Sauret *(because it was once owned by that French violinist), this Stradivari violin was made in 1683.*

greater resonance but less volume. The social status of the violin was further enhanced in 1626 when the ensemble known as the *Vingt-quatre Violons du Roi* was founded at the court of Louis XIII.

Stradivari

Without doubt, the greatest of all violin makers was Antonio Stradivari (1644–1737). Descended from an old Cremonese family, young Antonio was first apprenticed to a wood-carver. However, he soon became associated with Nicola Amati (1596–1684), the grandson of Andrea and the finest maker of the Amati family, who taught him the art of violin-making. Stradivari's earliest surviving violin is dated 1666. With the death of his master, Stradivari's fame began to spread and he soon became recognized as the finest violin maker of his day.

Stradivari's highest pinnacle was reached in 1715 when his now well-known, orange-brown coloured varnish, which dried to a light delicate elastic skin, began to appear. Although varnish cannot improve a violin's tone, it can affect it adversely. A hard varnish causes an instrument to produce a hard

ABOVE: *The Japanese violinist Kyoko Takezawa playing a Stradivari violin in Munich in 1993.*

sound, with little or no tone-colour. A thick oily varnish, on the other hand, inhibits the wood's vibrations and a varnish that is applied badly may well prevent the best tones from being realized. Sadly, the recipe for Stradivari's varnish is now lost.

Decline of Italian violin-making

Despite the fact that the violin had become the backbone of the emergent orchestras and operas of Europe by the 18th century, this period coincided with a general decline in violin-making in Italy. By the end of the century, France had become the centre of

ABOVE: *Two violins made by the two greatest Cremonese violin makers. On the left is the back and front view of Stradivari's* **Alard** *which was made in 1715 and is considered to be the finest Stradivari in existence. On the right is Guarneri's* del Gesù.

excellence in violin-making. One of the greatest French makers was Nicolas Lupot (1788–1824) who, taking Stradivari as his model, linked French and Italian workmanship. Another French violin maker was François Tourte (1747–1835) who revolutionized and standardized the design of the bow.

ABOVE: *Nigel Kennedy (born 1957) is one of England's most controversial violinists, and is shown here playing a Stradivari violin. His intense concentration, vitality and all-or-nothing approach make him one of the most likeable musicians on the stage today.*

🎼 Fritz Kreisler

One of the finest violinists and composers for the violin in the 20th century, Fritz Kreisler (1875–1962) was born in Austria but became an American citizen in 1943. As well as writing numerous short pieces for the instrument, he also added cadenzas to the concertos of Beethoven and Bach. In addition, he fooled the musical world by composing many works in an archaic style that he ascribed to various 18th-century composers such as Pugnani and Francoeur. In spite of many experts – who had been misled – being angered when Kreisler admitted to the hoax in 1935, these works continue to enrich the violin repertoire.

ABOVE: *This 19th-century photograph shows a Hardanger fiddle being played held against the chest. Despite its name, it is a violin and today, with the addition of a chinrest, the instrument is played in the manner of orchestral violinists.*

Playing techniques

Although the violin is basically the same as it was 300 years ago, playing techniques have improved, allowing new types of music to be written. Before the invention of the chinrest – by Louis Spohr in about 1820 – the violin was played in several different ways. It was held either at the chest, at the shoulder, to the right or left of the neck, or, in the case of folk music, cradled against the left upper arm.

By the late 18th century, performance styles had changed so much that the violin needed strengthening. Heavier strings and tighter string tension were needed to produce the stronger sound required to fill the new larger concert halls.

Vibrato

One of the characteristics of modern violin-playing is vibrato. Created by a controlled rocking of the finger that is stopping the string, vibrato adds intensity to the tone. In the 18th and 19th centuries it was considered solely as ornamentation. Such is its universal acceptance, however, that whereas pre-20th-century music was marked where vibrato was required, today it is marked where it is not required. The use of vibrato seems to have become fashionable in the 1930s, due to the influence of performers such as Fritz Kreisler and Jascha Heifetz (1901–87). Some players use it all the time, and some, it is said, use it to cover up bad intonation.

Jazz violin

One of the first great jazz violinists was Eddie South (1904–62), a classically trained black musician who had already formed a popular dance band in Chicago when he toured Europe and discovered gypsy fiddling in Bucharest. He arrived back on the Chicago jazz scene in the late 1920s. South worked with the guitarist Django Reinhardt,

ABOVE: *Jascha Heifetz, seen here in 1929, is remembered for his hard sound that could melt unexpectedly into the sweetest, most effortless legato. His nimble left hand and flawless bowing technique astonished all who heard him.*

and his version of *Eddie's Blues* (recorded in 1937) is regarded as one of the finest of its genre; South's piteous blue slides and scoops were ably invigorated by Reinhardt's potent

ABOVE: *The violin can be held in several different ways – under the chin or resting against the jaw, as shown here, or held against the chest.*

guitar. Reinhardt also had a famous partnership with Stéphane Grappelli (1908–97), whose jazz violin style had been inspired by South: the two played together as principal soloists in the Quintet of the Hot Club of France from 1934–39.

Jazz is also a medium in which the electric violin is used. The electric violin has no soundbox and has a solid body, with a set of pick-ups that transmit the sound to an amplifier. It is capable of producing many new sonorities, and various avant-garde jazz players and composers have experimented with the instrument. One of the foremost electric violinists is Jean-Luc Ponty (born 1942) who, as well as working with musicians such as Frank Zappa, has produced hitherto unheard tones, some of which blare out like an electrified jazz horn.

Folk violin

The violin is used in folk music almost all over the world. Folk violinists do not follow the conventions of orchestral violinists, in that the instrument is not always held to

the chin. Country band fiddlers also often perform very skilled acrobatics with their instrument, such as playing it upside down, backwards, behind their back or even under their legs. In North American folk dance music, the violin is held against the chest or even the waist, while in North Africa the performer plays seated on the ground

LEFT: This musician is standing outside the Geigenbau, a stringed instrument museum in the southern Bavarian village of Mittenwald. Today it is a technical school, and a dozen artisans still carry on the long tradition of violin-making in the village.

with the instrument resting upright against the left knee.

Variations on the traditional violin include the single-fret *mazanki* of the Wielkopolska region of Poland. Carved out of one piece of wood, the *mazanki* is usually played in ensemble with the *dudy*, a form of bagpipe. The Hardanger fiddle, or *Hardingfele*, of western and southern Norway, was invented in about 1650, and was improved during the 18th century by Trond Isaksen (1712–72). The instrument, which includes four sympathetic strings placed below the fingerboard and playing strings, is still played today.

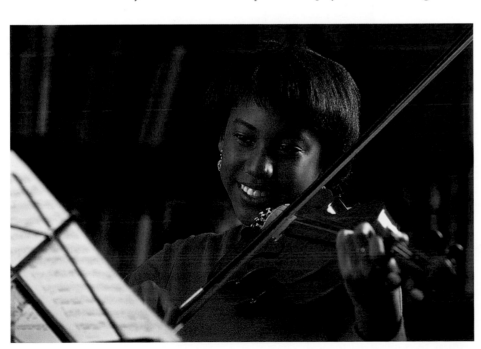

ABOVE: The violin is an extremely popular instrument among young people. Many students will learn the violin at school and carry on playing into adulthood.

ABOVE: Electric violins come in various sizes, including this MIDI of 1999.

Viola

The viola is a philosopher, sad and helpful; always ready to come to the aid of others, but reluctant to call attention to himself.

ALBERT LAVIGNAC (1846–1916)

The viola is the alto of the string section, and is pitched a fifth below the violin, whose fingering and bowing technique it shares. Fortunately, not many people share Wagner's view that it is "commonly played by infirm violinists or by decrepit wind players who were at one time acquainted with the violin". It came into being in northern Italy in the early 16th century and, by 1535, had become established as one of the three principal members of the new violin family. Known as the "instrument of the middle", the viola, with its dark, warm and rich tone, was used for both the alto and tenor registers. The strings were originally made of gut, but modern violas have

Key features

TYPE: stringed

TUNING: *c, g, d', a'*

NOTABLE PLAYERS OF THE VIOLA: Victor Lalo, Lionel Tertis, Paul Hindemith, William Primrose, Yuri Bashmet.

strings that are made of wire wound over gut or metal cores.

The main problem with the original viola was its size; some of the early models were so large that they could barely be played on the arm. The huge Andrea Amati tenor viola, for instance, had a body length of 47cm/19in. This problem was aggravated in the 19th century when some makers attempted to improve the viola's acoustics by making the body even longer. These improvements could only be effective if players had sufficiently long arms.

The perfecting of the Tourte bow, around 1785, opened a new era in string-playing. During the early 19th century the viola went through various alterations to increase string tension and carrying power, modifications that

LEFT:
The viola is slightly larger than the violin, and is pitched a fifth lower.

involved the introduction of heavier strings and the lengthening of the neck.

Repertoire

Before 1740 there were no known outstanding violists and consequently, virtually no repertoire for the instrument.

Although composers such as Bach, Handel and Vivaldi had given the viola important parts in fugues and concertos, it was not until the late 18th century that it began to be treated as a solo instrument.

One of the first composers to write a major part for the viola was Mozart, who, in his 1779 *Sinfonia Concertante* (K364), treated the viola and violin as equal partners. Paganini played the viola as well as the violin, and wrote caprices for the instrument. In the 20th century, mainly through the presence of outstanding players such as Lionel Tertis and Paul Hindemith, more solo viola works were written, including concertos by Walton, Bartók and the American composer

ABOVE: The composer Paul Hindemith (1895–1963) was an outstanding viola player. He had the distinction of being the first to play Walton's Viola Concerto in 1929.

Quincy Porter (1897–1967). Hindemith himself also wrote a number of works for the viola, including four concertos, four pieces for viola and piano, and two for unaccompanied viola.

Modern viola

Today's violas owe much to the work of the English viola virtuoso Lionel Tertis (1876–1975) who, in the 1940s, created an instrument that, although combining the fullness, depth and beauty of tone of a "full-size" viola, was still manageable by the player. More recently, Carleen Hutchins (born 1911), of the American Catgut Acoustical Society, has designed and built a whole new family of eight instruments acoustically scaled to the violin. Her viola, which

ABOVE: The viola section of the London Symphony Orchestra.

is rescaled to a body measurement of about 53cm/21in, has a spike and is played between the knees like a cello.

Viola d'amore

An instrument related to the viola, the viola d'amore was popular during the late 17th and 18th centuries. It is unfretted with 14 strings – seven playing and seven sympathetic strings tuned an octave higher. Although it fell out of use during the 19th century, it was revived in the 20th century by composers such as Janáček, who used it in his opera *Kátya Kabanová* (1921) and Prokofiev, who included it in the score of the ballet *Romeo and Juliet* (1935).

LEFT: One of the builders of the viola d'amore was Jacob Rauch who made this one in 1718.

BELOW: Despite its name, the viola da gamba is actually a viol. Unlike the viola, the viola da gamba has frets and is played between the knees like a cello.

Harold in Italy

One of the most important 19th-century works for the viola was Berlioz's *Harold en Italie*, a symphony with viola obbligato, written in 1834. Although it had been commissioned by Paganini, who had just acquired a Stradivari viola, when he saw the composition he declined to play it, complaining that it did not give him enough work to do, or adequately display his talents as a virtuoso.

Cello

The cello is like a beautiful woman who has not grown older but younger with time, more slender, more subtle and more graceful.

PABLO CASALS (1876–1973)

The violoncello, commonly referred to by its abbreviated name in English and German, is the bass instrument of the violin family, sounding an octave below the viola. The instrument originated in the 16th century. One of the earliest makers was Andrea Amati of Cremona, who built his *King Amati* in 1572.

One of the disadvantages of the original cello was its size. Early cellos were considerably larger than those of today, some having a body as long as 80cm/32in. This large size made it difficult to play rapid passages and so, in about 1660, experiments began in Bologna to create a smaller cello. At some time between 1707 and 1710 Stradivari decided on a length of about 75cm/30in, a length that has been standard ever since.

It took some time for the cello to become fully accepted, and it was not

RIGHT: A view of a cello player's bow action and fingering technique. This performer is using the modern overhand bow grip with his right hand, while the third finger of his left hand has reached a high note on the top A string.

until the latter half of the 17th century that composers began to score for it regularly. One of the earliest composers for the instrument was the Bolognese cellist Domenico Gabrieli (c.1655–90) who, in 1684, published his *Balletti, gighe, correnti, sarabande, a due violini e violoncello con basso continuo.*

Improvements

In the 18th century various improvements to the cello were carried out, including lengthening and thinning the neck and fingerboard, raising the bridge and introducing thinner and tauter strings, an innovation that produced a clearer and more responsive tone.

There were also improvements to the bow. Until the second half of the 18th century, cello bows were either straight or convex — like those of the viol and violin — and were gripped in the fist,

LEFT: The cello is a large instrument, and since it is supported by a spike and not the left hand, the strings can be stopped with the thumb as well as the fingers.

Key features

TYPE: stringed

TUNING: C, G, d, a

NOTABLE PLAYERS OF THE CELLO: Giuseppe Jacchini, Luigi Boccherini, Alfredo Piatti, Karl Davidov, Pablo Casals, Paul Tortelier, Mstislav Rostropovich, Jacqueline du Pré.

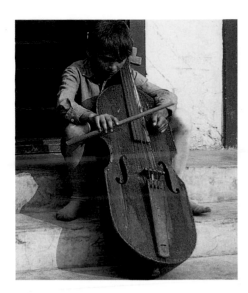

ABOVE: *A Romanian child playing a gardon by plucking the strings immediately after he has hit them with a stick.*

RIGHT: *The Portuguese cellist Guilhermina Suggia (1885–1950) played a Stradivari. She is remembered for her grace and style.*

with the palm facing upward, as for the viol, or downward. François Tourte allowed cello players greater control when he introduced his concave bow of pernambuco wood in the 1780s, and fixed it at a length of 72cm/29in, with the playing hair between 60cm/24in and 62cm/25in,

Method of play

Early cellists either sat with their instrument resting on the floor between their legs, or stood with it leaning against their body. Sometimes it was played resting on a stool, or even in a horizontal position. By 1700, it was usual for the player to place his cello between his knees and support it with his calves. This high posture permitted the player to draw the neck back towards him, so that the left hand could approach the strings from the side, instead of from behind, thereby making the entire compass of the instrument more accessible.

In the 17th century cellos were also played in religious processions, especially in northern Italy. The peripatetic cellists cut a hole in the back of their instrument through which a strap was passed, which was

Cello music

While it has never been as well provided for as the violin, some notable 20th-century works have been composed for the cello, including Elgar's Cello Concerto (1919), Kodály's Sonata for Cello and Piano, Op. 4 (1910), Webern's *Drei Stücke* (1914), Villa-Lobos's *Bachianas Brasileiras* (1916), part of which is written for eight or more cellos, Britten's Cello Symphony (1963) and Mauricio Kagel's *Match* (1964), in which the two cello soloists dress as table-tennis players and perform against each other.

hung around the player's neck, leaving him free to play with both hands – not an easy task.

Gardon

Originating from the eastern Carpathians, the gardon is a folk instrument similar to the cello, and is played as a rhythm instrument by Romanian gypsies. It used to be made out of a single block of wood, but the modern gardon has a body like that of the cello. It has three or four strings, all tuned to *d*. The player, who either sits or stands, hits the strings with a wooden stick or may slap the fingerboard. The strings may also be plucked.

ABOVE: *This painting of 1753 vividly shows the old style of playing the cello with the instrument grasped between the legs – there is no spike. The bowing technique shows the hand under the bow rather than over it, unlike the technique favoured by modern cellists.*

Double Bass

A composition without a bass
would be full of confusion and dissonance.

GIOSEFFO ZARLINO (1517–90)

The double bass is the largest and lowest-pitched stringed instrument of the orchestra. As well as being indispensable in the symphony orchestra – the average orchestra has eight – the double bass is also an essential member of jazz and dance bands, where its *pizzicato*-playing provides the rhythmical bass line. Today the bass generally has four strings, tuned in fourths, but this has not always been the case. During the 17th century five-string basses were used in Austria and Germany and in the early 18th century three-string basses were normal.

Size

The double bass has always been made in a number of sizes. The full-size instrument was used in the early Baroque period, but with the development of the overwound gut

Key features

TYPE: stringed

TUNING: *E', A', D, G*

NOTABLE PLAYERS OF THE DOUBLE BASS: Josef Kämpfer, Giovanni Bottesini, Serge Koussevitzky, Charles Mingus, Ludwig Streicher, Gary Karr, Barry Guy.

RIGHT: On the double bass the tuning pegs jut out at the back. Because of the high tension of the strings, a cog wheel mechanism is used for tuning.

ABOVE: A double bass player.

string, makers were able to reduce it to more manageable dimensions. The modern orchestra generally uses a three-quarter size instrument, with a body length of about 115cm/45in, and all-steel strings are commonly used. Jazz and dance bands also use the three-quarter size, although they sometimes play the "piccolo bass", which is fitted with thin strings and tuned an octave higher than the standard bass. In the 17th century half-size basses were carried in processions, suspended by a strap over the shoulder. At the other extreme, some gigantic basses have been built. These include Vuillaume's *octobasse*, which was built in 1849. Over 4m/13ft high and tuned an octave below the conventional bass, it was so big that it required two people to play it and the strings could only be stopped by operating a system of levers and pedals. Even larger was Paul de Wit's bass, 4.8m/16ft high, which he built for the 1889 Cincinnati Music Festival. One of the largest double basses built in Britain – if not the largest ever – was that constructed by Mr Martin, the landlord of the Blackamoor Lady in Leicester. Martin's instrument was so big that a hole had to be cut in his ceiling

ABOVE: *Vuillaume's* octobasse *(1849) was so big that the bow had to be held in place by a kind of oarlock.*

ABOVE: *Double bass strings are very long, so they vibrate well — the instrument is highly suited to playing* pizzicato.

through which the neck protruded, and it could only be tuned by going upstairs into the room above.

Virtuosi

Domenico Dragonetti (1763–1846), a Venetian, was considered the world's finest bass player of his time. He was a great friend and admirer of Beethoven and wrote several concertos and other pieces for the instrument. He freed it from doubling the cello part and assured its permanent place in the orchestra by pushing the playing technique to new heights. Such was Dragonetti's mastery over his instrument that once, while staying at a monastery, he stood in the corridor outside his room during the night and imitated a storm with his bass. The next day the main topic of the monks' conversation was the "thunderstorm" of the previous night.

Giovanni Bottesini (1822–89) extended the range of the double bass even further than Dragonetti, and was known in his day as the "Paganini of the double bass", particularly for his use of high harmonics. He toured Europe, Russia and the United States as a double bass soloist, wrote an important book on the instrument and composed a large number of works for it. A friend of Verdi, he conducted the first performance of Verdi's opera *Aida* in Cairo in 1871.

Bowing techniques

Methods of bowing for the double bass vary in different countries. Most players in Europe use the Bottesini, or "French" bow, which is shaped like a shorter, heavier cello bow and held overhand as for the cello. In central and eastern Europe, however, players prefer the "German" bow designed by Franz Simandl (1840–1912), which is derived from the old Dragonetti bow. Used underhand like a viol bow, it is also known as the "meat saw".

 Bass music

It was only in the 19th century that composers started to write distinctive double bass parts. Before this time the bass player shared the cello part, usually playing an octave below the cello. By the early 19th century the bass was becoming popular as a solo instrument and composers were writing more exposed passages for the instrument, such as that in Schubert's "Trout" Quintet of 1819. In Saint-Saëns's *Le Carnaval des Animaux* (1886), the elephant is represented by the double bass. Other composers for the double bass include Hindemith, Prokofiev and Darius Milhaud.

ABOVE: *This double bass player is using the German technique, whereby the bow is held from underneath — similar to viol technique.*

Harp

His harp, the sole companion of his way.

JAMES BEATTIE (1735–1803), "THE MINSTREL"

One of the largest of all orchestral instruments, the modern harp has 46 strings with a compass of six and a half octaves. It is played tilted back against the player's right shoulder and usually has double-action pedals, which allow the player to raise the pitch of the strings by either a semitone or a tone. The harp is unique in that the strings run perpendicular to the resonator, whereas in all other stringed instruments the strings run parallel. The strings are plucked with the fingers, as was the case with early harps, although by 2000 BC the plectrum had been introduced.

The modern frame harp is descended from two basic types: the bow or arched harp, and the angular harp.

Bow or arched harp

The earliest form of harp is thought to have developed from the hunter's bow. Bow harps first appeared in western Asia in about 3000 BC, where they were played in processions and at

LEFT: A beautifully decorated modern pedal harp made by Leffler of Germany.

banquets. They had a resonator at the base from which the strings were attached to a curved neck. Many of these harps, which were just over 1m/3ft long, were decorated with a bull's head motif.

The first Egyptian harps of which we know date from the Fourth Dynasty (2625–2500 BC). They were used alone to accompany singing as well as in larger bands, and varied in size from the hand-held shoulder harp, usually played by women, to the larger instruments that were played by men. One of these, over 2m/6ft in height, is seen on a wall painting in the tomb of Rameses III (c.1150 BC). Played with the resonator resting on the floor, this instrument is decorated with a carved human head. Today the arched harp survives mainly in Africa and East Asia.

Angular harp

The earliest evidence of angular harps is to be found in three marble statuettes of seated musicians which date from about 2000 BC. Usually played by women, these instruments were in the shape of an equilateral triangle with each side some 55cm/21½in long. The strings were attached to the neck, forming a 60° angle with the resonator that rested on the player's right thigh.

Although the angular harp had been introduced into Egypt by about 1500 BC, it was several centuries

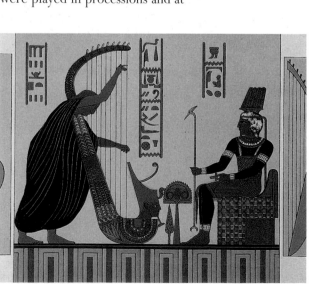

LEFT: This Egyptian mural from the tomb of Rameses III at Thebes (c.1150 BC) shows a harp with nine strings and a carved human face at the base of the resonator.

LEFT: An ancient Egyptian musician playing an arched harp. Played with the resonator resting on the floor, this six-stringed instrument is typically decorated with a carved human head.

Western Europe

The harp was known in western Europe by the 7th century. An 8th-century Anglo-Saxon manuscript depicts a frame harp, as does the 9th-century Utrecht Psalter. There is also a reference to the harp in Wace's 12th-century French poem, *Roman de Brut*. In the frame harp, the third side of the triangle, left open in the angular harp, is closed by the piece known as the pillar, so that the strings are enclosed within a frame. In early European harps, the pillar was usually curved.

before it gained full acceptance. It was played in an upright position, with the resonator held against the body and the neck resting in the player's lap.

Egyptian harpists evolved highly developed playing techniques, such as using the flat of the hand to dampen the strings. Another innovation was the sounding of stopped as well as open strings.

In Greece the harp never achieved the popularity of the lyre and was denounced by Plato as a "dreamy" instrument that was usually played only by women. The angular harp became popular in Imperial Rome where it was often played (again by women) in processions, sacrificial ceremonies and at the religious rites associated with the cult of Isis, which the Romans had adopted from the Egyptians.

ABOVE: This illustration of a harp player, entitled Gabinetto Armonico, *was drawn by Bonanni in the 18th century.*

RIGHT: A late 13th-century French illustration showing King David playing the harp.

Irish harp

The earliest evidence of the Irish harp, with its slender neck, pillar and resonator, is seen on relief carvings on 9th-century stone crosses. The instrument, which had a pronounced outward curve of the pillar, from which a low neck projected, was played held against the player's left shoulder. The harpist plucked the metal strings of the upper register with the long fingernails of his left hand. Early instruments were about 60cm/24in high and had up to 30 strings, but by the 16th century they had become larger and boasted up to 43 strings. Unlike earlier harps played with both hands, the new type was held against the body with one hand and played with the other. The Irish harp virtually died out in the late 18th century.

BELOW: A wooden Irish, or Celtic, harp. It has 22 strings with a flat soundboard on a round-backed resonator. The strings are tuned by means of pegs.

ABOVE: An Irish, or Celtic, harp decorated with gilt vine. This harp differed from other harps in that the strings were played with the fingernails instead of the fingertips.

Welsh harp

Known as the *telyn*, the Welsh harp is mentioned in poetry from the 10th century. Such was its importance that it was said to be one of the three indispensable possessions of a freeman. Unlike its Irish relation, the Welsh harp's strings, 31 or 34 in number, were made of horsehair or gut.

In the late 17th century the traditional Welsh harp was superseded by the triple harp, a chromatic instrument capable of producing all the notes in every key, and this remained the standard bardic instrument until the 19th century. Its diatonic strings were in the two outer rows, tuned in unison, allowing repeated notes to be played quickly using alternate hands. The strings in the inner row were tuned to the semitones. Held at the shoulder, the left hand generally played the treble and the right the bass strings.

Modern harp

An alternative to the chromatic harp was the hook harp, in which the pitch was raised a semitone by a series of U-shaped hooks set in the neck. The drawback with this system was that it was manually operated, so the player temporarily lost the use of one hand when tuning each string. This inconvenience was remedied in about 1720 by the invention of the pedal harp by Jakob Hochbrucker of Donauwörth and Johann Vetter of Nuremberg. The first pedal harps had five pedals that were connected to the hooks by wires passing through the hollow pillar. By depressing one of the pedals, all the strings of one note were raised by a semitone. The number of

ABOVE: An early 19th-century pedal harp player.

ABOVE: *Detail of the top area of a modern harp, showing the tuning pegs and chromatic shift mechanisms.*

pedals was eventually increased to seven – one for each note of the diatonic scale, and this has remained the number in common use today.

Refinements to the system – replacing hooks with levers or forks – were made by the French makers Cousineau and Erard in the late 18th century. Erard created the double-action harp, with pedals that can be set in two positions to raise the pitch of each string by either a semitone or a whole tone. The harp was considered

ABOVE: *A close-up view of three harp pedals.*

to be a suitable instrument for ladies to play, and many were sold for domestic use during the 18th and 19th centuries.

One of the more notable harp makers of the 20th century is Victor Salvi (born 1921), who made his first harp in 1954. Seeking traditional Italian carving and veneering skills, Salvi moved from New York to Genoa, Italy, where he began producing harps such as the *Orchestra*. Salvi's innovations include a stainless steel linking system and nylon bearings, eliminating the need for lubrication. By the 1970s Salvi harps were available in a number of different sizes, ranging from the 164cm/65in high *Angelica* to the 188.5cm/74in high *Electra*.

Repertoire

The first symphony to include a part for the harp was Berlioz's *Symphonie Fantastique* (1830). Before this it had mainly been used orchestrally for special effects, as in the operas of Handel and Gluck. An exception was Mozart's Concerto for Flute and Harp, which he wrote in 1778 as one of a series of works commissioned by a wealthy flautist.

At the end of Wagner's *Das Rheingold*, the gods enter Valhalla accompanied by an orchestra including six harps. Both Debussy and Ravel wrote chamber music for the instrument, each having been commissioned by rival harp makers. Following the folk tradition, the modern harp is sometimes used to accompany voices, as in Benjamin Britten's 1942 *Ceremony of Carols* as well as works by Falla and Webern.

ABOVE: *Although not all musical works include a part for the harp, the modern harpist is a key member of most large symphony orchestras.*

Electric harp

The first to use an amplified harp was the American harpist Lloyd Lindroth, who introduced it in 1964. He also later modified his harp to include a "wah-wah" pedal that "bent" the harp tone.

𝄞 Key features

TYPE: stringed

PITCH: concert

NOTABLE PLAYERS OF THE HARP: Turlough Carolan, Nicholas Bochsa, Elias Parrish Alvars, Sidonie Goossens, Marisa Robles.

Guitar

A guitar has moonlight in it.

JAMES M. CAIN (1892–1977)

The guitar's wide appeal as a folk instrument led to its current pre-eminent role in rock and pop music. The instrument has a long history and, although as a classical instrument it has hardly figured in the orchestra, its solo repertoire is extensive.

Gittern

The modern guitar is a descendant of the gittern, a small lute-like instrument that came to Europe via Moorish Spain in the second half of the 13th century. The gittern, which had four gut strings, was popular not only among minstrels but also with the aristocracy. During the 15th century, the instrument increased in length and the number of strings changed to three courses of two, tuned to *D, G* and *B*, with a single chanterelle tuned to *E*. The second string of each pair doubled at the octave.

Vihuela

In Spain the gittern became transformed into the vihuela, a flat instrument curved in at the sides, with five pairs of strings and a single chanterelle. Although it was rarely found outside Spain, Henry VIII of England was known to have had four "Spanish vialles". These possibly came into his possession though his marriage to his first wife Catherine, daughter of

RIGHT: A four-stringed gittern carved with hunting scenes, grotesques and the arms of Queen Elizabeth I.

BELOW: The classical guitar, made famous by Andrés Segovia, a great guitarist of the 20th century.

Ferdinand of Aragon. The vihuela was an instrument of courtly society, whereas the smaller, four-course guitar was used for more popular music, and by the end of the 16th century was famous all over Europe. By the mid 16th century music was being especially written for the guitar, and in 1586 Juan Carlos Amat brought out the first edition of his tutor, *Guitarra Española*. Within 100 years the guitar had become the instrument of choice even in Spain, and the days of the vihuela were numbered.

Renaissance guitar

The Renaissance four-course guitar appeared during the early 15th century. Played with a quill plectrum, the strings were strung over gut frets that were tied around the neck, and passed over a movable bridge before terminating at a fixed frontal string holder. It was a much smaller instrument than we know today, combining the small size of the gittern with the body shape of the much larger vihuela. In the late 17th century a fifth course of strings was added below the other four.

Modern guitar

The playing technique was simplified by removing one string of each pair, and the modern six-string guitar, which has a wooden resonating chamber with incurved sidewalls and a flat back, began to make its appearance in the 18th century. Early instruments were much narrower and more elongated than

ABOVE: This 17th-century painting by Vermeer shows a girl playing a five-course guitar made by Vaboam, whose trademark ornamental rose sound-hole can be seen.

those of today. Eminent makers included José Pages of Cadiz, René François Lacote of Paris and the London-based Lewis Panormo.

In the 19th century the body was broadened and the internal bracing changed to a fan shape. Fixed metal frets were fitted to the neck and the bridge was raised. These innovations were largely the work of the Spanish guitar maker Antonio Torres Jurado (1817–92), who also standardized the

ABOVE: Chuck Berry was an early rock 'n' roll singer who helped promote the popularity of the guitar. Many young people purchased a guitar to imitate their idols.

ABOVE: The guitar is an ideal instrument for street buskers. This unusual group from Santa Monica, California, consists of two guitars and a balalaika.

string length to 65cm/26in. Metal screws replaced the wooden tuning pegs and, during the 20th century, further modifications were made, including lengthening the fingerboard down to the sound-hole.

The guitar in rock music

Today the guitar is most widely used by popular music bands. The electric guitar, using pick-ups to amplify the sounds of the strings, was developed in the 1930s and the solid-body guitar was invented by Les Paul in the 1940s. As an aid to rock musicians, transposition is facilitated by a *capo tasto* that is fitted over the fretboard, stopping all the strings simultaneously. Modern electric guitars are strung with metal strings and played with a plectrum.

ABOVE RIGHT: The tres, indigenous to Cuba and the Dominican Republic, has three double courses of strings. It is often used to accompany dance.

MIDDLE RIGHT: The electric guitar is always played with a plectrum. The vibrations of the strings are picked up electronically so there are no sound-holes.

RIGHT: The bass guitar has four thick steel strings and is made in many varied shapes. It is mainly used in rock and dance bands.

LEFT: The acoustic guitar, still the instrument of choice for folk and classical players.

BELOW: The 12-string guitar has six double courses of strings. It often has gut strings for a softer tone.

Hawaiian guitar

A modification of the Spanish guitar, the Hawaiian guitar was introduced into the islands in the 1830s. It is believed that one Joseph Kekuku was the first person to place the guitar across his knees, in the manner of a fretted folk zither, and run a comb along the strings to produce the

BELOW: The Hawaiian guitar, played across the player's knees, is best known for the glissando *effect achieved by running a steel bar along its strings.*

glissandos for which modern Hawaiian music has become known.

In the early 20th century the Hawaiian guitar became popular in the United States and makers began to market models for which a steel bar was sold as an accessory for slide playing – hence the American term "steel guitar". Outside Hawaii, the use of the steel guitar is now almost solely restricted to country music bands, where the doleful sound is a feature of many songs about lost love. The player holds the steel bar in one hand, while the fingers of the other wear plectra that are used to pluck the strings. In the 1950s, pedals and knee levers were introduced as an aid to rapid alteration in tuning.

Dobro

The dobro is a guitar that has one or more metal resonator discs inside the body under the bridge. It was first produced by the National String Instrument Corporation of Los Angeles in 1925 to a design by John Dopyera, the son of a Czech violin maker. Three years later Dopyera left the company to set up – with two of his brothers – the Dobro Corporation. The idea for the resonator discs came from the banjo, which sometimes had a metal resonator in its back. The dobro was originally developed in response to the growing demand for a guitar that would produce a greater volume than the conventional instrument. Although occasionally used by rock musicians, the dobro is mainly used in country and bluegrass music, where it is often played, Hawaiian-style, across the knees.

The name "Dobro" was formed by eliding the first syllables of Dopyera

ABOVE: This 19th-century painting, The Concert *by Vincente Palmaroli, shows a Spanish woman playing her guitar to a small audience at home.*

Brothers – though it also, helpfully, means "good" in Czech.

Ukulele

In 1879 Portuguese sailors introduced their *machete de braca*, a cross between a guitar and a mandolin, into Hawaii, where it was transformed into the ukulele, a word meaning "leaping flea". For

ABOVE, FROM MIDDLE TO BOTTOM: The dobro is an acoustic guitar with metal resonator discs inside the body which add volume to the sound. It is used by rock musicians – most famously by Mark Knopfler of Dire Straits – and country and bluegrass singers.

The ukulele was advertised in 1916 as the most popular instrument of the day, its popularity being mainly due to its small size, light weight and low cost.

ABOVE: Two mandolins – English (top) and an Italian copy, both played by plucking the strings.

about 30 years the instrument remained relatively unknown outside the islands; its introduction to American popular music came in 1915 at the San Francisco Panama Pacific Exposition, where a group of Hawaiian performers enthralled the crowds with their music and in so doing created a new musical vogue.

The instrument reached a peak of popularity in the 1930s and '40s, in Britain mainly due to the music-hall artist George Formby, and in the United States due to the television

ABOVE: In Hawaii a small type of guitar is used to accompany the joyful vocal groups that are a feature of these wonderful islands.

Guitar music

The earliest surviving music for the four-course guitar is found in Alonso de Mudarra's *Tres libros de musica en cifras para vihuela*, published in 1546. In the late 16th century the Italian Melchiore de Barberis (born 1545) wrote four fantasias for guitar. Much of the music subsequently written for the classical guitar has been by Spanish and South American composers. Francisco Tarrega (1852–1909) was the first guitarist to use the improved design of Torres, for which he both composed solo works and transcribed the works of other composers. The classical repertoire also includes works by Manuel de Falla (1876–1946), Joaquin Turina (1882–1949) and the Mexican Manuel Ponce (1882–1948). Most popular of all is the *Concerto de Aranjuez* by Joaquin Rodrigo (born 1902), which was first performed in 1940.

star Arthur Godfrey. Its music is usually written in tablature – representing the player's finger positions rather than pitch.

Guitarillo

The Bolivian guitarillo has five double courses of gut strings and six frets. The instruments are often played in pairs by the Chipaya people to accompany

ABOVE: A guitarist in Buenos Aires playing with the aid of a capo tasto. Fitted over the fretboard, this device enables different keys to be played with the same chord positions.

the *waynus de cordero* and *tonadas del cordero* (songs in praise of sheep and cattle) at the *k'illpa* festival.

BELOW, FROM TOP TO BOTTOM: A Gibson Stereo electric guitar and an Epiphone mandolin with four double courses of strings, usually plucked with a plectrum.

Fiddles

They hadde menstrales of moch honours,
Fydelers, sytolyrs, and trompours.

THOMAS CHESTRE, "SIR LAUNFAL" (C.1400)

The first fiddles were almost as tall as their standing players. Held vertically, they had three strings and a round pegbox. Although all fiddles were generally made from a single block of wood, hollowed out and covered with a wooden soundboard, there were regional variations in shape. Three strings continued to be the norm until well into the 13th century, when five strings became general. Although gut was the usual material for strings, silk was sometimes used, and from the 13th century metal strings began to appear.

There were two distinct methods of playing the fiddle. In areas of Islamic influence it was held upright with the lower end resting against the player's knees or on the floor. The bow was held palm-up. In all other areas it was held approximately horizontally,

BELOW: The Cretan lyra is a short-necked fiddle with three gut or wire strings. The bow was once fitted with small bells to give rhythmic accompaniment.

sometimes supported across the chest with a strap, or vertically with the lower end against the player's chest or shoulder and the pegbox pointing down to the ground.

Kit

Used mainly by French dancing masters from the 16th to the 19th centuries, the kit was a small unfretted fiddle that was made in a great variety of shapes. When not in use the instrument was kept in a pocket in the teacher's coat-tails, a practice that gave it its nickname "pocket violin". The kit was made in four main forms: rebec,

ABOVE: A woodcut from Agricola's Musica Instrumentalis Deudsch *(1529) showing four fretted viol-type fiddles: bass, tenor, alto and descant. Each instrument has not only a round sound-hole in the centre of the resonating box, but also two f-holes by the neck.*

ABOVE: This 19th-century watercolour by Per Nordquist shows a man playing the nyckelharpa or keyed fiddle.

mandora, viola and violin – the last being the most common. Its name may be derived from the Greek kithara, or may be a reference to its diminutive size, like the kitten of the violin family.

Nyckelharpa

Used throughout Scandinavia for popular dance, festive and folk music, the nyckelharpa is a keyed fiddle. Fifteenth-century nyckelharpan had between seven and 12 wooden keys and from three to six strings, some of which were drones. The oldest surviving nyckelharpan date from the 16th century and are of two types. One has an elongated body in the shape of a figure eight, with a flat bottom and flat soundboard. The

LEFT: This 15th-century fresco by Fra Angelico at San Marco, Florence, depicts an angel playing a pear-shaped rebec.

century, when it was the recognized instrument of professional minstrels attached to noble households, and was played at courtly feasts and dances.

By the mid 16th century the rebec had been relegated to street musicians as people took up the increasingly popular violin. Indeed, such was the pejorative feeling against the rebec that in 1682 the French forbade musicians to exercise their trade unless they had served a six-year apprenticeship and had passed an examination; those who failed the examination were permitted to play only the rebec.

ABOVE: The rebec was introduced into Spain by the Arab invaders and, after undergoing various modifications, it evolved into the pear-shaped instrument of the early 11th century, which was played held propped against the shoulder.

second type is pear-shaped and the soundboard and neck are made in a single piece. More recently, the shape of this type has come to resemble that of the violin family.

Rebec

An adaptation of the Byzantine lyre and the Islamic two-stringed rabab, the rebec was a plucked lute that dates back to at least the 8th century. The rebec was a bowed string instrument with a vaulted back, carved from one piece of wood that tapered in such a way that there was no clear demarcation between the body and the neck. At first the instrument had only two strings – tuned a fifth apart – with a compass of ten tones. However, by the 15th century it had anything from one to five strings, the average being three.

Although as early as the 13th century both the French and English courts employed rebec players, the heyday of the instrument was during the 15th

ABOVE: When the bow reached Europe it was applied to instruments that had hitherto been plucked. For the first time, instruments such as this guitar-shaped fiddle were bowed, thus allowing them to produce a sustained sound.

Lyre

The lyre is welcome at the feasts of Jupiter.

HORACE (65–8 BC), "ODES"

The lyre is distinct from the harp in that its strings are attached to a yoke that lies in the same plane as the soundboard. There are two types of lyre: the box lyre, in which the resonator is a built-up wooden box, and the bowl type, which has a natural or artificially hollowed-out bowl as the resonator.

Origins

The lyre was played in Sumeria, since a representation of a lyre, standing higher than the seated player, has been found on a seal of about 3000 BC. Such lyres were asymmetrical, with the longer arm held away from the player. Plucked with the fingers of both hands, they had from eight to 12 strings that were fastened in a bunch on the lower left of the resonator before fanning out to the crossbar. Tuning was achieved by winding each string around a small rod tangential to the crossbar. Many lyres were carved with a bull's head and sometimes the strings emerged from a bull's body, perhaps giving a quasi-

divine voice to the instrument. From Mesopotamia, the lyre passed on to Syria and Israel. The Hebrew lyre, or *kinnor*, had strings of sheep gut and

LEFT: The main type of lyre used in ancient Greece was the kithara. It had a wooden resonator and a row of gut strings attached to a bridge and crossbar, but no examples have survived. The words "guitar" and "zither" probably derive from "kithara".

was probably the "harp" of King David. The Hebrews had two methods of playing the lyre. For the dance, a plectrum was used, while for accompanying the voice, the strings were plucked with the fingers. The Israelites used the lyre only to express joy; it was considered a sacred instrument and was never used for sad music. When the Jews were in exile they suspended their "harps" on the willows, unable to "sing the Lord's song in a strange land".

Egypt and Greece

Around 1360 BC huge lyres appeared in Egypt, often decorated with a duck's head as a sign that they were associated with the god Amun. They were played with a long plectrum held in the right hand; all the strings, which varied in number from 7–15, were struck with a sweeping movement, while the left hand dampened those that were not wanted.

Lyres appeared in Crete by about 1800 BC, from where they passed to the Greek

RIGHT: An artist's impression of some of the instruments used by the ancient Egyptians and Hebrews. The blue instrument in the centre of the picture is an Egyptian lyre.

ABOVE: A Roman woman using a plectrum on a form of lyre.

and louder, with a wooden sound-chest and arms. Held at a tilt, the kithara was the primary instrument of Greek classical drama, contests and official cults.

Rome

From Greece the lyre migrated to Etruria, where tomb paintings of the 5th century BC show instruments with six or seven strings, a heavy bridge and a small body with long arms. Although the lyre was known to the Romans from this time, it did not play an important part in the city-state's musical life. In Roman art, Orpheus was often depicted playing his lyre to pacify lions. In the early days of Christianity, this subject was replaced by that of Christ with a flock of sheep, signifying the "Good Shepherd".

mainland, assuming a horseshoe shape. The Greeks originally made their resonators out of tortoiseshell. Later other materials were used, but were made to resemble tortoiseshell. In Greece the lyre evolved into the more sophisticated kithara, which was larger

ABOVE: The 19th-century Italian mezzo-soprano Sofia Scalchi in Gluck's opera, Orpheus, *holding a replica of a Greek lyre.*

ABOVE: This painting by Madjera (c.1900) shows a Roman muse playing the lyre.

Medieval lyre

A six-stringed lyre was the main stringed instrument of northern Europe between the 5th and 7th centuries. Substantial remains of a lyre were discovered in the excavation of the Sutton Hoo ship burial, dating from before AD 625. Early medieval lyres were usually made from a hollowed block of oak, 3–4cm/ 1¼–1½in thick, to which a thin

ABOVE: An early 19th-century painting of Elizabeth O'Neil as Melpomene the Tragic Muse leaning on a lyre. This is a medieval lyre with tuning pegs on the crossbar, rather than the Greek method of rings and rods.

soundboard of maple or other fine-grained wood was attached. Ranging in length from 40cm/16in to 80cm/ 32in, these were an improvement on the classical lyre, in that the tuning was now achieved by pegs inserted into the top, as opposed to the rings and rods

used previously. The lower ends of the strings, which numbered five, six or seven, were secured to a short projection at the bottom of the resonator. The lyre was held in front of the body, resting on the player's knee, and the strings were played with a plectrum.

Bowed lyre

By the 11th century, the four-stringed bowed lyre, or *rotte*, had evolved. Instruments that are bowed require strings to be under a greater tension than plucked ones, so the frame of the lyre had to be strengthened. The former yoke was enlarged and the open arc considerably diminished, ultimately becoming little more than a hand-hole. Of the four strings, only one was played, the others acting as drones. Bowed lyres were generally played resting against the player's chest, shoulder or, as a sign of the fiddle to come, the chin. They were also played supported by the left arm in an upward slanting position, resting on the player's right thigh.

During the early Middle Ages a "figure-of-eight" lyre evolved in central Europe; it was three times longer than it was wide, but was doomed to failure as it was not able to withstand the strain imposed upon it by the bow.

ABOVE: This painting by John Strundwick shows an angel playing a rotte, a medieval type of lyre. In its early form it was plucked, but by the 11th century it was bowed.

LEFT: Lyres were introduced to Ethiopia from Egypt at a very early date. They have survived to the present day almost unchanged, as can be seen from this Eritrean box lyre.

crwth was played in the violin position. In addition to the four playing strings it had two drone strings, which were set individually to the left of the fingerboard. Its unique feature was the bridge, which had two feet: a short one that rested on the soundboard and a longer one that passed through one of the small circular sound-holes and rested on the back of the body, thus serving as a soundpost to transmit the vibrations to the back.

African lyre

Forms of lyre are still played (mainly as a solo instrument to accompany the player's singing) in parts of Africa such as Ethiopia, the Sudan, Kenya and Zaire. Some have a wooden resonating bowl covered with lizard skin. In the absence of a bridge, the plucked strings create a buzzing sound when they hit the soundtable. In Kenya, where it is viewed as a ritual object with healing powers, the lyre is played at weddings, both as an entertainment and as a blessing. In Buganda it sometimes appears in consort with flute, drum and tube fiddle.

BELOW: The crwth is a form of Welsh lyre. Unlike its ancestors, the crwth has sound-holes in the resonator.

ABOVE: A 16th-century Italian depiction of a lyre, the shape of which has come to serve as a universal symbol for music in Western civilization.

Although the plectrum-played lyre died out in the early Middle Ages, the bowed version survived into the 15th century, by which time it had been replaced almost everywhere by the fiddle. It did survive, however, in parts of Wales and East Africa.

Crwth

In Wales the lyre lived on in the form of the crwth, which is about 60cm/24in long, 30cm/12in wide and 6cm/2½in deep, the body, arms and crossbar all being made in one piece. Still in use in the 19th century, the

Lute

The lute is the most perfect of all instruments.

GIOVANNI LANFRANCO (1490–1545), "SCINTILLE DI MUSICA"

The lute is believed to have originated in Mesopotamia; the earliest depiction of a primitive lute-like instrument, which may have either two or three strings, appears on a terracotta plaque dating from the 17th century BC, now housed in Baghdad Museum. Always played by men, the prototype lute had a small ovoid body and a long fretted neck.

Africa and Asia

The instrument soon reached Egypt where, interestingly, it was played by women. Some of these two-stringed lutes were made with a tortoiseshell body and an animal-hide belly with six sound-holes. Sometimes the end of the neck, which was about 32cm/12¾in long, was carved with the head of a goose or falcon. Played with a plectrum, contemporary paintings show lutes with ovoid bodies and fretted necks that penetrate the whole length of the body. The strings

BELOW: An Italian lute built in about 1600 by Magno Tieffenbrucher of Venice, showing the sharp angle between the pegbox and neck.

were fastened underneath the belly, through which they issued through a hole and were secured by tuning pegs at the upper end of the neck. Over 3000 years later this type of lute still survives in north-western Africa.

The long-necked lute appeared in Greece in the 4th century BC, whence it travelled to Etruria and Rome, although it never achieved popularity in any of these areas. In the 5th century AD long-necked lutes were being played in Byzantium and Libya, but did not reach India until the 10th century.

Ud

The Western lute is directly descended from the Arab ud, a short-necked instrument with four strings, played with a plectrum. The ud first appeared in Mecca during the 6th century. Tuned in fourths, the instrument was improved when a fifth string course – and subsequently a sixth – was added. Although the ud was introduced into Europe by the Moors during their occupation of Spain (711–1492), it did not appear in other parts of Europe until the 13th century.

BELOW: The saz is a long-necked fretted lute originating from Iran and Turkey. It has eight to ten metal strings.

LEFT: The kora is a long-necked, 21-stringed, plucked lute-like instrument found in Senegal and neighbouring countries.

ABOVE: The lute has survived in various forms. In Morocco, because of the country's strong historic links with the Arab world, the instrument of choice is the ud.

RIGHT: The ud is the principal instrument of the Arab world. Its name means "wood" and "tortoise", referring to the material from which it is made, or to its shape.

Structure of the lute

The medieval lute was characterized by its vaulted body and flat soundboard. The body was constructed from a number of separate ribs, usually of maple or sycamore, shaped, bent and glued together. The strings were laid along the distinct neck and the fingerboard, which was tied with four gut frets. By 1480 the frets were being made of fixed metal, and over the years their number was increased to ten. One of the most notable features of the lute is the pegbox, which is placed

Lute music

The first half of the 16th century was the golden age for lute music, with more than 400 pieces being published all over Europe. The first music specifically written for the lute was Spinaccino's *Ricercai*, composed in 1507. Much lute music developed an international character that reflected the travels of the great lutenists of the day, such as Francesco Canova da Milano (1497–1543), Alberto da Ripe and the Hungarian Bakfark.

almost at a right angle to the neck. The lute's strings are arranged in paired courses. At first, European lutes had four courses of strings, but during the 15th century a fifth course was added and, in about 1600, a sixth. By 1630, ten and even 12 courses were common. Metal strings were a German invention and first appeared in Nuremberg in 1414.

ABOVE: A 15th-century illumination showing a lute player and two men playing the anvil as a percussion instrument.

ABOVE: This early 16th-century Italian lute has five courses of strings and ten frets.

By the beginning of the 16th century the lute had attained its perfection of form. In spite of the great size of its resonance cavity, it was remarkably light, since the ribs that made up the swelling, pear-shaped body were extremely thin. The strings were tied to the bridge, which was glued to the soundboard. The bent-back pegbox was also made as light as possible. The most famous lute-making centre at this time was in Bologna, the workshop of Laux Maler (1518–52) being one of the finest. Other craftsmen worked in Venice and Padua, and, although working in Italy, nearly all were German.

ABOVE: The lute is instantly recognizable by its characteristic swelling pear-shaped body and flat belly. This lute has six courses of strings, five of which are paired.

Playing methods

The medieval lute was a melodic instrument that was played with a quill plectrum. It played one line of music, with chords at cadences and phrase endings. During the 15th century, however, it began to be played with the fingertips, a development that allowed for the playing of several parts at once. The substitution of fingers for plectrum-plucking is a sign that the lute was becoming a solo instrument with a polyphonic style of playing.

Notwithstanding its popularity, the lute was in a sense the most inefficient musical instrument ever conceived; the bulbous form of its large body made it difficult to keep in position. This was such a problem that it was not unknown for the little finger of the left hand to be "glued" to the soundboard, thereby immobilizing the entire hand. The lute was also difficult to tune and the strings were often breaking. Indeed, in 1713, it was said that an 80-year-old lutenist had spent 60 of his years just tuning his instrument.

Theorbo

Believed to have been invented by the Florentine Antonio Naldi in the late 16th century, the theorbo was longer

ABOVE: *The theorbo is still occasionally seen today and one musician who has revived the instrument is Paula Chateauneuf, who is seen here performing in 1993.*

ABOVE: *Longer than the lute, the theorbo has a separate nut and pegbox for the unstopped bass strings. When the theorbo was introduced into England (1605) it was confiscated by the customs who, remembering the recent activities of Guy Fawkes, believed it to be a device to kill the king.*

than the conventional lute and had a separate nut and pegbox for its set of unstopped bass strings, which were known as diapasons. It was popular during the 17th and 18th centuries both as a solo instrument and as an accompaniment to singing.

Archlute

During the 16th century, in response to the lutenists' requirements for additional bass strings, a new series of bass lutes came into being. They were characterized by their open bass strings secured to a separate pegbox as with the theorbo, as opposed to the conventional lute whose bass strings were always stopped. The archlute resembled a smaller version of the theorbo, but had 13 or 14 double string courses, whereas the theorbo had single courses. Used both for solos and accompaniment during the 17th

ABOVE: *An engraving from Bonanni's Gabinetto Armonico of 1723 depicting an archlute player.*

and early 18th centuries, the archlute was plucked using the fingernails of the right hand. One of the last composers to write for the archlute was Handel, who gave it a part in his oratorio *Athalia* in 1733.

Balalaika

A descendant of the 16th-century *dombra*, the balalaika is a lute-like folk instrument of northern and central Russia. It has a triangular

BELOW: *Today the balalaika is internationally known, in no small part due to the tours in the 1960s and '70s of the former Red Army Ensemble, and its prominence in the score for the film* Dr Zhivago.

body, a long neck with four or five movable frets, three rib-fastened gut strings and a simple pegdisc. It has a flat back and a thin, slightly arched soundboard made from four strips of spruce into which the small sound-hole is cut. In the later years of the 19th century the St Petersburg musician Vassil Vassilyevitch Andreyev (1861–1918) designed balalaikas in six sizes, each with three strings. Andreyev's work transformed the balalaika from the realms of folk music into a popular instrument used in bands and orchestras.

ABOVE: The balalaika is often used to accompany the hectic folk-dancing for which the Russians are famed.

plantations the banjo slowly moved north, where it became a feature of black-faced minstrel shows. Through the influence of white banjoists in these shows, such as Joel Sweeney (c.1810–60) and Dan Emmet (1815–1904), the composer of *I Wish I Was in Dixie*, the banjo was rapidly introduced to American white urban culture, where it was increasingly played as a parlour instrument in the 19th century. It was exported to Britain and taken up by music hall entertainers and jazz bands. It has occasionally been used in 20th-century orchestral music, such as Kurt Weill's *Mahagonny* (1927) and Gershwin's *Porgy and Bess* (1935).

The modern banjo has five steel strings, although "classical" banjo players still use gut strings. The fifth of these – the "thumb string" – is short and is secured by a peg in the side of the neck at the level of the fifth fret. It is tuned to G and plays only that note, usually being sounded between beats.

BELOW: The modern banjo's tambourine-shaped body consists of a plastic membrane stretched over a circular frame, tightened by screws.

ABOVE: Side and front views of a balalaika, showing the distinctive triangular ribbed shape of the body. The balalaika has only three strings, and comes in a variety of sizes.

Banjo

A long-necked lute-type instrument, the banjo originated in West Africa and was introduced into North America by African slaves as early as the 17th century. From the southern

Banjo key features

TYPE: stringed

TUNING: *g', c, g, b, d'*

NOTABLE PLAYERS OF THE BANJO: Pete Seeger, Earl Scruggs.

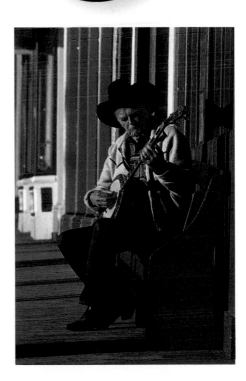

ABOVE: A musician sitting on his front porch in Nevada playing the banjo. The banjo became a popular instrument in the southern states of America.

Cittern

A citole in hir right hand hadde she.

GEOFFREY CHAUCER (C. 1340–1400), "THE KNIGHT'S TALE"

The cittern evolved from the citole, a plucked lute-like instrument played by 13th-century French troubadours. Made from a single piece of wood, the citole had a flat, pear-shaped body and a short neck, and was usually fitted with three single brass or steel strings that passed from a flat pegdisc to a frontal string-holder.

Shape of the citole

In different parts of Europe the citole assumed various shapes, all of which had a protuberance at the bottom to which the strings were attached. The Italian style was a "spade-fiddle" shape, with the shoulders swept upwards to form points. In France, the shoulders developed into wings and the oval sides became either straight or slightly waisted. The English and Germans preferred a citole of a "holly-leaf" shape with the

RIGHT: The flat-backed cittern was the most important plectrum-plucked instrument of the Renaissance, and its popularity is attested by numerous literary references.

ABOVE: This finely carved cittern is said to have been made by the great Italian stringed instrument maker Antonio Stradivari in 1700.

sides forming points at the intersections of concave curves.

During the 15th century a bridge was added to raise the strings off the soundboard, the pegdisc became a pegbox and the neck was fitted with 12 or more brass frets. The quill was abandoned and the four courses of strings began to be plucked with the fingers. The citole seems to have lasted longest in Spain, but by the early 16th

century it had become universally transformed into the cittern.

Early cittern

A characteristic of the cittern, which was very popular in the 16th and 17th centuries, was its unusual neck, which was half cut away from behind the fingerboard on the bass side. The resulting overlap formed a "channel", which facilitated very rapid shifts to and from the high positions that were so often required in the instrument's solo repertory.

Modifications

During its early years the cittern underwent many modifications, including increasing the number of courses of strings from five to 12. In 16th-century France and northern Europe the cittern eventually became standardized as a four-course instrument, with the top two courses of strings doubled and the other two trebled.

Towards the end of the 16th century a larger cittern with extra bass strings appeared. Called the *ceterone*, it was developed as a continuo instrument, its extra strings being secured to a separate pegbox, much like the theorbo. In the early 17th century a small English version of the cittern appeared. One person who enjoyed

ABOVE: *This 18th-century engraving shows a trio of musicians, with one playing a bass cittern. It had seven courses of single strings and a set of five extra bass strings that were fixed to a separate pegboard.*

ABOVE: *This early 17th-century painting by Wouter Pietersz Crabeth shows a cittern (left) being played in company with a lute and flute.*

ABOVE, FROM LEFT TO RIGHT: *Back and front views of a bell cittern, which became popular in Germany in the 17th century. The Neapolitan mandolin is distinguished from other lute-type instruments by the pronounced increase in depth of vaulting at the body's lower end.*

playing the *Englisches Zitterlein* was J. S. Bach's grandfather Veit, who, it is said, played it while working in his mill.

Demise of the cittern

By the mid 17th century in England and France, the cittern had degenerated into a barbershop instrument and was fast losing out to the increasingly popular guitar. By the mid 19th century the guitar had completely taken over and, apart from a few pockets in rural areas of Germany and Switzerland, the cittern had died out by the beginning of the 20th century.

Archcittern

During the 17th century Italian and French builders began to make larger citterns with two pegboxes. These archcitterns had from five to seven melody gut strings and six or seven off-board strings on the lines of the theorbo. Popular in the 18th century, they were about 1m/3ft long, and reportedly as loud as a harpsichord.

Hurdy-gurdy

One of the street musicians was an old lady who played upon a hurdy-gurdy.
She had been about the streets of London for upwards of forty years, and being blind,
had had during that period four guides, and worn out three instruments.

HENRY MAYHEW (1812–87), "LONDON LABOUR AND THE LONDON POOR"

Originally known as the organistrum, the hurdy-gurdy is a kind of mechanical violin able to sound two or more notes simultaneously while producing a continuous drone. Although it was built for use in churches and monastery schools to teach music and provide correct intonation for singers, by the end of the 13th century it had lost its ecclesiastical position to the newly developed portative organ.

Known from at least the 10th century, these early instruments, which had three strings, were up to 2m/6ft long. To play, they were set horizontally across two players' laps. One turned a handle to rotate the wheel that set the strings into vibration, while the other operated the keys that determined the pitch. For singers, the advantage of the organistrum over other conventional stringed instruments was that the stopping mechanism ensured an exact, invariable pitch, while the disadvantage was that only slow playing was possible.

Evolution

By 1300, the organistrum had become much smaller and was played by one musician. It now had a higher pitch, a range of over an octave, and could be played much faster than before. It became fully established as a minstrel instrument and was played suspended by a strap around the neck, in particular by blind musicians and beggars. Its use as a beggar's

BELOW: This replica of a six-stringed hurdy-gurdy clearly shows the keys and the handle.

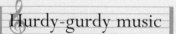

Hurdy-gurdy music

In 18th-century Germany, marches and polonaises were written for the hurdy-gurdy, and in 1786 Haydn wrote five concertos for the instrument. Mozart scored for it in a set of minuets (K601) and four German dances (K602), while Nicolas Chédeville (1705–82) adapted Vivaldi's *Four Seasons* for the instrument. Gaetano Donizetti (1797–1848) included two Savoyard songs with hurdy-gurdy accompaniment in *Linda di Chamounix* (1842) and it is interesting to note that itinerant Savoyards were still playing the instrument in the streets of London and Paris at the end of the 19th century.

instrument continued, for in the 17th century the French were referring to it as an *instrument de truand*, while those still writing in Latin called it the *lyra mendicorum*. Its name also changed in England, the name "hurdy-gurdy" first appearing in 1749. In Italy it was known as the *lira tedesca*, possibly signifying that the instrument had been imported from Germany.

The hurdy-gurdy as a "serious" instrument

In 18th-century France, where it was known as the *symphonie* (a name that could be applied to almost any

ABOVE: A 17th-century hurdy-gurdy player in Georges de la Tour's Le Vielleur.

instrument that could emit two or more tones simultaneously) or the *vielle*, the hurdy-gurdy achieved heights not reached elsewhere when it became accepted as a fashionable court instrument during the vogue for *fêtes champêtres*. The variation favoured by the aristocracy was the *lira organizzata*, an instrument that had two ranks of organ pipes and bellows housed in its body. There were many French virtuosi of the hurdy-gurdy, and many composers wrote music for it. The most notable of them were Henri Baton (died 1728), who redesigned the *vielle*, and his son Charles (died 1754),

who composed a number of suites for it and also wrote a history of the instrument in 1741. As with many other things associated with the aristocracy, the popularity of the hurdy-gurdy in France ended with the Revolution.

ABOVE: The neck of this six-stringed German hurdy-gurdy is finely decorated and is carved in the shape of a head.

ABOVE: Detail from Four Musicians, *painted in 1678 by Jacob Toorenvliet, showing a hurdy-gurdy player.*

ABOVE: The Blind Hurdy-gurdy Player *by David Vinckboons (1576–1632). Because it was easily portable, the hurdy-gurdy was widely used by travelling minstrels, pilgrims and especially by the blind, who could make a living from it even if they had learnt only a few tunes.*

Zither

It was an Abyssinian maid,
And on her dulcimer she played, Singing of Mount Abora.

SAMUEL TAYLOR COLERIDGE (1772–1834), "KUBLA KHAN"

The term "zither" is generically applied to any stringed instruments not classified as harps, lutes or lyres. It refers to instruments in which the resonator can be detached from the string-bearer without destroying the sound-producing apparatus. Evolved from instruments played over 2000 years ago, there are various forms of the instrument, ranging from the simple ground zither to the more sophisticated folk instruments that are played in southern Germany and Austria.

ABOVE: The harp zither is used by Austrian folk musicians.

Ground and trough zithers

The most primitive of the family is the ground zither, which is nothing more than a string stretched between posts in the ground, set over a bark-covered pit that acts as the resonator. The string is beaten by pieces of wood, and is used to accompany singing mainly to reinforce the rhythm of the music. Evidence of ground zithers has been found in neolithic excavations, and they are still played in parts of Africa and South-east Asia. A development of the ground zither is the trough zither, which is also found in Africa. This is usually plucked and consists of a hollowed-out piece of wood, sometimes elaborately sculpted, with a length of string laced back and forth over it.

Tube and raft zithers

The tube zither, as the name implies, is based on a wooden tube, usually cane. These are found in diverse parts of the world, ranging from New Guinea to eastern Europe. The strings are formed by detaching long fibres from the body of the tube

and raising them on bridges. Several tube zithers bound together form a raft zither, which is played in parts of Africa. The Nigerian version has a gourd resonator attached to the underside. Popular in Cameroon, the harp zither has strings made of raffia that run over a tall vertical bridge.

Psaltery

An ancestor of the modern European zither is the psaltery, a development of the Turkish *qanun* that reached Europe in the 11th century. Psalteries were flat boxes of various shapes, ranging from the early square or triangular to the wing shape of the 14th and 15th centuries. They could also have incurved sides and some were even semicircular, and they were often made with finely decorated cases. The psaltery was played with quill plectra or sometimes plucked with the fingers, either resting on the lap or leaning against the chest.

ABOVE: A wood cut, Die Hackbrettspielerin, *by Tobias Stimmer (1539–84). One of a series of nine, it depicts a courtier playing a medieval trapeze-shaped zither.*

ABOVE: Unlike most of the rest of the world, in Iran the zither occupies a pre-eminent place in classical music and is never used in folk music. It is played with two hammers.

Dulcimer

The dulcimer is virtually identical to the psaltery, but is played by striking the strings with small hammers, the instrument resting either on the lap or on a table. It probably originated in Persia, and is still played in modern Iran. The Hungarian version is a large concert instrument called the *cimbalom*, which features in Kodály's opera *Háry János* (1926). The dulcimer is also played in China, where it arrived from the West around 1800. It is called *yang ch'in*, or "foreign zither".

Ch'in

The indigenous Chinese zither is a plucked instrument with seven strings and no bridges, and is one of the oldest instruments in China. As such, it is a symbol of culture and civilization and is often depicted as an attribute of the sage, especially Confucius.

Scandinavian zither

Although unfretted box zithers were in use in Europe from at least the 12th century onwards, fretted zithers seem to have been developed from the 16th century in northern Europe. The concept was probably brought back to Europe by merchants who had travelled in the East.

Alpine zither

Most modern European zithers, which are popular in Austrian and southern German folk music, are board zithers. Laid flat on the knees or on a table, they consist of a shallow wooden box either with two curved sides or one curved and one straight. Usually the body acts as a resonator, although

BELOW: The ukelin is a kind of bowed zither used in North American folk music. It has a system of hoops along the side of the instrument; by threading the bow through different hoops, chords can be played.

sometimes a supplementary resonator is added. The 45 strings, of which five are melodic and the rest accompaniment, run parallel to the body along its entire length.

Several variations of the alpine zither have been invented, and various schools of playing have developed. The most common type today is the

ABOVE: The dulcimer is now restricted to the alpine regions of Austria and Switzerland. It can be played on its own, but is more often accompanied by guitars and accordions.

Salzburg form, with a semicircular projection on one side, which can be played in one of two tunings, the "Munich" or the "Viennese".

ABOVE: The zither has been used as a folk instrument in Scandinavia since the 16th century. In Sweden it is referred to as a lángharpa *and in Norway it is a* langspil.

Sitar

*The mark of a good sitar player is the ability to improvise extensively
without abandoning the laid down set of rules defining the raga.*

JAMEELA SIDDIQI

The sitar, a large, fretted, long-necked lute, is the best-known Indian instrument. Prominent in the classical chamber music formerly played at the Muslim and Hindu courts, tradition credits the invention of the sitar to the court poet Amir Khusrav (c.1253–1325). The name is an Urdu transcription of the Persian *sihtar*, or "three-stringed", Persian being the court language of northern India between the 13th and 19th centuries. The *tambura*, a long-necked lute and near relation of the sitar, is recorded in a late 16th-century contemporary account of court musicians in the reign of Akbar.

The sitar took on the outline of its present form as a classical solo instrument in the 18th century, when the use of a gourd for the shell and the adoption of the carvel-built ribs and heavy metal frets and strings became the norm. Usually accompanied by the tabla drums, the sitar has six or seven main strings, four of

RIGHT: The characteristic sound of the sitar is derived from the shimmering echoes of the sympathetic strings and the distinctive rectangular bridge.

which are played by a plectrum, the others being drones. In addition there are anything from 11–19 sympathetic strings, fitted on to a separate bridge. To the long hollow neck are fitted 20 brass frets that can be moved easily to conform to the scale of a particular *raag*. The convex neck allows the player to alter the pitch by pulling the string sideways across the fret, thus creating the sliding *portamento* that is so characteristic of Indian music.

Although several types of sitar are made, the most common is the *tarafdar sitar* (concert sitar), which is made in two main models: the single-gourd and the double-gourd. It is made of wood with a bulging gourd segment and is based on the large sitar of the 19th century, which was standardized to a length of about 122cm/48in. The wood used is usually toonwood (from the Punjab) or teak. The neck is a large

ABOVE: An Indian shop showing a row of sitars displayed for sale.

ABOVE: Sometimes referred to as the glory of all stick zithers, the vina is a type of sitar with its strings passed between two large gourd resonators.

ABOVE: *Ravi Shankar (born 1920) is the foremost player of and composer for the sitar.*

hollowed piece of wood, rounded at the back, and about 90cm/36in long and 9cm/3½in wide.

The sitar is always played with a twisted wire plectrum worn on the right index finger. The player sits on the floor with the left leg tucked flat beneath the right and the shell supported in the hollow of the right foot. Some players sit cross-legged with the raised right thigh supporting the neck of the sitar.

Surbahar

The surbahar is a bass sitar that produces a deep, dignified sound. The neck is wider and longer than that of the sitar but its frets are fixed. The soundtable is also much larger, with a diameter of over 40cm/16in. The instrument was invented in about 1820 by the sitar player Glunlam Muhammad of Lucknow.

ABOVE: *Played by both men and women, the sitar is India's most popular instrument.*

Vina

The name "vina" has become a generic term for stringed instruments in southern India, and the sitar is sometimes described as one. Originally, the vina was a type of stick zither with the fingerboard stretched between two gourds, but it underwent structural changes in the 16th century. The modern instrument is a kind of lute, with a hollow neck attached to a large hollow body and a soundboard made of wood. It has seven strings, three of which are drones, and there are 24 adjustable frets along the neck. It has a softer, sweeter tone than the sitar and is the principal instrument of classical southern Indian music.

ABOVE: *Illustration of a vina from* Oriental Drawings *(1806) by Charles Emilius Gold.*

Woodwind

✦ and ✦

Brass

Harnessing the Breath

Never let the horns and woodwind out of your sight:
if you can hear them at all, they are too strong.

RICHARD STRAUSS (1864–1949)

Wind instruments can be classed in two main groups: woodwind and brass. Technically known as "aerophones", wind instruments produce sound when the column of air inside them is set into vibration by either a reed or the player's lips. They depend for their tuning on the length of their pipe; the longer the pipe, the deeper the note that is produced.

Transposing instruments

Instruments with a fundamental note other than C are described as "transposing" instruments. This means that their music is written not at the actual pitch produced, but transposed by a specific interval upwards or downwards. The result is that the player can maintain the same fingering (or harmonics, in the case of brass)

ABOVE: *The woodwind section of the BBC Symphony Orchestra rehearsing in London.*

ABOVE: *The woodwind section consists of flutes, oboes, clarinets and bassoons.*

when playing instruments of different pitch. For instance, the B flat trumpet's written part sounds a tone below that which is written – if it is to play in the key of G major its part is written in A major. Other transposing instruments include the F horn and B flat clarinet.

Woodwind

Four distinct families of instruments make up the woodwind section of the modern symphony orchestra: flutes, oboes, clarinets and bassoons. Although today some of these instruments are no longer made entirely of wood, they still keep the appellation "woodwind", and can be divided into two types depending on

the shape of the bore, which is either cylindrical or conical.

Early woodwind instruments, such as the curtal, shawm and racket, were not only difficult to play in tune but also made harsh sounds. As such they were not popular, and in the mid 17th century Lully excluded them from his band. The then leading French woodwind maker, Jean Hotteterre (c.1605–90) and the court musician Michel Danican Philidor (c.1600–59) are credited with the design and production of new-style instruments, including the transverse flute and the three-section recorder. The shawm was redesigned to create the oboe, and the bassoon was a development of the curtal. The new instruments had a

ABOVE: B flat euphoniums are really tenor tubas, and are a major feature of brass and military bands. Although they are not a standard orchestral instrument, they are sometimes used to great effect. Holst, for example, wrote a part for the euphonium in his suite The Planets *(1916).*

Brass

A modern orchestral brass section usually consists of four horns, two trumpets, three trombones and a tuba. Brass instruments — which were originally used in hunting, for military functions or on religious occasions — became regular members of the orchestra in the 18th century, when court orchestras called on the resources of the military bands attached to the same household.

Mouthpiece

The cup mouthpiece can be dated back at least 3000 years, having been found on northern European *lurs. Lurs* were bronze conical trumpets built in two or more detachable parts, the smallest of which had the cup mouthpiece cast with it. The Etruscans, whose civilization can be traced back beyond the 8th century BC, were noted bronze workers whose horns and trumpets — which were played with cup mouthpieces — were eventually adopted by the Romans. Etruscan horns in the shape of three-quarters of a circle are seen in tomb murals from the 5th century BC. These were carried in funeral processions on the shoulders of white-robed officials, who held them by a crossbar as they played.

refinement and flexibility that enabled them to co-exist with Lully's violin orchestra, and he accepted them back into his band.

In the 1830s the woodwind instruments were redesigned again, this time by Theobald Boehm, who developed a new system of keys.

ABOVE: Besson & Co. were the foremost manufacturers of brass instruments in the 19th and early 20th centuries. Founded in Paris in about 1838, the firm opened in London in 1851. The makers were inventors and patentees of the "Prototype" system of manufacture, assuring the exact duplication of instruments, as well as marking the birth of modern methods of musical instrument manufacture.

ABOVE: A brass section: horns, euphonium, trumpets, trombones, tubas (and saxophones).

ABOVE: The modern trombone mouthpiece is deeper than its medieval counterpart.

Woodwind and Brass **143**

Flute

*The flute has now achieved such perfection and evenness of tone
that no further improvement remains to be desired.*

HECTOR BERLIOZ (1803–69)

Except for percussion, the flute is arguably the oldest musical instrument known, and ancient examples have been found all over the world, apart from Australia and New Zealand. Unlike the modern side-blown (cross or transverse) instrument, early flutes were end-blown (vertical) and were made of animal bones, such as a reindeer horn or sheep's tibia, pierced with a blow-hole and several finger-holes. The flute has been used as a decoy instrument throughout history, from the Pied Piper of medieval central European folklore to bird-catchers of the 20th century.

BELOW: The modern flute follows the improved design devised by the Bavarian goldsmith and musician Theobald Boehm in the 1830s.

Boehm's system used larger holes than hitherto; he also changed all the closed keys into open keys and cut the holes within easier control of the fingers. In 1847 he brought out an improved metal flute with 15 holes and 23 levers and keys. This system was so successful that it was adapted for the oboe, clarinet and bassoon.

Ancient Egypt

A 5000-year-old Egyptian palette from Hierakonpolis has been found that depicts a fox playing a flute, accompanying a dancing ibex and a giraffe. Egyptian flutes predating the pharaonic dynasties were made of cane or metal. Known as *m'ats*, and dating back to at least 2000 BC, they were 90–100cm/36–39in long. These early forms of flute had from two to six finger-holes and were played by being blown across the sharp top end of the tube. A descendant of the *m'at*, known as the *n'ay*, is still played today in some Islamic countries.

Early transverse flute

The transverse flute has been known in Etruria and Greece since at least the 4th century BC, since it is found depicted on Etruscan tombs and urns of that period as well as in contemporary Greek art. An early reference to the instrument and its method of playing appears in Apuleius's *Metamorphosis*, written in the 2nd century AD, which describes "tibia players who have their oblique instruments extended towards the right ear".

Western Europe

The earliest unambiguous reference to the use of the transverse flute in western Europe occurs in the mid 12th-century *Hortus deliciarum* of the Abbess Herrad of Landsberg. During the 14th century the flute spread to most parts of Europe, especially Spain, France and Flanders. The first extant

ABOVE: This painting by Dirck de Quade van Ravesteyn (c.1612) shows a woman playing a keyless cylindrical flute.

written reference to the instrument in England – "... and many flowte and lyltyng horn ..." – appears in Chaucer's *House of Fame*, written from 1378–80.

Although the main material used for making flutes was boxwood, some were made of other materials such as silver, and it is possible that the *flute traversaine* mentioned in the inventory of the Duke of Anjou's property in 1360 was made of this metal rather than wood. Henry VIII had three flutes made of glass, a material that was still being used by certain French makers in the early 1800s.

As international trade grew in the 19th century, flutes began to be made of harder woods, such as South American granadilla, pallisando or rosewood, and ebony from Africa. From the 1840s artificial materials were sometimes used, such as ebonite, a substance that is still popular today for instruments intended for beginners and schoolchildren. Wood is now rarely used, as silver and even denser metals, such as gold or platinum alloys, are considered to enable the player to produce a more expressive tone.

ABOVE: The newly fashionable one-keyed Baroque flute became a firm favourite with both professionals and amateurs, so much so that it was fashioned in the form of walking sticks. In mid 18th-century Dublin these were referred to as German Canes. Twenty years later Parisians were still able to buy flûtes en forme de canne.

ABOVE: This 1759 portrait by Gainsborough shows William Wollaston holding a one-keyed four-sectioned flute.

ABOVE: A depiction of a transverse flute of the early 18th century.

The flute in the orchestra

The transverse flute is believed to have been used for the first time in the orchestra in 1681, in one of Lully's ballets for the French court. By 1691 the flute had entered the French Royal Chapel band, and over the next 50 years, coupled with the advent of public concerts in France, Germany and England, it became an indispensable member of the orchestra.

In 1702 Michel de la Barre gave the world his *Pièces pour la flûte traversière avec la basse-continue* – the first music for solo flute ever published. In 1717 the instrument received a seal of approval when J. S. Bach scored specifically for the *flauto traverso*. Hitherto he had preferred the recorder, whose dulcet tones compared favourably with the shrill sound of the flute. As well as Bach, Handel was also a prolific composer for the instrument. Handel's set of 12 *Sonates pour une traversière, un violon ou hautbois avec basse-continue* (1730) still occupies a central place in the repertoire of many modern flautists. By the end of the 18th century the position of the transverse flute was secure, and it had completely replaced the recorder in the orchestra.

Boehm flute

Always a difficult instrument to master, many people have tried to improve the mechanics of the flute. One of its more important modifiers was Theobald Boehm (1794–1881), a flautist from Munich, who in the 1830s introduced a large-holed instrument that overcame the acoustic deficiencies inherent in earlier flutes. Boehm's changes were revolutionary inasmuch as they changed the hitherto closed keys into open keys controlled by rings. By 1847 he had increased the size of the tone-holes so much that they had to be closed by padded covers, worked by keys that both operated independently and interacted with others, and it is this type of flute that is played today.

ABOVE: The flute section of a youth band.

BELOW: The alto flute, a fourth lower than the concert flute, was invented by Theobald Boehm in the 1890s. It is a larger version of the standard flute, measuring 87cm/34in, and is specially adapted to allow the player to reach the more widely spaced holes.

The alto flute was said to be Boehm's favourite instrument due to its distinctive "song style"; it produces an unmistakable, full tone with a haunting sound in all registers, and is used to beautiful effect in three famous works composed between 1912 and 1916: Ravel's Daphnis et Chloé (1912), Stravinsky's The Rite of Spring (1913) and Holst's The Planets (1916). More recently, the alto flute has been used in Britten's works for the stage, in compositions by Boulez and Stockhausen, and in music composed for television.

Key features

TYPE: woodwind

PITCH: C

NOTABLE PLAYERS OF THE FLUTE: Charles Nicholson, William Kincaid, Severino Gazzelloni, Jean-Pierre Rampal, James Galway, Harvey Sollberger.

LEFT: *The bass flute is pitched an octave below the flute. Its tubing is 130cm/51in long, and it is bent back on itself near the mouthpiece to make it more manageable.*

Fife

Smaller than the flute, the fife has a narrower bore and hence a louder and shriller sound. Played to accompany marching and for giving signals during battle, the fife was used in the British army until the 1890s. Fife and drum corps continue to thrive in the United States, performing early American martial music.

Alto and bass flutes

Pitched in G and a fourth lower than the concert flute, the alto flute was developed in the 1890s. It proved popular in France, where its slightly melancholic, haunting tone was used to the full by Ravel in *Daphnis et Chloé* (1912) and by Stravinsky in *The Rite of Spring* (1913). The bass – or double bass – flute in C, pitched an octave below the standard flute, is now rarely found.

Piccolo

Pitched in C and an octave higher than and half the size of the concert flute, the piccolo evolved early in the 19th century. One of the first composers to write regularly for the piccolo was Beethoven, who used it in his Fifth and Sixth Symphonies.

BELOW: The piccolo is pitched an octave higher than the flute. Perhaps the first composer to use the piccolo to its full potential was Tchaikovsky.

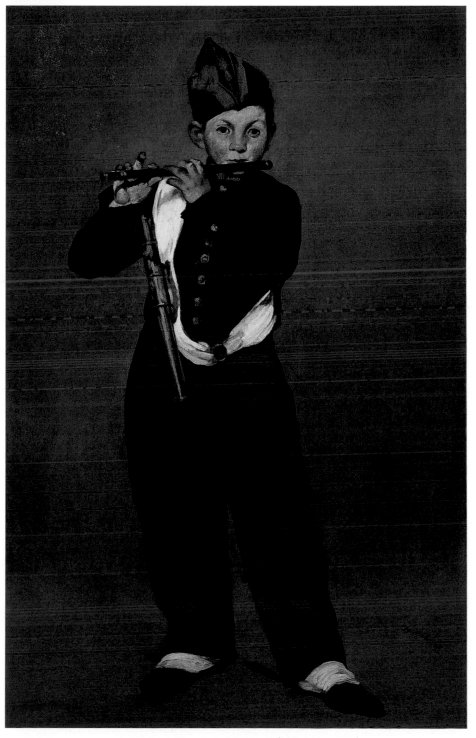

RIGHT: The well-known 1866 painting by Edouard Manet, entitled Le Fifre *("The Piper").*

Recorder

*Did buy a recorder, which I do intend to learn to play on, the sound
of it being, of all sounds in the world, most pleasing to me.*

SAMUEL PEPYS (1633–1703)

The recorder is a relatively simple instrument and can be traced back about a thousand years, for what looks like a duct flute with a tapering bore appears in an 11th-century French miniature. It is possible, therefore, that the Normans introduced the instrument to England, the only country, incidentally, where the instrument is called a "recorder" – mainland Europe preferring such terms as *flûte à bec* or *Schnabelflöte*. In England the name goes back to at least 1388, when the recorder is mentioned in the household accounts of the Earl of Derby, who later became Henry IV.

The recorder is relatively simple to play and was one of the most popular instruments of European Renaissance and Baroque music. A type of whistle flute with a wide tapering bore, it was originally made of a single piece of boxwood or ivory with a beaked mouthpiece. French 17th-century makers improved its construction,

*ABOVE,
FROM LEFT
TO RIGHT:
Three modern recorders
of varying pitches —
tenor, treble and descant.*

making it in three sections. Twentieth-century examples are made from many kinds of wood, or from plastic.

Early types of recorder

Until 1470, the recorder had six equidistant finger-holes and a thumb-hole. In Italy, in or about that year, an extra hole was added. Although Italian recorders continued to be built with a wide bore, in northern countries it was somewhat narrower. The two types can be clearly seen in two pictures: Caravaggio's *Lute Player* includes a wide-bore instrument in the composition, while Dürer's *The Men's*

Bath depicts a recorder with an extremely narrow bore. Another early illustration of the instrument is a woodcut of four recorders published in Sebastian Virdung's *Musica getutscht und ausgezogen* in 1511. The earliest known extant recorder was found under a 15th-century house in Dordrecht, and is presumed to be at least as old as the house.

The Renaissance recorder was built for playing in consort rather than as a solo instrument. Henry VIII was a recorder player and had many cased sets of between four and nine instruments. These would have been made together and tuned to match each other. Samuel Pepys and his wife

ABOVE: During the 16th and 17th centuries recorders were played in consorts of various sizes. This picture shows the very large, bassoon-like bass recorder.

Recorder music

The renewed popularity of the recorder in the 20th century led composers such as Benjamin Britten (*Noyes Fludde* and *A Midsummer Night's Dream*) and Hans Ulrich Staeps (*Sieben Flötentänze*) to score for the instrument.

ABOVE, FROM LEFT TO RIGHT: A selection of recorder-type instruments – one-keyed flute, bass recorder, double flagolet and boxwood recorder.

both played the flageolet, but he heard the recorder played at the theatre in 1668 and thought it superior.

In late 16th-century Germany recorder-like instruments, turned on a lathe, were known as *Kolomen*, while in France, by the mid 18th century, the recorder was known as the *flûte à neuf trous*. The ninth hole to which this name refers was an alternative hole for the little finger used by left-handed players of the one-piece instrument; the unused hole on the other side was sealed with a plug of wood or wax.

The recorder in the orchestra

By the 16th century recorders were being made in five different sizes: descant, treble, tenor, bass and contrabass, the latter between 2.5m/8ft and 2.8m/9ft long. In the 16th and 17th centuries they were widely played by groups of amateurs, but by the 18th century the recorder

had become an established part of the orchestra, and both Bach and Handel scored for it, the latter writing a number of sonatas for the *flûte à bec*. Around 1750, however, the recorder – which was known in France as the *flûte d'Angleterre* – was being discarded in favour of the transverse flute, which offered a greater dynamic range and better pitch control. By the 1790s the recorder had totally disappeared from the orchestra.

Twentieth-century revival

Were it not for the revival of interest by Arnold Dolmetsch (1858–1940), the recorder might now be only a museum piece. Dolmetsch pioneered the reconstruction of obsolete instruments, realizing that without them the music that had been written for them could not be heard. He made his first recorder in 1919, and presented a consort of four in a performance in 1926. His son Carl, a recorder virtuoso, made further

improvements that enabled the recorder to play effectively with a modern string orchestra.

The renewed popularity of the instrument led to the development of cheap plastic recorders which are particularly useful in schools, where the recorder is often the first musical instrument taught to children. It was first introduced into schools in the 1930s. In this way, the modern recorder has become widespread in most of Europe and the United States.

LEFT: The bass recorder, unlike its smaller counterparts, is blown via a curved metal mouthpiece called a crook. The bass recorder's sound is deep and resonating.

LEFT: This 17th-century German columnar alto recorder bears the device of two trefoils, with the stems curving to the right beneath the upper grill and on the base.

Key features

TYPE: aerophone woodwind

PITCH: C or F

NOTABLE PLAYERS OF THE RECORDER: Franz Brüggen, Rudolf Barthel, Amico Dolci, David Munrow.

RIGHT: Recorders were originally made from one piece of boxwood or ivory, rather than the three-piece instruments common today. Here we see a one-keyed flute and a boxwood recorder.

Oboe

The inimitable, charming sweet tone of the oboe.

JOHN BANISTER (1630–79)

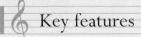

The English word "oboe" is a phonetic rendering of the French *hautbois*, meaning "high wood", which refers to the instrument's tone. It is not known who actually invented the oboe, but it was being played in Paris by 1670 and within ten years had spread to other European cities. It was developed as a woodwind instrument that could provide a tone quality suitable for indoor music, as opposed to the shrill sound of the shawm, which was regarded as fit only for open-air performances. Prototype oboes had two keys, and were first played in the band of Louis XIV's *Grande écurie* in 1657. One of the first compositions actually to specify a line for the oboe was Robert Cambert's opera *Pomone* (1671).

LEFT: The oboe's broad, sweet, plaintive and melancholic tone — which blends in so well with the violins — is an unmistakable feature of the modern symphony orchestra.

The oboe differed from the shawm in that whereas the latter was a one-piece instrument, the oboe was made in three sections connected by tenon-and-socket joints. The oboe's musical superiority over the shawm was assisted by the abolition of the pirouette, the turned wooden component into which the double reed was inserted. Instead, the reed was mounted on a staple clear of the body, facilitating a more delicate control of the reed between the lips. A greater compass was also attained by altering the size and disposition of the finger-holes to allow for a fully chromatic system of fork or cross fingerings through two octaves.

The oboe reached England in 1674, when a band of French musicians was brought over for a performance of John Crowne's masque *Calisto*. One of these instrumentalists was James Paisible (died 1721), who remained in London, entered the king's service, and became the first professional oboist in

ABOVE: An early 18th-century oboe as depicted by Johann Weigel.

England. The oboe soon became popular, and by 1695 the first printed tutor for the two-keyed oboe was published. One of the first to score for it was Henry Purcell (1659–95), who used it in all his larger works, including at least three obbligato parts for solo oboe.

The Horse Grenadiers adopted the instrument in 1678, and by the early 18th century almost every European band and orchestra included a pair of oboes. By the 1750s, players had begun to hold the instrument with the left hand above the right, as is standard today.

Nineteenth-century oboe

During the 19th century the original two keys were increased to eight and a speaker, or octave, key was introduced. This small aperture, which was placed above the finger-holes, greatly facilitated over-blowing, thereby giving the

Key features

TYPE: double-reed woodwind

PITCH: C

NOTABLE PLAYERS OF THE OBOE: Jacques Hotteterre, Giuseppe Sammartini, Johann Christian Fischer, Leon Goossens, Pierre Pierlot, Heinz Holliger.

instrument a wider compass. The two-keyed model was still being made up to the 1820s, with the four-keyed variety becoming popular in the 1830s. At about this time, the French makers began to develop the instrument in ways that differed from the simpler German and Austrian construction.

Frédéric Triébert

The most celebrated of the French oboe makers was Frédéric Triébert (1813–78). His contributions to the development of the oboe included narrowing the instrument's bore, resulting in a much more refined tone. The reed was made narrower and thinner, and the position and size of the finger-holes changed. The firm

Oboe music

An obbligato part for the oboe appears in Purcell's *Come Ye Sons of Art* (1694), and during the 18th century it became a leading solo instrument, featuring in concertos by Vivaldi and Albinoni. It was used extensively by Bach and Handel, and was particularly well understood by Mozart, who wrote an Oboe Concerto in C (K314). It was not prominent as a solo instrument in the 19th century, but in the 20th century oboe soloists came into their own with concertos by Richard Strauss, Ralph Vaughan Williams, Gustav Holst and many others. One of the major composers for the oboe is the player Heinz Holliger, whose *Siebengesang* of 1966 has an elaborate oboe part.

ABOVE: *A present-day oboe player.*

LEFT: *The* algaita *is a type of oboe played in West Africa, made from a single piece of wood covered in leather. The player presses his lips to the disc and uses his cheeks as an air reservoir so that the instrument can be blown continuously.*

of Triébert introduced both the "thumb-plate" and "Conservatoire" systems, which are still in use on modern instruments. After Triébert's death, his erstwhile foreman François Lorée continued to experiment with the instrument, developing a complicated key system known as the "plateau". Today, at least four systems of keywork are in use on the oboe.

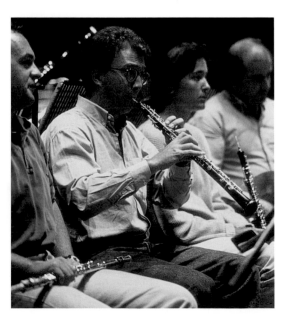

RIGHT: *The oboe is the principal instrument of the orchestra's woodwind section.*

Cor anglais

The cor anglais or English horn, the tenor version of the oboe, is a misnomer, for it is neither English nor a horn, and the origin of its name is a mystery. Played with a curved brass crook that carries the reed, the fingering and keywork of the cor anglais are the same as that for the

ABOVE: The cor anglais is used only in certain passages of music. This player has his oboe by his side, ready to be taken up when the music no longer calls for the cor anglais, or tenor instrument.

RIGHT: The straight cor anglais that is played today is based on Henri Brod's model of 1839. The origin of the name is unknown, but it is known that Haydn referred to the instrument as the cor anglé *("bent horn").*

oboe. The cor anglais of the mid 18th century was usually curved to a crescent or bent at an angle and covered in black leather. As the holes were of necessity farther apart than those on the conventional oboe, the curve or bend made the instrument both easier to hold and to play. The straight cor anglais that is familiar today, with its characteristic globular bell, is based on Henri Brod's *cor anglais moderne* of 1839. Brod got around the problem of reaching the widely spaced finger-holes by introducing keys with long levers.

Although the cor anglais was mainly used in French military music, both

ABOVE: The characteristic long curved brass crook that carries the reed of the cor anglais.

Bach and Purcell included the instrument in their orchestral scores, as have various later composers.

Oboe d'amore

A close relation to the cor anglais is the oboe d'amore, pitched in A. Known since about 1720, the distinctive feature of the oboe d'amore is the bulbous end joint that modifies the timbre by allowing the air to expand before it is forced through a smaller aperture. It was used by J. S. Bach in his *St John Passion* (1723) and about 60 other works, in order to achieve low notes then outside the oboe's range and also because it could cope with sharp keys. Due to the difficulties of playing it in tune, the oboe d'amore did not survive much beyond the 1750s, but it was revived in 1854 when the Belgian instrument maker Victor Mahillon reconstructed one for a performance of one of Bach's works in Brussels. Since then it has rarely been used; the most notable 20th-century work requiring the oboe d'amore is Richard Strauss's *Symphonia domestica* (1904).

Baritone oboe

The earliest baritone oboe known, which was pitched one octave below the regular orchestral oboe, was that made by Charles

RIGHT: The baritone oboe.

LEFT: The oboe d'amore, whose pitch falls between the oboe and the cor anglais, has a narrow bore and a bulbous end joint, resulting in a less strident tone.

experimentation, Heckel produced his heckelphone – however, it had taken him so long that Wagner had been dead for 20 years before the first one was produced.

Generically allied to the oboe and pitched at baritone range, the heckelphone was built in three sections, with a wide conical bore and bulbous bell, the large diameter of the instrument calling for a powerful double reed like that of a bassoon, which is carried on a curved crook. In 1905 Richard Strauss wrote an important part for the heckelphone in *Salome*, and since then its deep and powerful tone has been used freely as a substitute for the bass oboe.

RIGHT: This three-keyed fruitwood oboe with fishtail brass keys and trapezoidal covers was made by Andreas Kenisgperger.

Bizet in the 1740s, which now resides in the Paris Conservatoire de Musique. Bizet solved the problem of the excessive length of tubing by doubling the bore on itself and carrying the mouthpiece on a crook. He was also able to reduce the distance between the adjacent finger-holes by boring them obliquely through thickenings in the tube wall. Although Delius scored parts for the baritone oboe, today it is virtually a museum piece.

Heckelphone

In 1884 Richard Wagner asked the maker Wilhelm Heckel of Biebrich for a baritone double-reed instrument that would combine the character of the oboe with the soft but powerful tone of the alphorn. After much

ABOVE: The oboe section of the London Symphony Orchestra.

Clarinet

The many-keyed clarinet, which can sound so ghostly in the deep chalumeau register but higher up can gleam in silvery blossoming harmony.

THOMAS MANN (1875–1955), "DR FAUSTUS"

The clarinet was invented in the first few years of the 18th century by the renowned woodwind maker Johann Christoph Denner (1655–1707), or his son Jakob (1681–1785) of Nuremberg. It was the first reed-blown instrument to have a cylindrical rather than a conical bore. Denner's main achievement was in his practical use of the way that the scale of fundamentals could be made to sound a twelfth higher if a vent hole were pierced at the upper end of a cylinder. This hole was covered by what is now known as the speaker key.

Made of boxwood, the first clarinets were pitched in C and had six finger-holes and two keys. A third key was soon added to extend the range down a semitone and, more importantly, to make possible the playing of the "missing" *b'* at the break – even today,

amateur clarinettists still find this note difficult to produce. The body was divided into three sections, a feature that allowed the use of interchangeable joints of varying length to facilitate playing in different keys.

The first clarinets were played with a reed about 15mm/⅝in wide, tied to the mouthpiece with twine – the barrel of the modern instrument

ABOVE: *The first mention of the clarinet was in an advertisement by the Amsterdam publishers Roger & Le Cene in 1706.*

did not appear until the 1760s. At first it was common practice to play with the reed uppermost against the top lip. The modern style of placing it on the lower lip was adopted by the Paris Conservatoire in 1831, but did not become universal for many years.

Around 1750, when the fourth (A flat and E flat) and fifth (F sharp and C sharp) keys were added and the foot joint expanded into a bell, the clarinet became more accepted into the orchestra, having previously been used chiefly as a solo instrument, but it did not become firmly established until the mid 19th century. For a time it looked

as if it might replace the oboe and, although the latter has retained its position in the symphony orchestra, the clarinet has succeeded in ousting it from military bands.

In 1790 a sixth key, invented by Jean Lefèvre, was added to give an additional C sharp and G sharp, and the pear-shaped barrel disappeared. In spite of these improvements the instrument was still beset with problems of fingering and intonation, and for these reasons clarinets were built at different pitches. Although the "type" instrument was in C, there was also a B flat clarinet for playing in flat keys and A, B and D models that could be used for sharp keys.

Modern clarinet

In 1809 Iwan Müller (1786–1854), one of the finest clarinettists of his day, brought out the prototype of his 13-keyed model pitched in B flat, which was to become the standard instrument for the next hundred years.

ABOVE: *A 19th-century two-keyed clarinet.*

Key features

TYPE: single-reed woodwind

PITCH: B flat or E flat

NOTABLE PLAYERS OF THE CLARINET: Anton and Johann Stadler, Heinrich Baermann, Benny Goodman, Frederick Thurston, Gervase de Peyer, Woody Herman, Jack Brymer, Alan Hacker.

In 1817 its development was refined when Müller, who was the first to use pads over the countersunk tone-holes, invented the metal ligature. His tutor was published in 1826, and dedicated to George IV. As an instrumentalist Müller performed all over Europe, his style being described as brilliant and expressive.

The final major modification of the clarinet occurred between 1839 and 1843 when the clarinettist Hyacinthe

ABOVE: *A monk playing an 18th-century two-keyed clarinet.*

Eleonore Klosé collaborated with the maker Louis-August Buffet to simplify the fingering system, using the ring-keys Boehm had developed for his flutes.

Chalumeau

The clarinet was a modification of the chalumeau, a small woodwind instrument with seven holes. Chalumeaux were difficult to play and were never popular. Not only was it difficult to obtain the correct embouchure (lip technique), but they were restricted to a range of just over an octave. The sound of the chalumeau was also not to the liking of all, the Hamburg musician Johann Mattheson (1681–1764) describing the instrument's tone as a "dreadful evening symphony". The lower register of the clarinet is known as the chalumeau register.

Bass clarinet

The first bass clarinet was made in 1772 when Giles Lot of Paris produced one with a range of three and a half octaves. In 1793 Carl August Grenser of Dresden presented his *Klarinettenbass*, an instrument built in the form of a bassoon with nine keys. Various other attempts followed, but were all made redundant by Adolphe Sax's bass clarinet of 1838, which resembled a saxophone, with both bell and mouthpiece bent back. Although it has not always been part of the standard woodwind section, many works call for it, including Wagner's *Ring* and Franck's Symphony in D minor.

Clarinet music

One of the first composers to write for the clarinet was Jean-Philippe Rameau (1683–1764), who scored for it in *Zoroastre* (1749). Its inclusion in the Mannheim orchestra established it as an orchestral instrument, and as such it was used by Mozart, who also wrote three important works for the clarinettist Anton Stadler: the *Kegelstaff Trio* (K498), the Clarinet Quintet (K581) and the Clarinet Concerto (K622). With the improvements to the clarinet that were made in the early 19th century, composers such as Carl Maria von Weber (1786–1826) and Louis Spohr (1784–1851) began to write solos for it. One of the great works of the 20th century that features the clarinet is George Gershwin's (1898–1937) famous symphonic jazz poem, *Rhapsody in Blue*. This original work was written in 1923 in the unbelievably short space of ten days.

LEFT: *The bass clarinet has a compass from* D *to* f". *To accommodate its length and make it easier to play, it has a curved bell and has its reed mounted on a curved crook.*

ABOVE: *Hand positions on the bass clarinet.*

Saxophone

The saxophone is the embodied spirit of beer.

Arnold Bennett (1867–1931)

The saxophone is characterized by a fairly wide body made from a conical tube of thin metal, commonly brass, which is expanded at the open end with a small flare. It has 18–21 tone-holes of graduated size, all of which are controlled by keys. At the mouthpiece end are two speaker keys that enable the instrument to over-blow at the octave. The mouthpiece, which is fitted with a single reed, was originally made of wood, but is now commonly of ebonite or sometimes brass.

The saxophone was patented in 1846 by Adolphe Sax (1814–94). Although Sax's combination of a single bleating reed with a conical body was not entirely new, the saxophone was the first successful instrument of this type. The idea had first been used by William Meikle, a Scotsman who in about 1825 had produced a now virtually forgotten "alto fagotto", a modified small bassoon played with a clarinet mouthpiece.

Key features

Type: single-reed woodwind

Pitch: B flat or E flat

Notable players of the saxophone: Sidney Bechet, Marcel Mule, Johnny Hodges, Coleman Hawkins, Lester Young, Charlie Parker, John Coltrane, Stan Getz.

LEFT: The alto saxophone was invented in 1846 by Adolphe Sax as an attempt to introduce a more powerful group of instruments into military bands to form a link between the clarinets and tenor brasses.

The saxophone family consists of the sopranino in E flat, soprano in B flat, alto in E flat, tenor in B flat, baritone in E flat and bass in B flat. Larger saxophones are made more manageable by introducing a U-bend and tilting the bell slightly forward. From the baritone size downwards, the tubing is doubled by being folded at the upper end.

At the beginning of the 21st century many new models, with only minor differences, are still being brought out yearly. One more radical development was the plastic saxophone, in which all but the keys and mountings are moulded from synthetic materials, but this instrument has not been enthusiastically adopted by players.

Rise in popularity

Since its introduction into French infantry music, the saxophone has steadily gained favour in military bands. Bands such as Jullien's, which introduced the instrument to England in 1850, did much to make the instrument familiar to concert audiences, as did Sousa's band half a century later in America. The saxophone, which became established as a regular member of British military bands in the 1920s, is now also an

ABOVE: One of the most important roles for the saxophone has been in jazz.

ABOVE: *One of the finest exponents of the alto sax was Charlie Parker (1920–55), whose astounding technique meant that he was idolized by jazz fans everywhere.*

Georges Bizet's *L'Arlésienne* Suite (1872) includes a famous alto solo, and other composers that have featured the instrument include Ravel (*Bolero*), Prokofiev (*Romeo and Juliet*) and Vaughan Williams (Symphony No. 6). However, Simon Haram, one of the world's foremost saxophone players, is quoted as saying that saxophone players are like jackdaws – they have to steal a lot of stuff.

ABOVE: *The saxophone's popularity has spread all over the world. Here a Tanzanian musician is entertaining his audience.*

established part of the modern symphony orchestra. The alto instrument was the first to be so used, but Richard Strauss's *Symphonia domestica* (1902) called for a saxophone quartet.

Jazz saxophone

Since World War I the saxophone has become extremely popular in music of all kinds, and is now one of the most common wind instruments. Its playing

RIGHT: *The B flat soprano saxophone.*

technique is regarded as fairly simple compared with other reed instruments. Since the 1930s it has played a leading role in jazz bands, and it is in this medium that the instrument's potential has been most thoroughly exploited. Although today's jazz musicians mainly use B flat tenor

and E flat alto saxophones, between the 1930s and '60s, saxophone consorts of the four main types featured strongly in big bands, such as those led by Glenn Miller and Duke Ellington in the United States, Henry Hall in England and Bert Kaempfert and James Last in Germany.

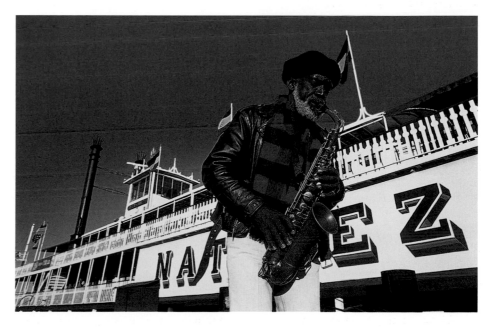

ABOVE: *The most commonly used saxophone is the tenor. This musician is playing for passengers boarding a Mississippi river boat.*

Bassoon

The wedding guest here beat his breast,
For he heard the loud bassoon.

SAMUEL TAYLOR COLERIDGE (1772–1834), "THE ANCIENT MARINER"

Often described as the clown of the orchestra, the bassoon is the bass of the woodwind section. As well as solo work, the bassoon adds colour to the orchestra, as it blends in well with all the other instruments.

In France the word "bassoon" came into use in 1613 to denote the double or bass curtal. Over the next 25 years it was transformed into the separately jointed instrument that is known today as the bassoon. First provided with three swallow-tailed keys – two for the thumbs and one for the little finger – by the mid 17th century the bassoon was being made in four separate sections: the butt, wing, bass and bell. Pitched in C, and made of maple or pearwood, it formed a continuously expanding tube of 2.4m/8ft, which

ABOVE: The bassoon is the bass member of the woodwind section of the orchestra, with the contrabassoon, supported on a spike, playing the lowest notes.

LEFT: The bassoon has a compass of about three and a half octaves. The tube, which is usually made of maple, is doubled.

ABOVE:
Pitched an octave below the bassoon, the contrabassoon has a metal bell as its last section.

was doubled to make it manageable. By 1730 a fourth key had been added, and by 1800 six were common.

During the 19th century many more improvements were made to the bassoon. One of the more notable modifiers of the instrument was Charles-Joseph Sax (1791–1865), who by 1825 had introduced covered tone-

holes. Sax continued his work and in 1851, with his son Adolphe, brought out a 23-keyed metal bassoon.

Another important figure in the history of the bassoon is Carl Almenraeder (1786–1843). A performer, teacher, bandmaster and composer, in 1825 he published a treatise in which he described how, by adding certain keys and relocating others, not only could the intonation be improved, but playing in all keys could be facilitated. By 1831 he had founded his own factory in Biebrich, near Wiesbaden, where by increasing the number of keys to 15 he was able to extend the bassoon's compass to nearly four octaves. On Almenraeder's death, his partner Johann Heckel (1812–77) continued to refine the instrument, which by 1843 had 18 keys and a chromatic range of over four octaves. Successive members of the Heckel

Key features

TYPE: double-reed woodwind

PITCH: C

NOTABLE PLAYERS OF THE BASSOON: Paolo Besozzi, Felix Rheiner, Georg Wenzel Ritter, James Mackintosh, Archie Camden, Simon Kovar.

family carried out many reforms to the bassoon, launching a famous model in the 1870s, and it is through their efforts that the instrument reached its present degree of perfection. French and Italian players tend to prefer an alternative French design by Buffet-Crampon, made in rosewood.

Music for the bassoon

An outstanding work in the bassoon's solo repertoire is Mozart's Concerto in B flat (K191) of 1774, and many chamber works for bassoon and strings were written around 1800. Hummel and Weber wrote bassoon concertos; Paganini wrote a Concertino for Bassoon and Horn. The bassoon achieved greater prominence in the 20th century, with solo works such as Elgar's *Romance* (1909) and orchestral

Archie Camden

One man who more than most helped to popularize the bassoon in the 20th century was Archie Camden (1888–1979). At the age of 15, Camden won a scholarship to Manchester where he studied under Otto Schieder, the principal bassoonist with the Hallé Orchestra. Young Archie was soon sitting alongside his master in the orchestra, and on Schieder's retirement in 1914 Camden was promoted to principal. He stayed with the Hallé until 1933, when he joined the BBC Symphony Orchestra, and in 1946 he became a freelance soloist. In 1962 he published his *Bassoon Technique*, the definitive bassoon tutor.

ABOVE: *The bassoon player of the orchestra of the Paris opera in 1868.*

RIGHT:

To encourage children to take up the bassoon, small faggottini *have been made. This one is seen side by side with a full-size instrument.*

parts like the opening of Stravinsky's *The Rite of Spring* (1913). Shorter compositions for the bassoon in the 20th century have often been given picturesque titles, such as Granville Bantock's *Dance of the Witches*, Gilbert Vinter's *The Playful Pachyderm* and André Bloch's *Dancing Jack*.

Curtal

In the 16th century the need for instruments of a bass register for use with choirs led to the creation of the curtal or dulcian, the immediate predecessor of the modern bassoon. More manageable than the bass shawm because of its doubled tube, the curtal

was named after a short-barrelled cannon of "curtailed" length. By 1600 curtals were being played over much of Europe, from Spain and Italy to Germany and England. Small high-pitched models were particularly popular in Austria and Spain, where they were often played in church ensembles. Court bands also included curtals, and composers such as Giovanni Gabrieli (1555–1612) began writing separate parts for them.

Curtals were made in one of two different ways. The more usual method was to bore two channels, connected to each other by a U-bend at the lower ends, into a single block of wood. The other method was to hollow out two sections of wood, then glue them together. In each case, the finished instrument was covered with leather. A slightly flared bell was fitted to the terminal end of the bore, while a short crook with a double reed was attached to the proximal end.

ABOVE: *Known since at least 1559, the curtal was less strident in tone than the shawm and as such was often dubbed the dulcian. This replica was made in 1971.*

Horn

The horn is perhaps the least efficient instrument of the brass family,
but it produces the most beautiful sound of all.

BARRY TUCKWELL (BORN 1931)

The horn is unique among orchestral instruments, not only in that the keys are operated with the left hand, but because it is also played backwards, with the bell facing towards the rear of the orchestra. It is the most expressive brass instrument in the orchestra, and also the most difficult to play. The normal position for the right hand is with all fingers close together against the far side of the bell and with the thumb close against them. The hand is cupped and can be straightened to sharpen various harmonics, while increased cupping of the hand flattens the harmonics.

ABOVE: Some horns had the tube coiled several times. This 19th-century painting shows two brothers playing horn and drum.

Although still popularly referred to as the French horn, most horns played in orchestras today are in reality the wider bore German horn. Both, however, evolved from the long, coiled *cor de chasse* of the French hunt, and by 1900 had come to resemble the modern instrument closely. F had become the standard pitch and rotary valves were the norm.

Animal horn

The first horns were, as the name implies, made from animal horns. In Africa they were made principally from the horns of antelopes, cattle horns being a poor substitute. One of the oldest types of horn is the Jewish *shofar*, or ram's horn. Made from a ritually killed sheep or goat, the *shofar* is the only musical instrument that has survived into the 20th century in the same form it had in antiquity. The small end of the horn is pierced with a long narrow passage that connects the proximal end with the main cavity of

LEFT: The learner needs a good ear, for the horn has the longest series of harmonics of any brass instrument, the number depending on the skill and lip strength of the player, who must also learn the varying degrees of hand-stopping.

the bore. Two pitches are possible, and are often, but not always, a fifth apart. The *shofar's* use as a martial instrument is documented in the story of the capture of Jericho, when its powerful sound is said to have caused the city walls to fall down. It is still used today in Jewish religious ceremonies such as Rosh Hashanah (the Jewish New Year) and Yom Kippur (the day of atonement).

Hunting horn and post-horn

The horn has been a part of European hunting life since Saxon times. By the 17th century there were two types: in Germany the preference was for a curved shape, while the English hunt

Key features

TYPE: brass aerophone

PITCH: F

NOTABLE PLAYERS OF THE HORN: Denis Brain, Barry Tuckwell.

ABOVE: The shofar is an early type of horn still used today to mark the Jewish occasions of Rosh Hodesh (the first day of the month) and Rosh Hashanah (the New Year).

ABOVE: Before valves were introduced, horns were very simple instruments consisting solely of a coiled tube and a large bell into which the hand was inserted.

preferred a straight horn, which could give a more penetrating call. When postal services began to operate in the 15th century, the courier would announce his arrival and impending departure by a distinctive call on a small brass horn.

From crooks to valves

The main problem of the early horns was that, without hand-stopping, they could play only one set of harmonics. One solution, put forward in about 1750 by the Dresden instrument maker Johann Werner, was the slide crook. As each crook was a separate coil of tubing of the correct length for each tonality, by fitting on the appropriate crook the horn could be played in all keys. Useful as this was,

the drawback was that the player had to carry a full set of up to 13 crooks, one for each key, which they had to fit as and when required. Composers allowed for this and, when the music modulated, they gave time for the horn players to change coils before they made their first entry in the new key.

In 1815 the invention of the valve revolutionized the playing of the horn. With the two valves with which the horn was originally fitted, only two extra crooks were now needed. At this time composers wrote for specific orchestras, and it is said that Beethoven wrote the horn solo in the slow movement of his Ninth Symphony for the fourth horn player in the orchestra, as he was the only one playing an instrument with valves.

Double horn

One of the perennial problems for horn players is hitting the wrong note in the high harmonics, where they lie close together. To address this problem in 1898 Fritz Krupse of Erfurt

ABOVE: The double horn enables the player to change the pitch from F to B flat by depressing an extra valve.

RIGHT: An 18th-century German post-horn made in three coils of tubing.

designed a double horn. As its name implies, this is two horns in one, each with its own set of valves but sharing the same mouthpiece and bell. It is pitched in F and B flat, the playing choosing his pitch by depressing an extra valve. The advantage of the double horn was that the twelfth harmonic in F became the ninth in B flat and was, therefore, much safer to play.

Horn music

Mozart wrote four horn concertos, which is all the more remarkable when it is remembered that in his time the horn did not have valves and that pitch depended solely on hand-stopping. Another composer who used the horn to full effect was Richard Strauss. Hindemith and Tippett both wrote sonatas for four horns, and Thea Musgrave wrote a Horn Concerto in 1971. The most ambitious of all works for the post-horn is the popular *Post-horn Galop*, which was composed in 1844 by Koenig, the principal cornettist in the famed Jullien military band.

Trumpet

The quality of tone of the trumpet is noble and brilliant.

HECTOR BERLIOZ (1803–69)

ABOVE: *The Greeks compared the sound of the trumpet to that of an elephant, and elephants are still said to "trumpet".*

The trumpet has a narrow, mainly cylindrical bore and is lip-vibrated. Forms of the instrument are found all over the world, and with rare exceptions they have traditionally been played by men. They have often been associated with magic and ritual, and with official or military ceremonies.

Egypt and Israel

The ancient Egyptians used metal trumpets 50–60cm / 20–24in long and made of silver or bronze; they were sacred and were played only in the worship of Osiris. On their return from exile in Egypt, the Israelites adopted the Egyptian trumpet. It became part of the insignia of the Hebrew priests, who used pairs of silver trumpets to be played in certain rites of the temple.

Etruria and Rome

A forerunner of both the trumpet and the alphorn, the Etruscan *lituus* evolved from a curved animal horn attached to a slender wooden cylindrical tube terminating in an upturned bell. The Romans modified the *lituus* by discarding the bulb bell, thus creating a straight wide-bore bronze trumpet about 1.2m/4ft long. This was known as the *tuba*, and was played with a long detachable conical mouthpiece. As well as being used in the civilian arena, this instrument was also played by the cavalry, who used it bent into two folds like a modern bugle, making it easier for a mounted man to play.

Post-classical trumpet

Early post-classical trumpets were made in the same form as the straight Roman instruments with detachable mouthpieces. They were held halfway down with the right hand, while the left hand held the mouthpiece. In the 11th century, the Spanish adopted the straight-tubed Arab *nafir*, which they called the *trompeta morisca*. The crusaders took over the Saracens'

ferocious *cor sarrazinois*, calling it a *buisine*, a term that is an etymological ancestor to *Posaune*, the modern German name for the trombone. The *buisine*, made of brass, copper or silver, terminated in a wide bell.

Medieval Europe

Such was the importance attached to the trumpet in early medieval Europe that the right of owning one was restricted to the aristocracy. Later, because of its noble associations, it became the instrument of the cavalry, a branch of the army that was originally formed from the nobility, where trumpets were used both to sound military signals and to help maintain morale. One such occasion

ABOVE: *This 15th-century French miniature depicts the Bible story of the fall of Jericho. The event is signalled by the trumpets of Joshua, which had very long bores.*

Key features

TYPE: brass aerophone

PITCH: B flat, C or D/E flat

NOTABLE PLAYERS OF THE TRUMPET: Giovanni Pellegrino Brandi, Valentine Snow, Louis Armstrong, Dizzy Gillespie, Miles Davis, Wynton Marsalis.

was the night before the Battle of Agincourt (1415), when the opposing armies were "serenaded by the continuous sound of the trumpets".

Trumpet players were attached to the more important European courts and, as the 14th century progressed, long trumpets appeared with banners displaying the seigneurial arms suspended from the bell to the boss. Such was the prestige of the instrument that, when Charles VI entered Reims in 1380, he was preceded by over 30 trumpeters.

Slide trumpet

It was when trumpets began to be played in ensembles with other instruments that problems of pitch

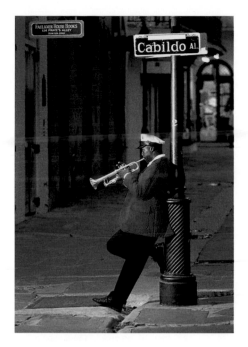

arose. One solution was the slide trumpet, which not only allowed the trumpeter to adjust his pitch easily, but also gave him the first opportunity to play a chromatic scale on an instrument that was otherwise only playable in harmonics. The slide trumpet had an elongated mouthpiece, sometimes over 50cm/20in in length, that was held by the left hand, while the right hand drew the body of the instrument in and out like the slide of a trombone.

A variation on the slide trumpet was designed in the late 18th century by the English trumpeter John Hyde. Hyde's trumpet, in F, had a U-shaped slide that replaced the bend nearest the player and could be pulled out when needed and returned by a spring. Although not fully diatonic, the slide did allow the player to temper the 11th and 13th harmonics that were out of tune with the normal scale.

Keyed trumpet

The various attempts by instrument makers and players to improve the trumpet by altering the pitch with circular tuning bits and crooks only raised the pitch of the whole instrument, which still played only

LEFT: A trumpeter playing in the streets of New Orleans, Louisiana.

harmonics. There were several attempts during the 18th and early 19th centuries to create a trumpet that could play a chromatic scale.

One successful innovator was the Viennese instrument maker Joseph Felix Riedel, who made a 15-keyed trumpet to the plans of Anton Weidinger, a trumpeter at the Viennese court. Although the keyed trumpet became popular in Austrian and Italian military bands, it was soon overtaken by the valved trumpet, which began to appear in the 1820s.

Modern trumpet

Although most 19th-century trumpets were in F, military bands preferred E flat trumpets, while in the 1880s trumpets in A, B flat and C started to be produced. During the 19th century various special types of trumpet were made, such as the "Aida" trumpet and the "Bach" trumpet. Today, however, most trumpeters' instrument of choice – whether they are orchestral, jazz or pop musicians – is generally the B flat trumpet, although orchestral musicians occasionally use trumpets pitched in D.

ABOVE: A Ganter rotary valve B flat trumpet. This rotary valve trumpet has a hand protector on the tubing to protect the surface against wear while it is being held.

Trumpet music

Although by the 1560s trumpets were being played between acts in the theatre, they were not formally introduced into the opera band until Monteverdi scored for the instrument in *Orfeo* in 1607. By the mid 17th century they were becoming a regular part of the orchestra, used in works by Pietro Cavalli (1602–76) and Giovanni Legrenzi (1626–90). Purcell's *Dioclesian* (1690) used trumpet fanfares, while Alessandro Scarlatti (1660–1725) frequently included trumpets in his operas. The valved trumpet, developed in the 1820s, was introduced to the orchestra by Gioacchino Rossini (1792–1868), who used it to wonderful effect in *William Tell* in 1829.

Trombone

The trombones are too sacred for frequent use.

FELIX MENDELSSOHN (1809–47)

The trombone, with its telescopic slide, is the most distinctive member of the orchestral brass section. Invented in the mid 15th century as an answer to the demands of late 14th and early 15th-century composers who were increasingly writing for low pitches, the first trombones were a development of the large S-shaped trumpets that were being built by Flemish makers for the Burgundian court. The instrument's first name was the *trompette-saicqueboute* – the "push-pull trumpet". Different countries abbreviated this descriptive name in various ways: in England it was called the sackbut (first recorded in 1470), in Italy the *trombone* and in Germany the *Posaune*.

These early instruments, which had a softer and mellower timbre than those in use today, were often used –

sometimes coupled with cornetts – as an accompaniment to a single voice, especially in Venetian churches.

Indeed, by the early 18th century the trombone was rarely heard outside ecclesiastical establishments. It did not become a conventional part of the orchestra until the late 18th century. The first classical composer to score for the trombone regularly was Beethoven, who used it for the first time in his Fifth Symphony in 1808.

ABOVE: A trombonist performing in a New Orleans jazz club.

Trombone variations

Although there have been various cosmetic modifications, the principle of the trombone's telescopic slide has remained virtually unchanged. By the 17th century trombones were being made in three sizes: alto in F, tenor in B flat and bass in E flat. During the 17th century various attempts were made to produce ever-larger trombones. One such, built in 1615 by Hans Schreiber, was twice as long as the tenor and consequently pitched an octave lower. Other contemporary contrabass trombones built in Germany include those of Isaac Ehe (1612) and Jan Brueghel (1620).

The double-slide trombone briefly appeared in Nuremberg in the early 17th century and re-emerged in France in the 19th century. Although the basic idea was admirable – to be able to obtain all seven positions with greater ease by diminishing by half the distance between positions – it was found

BELOW, FROM LEFT TO RIGHT: Mutes for brass instruments come in a variety of sizes – trombone mute, French horn mute, trumpet mute, trumpet cup and piccolo trumpet mute.

ABOVE: The trombone has seven slide positions; the farther out the slide, the lower the fundamental. The seventh position is like depressing all three trumpet valves.

ABOVE: *The trombone has a distinctive, large bell.*

to be impracticable as it proved impossible to make the tube airtight.

The valved trombone was first produced in Vienna in about 1818, and achieved its peak of popularity in the mid 19th century. It was, however, not able to compete with its slide counterpart, and by the end of the 20th century its use was restricted to Latin American, eastern European and Asian bands.

B flat and F trombones

The bass trombone, pitched in G, was so long that the slide had to be operated by a wooden handle.

Although it is still sometimes found in English brass bands, by the 1970s the G trombone had been virtually replaced by the B flat and F trombone, which was introduced as early as 1839 by the Leipzig maker C. F. Sattler. The F trombone consists of a B flat tenor instrument with an F attachment, made of about 1m/3ft of coiled tubing, and brought into play by a rotary valve operated by the player's left thumb.

Modern trombone

Today the trombone is made with one of three bores: France prefers

a narrow bore, England a medium and the United States and Germany a wide bore. The wider the bore, the warmer and richer the sound. It is only necessary to compare the tone of a pre-World War II narrow bore "peashooter" with that of a modern B flat and F to appreciate the difference.

Key features

TYPE: brass aerophone

PITCH: B flat

NOTABLE PLAYERS OF THE TROMBONE: C. T. Queisser, F. A. Belcke, A. G. Dieppo, Glenn Miller, Tommy Dorsey, Albert Mangelsdorff, Christian Lindberg.

ABOVE: *The valved trombone has never been a widely popular instrument and today it is used more in novelty than serious music.*

Bent Sørensen

The Danish composer Bent Sørensen (born 1958) wrote a trombone concerto for the Swedish virtuoso Christian Lindberg. The work is described as a *"pianissimo"* rather than a "roaring" concerto and is influenced, as is most of Sørensen's work, by his fascination with birds, bells and jazz. Another solo trombone composition by Sørensen is *The Bells of Vineta*, a piece that imagines the ringing bells of the church, threatened by coastal erosion, sinking into the sea.

Tuba

The tuba is certainly the most intestinal of instruments,
the very lower bowel of music.

PETER DE VRIES (BORN 1910)

The tuba is the bass of the orchestral brass section. English and German orchestras generally use a tuba in F, while those in Italy and the United States prefer the larger CC or BB flat types. In France, the instrument of choice is a very large bore six-valved tenor tuba in C, which was a development of the five-valved tuba used at the Paris Opera House between 1880 and 1892, and which Ravel included in his orchestration of Mussorgsky's *Pictures at an Exhibition* written in 1922.

The orchestral bass tuba was patented by Johann Gottfried Moritz in 1835, and Berlioz enthusiastically asked his publishers to substitute tubas for the ophicleides specified in the score of his *Symphonie fantastique* (1830). In 1832, A. G. Guichard of Paris brought out his newly invented three-valved *ophicleide à pistons* in E flat, and three years later Wilhelm Wieprecht, the bandmaster of the Prussian Dragoon Guards, introduced a five-valved bass tuba in F as a

RIGHT:
The E
flat tuba is
the bass brass
instrument.

replacement for the bass trombone. It was not long before these early tubas had totally replaced the serpent, bass horn and ophicleide. Although today the word "tuba" refers only to the bass instrument, originally the name was applied equally to the whole range. In 1852, for instance, Schubert did not distinguish between the cornet, flugelhorn or tuba. The E flat tuba is still sometimes referred to as a "bombardon".

By the mid 19th century the Bohemian instrument maker Václav

Cerveny had began building tubas with rotary valves, a modification that soon became standard on Austrian and German instruments. In other countries, however, tuba players preferred to retain the piston valve.

Over the years, various large tubas have been produced, including Adolphe Sax's sub-bass in E flat and the sub-contrabass in B flat (1855). Among other giants was Cerveny's *Kaiserbässe*, which was 2.4m/8ft high and had a tube length of almost 13.7m/45ft.

Since World War II tuba players have improved their technique and steadily pushed the range upward. Another important influence is the rise in popularity – especially in the United States – of the brass quintet. Composers who have produced pieces for this ensemble

ABOVE: *Two well-worn rotary valve tubas*
being played in Ghana.

Key features

TYPE: brass aerophone

PITCH: F, E flat, B flat or C

NOTABLE PLAYERS OF THE TUBA: William Bell, Howard Johnson, Philip Catelinet, John Fletcher, Roger Bobo.

have treated the tuba as a tenor instrument and many write for it in the same way as for the cello.

The instrument that is known today as the B flat euphonium is really a tenor tuba and until the late 19th century it was uncommon to find anything bigger in orchestras. It was for this instrument that Holst wrote a part in *The Planets* (1916). The first true bass tubas were in F, as used in orchestras, or E flat, as used in brass bands. The BB flat, with its orchestral version in C, is now the normal brass and military band bass and was introduced into the orchestra by Wagner when he scored for a *Kontrabass* tuba in *The Ring* (1876).

Wagner tuba
Invented by Johann Moritz for use in Wagner's *Ring*, Wagner tubas were intended as a bass voice that is a cross between the horns, trumpets, trombones and bass tubas. Built in B flat and E flat with four valves, they were designed to be played by horn players; they have horn mouthpieces and are keyed using the left hand.

Helicon
As the large tubas were rather unwieldy, some builders designed

ABOVE: Two tuba players in a youth band.

them in circular form, resting the bell on the player's left shoulder with the tube passing under the left arm. Such instruments were known as helicons. The disadvantage was that due to the shape, much sound was lost when it was projected to one side. John Philip Sousa (1854–1933) modified the instrument by having the bell project forward over the player's shoulder and, through association, the instrument became widely known as the sousaphone. Today, sousaphones are often made with a fibreglass bell in an attempt to keep the weight down.

ABOVE: The euphonium is a tenor tuba and is mainly found in brass and military bands.

ABOVE: Sousaphones in a Chilean police band, showing the bells facing forwards.

BELOW, FROM LEFT TO RIGHT: These tuba and euphonium mutes are much larger than other brass mutes.

ABOVE: An unusual view of the bell of a B flat euphonium.

Tuba music

Since World War II, composers of classical, jazz and avant-garde music have all used the unique character of the tuba, which was given a high profile in popular music with George Kleinsinger and Paul Tripp's *Tubby the Tuba* of 1948. Vaughan Williams's Tuba Concerto was written in 1955. Hindemith, Gordon Jacob, Alex Wilder and Malcolm Arnold have all written solo works, and Walter Hartley and Barney Childs have composed works for tuba ensembles.

*The two Ajax showing off with a swagger their double thorax
amid immense blasts from Sax's horns.*

JACQUES OFFENBACH (1819–80), "LA BELLE HÉLÈNE"

The invention of the valve at the beginning of the 19th century transformed the design of brass instruments. Instead of using a set of crooks to change the key of a horn, the player could produce a full range of tones by operating a system of valves to change the length of the tubing in the instrument.

LEFT: The cornet is the "violin" of the brass band, and a virtuoso player can truly make the instrument sing.

Cornet

After the horn, one of the earliest valved instruments was the cornet. In the 1820s when Jean Hilaire Asté (known as Halary) applied first two, then three valves to the little *cornet de post* – a post-horn with tuning slides and crooks in straight rather than circular form – the instrument became known as the *cornet à pistons*. In England the first manufacturers of the new instrument were Pace and Köhler of London, who called their creation the cornopeon (the "horn of

triumphant songs"). By the mid 19th century, however, the usual generic term for the instrument had become "cornet". Although at first a wide variety of crooks was available, ranging from B flat down to F, by about 1850 B flat was becoming the norm.

The cornet differs from the trumpet in that it has a conical rather than a cylindrical bore. The other essential difference is in the mouthpiece: the cornet's is much deeper, which makes

the instrument more flexible and less tiring to play for long periods.

Saxhorn

In 1842 the Belgian instrument maker Adolphe Sax (1814–94) moved to Paris where, under the patronage of Berlioz, he set up a brass and woodwind workshop. In the early 1840s, Sax produced a family of five conical-bore brass instruments, subsequently extended to ten. Although the principle behind the saxhorn was not entirely new, the proportions

♪ Cornet key features

TYPE: brass aerophone

PITCH: B flat or E flat

NOTABLE PLAYERS OF THE CORNET: George Macfarlane, Hermann Koenig, Jules Levy, Howard Reynolds.

ABOVE: Cornets can be made in silver instead of brass, such as this B flat cornet.

Eric Ball

Most of the music written for the saxhorn has been for brass bands. One of the most prolific composers for the medium was Eric Ball (1903–89), whose output included many arrangements and transcriptions as well as original compositions such as *Resurgam* (1950), a wonderful tone poem that depicts the events of Good Friday and graphically portrays the Romans knocking the nails into Christ's hands and feet at the Crucifixion.

adapted by Sax made his instruments superior. Built in upright form, they were generally pitched either in E flat or B flat and were fitted with three vertical valves on horizontal tubing. On early saxhorns these were fitted with Wieprecht's *Berliner-pumpen* valves, but later instruments were provided with slender Perinet valves.

Sax's breakthrough with the saxhorn came in 1843. After a public contest

ABOVE: The piston valves of a B flat cornet.

between an authorized military band and a smaller group, led by the inventor, playing Sax's instruments, the latter were officially adopted and Sax secured a virtual monopoly as supplier of instruments to the French army. The fury this engendered among the more established Paris instrument makers led to attacks on his business and lawsuits that resulted in Sax's financial ruin, but not before the name "saxhorn" had passed into common usage.

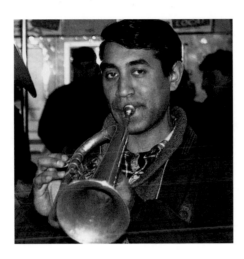

ABOVE: A rotary-valved flugelhorn player busking on the Paris Métro.

Distin family
The earliest performers on Sax's instruments included the Distin family. Led by John Distin, who had served at Waterloo as a member of the band of the Grenadier Guards and had subsequently been principal trumpet in the private band of King George IV, the band also included John's three surviving sons. In 1846 Distin established a music shop in London and became Sax's British agent. Four years later the Distins began to manufacture their own saxhorn-type instruments, and also started to publish *Distin's Brass Band Journal*.

Saxhorns became especially popular in British brass bands. The first group to be completely equipped with them was the Mossley Temperance band,

ABOVE: The Distin family playing the set of six coiled circular horns that Sax built for them in 1845. Sax later redesigned his horns with the bell pointing upwards.

which achieved success in the Belle Vue Contest of 1853. The tenor saxhorn in E flat, these days known simply as the tenor horn, is still used in brass and military bands.

Over-the-shoulder horn
Introduced by Alan Dodworth, over-the-shoulder horns were especially popular during the 1850s and '60s in the United States. The advantage of this type of instrument was that the sound of the larger instruments went to the rear of the band rather than up into the air. During static performances some bands had the over-the-shoulder horn players facing backwards, so that the sound was projected in the same direction as all the other instruments.

RIGHT: Over-the-shoulder horns were popular in the mid 19th century with American bands. Today they are found only in living-history bands.

Alphorn

He that blows best, bears away the horn.

PROVERB

The alphorn, as its name implies, is an instrument found in mountainous districts, not only in the Swiss Alps, but also in the Carpathian Mountains of Poland and Romania, as well as in Lithuania and Scandinavia. The instrument is distantly related to the Etruscan *lituus*, whose name survived into the mid 19th century in the Swiss canton of Unterwalden, where the horns were called *liti*.

Construction

No matter where it is found, the alphorn is almost invariably made of wood. It has a conical bore, and the oldest form is the straight expanding tube with a slight flare at the end, while alphorns constructed

ABOVE: *Brightly painted bells of a collection of Swiss alphorns.*

ABOVE: *A 1661 engraving of an alphorn.*

in more recent years usually have an upturned bell.

Although ash, lime and hazel have been used in the manufacture of alphorns, the wood of choice was usually a young fir growing out of a mountainside and curving upwards from its roots, thereby giving a natural upturned bell. After seasoning, the long poles were longitudinally halved using an axe or saw, then hollowed out and glued back together. In Switzerland the method of making the alphorn changed in the 19th century, when the bore was formed from a single log by burning out the centre. The bell was made separately and added to the end. By about 1850 the total length of the alphorn had become standardized at about 3m/10ft, but modern Swiss instruments range from 1.5m/5ft to 4m/13ft in length and are made in two detachable sections.

Switzerland

Originally a herdsman's instrument, the Swiss alphorn can be traced back to the 14th century, when it had an average length of about 1.5m/5ft. Because of its superior carrying power, it was used as a signalling instrument to warn villagers of danger, and, in later years, to summon them to church. It is this use of the alphorn that was quoted by Beethoven at the end of his *Pastoral Symphony* in 1808. In 1826 an innovation occurred when Ferdinand Huber of Switzerland had three alphorns made of different sizes and tuned to different keys, for use in two and three-part ensemble performances.

In modern Switzerland the alphorn is now principally used to entertain tourists, if possible siting it where it will set up an echo on the opposite side of a valley. It is also used to call

LEFT: This Norwegian alphorn is not as long as its Swiss relatives, and can be held up by the player.

cattle down from the mountains, and a traditional melody played for this purpose is known as a *ranz des vaches* (which means something like a procession of cattle). Different tunes of this type exist in each district, of which the Gruyère version is one of the most famous. The tunes are characterized by short motifs frequently repeated, giving them

a mesmerizing effect. They now have words and are sung in the manner of folk songs, but the intervals used indicate that they were originally composed for the alphorn, which can play only harmonics.

Northern Europe

In Lithuania, alphorns were used both for signalling and in folk music, and

were played in processions and at weddings. In the western Carpathians they are played only by women and children, and among the Mari people of the Urals 1.5m/5ft wooden alphorns are especially made for the spring festival. The Polish version of the alphorn is the *trombita*; made of pine, it can be up to 4m/13ft long. A feature of the instrument is that, while the bells of most alphorns rest on the ground, the bell-end of the *trombita* is supported on a post.

In Moldova and Romania the alphorn is called the *bucium*, of which there are five kinds that vary in length from 1.5m/5ft to 3m/10ft. They are either straight or curved and are bound with bark, roots or gut. Although they are usually made of wood, in the north of Romania the *bucium* is often made from metal, sometimes with the tubing coiled back on itself.

ABOVE: What more epitomizes Switzerland than an alphorn player in his local costume, the sound resonating across the valleys?

Pipes

Into the street the Piper stept, Smiling first a little smile,
As if he knew what magic slept, In his quiet pipe the while.

ROBERT BROWNING (1812–89), "THE PIED PIPER OF HAMELIN"

Simple blown instruments, consisting of cylindrical or conical tubes without mechanism, have evolved in many cultures and are widely played as folk instruments.

Aulos

The best-known double pipe is the aulos, an ancient Greek reed instrument that dates from at least 2800 BC. Each pipe consisted of a slender cylindrical tube made out of cane, wood or ivory, about 50cm/20in long, with from three to six tone-holes. Two pipes were played as a pair, the musician holding one in each hand.

At the proximal end of the pipe was a bulb of wood or ivory that served as the staple for the reed. As the whole reed was taken into the mouth, it is unclear from illustrations whether auloi were single or double-reed

ABOVE: *A variation on the aulos was when one pipe terminated in a bell. The aulos was mentioned by Homer as an instrument of the countryside.*

instruments, all the original reeds having long since disintegrated. In order to support the lips and cheeks, male players – who apparently blew harder than their female colleagues – wore a *phorbeia*, or leather mouth-band tied around their heads.

The aulos was played on many different occasions. It was part of the orgiastic cult of Dionysus, and was used to accompany choirs and at marriages and funerals, at which it was played in processions. It was also played in celebration of famous people or victorious athletes, as well as in musical contests between performers, such as those held at the Pythian games at Delphi.

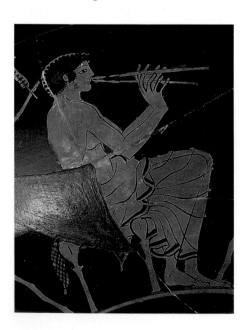

LEFT: *A pupil learning to play the aulos. This early 5th-century BC vase painting depicts an aulos in which the left pipe is longer than the right.*

Pan-pipes

The pan-pipes consist of a set of vertical tubes of different resonating lengths joined side by side. The tubes are stopped at the lower end while the player blows across the upper ends. They are made from various materials and are found all over the world. In most societies the pan-pipes have always had a lowly status, and are often portrayed as a characteristic instrument of herdsmen.

Classical Greek pan-pipes, known as a *syrinx*, consisted of a set of tubes all of the same length; each tube was

Aulos music

Auletes competed at the Pythian games by composing and playing the Pythian *nomos*, a solo performance that was descriptive of Apollo's legendary victory over the Python of Delphi. The music was presented in five sections, which had to illustrate the different stages of the battle. The winner in 586 BC was Sacadas, who created "sounds like those of the trumpet and gnashing like that of the serpent as it grinds its teeth after being pierced by arrows".

were bored. The pipes were held in both hands and moved from side to side as the player blew across the top.

Bladder pipe

Known from the 9th century, the bladder pipe was played by blowing through a short blowpipe into an animal bladder in which a reed was enclosed. This bladder served, like the bag of the bagpipes, as a wind reservoir. Out of the bladder came the chanter, with a varying number of finger-holes. Although the bladder pipe became virtually obsolete during the Renaissance, a descendant of the instrument survives in Poland, where it is still played in rural districts.

blocked with wax to the depth necessary to give the required notes. By the Hellenistic period, however, especially in Etruria and Rome, the tubes were graded in length. The pipes were usually stuck together with wax and the assembly was reinforced by a cloth binding or a wooden frame.

ABOVE: An area where the pan-pipes are still found is South America, where they are an integral part of Bolivian and Peruvian folk music. Some of these pipes are very large.

Occasionally pan-pipes were made from a solid block of wood, ivory or other material into which the holes

ABOVE: This representation of a bladder pipe is from Agricola's Musica Instrumentalis Deudsch *of 1529.*

Picco pipe

One of the more unusual musicians who toured Europe in the 1850s was Picco, a blind Sardinian minstrel who played a three-holed pipe only 8.5cm/3⅓in long, which he called his "pastoral tibia". Picco, who evoked "strains that would charm Apollo", played not only simple folk tunes but also variations on the *Carnival of Venice*, and was said to manage a range of three octaves. His popularity led to the commercial production of "Picco" pipes. Another person who played a small pipe in the mid 19th century was the Hungarian Kransky Baschik. Even smaller than Picco's pipe, Baschik's instrument could be played in octaves and thirds.

RIGHT: According to the legend surrounding the pan-pipes, one day the god Pan was pursuing the nymph Syrinx who fled to the river and, in an attempt to escape from her pursuer, transformed herself into a reed. Unable to distinguish her from the other reeds, Pan cut several at random and formed them into what are now known as pan-pipes.

Cornett

The sound of the cornett is like a ray of sunshine piercing the shadows.

MARIN MERSENNE (1588–1648)

LEFT: *A late 16th-century six-holed, curved cornett.*

Spelt with a double "t" to differentiate it from the 19th-century valved instrument, the cornett's origin can be traced back to at least the 9th century, when holes were pierced in cow and goat horns so that tunes could be played on them. The instrument was certainly known in 14th-century France, for romances of the period mention the *cor à doigts*. It was a wooden lip-vibrated wind instrument with finger-holes and a cup-shaped mouthpiece that was customarily played at the side of the mouth. The soft tone of the instrument made it – along with trombones – an ideal accompaniment for voices in churches, but it was also used to accompany dancing, both indoors and outdoors.

Construction

By the 13th century the cornett had five finger-holes and a bell made of animal horn. A later version had six finger-holes on the upper side and a thumb-hole on the underside. It was fitted with a separate mouthpiece, commonly made of ivory, bone or horn.

By the 16th century slender curved cornetts, which got their name from the Italian word for "little horn", were being carved from roughly shaped blocks of hard, close-grained wood. The blocks were halved lengthways and channels gouged into each half to make a cylindrical bore when they were glued back together. Finally, black leather was glued over the wood to seal any possible leaks.

Use of the cornett

Classified as valveless trumpets, medieval cornetts were made both straight and curved. The Germans preferred the former, while most of the rest of Europe settled for the latter. There were three main sizes of cornett: the small treble (cornettino),

ABOVE: *A 17th-century illustration of a cornett player by Weigel.*

ABOVE: *This 19th-century painting by John Spencer shows an angel playing a cornett.*

the treble and the tenor. In its heyday – between 1550 and 1650 – the treble cornett was used more than any other wind instrument for virtuoso-playing.

Cornetts were used with trombones and organs to accompany choral music, especially in Venice where, in 1600, they formed the nucleus of the band led by the composer and organist Giovanni Gabrieli (c.1553–1612). Some Italian curved cornetts were very ornate, with the bell end carved in the shape of a beast's head. In England, cornetts were used to support the treble voices of the choir of the Chapel Royal, while in France cornetts and trombones were the usual instrumentation for ceremonial music up to about 1650.

RIGHT: A mid 16th-century German engraving of a woman holding a cornett.

Decline

The cornett was tiring to play and presented problems in getting a good embouchure; in spite of Mersenne's remarks, it was often not played well. The higher register was similar to that of a trumpet and the lower like a trombone, while the indistinct wailing sound of the middle register was very unattractive when played in isolation. When used with other instruments the cornett could achieve special effects, however it began to fall out of use from about 1650. It was inevitable that the finest players of the instrument would start to turn their attention to the developing oboe.

By the end of the 18th century the cornett was no more than a rare curiosity. One of the last pieces written especially for the instrument was Matthew Locke's *Music for his Majesty's Sagbutts and Cornetts* (1661), while the last composer actually to score for the cornett was Christoph Willibald Gluck (1714–87), who used it in his *Orpheus*, composed in 1762. The last bastion of the cornett was in German *Turmmusik*, in which it lasted well into the 19th century. It was revived in the 20th century by early music specialists.

ABOVE: This 15th-century painting shows three English musicians on a balcony (top right) playing cornetts to accompany a dance.

ABOVE: Replica cornetts are made for living-history groups by Otto Steinkopf of Berlin (straight cornetts) and Christopher Monk of Surrey, England (curved cornetts).

Bugle

*The diabolical clamour produced by the call to arms
sounded by the bugles and drums.*

ALEXIS DE TOCQUEVILLE (1905–59)

The word bugle is derived from the Latin *buculus*, meaning "bullock", a reference to the fact that the first bugles were made out of short cattle horns. Originally the bugle was a hunter's instrument, but by the 15th century town watchmen and soldiers had begun to use it. Made of brass, copper or silver, the bugle retained its horn shape into the 18th century, when it began to be made with an upward-pointing bell.

In the 18th century the shape evolved into a large semicircle, which was held to the body by a leather harness. This form, called in German *Halbmond*, was introduced during the Seven Years War (1756–63) as a distinguishing instrument for the Prussian *Jäger* battalions. In the early 19th century the tubing began to be arranged in an elliptical coil, and in 1814 it was adopted as the badge of the British Light Infantry. The regular infantry B flat bugle, with twice-wound tubing and a small bell,

ABOVE: A silver-plated bugle. As a protection against loss, the mouthpiece is attached to the instrument by a chain.

was first authorized in 1858. In the United States this type is known as a cavalry bugle.

Keyed bugle

In the early 19th century Joseph Haliday (1772–1857), the bandmaster of the Irish Cavan Militia, transformed the bugle into a keyed instrument. Haliday subsequently sold the patent to the Dublin instrument maker Matthew Pace, who made the first keyed bugle as a compliment to the Duke of Kent, the then Commander in Chief of the British army. Henceforth the instrument became colloquially known as the Royal Kent Bugle. The earliest instruments had five keys, but a sixth was soon added and later examples had up to 12 keys.

When the keyed bugle was played by the band of the Grenadier Guards at a military review held in Paris after the battle of Waterloo in 1815, the Russian Grand Duke Konstantin was so impressed with the instrument that he

ABOVE: A bugle major of the Royal Sappers in 1823.

ABOVE: The flugelhorn is a cross between the cornet and bugle. It is mainly seen in brass bands and some jazz combinations.

ABOVE: A 19th-century brass bugle.

commanded John Distin, the band's chief musician, to have one of the new instruments made for him. Distin, who was later to manufacture instruments himself in London, approached the Paris instrument maker Jean Hilaire Asté (Halary). In 1821 he took out patents to cover three forms of keyed bugle: the clavi-tube, quinti-tube and ophicleide. In its various forms, the keyed bugle was the first fully melodic treble brass instrument and immediately became popular for solo work, until superseded in the middle of the century by the flugelhorn and the cornet.

Ophicleide

A much more efficient bass instrument than the serpent or bass horn, Asté's ophicleide of 1821 – named from the Greek for "keyed serpent" – was made of metal, the long tubing bending back on itself, with nine keys covering the large tone-holes. It was often unkindly called the "chromatic bullock". The first composer to score for the ophicleide was Gaspare Spontini (1774–1851), the *Generalmusikdirektor* to the king of Prussia, who used the instrument in his opera *Olimpie* in 1819. It soon entered many orchestras and bands, including the one led by the famous French bandleader Louis Jullien, who used it to augment the trombones.

With the invention of valves the construction of brass instruments was revolutionized, and in 1832 the Parisian brass instrument maker A. Guichard brought out his three-valved ophicleide, which had tuning slides for C and B flat. Although the ophicleide was eventually replaced by the tuba in the middle of the 19th century, it survived, especially in Italy, into the early 20th century.

ABOVE: A mounted bugler blowing a large-bell instrument.

ABOVE: This 19th-century French comical caricature shows a young boy learning to play the ophicleide, the largest wind instrument of the time.

Bagpipes

*Twelve Highlanders and a bagpipe
make a rebellion.*

PROVERB

Nobody is ambiguous about bagpipes – they either love them or hate them. They probably originated in Sumeria and perhaps independently in Greece. They were known by the Romans, and Arab references to the instrument date back to the 11th century. Their main characteristic is the continuous sound that is achieved using the air reserved in the bag, so that the player can breathe while playing. To articulate the melody, and ensure that each note is not tied to the next, the piper interpolates a grace note before each note of the melody. Most bagpipes have a limited range, with a compass of about nine tones.

The bag is inflated by air from the mouth or a set of bellows operated by the player's arm. The blowpipe, reeded chanter and drones, which are usually tuned in octaves and fifths, are inserted through the sides of the bag. Early bags were made from either the whole skin of a small animal, or the stomach or bladder of a larger one. Whole skin bags usually have the chanter inserted into the natural neck and the drones and blowpipe into the forelegs. Modern bags are usually made of tanned sheepskin cut to shape.

Scottish Highland pipes

The distinctive feature of the Highland bagpipes, with their loud and

BELOW: Believed to have been introduced to Scotland by the Romans, the Highland pipes have been used as a martial instrument from at least the 15th century.

penetrating tone, is the long blowpipe that allows the player to stand erect rather than leaning forwards. There are three single-reed drones, two tenor and one bass, and a double-reed chanter. Scotland is the most active of pipe-playing countries, and Scottish pipes have been exported to France and India.

Northumbrian pipes

Although bagpipes were once common in England as well as Scotland, today they are found only in Northumberland, where the bellows-operated small-pipes, intended for

indoor use, are played seated with the drones lying across the knees. A feature of these pipes is that the chanter has a closed end, enabling the piper to play staccato and repeat a note without interpolating grace notes.

Kathryn Tickell (born 1967) is recognized as one of the leading Northumbrian pipers of the present generation, and has been appointed the official piper to the Lord Mayor of Newcastle upon Tyne.

Irish pipes

The mouth-blown Irish war-pipe fell into disuse in the 18th century when it began to be replaced by the Scottish Highland pipe, although a new version was made during the 20th century. The bellows-blown union pipes, which are played seated, were probably introduced in the early 18th century. The modern pipe, which has a double-bore chanter with two reeds, has become so complex that it is often referred to as the "Irish organ".

Musette

Originally a pastoral instrument, the French bellows-blown musette

LEFT: A 14th-century English bagpipe with a single drone and chanter. This instrument pre-dates the Northumbrian pipes – it is not bellows-operated. Instead, the player inflates the bag by means of a blowpipe.

ABOVE: The Irish union bagpipes were introduced in the 18th century and, unlike the Scottish variety, they are played in a sitting position.

In some parts of Latvia and Estonia bags were often made of sealskin or a seal's stomach, which were unaffected by dryness or damp. In the 18th century the playing of such instruments was discouraged, as it was thought that they led to disorder and crime. They did, however, survive into the 1940s and have since been revived by several folklore groups.

In south-eastern Europe the end of the chanter was sometimes carved into the shape of an animal's head. The Czech *kozial*, commonly called "wedding pipes", can be traced back to the 14th century, while the Bosnian and Croatian *diple* is played outdoors on festive occasions. The bellows-blown Hungarian *duda*, which terminates in a cow's horn, has a small finger-hole opposite the thumb-hole, which raises any note by a semitone, thereby allowing modulations.

ABOVE, CLOCKWISE FROM TOP LEFT: Four different types of bagpipes – Irish Uilleann pipe, French cornemuse, Italian calabrian and French musette.

was popular in the 17th century at court, where it was used to accompany dancing. By the 18th century, with its ivory pipes inserted into a bag of matching silk and velvet, the musette had become a fashionable and delicate "toy" of the nobility and as such disappeared in the wake of the French Revolution.

Zampogna

Native to southern Italy and Sicily, the *zampogna* has two drones and two chanters arranged for playing harmony. At Christmas in the streets of Naples, two-man teams called *zampognari* serenade images of the infant Christ set up at the roadside.

Eastern European pipes

Today there are two main types of pipes in Poland: the bellows-operated *dudy*, whose drone pipe folds back on itself and terminates in a curved bell, and the *dudy zywieckie*, which is mouth-blown and played solo or with a violin.

Indian bagpipes

The traditional Hindustani *masak* is the simplest bagpipe of all. It consists of a single-reed cane pipe and a blowpipe tied into a whole goatskin. Another

ABOVE: The Italian single-drone bagpipe, the zampogna, *is native to southern Italy and Sicily. Both Handel and Bach alluded to the instrument.*

Indian bagpipe, the southern Indian *bajana scuti*, was used mainly to accompany devotional music until replaced in the mid 19th century by the harmonium.

♪ Bagpipes music

Until the 19th century there was no written music for the Highland bagpipes, as it was mainly transmitted by aural tradition. Although written music is now used, the many types of grace notes that feature in bagpipes music mean that the notation only approximates to what is to be played. Apart from traditional folk tunes, some pipe majors write special tunes in celebration of important events.

Mouth Organ

A cherub in a box.

ANONYMOUS

The concept behind the modern, horizontally held mouth organ came from Christian Friedrich Buschmann (1805–64) of Berlin, who realized in 1821 that melodies could be played on a set of pitch-pipes that he had made for use when tuning an organ. Various other people experimented with the idea, and the first instrument that looked like the modern harmonica was produced by Christian Messner, a young German clockmaker who began to construct similar instruments to Buschmann's, which he sold at country fairs and inns. At about the same time the first commercially produced mouth organs appeared in Vienna, one of which was Ernst Schmidt's apollolyra, with its 44 reeds controlled by keys.

Harmonica

In Tossingen, Christian Weiss and Matthias Höhner (1833–1902) started manufacturing harmonicas in the mid 1850s. Although their early models were all handmade, Höhner soon adapted the new methods and techniques of mass production and it was not long before his business had grown beyond all expectations. By 1879 he had made over 700,000 harmonicas – of which over 60 per cent had been exported to the United States.

Although harmonicas are made in various sizes and compasses, all consist of a set of free reeds mounted in a grooved metal box, which is moved from side to side in front of the player's mouth. Sounds are produced by both blowing and sucking and, if the instrument is diatonic, only one key can be played on any one model. The chromatic harmonica, which is used as a performing instrument, was first produced in the early 1920s.

Although virtuosi such as Larry Adler (1914–2000) have given the harmonica a wider appeal, the instrument has always been considered as more of a toy than a serious instrument. Since World War II, however, several symphonic composers have scored for it. In the 1960s the mouth organ became popular with folk singers such as Bob Dylan and

LEFT: *A modern harmonica made by Höhner. The sound is produced by both blowing and sucking air through the rows of reeds inside the instrument.*

Donovan. To keep their hands free to play the guitar, they held the mouth organ in a frame worn around the neck.

Melodica

Another type of mouth organ is the melodica, an innovative vertical form of the instrument produced from 1959. The two main types are the piano melodica, which has a miniature keyboard played with one hand, and the soprano melodica, which is operated by a series of push keys, one hand playing the diatonic and the other the chromatic tones.

ABOVE: *The harmonica has always been very popular among young people. This photograph shows a class of girls being taught to play the famous Höhner harmonica.*

BELOW: *The modern chromatic Chinese sheng has 17 pipes and is played polyphonically in triads. It is now a regular feature of the Chinese orchestra.*

ABOVE: *The piano melodica has a miniature piano-like keyboard, which is played with one hand while blowing into the mouthpiece.*

Sheng

The modern mouth organ has evolved from the classical Chinese *sheng* that dates back to the Chou dynasty (1122–221 BC), and consists of a gourd into which are inserted a short blowpipe and up to 36 bamboo pipes of varying length, each with a finger-hole and a free reed cut from a length of bamboo that vibrates when the finger-hole is closed. The pipes are arranged in an incomplete circle representing, according to popular legend, the folded wings of the mythical phoenix.

A new type of mouth organ, the *paisheng*, appeared in China in the 1960s. It is the size of a small piano, complete with keyboard, and has a range of four octaves. Used in the concert hall, the player sits in front of the instrument at the keyboard and fills the wind-chamber by blowing through a long blowpipe.

ABOVE: *Bob Dylan was one of the youth idols of the 1960s. He usually wore his mouth organ in a frame around the neck so that he could play the guitar at the same time.*

Didgeridoo

The spectrum of sound which can be produced by the didgeridoo evokes association with sounds perceived in the womb.

Dr Wolfgang Strobel

The didgeridoo is an end-blown straight natural trumpet used by the indigenous peoples of Australia. Depending on the region, didgeridoos are made of various types of eucalyptus wood, such as yellow box gum tree, bloodwood, Red River gum, stringy bark or woollybutt. To be suitable for making a didgeridoo, the trunk or branch must have the right diameter (7.5–15cm/3–6in), length (1.2–2m/4–6ft) and, of course, have been hollowed out by termites. As the didgeridoo builder cannot see that the trees are hollow from the outside, he peels off a piece of bark and taps the tree with his knuckles. Once a tree is selected, it is chopped down and the bark is peeled off.

The next stage involves using long chisels to scrape out any layers of wood that have not been devoured by the termites. The builder then thins the end of the interior walls to a depth of 30–40cm/12–16in to make a funnel shape. Although the didgeridoo is played without a separate mouthpiece, a rim of beeswax or eucalyptus gum is sometimes fitted to the mouth end.

Decoration
Didgeridoos are decorated only for special occasions;

LEFT: A didgeridoo is made from a scraped-out tree trunk or branch. By means of circular breathing, a player can produce a continuous sound.

generally they are plain. When they are decorated, the motifs are subject to religious taboo and are seen only by the initiated. The decoration is removed immediately after the ceremony and in some cases the didgeridoo is destroyed. On the other hand, some musicians decorate their instruments with totemic decoration, in which case the motif is down to the artist's imagination and has no religious significance.

Method of play
Didgeridoos are played by men and boys, often together with clapping sticks, to accompany singing and dancing as well as for funeral ceremonies. Although it is known for players to perform standing and sometimes moving around with the dancers and singers, the best position for playing the didgeridoo is seated with one leg bent to the side and the other stretched forward, with the foot helping to support the instrument. Sometimes, for added effect, the end is inserted into a tin-can resonator. Other performers prefer to support it off the ground between their feet. It is a very difficult instrument to play, and virtuoso players are recognized and highly valued members of society.

The pitch of the didgeridoo varies according to the length of the tube. To

ABOVE: Didgeridoos are now being mass-produced for tourists in workshops like this one.

ABOVE: *A native Australian playing a didgeridoo in Sydney, Australia.*

Gondwanaland, formed in 1978, features an electronically amplified didgeridoo whose unique rhythmical sound forms a bridge across thousands of years of musical history. The band uses no less than ten different didgeridoos played by Charlie McMahon, each of which is tuned to a different key.

McMahon has also played the didgeridoo with the London Philharmonic Orchestra, and invented an instrument that he calls the "didgeribone". As its name suggests, it is a cross between a didgeridoo and a trombone, and consists of two wooden tubes placed one inside the other. The inner tube slides in and out to create different tones, as with a trombone.

produce the characteristic continuous drone, frequent breaths are snatched though the nose while the air, which is stored in the cheeks, is continuously expelled down the tube. Although generally only one tone is available, a good player can produce another tone a fourth higher. Changes in the shape of the mouth can be made to change the timbre, and the tongue is used to give vibrato effects and achieve rhythmic patterns. Voiced sounds, which may imitate bird and animal noises, are superimposed on the fundamental drone.

Popular music
The didgeridoo is also used in pop music. The Australian band

ABOVE: *A selection of painted didgeridoos.*

ABOVE: *Today some Australian pop bands, such as the Marshall Whyler band, include a didgeridoo in their instrumentation.*

✳ Percussion ✳

Rhythm and Drama

The percussion acts as a central heating system.

IGOR STRAVINSKY (1882–1971)

Percussion in music is universal. There is not a country in the world that does not make percussion instruments of some kind to provide a rhythmic backbone for its music. Drums are probably the world's oldest musical instruments, but percussion is used for many effects that are not simply rhythmic: many instruments, such as cymbals, shakers and jingles, make more continuous, but exciting, noises, while a single stroke on a gong may create a dramatic climax to a musical work.

There are two main types of percussion instruments: those that are tuned to a definite pitch, such as timpani, xylophone or tubular bells, and those whose pitch is indefinite, such as the triangle, bass drum or

ABOVE: Russia is a country of large bells; these two men are erecting three bells.

tambourine. Orchestral percussionists play an ever-increasing number of instruments as composers search for original musical effects, and each player may need to play ten or more instruments in a single work. To manage a large percussion section, professional players have to master a range of techniques, as well as making purely practical arrangements to enable them both to reach the instruments and read the music on the concert platform without tripping over each other. The most specialized percussionist in the orchestra is the timpanist.

Magic and myth

Long before the drum became a musical instrument, its noise-making qualities were no doubt credited with the powers of making thunder and chasing away devils, not to mention frightening the enemy. In ancient Greece soldiers beat on shields made of tightly stretched ox-hide – a custom perpetuated by Zulu warriors well into the 19th century.

Like so many other musical instruments, the earliest use of the bell was in magic and ritual. Its power to ward off evil is illustrated in the *Book*

BELOW, FROM LEFT TO RIGHT: The jingle stick and tambourine are two forms of the same instrument. They can be struck to produce a percussive sound, or shaken to prolong the ringing.

BELOW, FROM LEFT TO RIGHT: A ridged guiro, wooden beater and wood block. The guiro can be struck or scraped and the wood block is struck to produce a short, untuned note.

of *Exodus*, written between the 9th and 5th centuries BC, when Aaron is instructed to wear bells of gold when he goes into the "holy place". Among the Bobati people of Zaire, bells were rung as a guard against evil influences entering the chief's body whenever he drank or smoked. In East Africa the Teso people wear bells around their ankles to appease the spirit of the storm, while the Bakrewi attach bells to the entrances of their houses to ward off evil.

Religious significance

Rattles often have a magical and religious significance, and a rattle or shaker is one of the accoutrements of

ABOVE, FROM LEFT TO RIGHT: *An orchestral percussion section showing timpani, congas, bass drum, gong, cymbals, claves, glockenspiel and tambourine.*

ABOVE: *The cog ratchet rattle has been used for many years and for many reasons — from scaring birds off the fields to supporting a favourite football team.*

the shaman. In China the thunder god Zin Shin was surrounded by a revolving wheel to which alternate barrel drums and kettledrums were fixed, the god striking them with a drumstick held in one hand. Ancient Japanese belief connected the playing of percussion with the invention of music, the myth being that the gods beat the measure upon "the mother of all the castanets".

Ever since their invention, drums have been used in rituals. Some were classed as sacred objects, while others were status symbols and emblems of royalty. In ancient Mesopotamia the hide of a sacred bull was used as the drum head, while a seal of the third millennium BC shows the goddess Ishtar standing before an altar that

looks like an upturned hourglass drum. The practice of using the drum as an altar has been carried into modern times, with soldiers in the field using an upturned drum as the focus of acts of worship.

Ancient scrapers were made from animal bones or ridged gourds, and have survived into modern times in folk instruments such as the guiro of Venezuela, a hollow gourd with a serrated surface. Related to the scraper is the cog rattle or ratchet, which was used in medieval religious ceremonies during Holy Week. Ratchet rattles are still used in some German festivals, particularly in the South. The cog rattle's tribal attributes re-emerged in the mid 20th century when it was taken up by football supporters.

ABOVE: *Maracas are hollow gourds filled with seeds. They are used in Latin American dance music, shaken to provide the rhythms.*

ABOVE: *A rainstick is a wooden or plastic tube containing pellets that make the sound of rain when the tube is turned over.*

ABOVE: *A selection of hand shakers. At the top are a ganza and a multi-guiro, and at the bottom is a torpedo. They can be struck with beaters as well as being shaken.*

ABOVE: *A native American shaman beating an octagonal buffalo-hide frame drum in the fields of Washington State.*

Timpani

When drums speak out, laws hold their tongues.

THOMAS FULLER (1608–61)

The timpani are the most important members of the Western orchestral percussion section. They can uniquely be tuned to a definite pitch and are used both as rhythmic and as melodic instruments.

Early kettledrums

Large kettledrums were developed during the 14th and 15th centuries in Germany. They were played as a pair, slung on either side of a horse. Such was the prestige of owning kettledrums in Germany and Sweden that they became the preserve of the aristocracy; no one under the rank of baron was permitted to own them. Kettledrums entered certain cavalry regiments that were owned

ABOVE: *This 17th-century engraving by Weigel shows a pair of early kettledrums from Germany being played with two wooden sticks in an outdoor setting.*

and to a large extent manned by the nobility. By the early 1600s they had followed the trumpet into church music and shortly thereafter into the orchestra.

Tuning

Before the military kettledrum was able to play a full part in the modern orchestra, it had to undergo various radical changes. Early kettledrums were expected only to contribute the tonic and the dominant of a tonality, which rarely changed. However, from the late 18th century composers such as Beethoven wrote music that expected the drummer to modulate right in the middle of a piece of music, a process that even for the most experienced players took one or two minutes.

LEFT: *Pedal-operated timpani are a main feature of the symphony orchestra. Pedals can change the tuning much faster than the old system of hand-tuning screws or taps.*

At this time the instruments were tensioned using square-topped screws turned with a loose key. The first advance was to replace the screws with taps. They were quicker and quieter to operate, but the timpanist still had to stop playing to re-tune, and the composer had to allow for this each time his score called for a key change.

There were various other attempts to make the life of the timpanist easier. These ranged from Gerhard Cramer's central screw (1812), which operated all the other tuning screws simultaneously to a method of rotating the barrel of

ABOVE: *A 19th-century kettledrummer of the French Lancers. Carried on either side of the horse, the drums are dressed with banners bearing the regimental crest.*

the drum itself, devised in 1821 by J. Stumpff of Amsterdam.

Adolphe Sax endeavoured to build a kettledrum with holes of different sizes in the shell. These were covered by keys that could be opened to produce different pitches. Sax also tried doing away with the shell altogether. Although this was intended to reduce the weight of the drums, the resulting framework was so heavy that the instruments weighed more than ordinary ones!

Pedal system

Modern orchestral timpani are tuned by a pedal that acts on a central screw, allowing the drummer to change tonality while continuing to play with both hands. This method was developed in the early 1880s by Carl Pittrich, a player in the Dresden Orchestra. Although Pittrich was not the first to produce pedal timpani, his were the first successful models. The Americans William Ludwig and Robert C. Danly brought out their balanced-action mechanism, with the pedal held by a spring, in 1925. Pedal timpani are known as "machine drums", and they have allowed composers like Bartók to include *glissandos* in their timpani parts.

Even with machine drums, a separate drum is needed for each different note when they follow each other in quick succession. The modern orchestral set consists of at least five pedal timpani in graduated sizes, giving a range of about two octaves. The large bowl-shaped resonating chambers are made from copper. Fibreglass is a much lighter, cheaper alternative, but gives an inferior tone. Plastic heads have now replaced calfskin.

India

Kettledrums in India are chiefly used in the *nahabat*, the noisy band that plays at state ceremonies and in processions. These bands often include a pair of silver kettledrums over 150cm/5ft in diameter and weighing about 205kg/450lb, which are mounted on an elephant. Each drum has its own player, who strikes the drum head with a silver stick. The small pairs of hand drums called *tabla* and *bayan* are miniature versions of the kettledrums.

Nakers

An early form of kettledrum is the nakers, a pair of small drums up to 25cm/10in in diameter, one pitched higher than the other. They were adapted from the Arab *naqqara* during the crusades of the 13th century. In Europe, these portable drums were used both for military music and in consort with trumpets and pipes.

ABOVE: *Drums are known in every part of the world. In India there are many types of folk drum, including the small kettledrum that is played strung around the neck.*

ABOVE: *The 15th-century Italian musician on the left is playing the nakers — small drums with barrel-shaped wooden, metal or clay bodies covered with animal skins.*

ABOVE: *A set of modern pedal-operated orchestral timpani with plastic heads.*

Side Drum

There is no instrument the sound of which proclaims
such vast internal satisfaction as the drums.

GEORGE MEREDITH (1828–1909)

The side drum gets its name from its playing position in military bands, where it is slung from the shoulder and worn on an angle at the player's side. It consists of a cylindrical shell of wood or metal covered at each end with a head of calfskin or plastic. Although the depth of the shell varies according to the purpose of the instrument, modern marching-band side drums usually have a depth of about 30cm/12in.

The orchestral side drum or snare drum is 10–30cm/4–12in deep with a diameter of 35–40cm/14–16in. In the 19th century, however, it was much deeper, at about 50cm/20in. It is played with wooden sticks, usually of hickory or ebony, with slim, rounded heads known as "acorns".

ABOVE: This 15th-century Italian painting shows an angel playing the side drum by hitting the snare head.

RIGHT:
Although
the side drum is generally
played with wooden sticks,
for special, softer effects
orchestral and jazz drummers
sometimes use wire brushes
instead. Evocative names
for particular rhythmic
ornamentations include
"paradiddle",
"flamadiddle" and
"ratamacue".

Snares

Giving the drum its characteristic timbre, the snares consist of eight or more strings of gut or thin wire coiled on a silk core, stretched across the lower head. Today an open coil of wire is often used, particularly by jazz players, which instead of producing a sharp rhythm adds a buzz to the sound. The snares must be at the right tension to produce the best sound and are tightened by screw devices.

One problem with snares in the orchestra is that the side drum easily

picks up sympathetic vibrations from other instruments, which can cause the snares to buzz very audibly. To resolve this, a quick-release lever allows the drummer to release the snares almost instantaneously when the drum is not being played. Playing the side drum with the snares released gives a tom-tom effect.

Tabor

An early version of the side drum was the 12th-century French tabor. This was a small and light cylinder drum, which was buckled on to the chest or left arm. The outside of the upper membrane was fitted with a snare, and it was this that was hit rather than — as is customary now — the membrane itself. Tabors,

RIGHT:
The tabor
was played
to accompany
dancing, and
would have been
accompanied
by bagpipes.

ABOVE: A regimental side drummer of the Fifteenth Kings Regiment of Light Dragoons ("The Hussars") in 1768.

which were used to keep time for dancing, were beaten by musicians who usually simultaneously played a three-holed pipe.

The name "tabor" is also given to a long, narrow drum, with or without snares, which is sometimes used in orchestral music and is otherwise known as a tambourin.

Military side drum

The side drum came into fashion in the late 18th century when Janissary bands, which imitated the Turkish music played by the Ottoman sultan's bodyguard, became popular in Europe. A feature of these bands, which says more about the moral values of the day than about musical taste, was that side drums were usually played by young black men, who dressed in the most

exotic manner and performed incredible acrobatic feats with their drumsticks as they played.

Playing technique

The main difficulty of playing the side drum is that the initial sound is of short duration. A longer sound is obtained by the roll, which is a rapid reiteration of strokes. This is a very skilled act and it requires a great deal of practice to produce an even roll with two strokes from each hand. It is much easier to play a roll on a drum with modern snares, as the traditional type make a snap rather than the contemporary buzz.

ABOVE: This side drum has been turned upside down to show its wire snare.

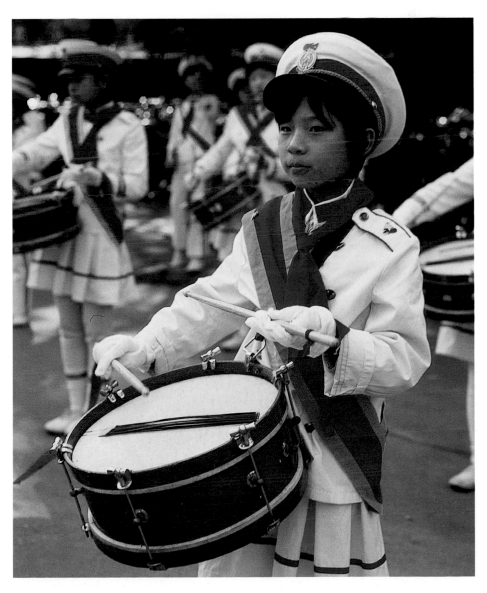

ABOVE: A member of a Chinese girls' band playing a shallow side drum in Beijing.

Bass Drum

A drum is a woman.

DUKE ELLINGTON (1899–1974)

The bass drum, the largest orchestral drum of indefinite pitch, remained a rarity in Europe until the 18th century, when it became well known through the Turkish Janissary bands that were fashionable at the time. The orchestral bass drum is played from a standing position, supported on a stand or a swivel frame which can be adjusted to suit the percussionist. It is struck with a large felt-headed stick, and the usual technique is to strike the drum with a glancing blow midway between the centre and the rim. Sometimes a double-headed beater is used, played with a rapid oscillatory movement of the wrist. This technique is called for in Dukas's *L'Apprenti sorcier* (1897) and Stravinsky's *The Firebird* (1910) to produce a bass drum roll.

LEFT: A rod-tensioned orchestral bass drum. The instrument is struck with a felt-covered beater and damped with the other hand.

Davul

The bass drum played in the modern orchestra is a descendant of the 14th-century Turkish davul. Introduced into Europe in the 18th century with other Janissary instruments, the davul was played with two different beaters: a heavy, spoon-shaped club and a light stick. The davul is still played, accompanied by a shawm, by buskers in modern Istanbul. In Europe it was first played in military bands, and was beaten on one head with a solid club and on the other with a switch of birch twigs in imitation of the Turkish style. It was introduced into the orchestra by Michael Haydn (1737–1806) in his *Turkish Suite* (1777) and was also used in Mozart's *Die Entführung aus dem Serail* (1782) and in Joseph Haydn's *Military Symphony* (Symphony No. 100) of 1794. In the scores for these works, the use of the two different beaters was distinguished by the direction of the stems of the notes. Today, this distinction is lost if felt-headed or lambswool beaters are used for both heads.

Military bass drum

The military bass drum, which consists of a cylindrical shell of wood or, more commonly today, metal or laminated wood, has a diameter at least twice as great as its depth. The average parade bass drum has a depth of about

ABOVE: The orchestral bass drum is often supported on a tilted stand facing the performer.

ABOVE: *An orchestral bass drum, seen from the player's perspective.*

ABOVE: *Rock and pop groups, such as this 1950s band, often include a drum kit with a bass drum that is struck with a foot pedal.*

Giant bass drum

The British firm of Distin & Son built a giant bass drum with a diameter of 240cm/8ft for the 1857 Crystal Palace Handel Festival. It was broken up in the late 1950s. One of the largest bass drums in existence today is in Disneyland in California. Built in 1961 by the Remo Company, it has a diameter of 320cm/10½ft, but it is never played.

30cm/12in and a diameter of about 70cm/28in. It is carried with the shell resting against the player's chest and the two heads facing sideways, and is played with hard felt beaters. The heads, which were originally of calfskin, are now more commonly made of plastic, which avoids the problems formerly experienced by drummers when marching in wet weather. The heads are lapped on to hoops placed over the open ends of the shell and secured by counter hoops. The tension of the heads is adjusted by thumbscrews, rods or rope.

The military bass drum player sets and maintains the marching tempo, as well as signalling to the rest of the band to stop playing using two fast successive beats called a "double tap".

Gong drum

Orchestras used to have their own kind of bass drum known as the gong drum. The advantage of this over the double-headed bass drum was that as it had a single head, so it was easier to stop vibrations and thus play short notes. On the other hand, as single-headed drums have a definite pitch, it had to have a very large head. Today the gong drum has largely been abandoned in favour of a double-headed drum with a diameter of about 150cm/5ft and a depth of about 50cm/20in.

ABOVE: *A band bass drum with a royal crest painted on the shell.*

Other Drums

You're not supposed to rape the drums,
you make love to them.

BILLY HIGGINS (1936–2001)

A drum can be any hollow body over which a membrane, or head, is stretched. When the head is hit, the ensuing vibrations are amplified by the body. Thousands of different drums – both pitched and unpitched – have evolved all over the world, to provide a rhythmic foundation for music and dance, to send signals, work magic or stir up emotions in battle.

ABOVE: A trio of Cuban conga players.

Tambourine

This ancient instrument, which has remained virtually unchanged since Roman times, consists of a shallow hoop, usually covered with a parchment head. Circular metal jingles set into the hoop sound continuously when shaken or briefly when the head is struck or rubbed with the thumb.

Tom-toms

Unsnared small drums with wooden shells and double heads, tom-toms are usually double-tensioned. The smaller ones are clamped together in pairs, and the drums are supported on legs or attached to the bass drum of a drum kit. Although tom-toms are usually of indefinite pitch, they can be tuned roughly within the range of E to B flat. Sets of chromatic tom-toms are now made.

ABOVE: Congas are made in a wide variety of sizes; this one is a medium conga.

Bongos

Usually played in pairs, bongos are found in most Latin American countries. In Cuba they are made from short sections of hollow tree trunks with drum skins nailed over the larger ends, then held near a source of heat so that they become taut. Factory-manufactured bongos are made in pairs and are held between the knees. There is usually an interval of about a fourth between the two small drums. Bongos are the highest-pitched hand drums of Latin America, and are widely used in popular music.

Congas

Conga drums or "tumbas" are the lowest-pitched Latin American drums. They are single-headed drums with a long tapering wooden shell. Like the bongo, the conga has a depressed rim that leaves the head free for finger-style playing.

ABOVE: The tambourine is an instrument of the dance and has been so since at least the 17th century when it was played by the singer and dancer Barbara Campanine.

RIGHT: Although bongos are authentically played with the fingers or hands, wooden sticks can be used for a louder sound.

Timbales

Built with shallow shells made of brass or copper, single-headed timbales are supported on an adjustable stand and are played in pairs with thin wooden sticks. They are of Latin American origin. Although each one of a pair is of the same depth, they each have a different diameter that can range from 23cm/9in to 36cm/14in. Timbales give a bright, penetrating sound that is metallic with a pronounced ring.

ABOVE: The timbale drum is predominantly used in Latin American dance music.

Tabla

The Indian tabla is an instrument consisting of two small, single-headed hand drums, the *tabla* and the *bayan*.

ABOVE: The Indian tabla player uses every joint and knuckle of his fingers and thumbs to produce a wide variety of sounds on the two drums (tabla and bayan).

They produce a mellow, round sound of well-defined pitch. The *tabla* is the higher-pitched of the two, with a wooden shell and a diameter of about 15cm/6in. The head is made of three layers of skin, with a central black patch of a paste of flour and iron filings made according to an ancient recipe. The *bayan*, the bass drum, has a metal shell and a diameter of about 23cm/9in. It also has a black patch on the head.

There is also an Arabic drum called a tabla, which has an egg-cup shape and is made variously out of wood, earthenware or metal. It is either laid horizontally across the left knee or held under the left arm, and is beaten with the hands.

RIGHT:
Steel drum pans can be played on the march, hung around the neck, or, as in this case, resting on a stand.

Steel drums

Originating in Trinidad in the 1930s and '40s, steel drums were first developed as instruments for use in processional and carnival bands, and were originally made by cutting down

RIGHT, CLOCKWISE FROM TOP LEFT: The drum kit consists of a ride cymbal, floor tom, two toms, snare drum, crash cymbal, hi-hat cymbal and bass drum.

ABOVE: Steel drum bands take part in many festivals. Here a band in the Virgin Islands is seen playing at an Easter sunrise service.

oil drums. A steel drum usually has a range of two octaves, and there are five steps in tuning it. First the head is pounded into a concave shape, after which the units are marked out by grooving with a steel punch. It is then tempered by burning, and the barrel is cut to the required length. Finally, the drum is tuned using a small hammer. Struck with a rubber-headed panstick, the tenor, or "ping-pong", plays the tune while the rhythm, guitar and bass pans provide the rhythm.

Drum kit

Dance, pop and jazz-band drummers generally sit at a drum kit that includes a variety of percussion instruments, including a bass drum of about 60cm/24in diameter that is played with a foot pedal. Other parts of the drum kit, such as the snare drum, cymbals and blocks, are played with sticks or brushes.

Cymbals and Gongs

*One single cymbal clash by Bruckner is worth all
the four symphonies of Brahms with the serenades thrown in.*

HUGO WOLF (1860–1903)

The cymbals are possibly the most spectacular percussion instruments of the orchestra. Generally made from copper or brass concave plates, the dramatic activities of the extrovert cymbalist never fail to attract the audience's attention.

Ancient cymbals

Cymbals were known in ancient Israel, where they were played during the dedication of the Ark. In Egypt small cymbals, only about 15cm/6in in diameter, were used from about the 8th century BC. From there the cymbals travelled to Greece, where they were originally used as a ritual instrument associated with the cult of the goddess Kybele. They passed into

ABOVE: Orchestral cymbals are held in the centre by leather hand-grips that pass through holes in the circular plates.

martial use and subsequently into the Greek theatre. The Greek *kymbala*, from which the modern name is derived, spread to Etruria, and so on to Rome and its empire.

Orchestral cymbals

The cymbals were almost forgotten in the West until the introduction of "Turkish" music in the second half of the 18th century. So unusual were cymbals at this time that when the French composer André Grétry (1741–1813) scored for them in his *L'Amitié à l'épreuve* (1770), it had to be explained to the performers how they were to be played. Nine years later Christoph Willibald Gluck used cymbals in *Iphigénie en Tauride* while, in the last quarter of the 18th century, the "clashpans" found their way into European military bands.

Cymbals began to be used regularly in orchestras in the early 19th century. Some composers used them simply as noisemakers, but others realized their full potential. One such composer was Berlioz, whose *Grande Messe des Morts* (1837) required ten cymbals, while his symphony *Roméo et Juliette* (1839) called for two "antique cymbals" tuned a fifth apart. Made of thick bronze and copied initially from those discovered in the ruins of Pompeii, antique cymbals or *crotales* are capable of being tuned to a definite pitch. They are sometimes arranged in a chromatic series and played with sticks. Other composers who have used the antique cymbals include Claude Debussy in *Prélude à l'après-midi d'un faune* (1892) and Igor Stravinsky in *The Rite of Spring* (1913).

Special effects

Cymbals are not just clashed together, but are capable of achieving many

ABOVE: As well as being crashed together loudly, cymbals can be slid lightly across each other to produce a soft note, or struck with a drum stick.

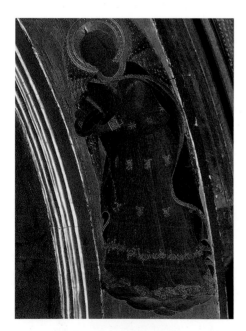

ABOVE: This 15th-century painting shows a player holding a pair of cymbals vertically by their handles, the prevailing mode of playing in the West.

ABOVE: Orchestral cymbals are heavy, and care is needed when preparing for an entrance.

in pairs to the thumb and forefinger or middle finger of each hand, are played in many countries, especially Egypt. Finger cymbals of a different type, like thimbles, are worn by Chinese dancers on the thumb and middle finger of each hand. Both kinds are also widely used in Western orchestral music.

ABOVE: Finger cymbals are attached in pairs to the thumb and forefinger or middle finger of each hand. These are still played in many countries, including Egypt and Greece, where the dancers prefer the two to be about a semitone apart.

effects. In the "slide", the edge of one cymbal is slid across the other, giving a quiet, sustained effect. The faces of the two cymbals can also be scraped together in a "roll *a due*". In his Five Orchestral Pieces (1909) Schoenberg asks that a cello bow be drawn over the edge of the cymbal, while Bartók's Sonata for Two Pianos and Percussion (1937) calls on the percussionist to stroke the edge of the cymbal with the blade of a penknife. In Debussy's *La Mer* (1905), a coin is scraped across the surface of the cymbal.

Modern cymbals

Since World War II, orchestras have come to prefer thinner cymbals with a lighter sound than the 19th-century instruments. Modern cymbals, made of an alloy of copper and tin, are usually considerably larger than earlier ones, and range between 30cm/12in and 65cm/26in in diameter, the most common being about 40cm/16in.

Finger cymbals

Usually made of brass or silver, finger cymbals originated in Asia as dancers' accoutrements, and they are still used this way. Miniature cymbals, attached

ABOVE: Bangladeshi dancers performing a traditional Manipur dance using small cymbals.

Hi-hats

Sometimes the cymbals are operated by a foot pedal. Originally, pedal cymbals were merely a pair of matched plates attached to wooden jaws held open with a spring, the player clashing the two together with the foot. Today, however, pedal cymbals – which are known as hi-hats (in dance bands) or choke cymbals (in orchestras) – are mounted on top of a stand so that they can be either played with the foot or clashed with a stick. They are occasionally found in the orchestra, but are a more common feature of small bands.

Jazz and pop bands

Since the 1920s, jazz bands have preferred Chinese-made cymbals because they make a louder clash with a shorter period of resonance. They have an upturned rim and a squared-off central section. Pop bands use various types of cymbals, such as the snap cymbal (which produces a quick splash of sound), the sizzle cymbal (which produces a sizzling sound due to the loose rivets inserted into the rim) and the ride cymbal (in which a constant reiteration of strokes does not build up into an echoing roar).

Indian cymbals

Various types of cymbals are used in India. The *cakva* of Maharashtra are about 9cm/3½in in diameter. Held by

ABOVE: *Hi-hat cymbals are played mounted on a column and either struck with a stick or clashed together by a foot pedal.*

ABOVE: *Cymbals are an important part of the modern drum kit.*

ABOVE: *In the 18th and early 19th centuries regimental bands often gave the cymbals to black musicians in the belief that they added "colour" to the band.*

cloth handles, they are used in dancing and folk-singing. The *bartal*, on the other hand, is a large and heavy metal cymbal native to Assam. When clashed, the deep resonant tone of the *bartal* can be heard for over 15 seconds.

Another type of Indian cymbal is the *ilatalam*, which is mainly used in temple music, dance dramas and shadow-puppet plays. Found in the Kerala region, these flat instruments, made of brass and 12–15cm/5–6in in diameter, are played in two distinct ways. One method is to clash a pair horizontally together and then slip the edge of one against the rim of the other to obtain a prolonged ringing sound. The other method is to hold them vertically in the hollow of one hand and clash them by contracting the fingers towards the palm.

ABOVE: The tam-tam is a shallow suspended bronze gong with a long and colourful reverberation. Those with a shallow rim are from China, while those with a deeper rim come from Burma.

Gong

For those of a certain age the gong will forever be associated with the opening credits of Rank films, in which a gigantic gong is struck by a muscular man. The player on the soundtrack of this famous sequence was the eminent percussionist James Blades.

Gongs are usually made of thin bronze with a turned edge, but may also be made of silver (Tibet), iron (Africa) or bell metal (India). They are found in various sizes. Those that are bossed have a definite pitch, while those that are unbossed have indefinite pitch. In the orchestra the unpitched gong, or tam-tam, needs to be at least 100cm/39in in diameter to produce a deep enough fundamental.

Apart from the *chempung* of Sumatra, which is played resting on a bed of banana leaves, gongs are generally freely suspended and are struck in the centre with either a beater or the fist.

Gong chimes

The Chinese *yun lo* is a set of small bronze gongs suspended vertically in an upright frame in three rows of three, with a single one at the top. Although they are all of the same diameter, they vary considerably in thickness. Originally they were Confucian and Buddhist cult instruments. Today, however, their

ABOVE: Detail of a traditional Chinese gong, showing the mallet striking the centre of the instrument.

use is restricted to funeral processions. Sets of tuned gongs are also made in the West for orchestral use, with a range of up to four and a half octaves.

ABOVE: The gong plays an important role in many religions. Here a monk is about to strike a gong suspended in a Chinese temple.

ABOVE: A tam-tam mallet.

RIGHT: The gong is an Asian instrument with its origin in 6th-century China, where it was used to ward off evil spirits. Until the beginning of the 20th century Chinese servants preceded their masters and mistresses beating a single gong, the rank of the personage being indicated by the number of strokes.

Castanets

*My feet were alright
but I could not manage the castanets.*

MIKHAIL GLINKA (1804–57)

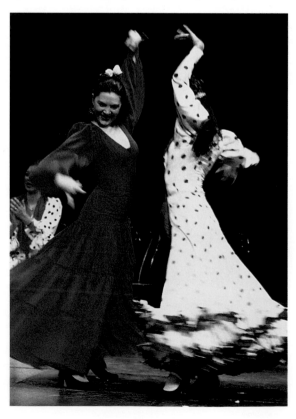

LEFT: Castanets have been used to accompany dancing from the earliest times. They came to Spain with the Arabs, but did not spread to the rest of Europe until the 16th century.

Castanets are percussion instruments of indefinite pitch that are either clicked rhythmically or sounded in a sustained roll. The name of the instrument comes from the Latin *castanea*, meaning chestnut, the wood out of which they were traditionally made. Today, however, other hardwoods, such as boxwood or walnut, are preferred. Each castanet is made from a single piece of wood, cut in half and hollowed out in the centre to form a hemispheric cavity. The two halves are united by a cord that is looped over the thumb for playing.

Ancient castanets

Clappers have been known for over 5000 years; in their most primitive form they were simply two sticks beaten together. Examples have been found made of wood, ivory or metal, and clappers originated both as a substitute for hand-clapping to accompany dance and as a noise to dispel devils. Hinged clappers, operated by one hand, have been traced back to the early third millennium when they were used by dancing girls in Sumer.

Vessel clappers, made from materials such as hippopotamus teeth, began to appear in Egypt from about 2000 BC. In some of these instruments the natural hollow inherent in the material formed the vessel, but in others the cavity was enlarged to increase the volume of sound. A hole was pierced in each shank to tie a pair together. Such instruments were always played by women to accompany dancing. These clappers evolved into prototype castanets, which made their first appearance – even though they were much longer than today's – in popular music-making in Greece and Egypt in about 500 BC. In a modified form they are still used by Copts in religious services. Castanets are also known to have been used in ancient Rome.

Spain

In Europe the castanets are primarily a dance instrument associated with flamenco in Spain, where they are believed to have been introduced while it was a Phoenician colony. Certainly a popular folk instrument, the castanets have

RIGHT: What would a Spanish dance be without the rhythmic sound of the dancers' castanets?

virtually become Spain's national instrument. Although they are traditionally made of wood, it is recorded that during the Roman occupation the dancers of Cadiz played castanets made from metal.

Often used with a guitar to accompany dances – especially the

saraband — Spanish castanets consist of two almost circular discs, hollowed in the centre of the striking side and connected by an ornamental cord. The two castanets of a pair are of different pitches. The lower-pitched one (the *macho*, or "male") is held in the left hand, while the higher-pitched one (the *hembra*, or "female") is held in the right hand. The cups are held downwards and are manipulated by the fingers, using the middle two fingers of the left hand and all four fingers of the right hand. By 1588 both the dance

RIGHT: Orchestral castanets are attached to a handle. The player shakes the handle, striking the shells on the free hand.

and the instrument had spread northwards into France, for in that year it is reported that the Duc de Richelieu, with castanets on his fingers and bells on his shoes, danced the saraband at a court ballet.

Orchestral castanets

True castanets are difficult to master and most modern orchestras use pairs, sometimes made of Bakelite, attached to long handles for ease in clicking. Many composers have scored for castanets in their Hispanic works, such as Georges Bizet's ever-popular opera *Carmen* (1873), Emmanuel Chabrier's *España* (1883) and Jules Massenet's *Le Cid* (1885).

Other composers have used the castanets to create special effects. Richard Wagner used them to create a great emotional impact in the lead-in to the "Venusberg" music in *Tannhäuser* (1845). Richard Strauss scored for them in the "Dance of the Seven Veils" from *Salome* (1905), and Benjamin Britten used them to imitate the sound of a night bird in *Let's Make an Opera!* (1949). The *castagnettes de fer*, for which Darius Milhaud scored in *Les Choëphores* in 1915, sounded like small cymbals or clappers.

LEFT: Castanets are not the sole preserve of Spanish folk music. As this lithograph of 1840 shows, they are also found in Italy.

Triangle

*Triangles and similar non-musical instruments
are forbidden to cornettists, be they master or apprentice.*

STUTTGART REGULATION OF 1721

The triangle was originally used as a folk instrument, and its value as an orchestral instrument was first realized in 1710 when it was employed by the Hamburg Opera. Seven years later it had entered the Dresden Opera. In both cases it was probably used to accompany folk-dancing.

Ancient triangle

The triangle is a descendant of the Egyptian *sistrum*, which was used in the worship of Hathor and Isis, and to ward off evil spirits. There were two main forms of the *sistrum*: the metal arched version and the faience "shrine" *sistrum*, which had as a central feature a head of the goddess Hathor. The metal version was shaped like an inverted U and was often made of silver with

ABOVE: *This 18th-century English scene shows a small boy playing the triangle, accompanied by a tambourine and flute.*

ABOVE: *The method of playing a triangle was described by Jacques Cellier: the triangle hung from the left thumb and was struck by a steel stick held in the right hand.*

a straight wooden handle protruding from the bottom. Loose-fitting metal rods or wires jingled when shaken, and small loose metal discs were hung on the rods to create additional sounds.

European folk triangle

In medieval Europe triangles were used for religious purposes and dance music. In northern Europe these early instruments, larger than they are today, were of trapezoid form and usually had a series of loose rings, or jingles, threaded on to the lower bar. Before 1660 three rings were standard, whereas after this date as many as five appeared. By the 19th century the rings had disappeared completely. Italy and Bohemia favoured a stirrup shape devoid of rings.

For many years the "lowly" triangle was frowned upon and considered a

beggar's instrument, chiefly in use among vagrants and gypsies. Such was the musical snobbery of the early 18th century that cornett players in Stuttgart were actually forbidden to play the "paltry instrument".

The triangle in the orchestra

As an orchestral instrument the triangle was first scored for in about 1750 in an overture by Johann Friedrich Fasch (1688–1758). When the fashion for Janissary music arose in the mid 18th century, the triangle was substituted in the orchestra for the Turkish crescent, or bell tree (otherwise known as a "jingling Johnny"), which was used by military bands to create exotic effects with the cymbals and bass drum. Mozart scored for it in *Die Entführung aus dem Serail* (1782), Haydn

ABOVE: *So that it is always in reach, the orchestral triangle is usually suspended over one of the side drums.*

in his *Military Symphony* (1794), and Beethoven in his Ninth Symphony (1823). Originally used only to provide rhythm, in the mid 19th century the triangle claimed its place as an indispensable member of the orchestra when Liszt raised it to the rank of a solo instrument in his Piano Concerto in E flat of 1853.

Many composers have since used the triangle to great effect, but none more picturesquely than Edward Elgar. In the eleventh of his *Enigma Variations* (1899) it is used to depict the tinkle of the medal on the collar of the bulldog Dan as he shakes himself after a plunge into the River Wye.

Construction

The modern triangle is a steel rod bent in the shape of an equilateral triangle, left open where the ends meet so as to allow the whole length to vibrate. It is usually suspended by a thin thread or wrist strap, so as not to interfere with the vibrations. The triangle is beaten with a rod of the same material. Although the sound it makes is not loud, because of its enharmonic overtones its indefinite pitch can be heard above the full orchestra. Were the gap closed to make a complete triangle, it would have a definite pitch. Orchestral percussionists generally use a range of triangles in different sizes.

ABOVE: The blurred beater in this picture indicates that this orchestral performer is playing a rapid trill on the triangle.

ABOVE: Although the triangle is traditionally struck on the bottom bar, for special effects it can be struck almost anywhere.

ABOVE: This late 15th-century painting shows angels playing open tambourine and triangle.

Xylophone

I must own that the skill of Michael Guzikow [Polish xylophonist] beats everything that I would have imagined, for with his wooden sticks resting on straw he produces all that is possible with the most perfect instrument.

Felix Mendelssohn (1809–47)

The xylophone was introduced into the orchestra in 1874 when the French composer Camille Saint-Saëns scored for it in *Danse Macabre*, intending it to represent the rattling bones of the dead. Although little original orchestral music has been written for the xylophone, it has a small but useful solo repertoire.

The xylophone is a set of tuned wooden percussion blocks, which are laid in a row parallel to one another and are played by being hit with sticks or knobbed beaters. Tuning is achieved by reducing the length of the block to raise the pitch, or filing the underside at the centre of the block to lower it. As no vibrations occur at the ends of the blocks, they are either placed on straw ropes or pierced and fixed to a frame, without impairment of tone. Up to the 1920s xylophones in Germany were built using the former method, a feature that caused them to be called *Strohfiedel* ("straw fiddles").

The modern xylophone owes much to the work of Hermann Winterhof who, in 1927, invented the "arcuate notch". This is an arc cut on the underside of each key, both to improve the quality of tone and to give greater definition of pitch. Modern instruments are built in various sizes capable of playing up to four octaves, with rosewood keys arranged in two

ABOVE: The xylophone has tuned wooden bars with tubular resonators suspended underneath, and is played with wooden, rubber or plastic beaters.

rows like those on a piano keyboard. Suspended under each key is a tubular metal resonator that gives the instrument its characteristic sound.

Europe

The xylophone has been known since at least the early 16th century, when Hans Holbein painted his *Dance of*

Death showing Death carrying a xylophone suspended horizontally, like a tray, from a cord around his neck. However, the instrument did not become popular until the 1830s, when the Polish xylophonist Michael Joseph Gusikow brought it to the attention of the public with his concerts. Gusikow gave the instrument an enduring popularity in folk music.

Asia

The xylophone is believed to have originated in South-east Asia. One Asian version is the *mokkin* of Japan,

ABOVE: The marimba was developed in the United States around 1910. It is similar to the xylophone but is pitched an octave deeper, giving it a characteristic mellow sound.

ABOVE: *The marimba can be played with four beaters instead of two. Playing in this way produces soft, deep chords.*

ABOVE: *The* rang nat *is a type of metallic xylophone — known as a "metallophone" in Java and Bali — used in Javanese Gamelan bands. Also seen in this photograph are some gong chimes, or* khong vong yai.

which, although it has between 13 and 16 keys, is used as a rhythm rather than a melody instrument, chiefly in *kabuki* music. In Burma the *pattala* has up to 23 keys, which are finely tuned

by fixing wax pellets to the undersides. The xylophones and metallophones of Indonesian percussion orchestras are many and varied, ranging from single-octave models to large multi-octave

instruments that are played using two beaters. As early as the 7th century, Balinese *gambang* players were using four beaters, two in each hand, held to form a V.

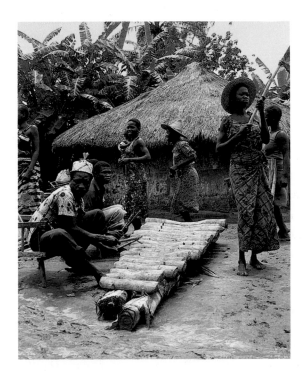

ABOVE: *In Zaire and other central African countries, xylophones are made by placing logs sliced into increasing sizes over a base of two long logs.*

Africa

From Asia the xylophone migrated to Africa. Here the simplest form is the pit or ground xylophone which, as the name implies, is a pit in the ground over which the ends of wooden bars are placed on bundles of grass. This primitive instrument is still played in parts of the continent, an example being the eight-keyed *ndara* of Uganda. The log xylophone, found in East and West Africa, as well as in Indonesia and Papua New Guinea, is composed of a few keys placed across the outstretched legs of the player. In a more developed form, gourds are suspended from the keys to augment the sound. In Nigeria a small portable version has ox-horn resonators.

Bells

Gay bells or sad, they bring you memories
of half forgotten innocent old places.

W. B. YEATS (1865–1939)

In one form or another, bells are known all over the world. Ancient Egyptian priests wore small closed silver bells as protective amulets when they were in the temple, a practice continued in the Christian church: as late as the 11th century, Archbishop Lanfranc of Canterbury wore a cope edged with 51 bells.

The practice of fitting animals with bells to ward off evil dates back to at least 520 BC, when they are mentioned in the *Book of Zachariah*. In Siberia small bells are still fitted on to the yokes of horse-drawn vehicles to scare off wolves and devils.

Ancient Greek soldiers attached bronze bells to their shields in an effort to terrify the enemy. It must have been an awesome sound for, owing to the density of bronze, their bells would have clanged rather than emitting the clear ringing tone that is expected today. The Greeks also issued bells to watchmen and sentinels for use in alerting the population in times of danger.

The custom of ringing a "passing bell", with the object of keeping evil spirits away from the dead, dates back to at least the 8th century. The Bayeux Tapestry, made in the late 11th century, clearly shows two boys, each carrying a pair of hand bells, accompanying the coffin of Edward the Confessor for exactly this reason.

Casting

Early bells were cast using the *cire perdue* or "lost wax" method. A clay or brick model of the inside surface of the

ABOVE: *A late 7th-century BC bronze bell found in Bologna, Italy.*

bell was made. Over this, a layer of wax was built up to the shape and thickness of the finished bell. Once the wax had set, it was covered by another layer of clay and the entire mould was thoroughly baked. As the clay hardened the wax melted and drained away, leaving a vacant space into which the bell metal was poured to form the actual bell. The Whitechapel Bell Foundry in London, which still casts church bells and a five-octave range of hand bells, was founded in 1420.

Some early bells were not cast but made from thin iron plates hammered into circular or rectangular sheets and riveted together before being dipped into molten copper to seal the joints.

ABOVE: *The bells of the Church of San Francisco in Córdoba, Spain. Bells are traditionally hung high in church towers so that they can be heard over great distances.*

Church bells

Early church bells were of a long, thin beehive shape. During the 12th and 13th centuries, however, the form of the bell evolved into a slightly conical sugar-loaf shape, which by the beginning of the 14th century had reached the fatter, wider appearance that is familiar today.

One of the earliest references to ringing church bells in England is found in Rutland. Here, in the church of St Andrew in Stoke Dry on the early 12th-century south pillar of the Romanesque chancel arch, is depicted a man pulling on a bell rope. Although it was not until the 16th century that bells regularly began to carry inscriptions, at Littleborough,

Nottinghamshire there is a bell made in about 1170 that bears the inscription "Santa Maria".

The mechanics of the church bell are relatively simple. The crown of each bell is fixed to a headstick of metal, which is in turn attached to a large wheel. The rim of the wheel is grooved to hold the bell rope which, when pulled, raises the bell, causing it to swing until its mouth is high enough for the clapper to strike it.

Change-ringing

Britain differs from the rest of Europe in that church bells are rung in changes. A change is the ringing of a set of bells in all possible combinations. Thus a set of three bells contains six changes (123, 231, 213, 321, 312 and 132). Each set of changes constitutes a peal. A peal of three bells consists of six changes, while a peal of four bells contains 24, one of eight bells contains 40,320 and so on.

ABOVE: The custom of fitting animals, such as horses and cows, with bells was originally to ward off evil, although on a more practical level it is also useful for the farmer to be able to hear them moving around.

ABOVE: The earliest known carving (12th-century) of church bell ringers.

ABOVE: An engraving of an 18th-century French bell foundry showing a bell being hoisted from its casting mould.

Hand bells

Hand bells, as the name implies, are relatively small bells fitted with a handle that enables them to be held in the hand for ringing. The oldest known hand bells come from China and date from about 1600 BC. Chinese hand bells were, however, in existence before this, for there are earlier written references to their use in religious music. In 9th-century Japan small hand bells struck with hammers were used to accompany the singing of *goeka*, a kind of Buddhist plainsong. This tradition lives on, and at the beginning of the 21st century there are many enthusiasts who form several thousand *goeka* societies in Japan, and hold regular conventions.

Modern Western hand bells are normally made in sets numbering between six and 60, covering a range of up to five octaves, and are usually rung by groups of between four and 15 ringers. Generally each player holds one or two bells in each hand. Sometimes, however, the bells are laid on a table and are lifted and rung as they are required.

By the mid 19th century almost every village in England had its own hand-bell team that played at local fairs, entertainments and during the Christmas season. In the 20th century, hand-bell ringing again became popular, this time in the United States. In 1954 the American Guild of English

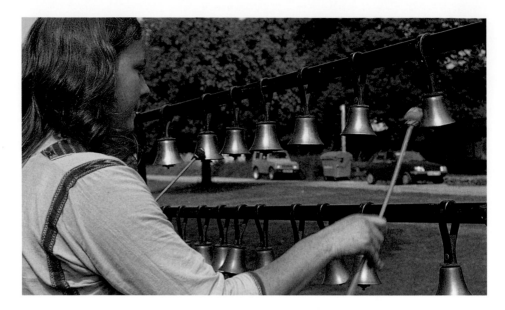

ABOVE: *A modern handmade set of bell chimes.*

Hand-bell Ringers was founded and today there are more than a thousand teams representing over 10,000 ringers.

Bell wheel

One of the earliest ecclesiastical uses of small bells is the bell wheel, or *Zimbelstern*, examples of which are recorded from the 10th century. Mainly found in France, Germany and Spain, and to a lesser extent in Britain, this contraption consisted of a number of small silver bells attached to a large wheel. The wheel was originally revolved by means of either a rope or a hand-crank, but by the 13th century clockwork was also used, and some were attached to the church organ and operated by a stop.

One of the finest bell wheels was the "Star" of Fulda Cathedral in Germany. This wonderful creation, which was suspended from the nave ceiling, was 7.3m/24ft in diameter and had no less than 350 bells attached to its 14 rays. In 1781 tragedy struck when its rope broke, causing it to crash down upon the assembled congregation. Since its restoration, it still has 150 of its bells and is operated by a treadmill.

Bell chimes

Although tuned sets of bell chimes have been in existence for at least 3000 years, it was not until the 11th century that they reached Europe. The first depiction of the instrument, in an illustrated Bible of about 1070, shows a musician hammering a seven-bell chime with one hand while tapping a frame drum with the other hand. During the 13th century some chimes, which were connected to town clocks, were mechanized, the time being sounded by bells that were struck by hammers operated by a cogwheel.

LEFT: *Hand-bell groups were very popular in the 19th century. One such band that toured extensively was the "Swedish Bell Ringers".*

Carillon

The art of making bell chimes was perfected in the Low Countries and northern France, where the bells were suspended from a framework inside a tower. Hammers were automatically released by iron pegs set into a large wooden barrel (later a metal cylinder) that was turned by weights and pulleys. As the barrel revolved, the pegs tripped levers that were in turn connected to the hammers by wires.

ABOVE: *The carillon at the church of Corneille sur Risle, France.*

ABOVE: *A 13th-century illumination depicting a man playing a bell chime with crudely made hammers. By his side is another musician playing a viol in the style of the period.*

Two of the earliest town clocks fitted with bells were the one in Mons (1328) and the astronomical clock in Strasbourg Cathedral (1354). The latter's pegs were fitted in such a way that the bells could play several tunes.

From about 1500 a keyboard was added to the Antwerp carillon, making it possible to play the bells manually. During the 16th century the compass of the carillons extended downwards, involving larger, heavier bells. As these were impossible to play by hand, a pedal board was added. The number of bells continued to increase and, by 1612, St Paul's church in Liège boasted a carillon of 24 bells.

As the popularity of the carillon grew, so did the demand for longer and more varied tunes. Once the cylinder had made a single complete revolution all its music had been played, so to accommodate longer tunes larger cylinders were made, some reaching over 2m/6ft in diameter.

The most famous carillon builders of the 17th century were the Van der Gheyn family and the Hemony brothers, Pierre and François, who came from Lorraine but worked in Amsterdam. In 1655 Pierre Hemony built the largest carillon yet, a machine containing 52 bells. He was such a perfectionist that he required his bells to contain the overtones of three octaves, two fifths, a major third and a minor third.

Today the world's foremost builder of carillons is the British bell foundry Taylor & Co., in Loughborough. Their creations have been installed in bell towers all over the world, including their home town, where a 47-bell carillon was built in 1923 as a memorial to those men of the town who died in World War I.

ABOVE: *These traditional Swiss cow bells are accompanying a procession of alpine singers.*

Bells in the orchestra

Bells have been used in orchestras since the 18th century. One outstanding use of bells took place in 1882 at the first performance of Tchaikovsky's *1812 Overture*. Although the ambitious Tchaikovsky had wanted to have all the church bells of Moscow peal out in the grand finale, the city fathers deemed the idea impractical so the composer had to be content with the bells of Uspensky Cathedral, in which the concert took place.

Many 19th-century composers, however, preferred to use other instruments to imitate the sound of the bell. Rimsky-Korsakov, for instance, used a combination of triangle, cymbal and gong combined with *pizzicato* and sustained chords from the strings and wind in his *Russian Easter Festival*

LEFT: Orchestral sleigh bells recreate the sound of the bells placed around the necks of sleigh-pulling Russian horses.

overture in 1888. Generally, however, modern orchestras use tubular bells, but since the 1970s synthesizers and other electronic instruments have been increasingly used to imitate bells.

Tubular bells

Tubular bells originated in South-east Asia. When they became known in Europe the chimes were at first made of bell metal, but this proved expensive. In 1886, after various experiments, a British instrument maker, John Hampton of Coventry, produced tubular bells made of bronze. Today chimes are usually made of brass. Ordered in graduated lengths to give a range of up to two octaves, they all have the same diameter and are suspended from a frame.

ABOVE: Modern orchestral tubular bells.

ABOVE: By the 16th century some bell chimes were connected to a keyboard, thereby making it possible to play the bells manually.

ABOVE: Tubular bells are sounded by being hit at the top with hard mallets. A foot pedal operates a felted damper to stop the sound when required.

ABOVE: Tubular bells mallets.

Glockenspiel

The European concept of the glockenspiel originated in the Netherlands, where it was introduced from Indonesia in the second half of the 17th century. The European instrument was originally a miniature carillon, and its earliest known use was in 1739 when Handel used one in a production of *Saul*. Today it is more commonly made of a series of graduated steel bars, arranged in two rows like the black and white keys of a piano, and played with moderately hard beaters.

ABOVE: The modern glockenspiel has steel bars covering two and a half octaves.

The keyed glockenspiel, in which small metal hammers strike the bars from below, arrived in the orchestra before what is now the standard instrument took its place in the mid 19th century, and Mozart, Tchaikovsky, Saint-Saëns and many other composers included it in their scores. Nearly all these parts are now played on the conventional glockenspiel, which has a superior tone and dynamic range.

Bell-lyra

The portable glockenspiel was designed in the 19th century specifically for German marching bands. Originally a single row of metal cups, it is now made with a series of metal bars arranged like a piano keyboard that are hung in a lyre-shaped frame set on a wooden handle. Tapped with a metal beater, it is carried in front of the player, level with the head.

Celesta

Similar to the keyed glockenspiel, the celesta resembles an upright piano. The metal bars are struck by felt-covered hammers activated by a simple piano mechanism, and there is a sustaining pedal. It was invented by Auguste

Mustel of Paris in 1886 as an improvement on the "dulcitone", an instrument consisting of a series of tuning forks operated by a keyboard, which he had constructed some 20 years earlier.

According to legend, Tchaikovsky was walking down a street in Paris when he heard a celesta being played. He was so enchanted by the sound that he used it to represent the Sugar-plum Fairy in *The Nutcracker* (1892). Béla Bartók scored for the celesta in his *Music for Strings, Percussion and Celesta*, which was published in 1936.

ABOVE: The celesta is played like a piano but has a bell-like sound. Although mainly used in classical orchestras, it is also occasionally used in popular music.

Vibraphone

The vibraphone is a cross between the glockenspiel and the xylophone, and was invented in the United States in 1921. Beneath the alloy bars are tubular resonators fitted with resonating lids that are made to vibrate by means of an electric motor. The vibraphone produces a bell-like sound and has been scored for by composers such as Benjamin Britten and Luigi Dallapiccola (1904–75). It quickly became popular as a jazz instrument, first played by its leading exponent Lionel Hampton (1909–2002).

ABOVE: The vibraphone has a foot pedal that opens and closes the resonating tubes.

Bells music

Among the earliest composers to score for bells were Nicholas Dalayrac (1753–1809) in his opera *Camille* (1791), and Luigi Cherubini (1760–1842) in *Elisa* (1794). Rossini called for a bell in the second act of *William Tell* (1829), and Giacomo Meyerbeer (1791–1864) demanded a specially made large bell for *Les Huguenots* (1836).

Keyboards

Harpsichord

One should have an easy manner at the harpsichord and
avoid either staring fixedly at any object, or looking too vague.

FRANÇOIS COUPERIN (1668–1733), "L'ART DE TOUCHER LE CLAVECIN"

The harpsichord can be dated back to at least 1397, when there is a record in Padua of the invention of an instrument called a *clavicymbalum*, a name that was translated as "virginal" in England. It did not become known as the harpsichord, from the Italian *arpicordo*, until 1607. The new instrument was the first to use a mechanical plucking action to activate the strings; this system was also used in the virginal and the spinet.

Mechanism

The harpsichord is a mechanized version of the psaltery. Each key operates a wooden rod, or "jack", on which is mounted a quill plectrum. As the key is depressed, the jack rises and the plectrum plucks the string. The jack is

LEFT: A harpsichord made in 1756 by Jacob Kirckman of London. The interior surfaces are decorated with holly and walnut marquetry, while the case is veneered with burr walnut.

so constructed that on its way down, when the key is released, the plectrum is pivoted back and avoids the string. As the jack descends a felt damper quietens the string.

Because the strings run at right angles to the keyboard, it is possible to mount more than one jack on each key, and more than one string to each note, each with its own jack. Each set of strings is called a "choir". By moving the jacks to one side, using a stop, one or more choirs can be left unplucked, so that the volume of sound produced is reduced. Apart from this facility, the player has no control over the level of sound, as the string is always plucked in the same way. However, additional

stops modify the sounds in other ways, such as the "harp" stop that mutes some strings to give a *pizzicato* effect, or the "lute" stop that operates extra jacks nearer the ends of the strings to give a nasal sound.

Two-manual harpsichord

From the 1670s, the development of double manuals allowed performers to change from louder to softer passages without interrupting their playing. The lower manual worked two choirs, while the upper manual worked a single choir for quiet passages. In French harpsichords, the two mechanisms could be coupled to operate all three choirs together for maximum volume.

ABOVE: A beautifully decorated harpsichord.

Key features

TYPE: keyboard

PITCH: concert

RANGE: *c'* to *c''''*

NOTABLE PLAYERS OF THE HARPSICHORD: Wanda Landowska, Arnold Dolmetsch, Thurston Dart, Christopher Hogwood.

Styles

The earliest surviving instruments are Italian, including one dated 1515. They have single manuals and separate outer cases, and may have had only a single set of strings.

Flemish harpsichords, principally made by the Ruckers family of Antwerp from the mid 16th to late 17th centuries, were played all over Europe. They were beautifully decorated with printed papers, and in some instruments the paintings inside the lid were by Rubens. Many Ruckers harpsichords were later rebuilt for the French market by Pascal Taskin, who inherited the French firm of Blanchet, the royal harpsichord makers.

The major English makers of the 18th century were Burkat Shudi (1702–73), who was joined in 1761 by John Broadwood (1732–1812) and Jacob Kirckman (1710–92). While French instruments were elaborately painted and gilded, English harpsichord cases were relatively austere, but were finely veneered in walnut and sycamore or, later, in satinwood and mahogany.

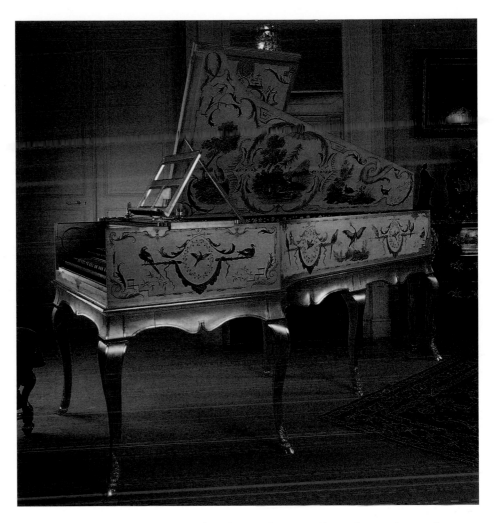

ABOVE: Harpsichords are often beautifully decorated, with gold panelling and painted scenes.

Innovations

During the 18th century there were many attempts to modify and improve the harpsichord. Jean Marius's *clavecin brisé*, or folding harpsichord of 1700, was made in three hinged sections. The century also saw ever-larger harpsichords with three and even four registers, together with a complex system of stops to provide different tone-colours. In 1769 Shudi patented the "Venetian swell", a device that opened and shut like a Venetian blind over the strings and soundboard, to produce *crescendos* and *diminuendos*. The quill plectrum was replaced by one made of hard leather.

Decline

In 1768 Johann Christian Bach's London recital made the piano instantly fashionable and ended the supremacy of the harpsichord. Although the harpsichord was still being built in Dublin as late as 1824, it was soon overtaken by the new, more expressive instrument. By 1837 it was almost extinct, for when in that year the pianist Ignaz Moscheles gave a "historical" recital in London, he had difficulty in finding a harpsichord on which to perform.

The modern revival began in the 1880s, when the French piano makers Erard and Pleyel built copies of 18th-century harpsichords, and in London Arnold Dolmetsch began to present recitals of Renaissance and Baroque music on antique instruments.

ABOVE: Detail of a modern harpsichord keyboard built by Colin Booth in 1993.

Virginal

*To teach men's daughters on the virginal is
as harmless a calling as any man can follow.*

SOLOMON ECCLES (1618–83)

Although virginals were the most popular keyboard instruments in Elizabethan households, the name is not, as many believe, a compliment to the "Virgin Queen". Descended from the psaltery, the instrument has been known since at least 1460, 50 years before Elizabeth's birth. The etymology of the word "virginals" (like "scissors", it is often used in the plural) is uncertain. It may be from the Latin *virga*, meaning "rod" or

ABOVE: *A 16th-century engraving showing a woman playing a virginal.*

Key features

TYPE: keyboard

PITCH: concert

RANGE: *c'* to *c''''*

ABOVE: *A 1976 replica of a 1623 Ruckers virginal from Antwerp. Apart from their musical quality, instruments from Antwerp are notable for the elaborate decoration of their interiors with printed paper and painting.*

"jack", or may even be a reference to the young ladies who most commonly played the instrument.

By 1500 virginals were being played throughout Europe. They are mentioned in a proverb that was inscribed on the walls of Manor House, Leckingfield, Yorkshire, in about 1500, while on the other side of Europe the court organist at Buda played the virginal to entertain the prince at mealtimes in 1501. Henry VIII is known to have purchased five virginals in 1530, while in 1549 the Innsbruck court bought an instrument made by an organ builder from Königsberg. Virginals were extremely popular as domestic instruments in the

Low Countries, England, Austria and Germany. In England they eventually gave way to the spinet and in Germany to the clavichord.

Shape

Strung with 32 metal strings lying parallel with the keyboard, the virginal had the form of a clavichord coupled with the sound of a harpsichord, since the strings were plucked. Each string was longer than that of its neighbour, forming a triangle inside the case, with the long bass strings at the front. In Flemish virginals the keyboard was placed either to the right or left of the centre of the long side, a feature that determined the timbre of the instrument. When it was placed to the right, the strings were plucked nearer their centre, and this produced a nasal tone that was described as "grunting

ABOVE: *Detail of the inside of a virginal with delicately painted flowers and embellishments. The highest standards of craftsmanship went into the lavish decoration of the domestic instruments.*

without a lid. Flemish virginals, which were chiefly made in Antwerp, had recessed keyboards made of thicker softwood and were furnished with a lid. English virginals, all surviving examples of which were made between 1640 and 1680, combined features of both the Italian and Flemish styles. They were exceptionally deep and featured a vaulted lid.

Double virginal

An extremely popular form was the double virginal, invented in Antwerp. Nicknamed the "mother and child", it combined a large keyboard cheek by jowl with a smaller one half the size. The smaller one was set in a recess between the soundboard and the bottom of the case, usually to the left of the larger keyboard. Although it could also be played on its own, during performance the "child" could be withdrawn and placed on top of the "mother" so that the latter's keyboard played both instruments, the "child" sounding an octave above the "mother". These were built in the late 16th century, and in 1584 a Leipzig musical instrument dealer named Krause had in his stock *"1 neu Instrument mit 2 Clavieren"* ("one new instrument with two keyboards").

like pigs". This form was called a *muselar*. With the keyboard to the left, in the form called a *spinett*, the sound was brighter.

There were three main centres of virginal-making: Italy, Belgium and England. Italian-made virginals, which were characterized by a projecting keyboard like the contemporary Italian spinet, were made of cypress wood

Spinet

Called upon one Haward, that makes virginalls, and did there like of a little espinette, and will have him finish it for me: for I had a mind to a small harpsichon, but this takes up less room.

SAMUEL PEPYS (1633–1703)

LEFT: *A typical early English example of a bentside spinet built in London in about 1770. This compact harpsichord, whose keyboard occupies much of the case, is made of walnut, with Italian-style interior trim in cypress.*

The spinet, a small version of the harpsichord, is believed to have got its name from either the Italian word *spina* or the French *épinette* ("thorn"), both references to the plectra with which the instrument's strings are plucked. Another theory is that it is named after one of the early builders of the instrument, the Venetian Giovanni Spinetti, one of whose surviving instruments is dated 1503.

The spinet has the same action as the harpsichord, but is built on a smaller, domestic scale. It was popular in France from the late 15th century. As well as being mentioned in an Avignon contract of 1503, the instrument is also included in the household accounts of the Countess of Angoulême in the mid 1490s. Although early instruments were built of thin cypress wood, without a lid, by the 18th century the cases were being made of thicker wood, such as Brazil or pine, and were complete with lids. Smaller spinets, termed "spinettinos", were also made.

The spinet was not introduced into England until Charles II's return from France at the Restoration in 1660. It soon proved very popular, and by the end of the century an English school of spinet-building had developed, and the instrument was beginning to replace the virginal. Most English spinets had a compass starting with G, whereas continental spinets tended to begin on F.

For those who could not afford a harpsichord or did not have room for one, the spinet was the next best thing. It flourished longer in England than anywhere else, only disappearing when it was replaced by the square piano in the early 19th century.

Shape

The spinet's single set of strings is arranged across the instrument (in

Key features

TYPE: keyboard

PITCH: concert

RANGE: *c'* to *c''''*

ABOVE: *This finely decorated 16th-century polygonal spinet was built by the Italian maker Annibale dei Rossi. He and his son Ferrante were recorded in 1595 as improvers and modernizers of clavichords.*

contrast to the harpsichord where the strings are set at right angles to the keyboard). The oblique stringing of the early models produced a trapezoid shape, while the characteristic Italian spinet of the 16th and 17th centuries was five or six-sided, with a keyboard projecting from the long side.

Small spinets of the Italian pattern were most popular in France in the 16th and 17th centuries. These were usually about 80cm/32in (tuned to an octave above concert pitch) or 102cm/40in long (tuned to a fourth above concert pitch).

In Germany there were rare cases of wing-shaped spinets being made with two manuals for use by organists and teachers.

In 1631 Girolamo Zenti invented the bentside or "leg of mutton" spinet, a development that achieved great popularity in England. So named because of its wing shape, it was made in the shape of a triangle with unequal sides, with the keyboard set into one of the shorter sides. It was a conveniently compact shape, being both shorter and narrower than a harpsichord of equal range.

ABOVE: *An engraving entitled* Dame am Spinett *by Johann Sartorius.*

Double-strung spinet

As a rule the spinet was not capable of changes of tone-colour or volume. An attempt to rectify this was the double-strung spinet. Examples of this rare type are the two-manual octave spinet built by Israel Gellinger, and Cristofori's *"cembelo traverso"*. Variations were obtained in these instruments by moving the keyboard in or out, so that both or only one set of jacks would be lifted when the keys were depressed.

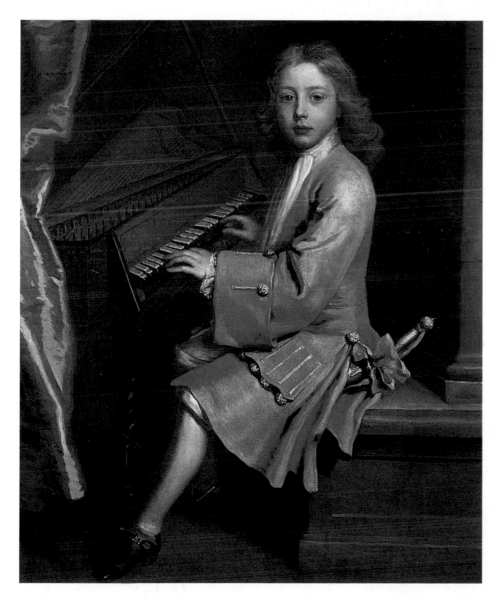

ABOVE: *An 18th-century painting of a young man playing the spinet by Jonathan Richardson (1665–1745). Like the harpsichord, the "natural" keys of the spinet are black and the "accidentals" are white.*

ABOVE: *This spinet was made by one of the main English keyboard makers of the 18th century, Thomas Hitchcock of London.*

Piano

The pianoforte is the most perfect of all musical instruments: its invention was to music what the invention of printing was to poetry.

GEORGE BERNARD SHAW (1856–1950)

The months of May and June 1768 saw the turning point in the history of the piano. On May 19, Henry Walsh gave the world's first public performace for solo piano in Dublin; two weeks later, on June 2, at the Thatched House, St James's Square, London, Johann Christian Bach (1735–82) – J. S. Bach's youngest son – performed on a square piano. These were not the first occasions that the instrument had been heard in public, for a year earlier Charles Dibdin had used a piano to accompany a song sung during the interval of a production of *The Beggar's Opera* at Covent Garden, London. However, the kudos given to the piano by Bach's recital made the instrument fashionable overnight.

Bartolomeo Cristofori

The pianoforte was invented around 1709 by Bartolomeo Cristofori (1655–1731), a harpsichord builder and keeper of the royal musical instruments in Florence. The early Cristofori pianos, which looked and sounded like contemporary harpsichords, had a range of four octaves, half that of a modern grand. Indeed the very name, *gravicembalo col piano e forte*, implied that it was considered merely as another type of harpsichord, there being no real desire at the time to create an entirely new instrument. Surviving Cristofori pianos, with their thin strings and

LEFT: An ornate 19th-century grand piano built by Joseph Schneider.

hard hammers, do in fact sound very like harpsichords.

The main difference between the piano and the harpsichord was that the strings of the former were struck

ABOVE: This sturdy grand piano was presented to Ludwig van Beethoven by the London firm of John Broadwood & Sons in 1817.

by hammers rather than being plucked by quills, as in the harpsichord. When the piano key was pressed, the hammer struck the string and immediately came away, allowing the string to vibrate and sound until the key was released, activating a damper to silence it. The earliest music published specifically for the piano was a sonata composed by Lodovico Giustini in 1732, the year after Cristofori's death.

Square piano

Actually an oblong shape similar to the clavichord, the square piano was first made in 1742 by Johann Sacher, a Bavarian instrument maker. Although these instruments took up less space and were cheaper to produce than grand pianos, the main problem was that the bass strings had to be short and were therefore weak in tone as well as volume.

In Britain, square pianos were made by Johannes Zumpe from 1760, and it was one of his instruments on which J. C. Bach gave his London recital. An early French builder of square pianos was Sébastien Erard (1752–1831) who introduced various improvements to the Zumpe design including the *agraffe* in 1808, a device that improved the tension of the strings, and, in 1821, the double escapement action that

ABOVE: *Franz Liszt playing a piano built by Ludwig Bösendorfer.*

ABOVE: *This 1726 Cristofori piano represents the climax of the Italian's work. It is double-strung and has a four-octave compass as well as a synchronized damper.*

ABOVE: *This square piano built by Adam Beyer of London in 1777 is decorated with two sorts of mahogany.*

increased the speed at which notes could be repeated.

Although upright pianos gradually became more popular in European homes during the 19th century, square pianos survived for many years, particularly in the United States, where they grew large and elaborate.

The piano in the home

By the end of the 18th century the piano had become more than just a fashionable toy, and was a living force

in culture and entertainment in the homes of the wealthy. As a sign of the piano's increased popularity as a domestic instrument, in 1797 James Harrison launched his *Piano-Forte Magazine*. Each issue included a note, signed by Harrison, promising a new piano to any reader who purchased the entire 250 numbers and could produce the signed certificates that were included in each issue.

Frédéric Chopin

Without doubt one of the greatest composers for the piano who ever lived was Frédéric Chopin (1810–49), the son of a French father and a Polish mother, who moved to Paris in 1831. His music was a kaleidoscope of three distinct traditions: German classicism, Italian *bel canto* and Polish folk music, and he composed almost exclusively for the piano. No other composer has enjoyed such lasting and continuous popularity with so many people, and his music is still found on almost every piano in the world. Chopin can truly be said to have dipped his pen in moonbeams and flooded the world with melodies.

ABOVE: *The First Piano Lesson by Jules Alexis Meunier (1863–1942) depicts an early 19th-century young lady receiving piano tuition from her teacher.*

Upright piano

Larger than harpsichords, early horizontally strung pianos took up a lot of floor space, and to address this problem Domenico del Mela of Gagliano built the first vertical piano in 1739. The piano was simply turned upright on a stand, with the strings and soundboard towering above the keyboard. About 1800 it was realized that the soundboard could be dropped towards the floor, placing most of the string length behind the keyboard in front of the player's knees, thereby decreasing the overall height of the instrument. The strings were tuned at the top and the hammers arranged to strike from the front. In 1811 the "cottage" piano appeared in London. It was just over 1m/3ft tall, with diagonally arranged strings.

In the 1830s the problem of the short bass strings was solved with the invention of the overstrung piano, in which the shorter strings ran vertically and the bass strings crossed obliquely over them allowing for greater length. This method of stringing soon became the norm for all pianos and is the method still used today.

ABOVE: Der Appollosaal, Berlin, is one of the centres in the reinstated German capital where piano recitals are given on a fairly regular basis.

Sound

As the 19th century dawned, there were two distinct piano sounds. There was the light action and sensuous tone of German and Austrian instruments, on which musicians such as Mozart had performed, and there was the firmer action and stronger tone of English instruments, particularly those made by John Broadwood. It was one of the latter that Beethoven used, for as his deafness increased he could no longer hear what he was playing on a Viennese instrument.

Pedals

In 1759 Weltmann in France had invented a piano-harpsichord combination with knee levers that were used to effect registration, but pedals were introduced by John

ABOVE: Upright pianos have two pedals. The left one is the "soft" pedal and the right the "sustaining" pedal.

Broadwood, the pre-eminent British maker, in 1783. There were usually two pedals to operate two stops, *forte* and *una corda*, but many experiments were made with other devices to modify the tone. Some pianos had as many as four extra pedals. The *forte* or sustaining pedal lifted the dampers so that the sound was sustained after the key had fallen back, while the *una corda* or "soft" pedal shifted the action sideways so that the hammers struck only one string for each note. One special stop created a bassoon effect

LEFT: This small upright piano was built by the renowned firm of Clementi of London in 1825. The instrument is veneered in rosewood with pleated silk panels in the front.

with a strip of parchment passed through the strings, and in deference to the craze for "Turkish music" some pianos were built with small drums, bells, cymbals and triangles inside the case, all controlled by pedals.

Strings

The instrument on which J. C. Bach had played in 1768 sounded very different from a modern piano. Beethoven and Mozart would not recognize their music now, as the "modern" piano sound did not begin to appear until about 1850. The strings of early 19th-century pianos were still quite light and thin and at much lower tension than today's models, in which the strings are so rigid and tense that they behave more like bars. This thinness gave the instruments more harmonic overtones than a modern piano, a characteristic that gives early pianos an "out-of-tune" tone quality, reminiscent of ragtime pianos of the 1920s. To increase the volume of sound, makers increased the thickness of the strings. This meant that the tension also had to be increased to maintain them at the same pitch.

ABOVE: *Instruments by Erard, one of the great makers of pianos (and harps) were used by players from Beethoven to Ravel. Built in 1866, this is an early example, veneered in costly Amboyna wood.*

ABOVE: *Piano fingering is very important, both to reach the notes and to interpret the music. There are nearly one hundred keys but only ten fingers to play them with.*

Frame

Added tension in the strings meant that the frame had to be reinforced. Although the first iron frame appeared as early as 1800, it was not until 1828 that Adolphus Babcock of Boston produced the first square piano with a full iron frame, cast in a single piece. The first iron frame for a grand piano was made in Boston in 1843 by Jonas Chickering. In the 1860s Steinway's cast iron frames were first seen in Europe, and almost all makers followed suit.

Unusual sounds

During the 20th century many new sounds and colours were brought out of the piano. Erik Satie (1866–1925) put sheets of paper between the strings for a performance of *La Piège de Meduse* in 1914. John Cage altered the tone of the piano by attaching objects such as paper, nails and milk bottles to the strings. One composer, David Bedford (born 1937), asked a performer to scream inside the piano to make the strings vibrate, while La Monte Young (born 1935), for reasons best known to himself, asked the pianist to bring a bale of hay and a bucket of water on to the stage for the piano to eat and drink.

ABOVE: *An inside view of a modern Steinway grand piano.*

ABOVE: *By the end of the 19th century there was a piano in almost every middle-class home. Singing around the piano was an enjoyable family activity.*

Organ

When the full Organ joins the tuneful Quire
Th' Immortal Pow'rs incline their Ear.

ALEXANDER POPE (1688–1744)

The organ is without doubt capable of producing the greatest effects, and is truly worthy of Mozart's praise as the king of instruments. Devised in Alexandria in the 3rd century BC, by the 2nd century AD the organ had become one of the main instruments of Rome and was heard in almost all aspects of Roman entertainment, including the theatre, games, gladiatorial contests, circus and banquets. Even Nero is believed to have played the organ.

Water organ

The direct ancestor of the modern pipe organ is the hydraulis, or water organ, believed to have been invented by Ctesibius, an Alexandrian engineer who is also credited with the invention of the water-pump, water-clock and water-powered artificial singing birds.

Although water was not the motive force in the hydraulis, it acted to maintain an even pressure of air, which was supplied by a hand-pump. The sound was produced through a set of bronze pipes, graded in length like the contemporary pan-pipes; indeed, the hydraulis was sometimes described as a *syrinx* played with the hands. Originally there was only one row of pipes, but by the 3rd century AD the instrument was being built with four, six or even eight ranks of pipes. It was said to be so loud that hydraulis players had to plug their ears. Ctesibius can truly be called the "Father of the Organ", for his basic conception of the provision

of a continuous wind supply to an array of tuned pipes controlled from a keyboard remains unchanged to this day.

The main drawback of the water organ was that it required precision engineering and needed constant

LEFT: This beautifully painted positive organ was built in about 1600.

maintenance, as it was prone to corrosion. By AD 200 the water tank had been eliminated in favour of a windbag inflated by bellows and compressed air.

Church organ

The European "organ revival" of the 10th century came about because the instrument was reintroduced from Byzantium. Between the 10th and 13th centuries the organ became almost exclusively a church instrument in western Europe. Organs were erected in places such as Cologne Cathedral (AD 950), where one was used "for purposes of teaching the

LEFT: A 4th-century illustration of a water organ, or hydraulis. The player stood at the keyboard while his assistant operated the long lever that worked the pump. Under the pipes was a keyboard that operated perforated sliders. When a key was pressed, a slider was pushed into position to release pressurized air from the wind canal and thereby sound the note. When the key was released, a spring pulled the slider back, shutting off the air supply and stopping the note.

science of music", and the Benedictine Abbey in Bagas, Spain (AD 972), where the instrument was placed near the entrance. At the consecration of the Bagas organ special mention was made of the fact that it could be "heard from afar", which has led to the theory that it was used for summoning the congregation, much like modern church bells. In England, an organ was built at Winchester in about AD 990.

By the 10th century, foot-operated bellows began to appear and the sliders, which all looked the same and therefore had the name of each note written on them, terminated in handles. For several centuries these relatively small organs constituted the typical church organ. By the 13th century all instruments other than organs were excluded from various churches in Spain, Italy and France. In the 15th century many new churches were built, most with an organ as part of the regular furniture.

ABOVE: *The beautiful and ornate organ in Roskilde cathedral, Denmark, was built in 1554. This is an organ of the type known as "swallow nests", because they were suspended against a church wall.*

ABOVE: *Grinling Gibbons decorated the interior of the church of St James, Piccadilly, in London in the 1680s. One example of his craftsmanship is the gilded organ case that is surmounted by musical angels.*

During the 13th century the sliders began to be replaced by keys. The early keyboards had wide keys that decreased in width from the wide bass keys to the narrower treble keys.

During the 14th century, with full chromaticism and larger compass, the keyboard began to take on its modern appearance, with the accidentals (the "black" notes) in an upper row.

In the 14th century the organ compass, which hitherto had not exceeded two octaves, increased until a chromatic compass of three octaves was achieved. By now, organs were becoming common and were no longer restricted to the major churches. By the end of the century some of the larger and more important churches, such as Meaux, Leyden and Westminster, had two organs: a great organ in the west end and a smaller positive organ in the choir.

Classical organ

Two manuals began to appear in the 14th century, enabling the same organist to control both the main organ and the small positive organ. This led to the rapid development of the organ and its performing potential, which ensured its pre-eminence in Europe until the mid 18th century.

A large organ may have thousands of pipes, divided into groups, or stops, each of which is brought into play by pulling out a knob on the console. Each pipe produces a characteristic sound, depending on its shape, whether it is made of wood, tin or an alloy, and whether it is a flue or reed-pipe. In early organs all the pipes were open flues but during the 16th century reed pipes, with resonators of brass or wood, came into use. Various types of reed are used to create distinctive sounds, some imitating orchestral instruments or the human voice.

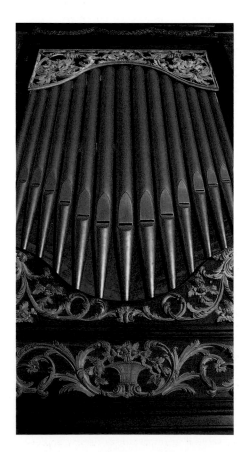

ABOVE: Detail of the pipes of the English house organ pictured above right.

RIGHT: Built by John Byfield of London in 1766, this is an outstanding example of an almost unaltered English house organ, with original glass doors and superb limewood carvings. The case is solid mahogany.

A series of up to five five-octave manuals and a 32-note pedalboard control valves that release air from the wind-chest into the various sets of pipes. The sets and their relative manuals are usually known as the Choir, Great, Swell, Solo and Echo.

Noted organ builders

During the late Renaissance, organ-building reached new heights of refinement. Organs were sumptuously decorated with inlaid wood, ivory and gold. The organ in the palace of Frederiksborg in Denmark, built in 1612 by Esaias Compenius, has solid silver stops shaped like human faces.

In Britain the period of the Commonwealth (1642–60) saw the Puritans execute the "speedy demolition of all organs". At the Restoration an influx of Dutch and émigré English builders arrived. The most noteworthy was Father Bernard Schmidt (died 1708) who introduced the "echo" organ in 1684. It was Schmidt who built London's Temple Church organ (1682–84), an instrument that was regarded as "a luxury unique in England", as well as organs for Westminster Abbey and St Paul's Cathedral. John Snetzler arrived in Britain from Switzerland around 1740. His work includes the organ used in Dublin for the first performance of Handel's *Messiah* in 1742, and that for the Lutheran Savoy Chapel in London.

Gottfried Silbermann (1683–1753) was a friend of J. S. Bach. He was

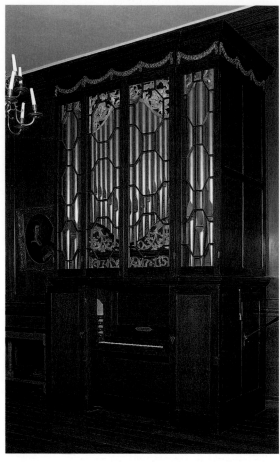

influenced by Casparini, who had built organs in northern Italy, especially Venice, and he also trained in Paris. He built a total of 45 organs in Saxony, all carefully sited for the best acoustical effect, and they remain unsurpassed. Silbermann's organs have a distinctive silvery sound, praised by Mozart as "magnificent beyond measure".

Portative organ

Emerging in the 13th century, the small portative organ was used mainly for secular purposes but also found its way into religious processions, in which it was carried suspended from a strap around the neck. It was positioned at right angles to the body for playing, allowing the player to operate the bellows with the left hand and the keys with the right. Like many "folk" instruments of its time the portative organ was fitted with drones – two tall pipes (bourdons) at the treble end.

ABOVE: *This marble relief depicts, among others, a putto playing a portative organ; the right hand plays the keys and the left hand operates the bellows.*

Positive organ

By 1425 the positive organ was being used in churches that either could not afford a large fixed organ or needed an additional chamber-size organ for occasional use such as for a service in a side chapel. It was distinct from the portative organ in that it was "moveable" rather than portable. It usually had two rows of flue pipes, a single manual and no pedalboard. An assistant was needed to operate the bellows while it was played.

Fairground organ

Gavioli of Paris started building fairground organs around 1870 to imitate a military band. One of the largest ever built had 104 keys, with large figures on each end of the front operating a bass drum and a side drum. Made by Charles Marenghi of Paris, this monstrous construction was said to reproduce the sounds of over 1200 instruments and was illuminated by hundreds of varicoloured electric lamps.

Cinema organ

Organs built by the American Wurlitzer Company in the early 20th century were designed to replace a small orchestra and to provide the perfect accompaniment to silent films. Every possible percussion instrument was imitated, including drums, telephone bells, surf, horses' hooves and even police sirens. In the United States the cinema organ died out with the advent of sound films, but in Britain it was retained and used to give short recitals before the films began.

BELOW: *An elaborate Dutch fairground organ, still a feature of many carnivals.*

French organ

In the 19th century many old organs were enlarged and improved. In France, Aristide Cavaillé-Coll, who pioneered electrically powered pneumatic tracker action, created flexible and expressive organs that inspired French composers to write a flood of large-scale secular works for solo organ. The organ symphony originated with Charles Widor (1844–1937), professor of organ at the Paris Conservatoire and organist at Ste Sulpice (1869–1933). César Franck (1822–90) was another leading figure in the French organ world and Widor's predecessor at the Conservatoire. He was organist at Ste Clotilde (1859–90) and wrote several pieces for the instrument, including *Six Pièces* (1862), *Trois Pièces* (1878) and *Trois Chorales* (1896). Franck's style is easily recognizable through its harmonic idiom and method of construction.

ABOVE: *A three-manual Wurlitzer cinema organ, looking like the deck of a jet aeroplane. The hands are kept busy with the stops and the feet have to master all the pedals.*

Accordion

*The accordion is an instrument with
the sentiments of an assassin.*

AMBROSE BIERCE (1842–1914)

The accordion is a hand-
held free-reed aerophone,
in which the sound is
produced by tempered steel
reeds that vibrate when
air is forced through
them by a set of
bellows. On one side of
the bellows there are rows
of buttons or a keyboard
on which the melody is
played, while on the other
side there are buttons for
the bass notes and chords.

Early accordions

In 1821, Christian Buschmann
(1805–64) of Berlin patented his

*LEFT: The long rows of buttons for
the right hand of the accordion
produce the melody, and the
buttons for the left hand play
the bass notes and chords.*

Handäoline, an instrument
that was worked by lever-like keys.
Seven years later, Cyrillus Demian
(1772–1847), a Viennese musician,
brought out his *Akkordion* (German for
"harmony"), which, although similar in
principle to Buschmann's instrument,
had accompanying chords. Made in
rosewood with inlays of
ivory and mother-of-pearl,
the instrument was copied by
various other musicians, who,
not being able to use the
copyrighted name, referred to
their versions by the generic term
Handharmonikas. One of the most
important advances in the history of
the accordion occurred in 1852 when
Monsieur Busson of Paris introduced
piano-type keys to the instrument.

accompaniments in all keys,
the piano accordion was still an
instrument of the people, its use
being restricted to popular and
rural entertainment in cafés, dance
halls and music halls. By 1931,
however, the accordion was
beginning to be taken seriously,
for in that year a music school for
accordionists was established in the
German town of Trossingen, a
location chosen for its vicinity to the
famous Höhner accordion factory.
The British College of Accordionists
was founded in 1936.

*ABOVE: The piano accordion has become a
folk instrument in most of Europe. Sweden
is no exception.*

Piano accordion

Although by the beginning of the 20th
century the bass keyboard had been
sufficiently developed to provide

*ABOVE: In 1852 Monsieur
Busson of Paris introduced piano-type keys
to the accordion. The advantage of the new
instrument was that it could be played
informally by ambulant performers. This
diminutive instrument is one of Busson's
first and does not have the chord and bass
keys of the more developed types.*

ABOVE: *A busker playing a piano accordion in Prague's Golden Lane.*

Modern accordion

Today's instruments have up to 140 basses actuated by seven rows of buttons and a keyboard compass ranging from two to four octaves. The usual 120-button Stradella fixed-bass keyboard, first developed by the Italian Mariano Dallape in 1876, consists of two rows of bass notes and four rows of chord buttons. Some models have a converter switch that enables chords to be played in any inversion. In Italy, a small variant of the accordion, the *organetto*, has almost replaced the *zampogna*, a type of bagpipe whose repertoire it shares.

Bandoneon

In Argentina, Uruguay and Brazil, South American tango bands often feature the bandoneon, a double-action square-shaped type of accordion. Invented in the 19th century by

ABOVE: *The double-action bandoneon is used in the tango bands of Latin America. This example was made by Wilhelm König in 1914.*

Accordion music

In 1948, when the Trossingen school became an official state academy, the first principal was Hugo Herrmann who, in 1927, had written *Sieben Neue Spielmusiker*, the first original composition for the solo accordion. Although the accordion is mainly played as a solo instrument or as part of the instrumental line-up in folk bands, many major composers have scored for it. These include Sergei Prokofiev (1891–1953) in *Cantata for the 20th Anniversary of the October Revolution* and Paul Dessau (1894–1979) in *Die Verurteilung des Lukullus*. Roberto Gerhard (1896–1970) also used the accordion in various works such as his Nonet and Concerto for Eight.

Heinrich Band of Krefeld, Germany, the early models had more than 88 notes. Today's instruments, however, are usually restricted to 71.

Concertina

Based on much the same principle as the accordion, the concertina, invented by Charles Whetstone (1802–72) in 1829, consists of two hexagonal casings, each containing a small button keyboard. The casings are connected by bellows that, when extended or contracted, cause a flow of air to activate the free reeds of the instrument when one of the keys is pressed.

There are two main types of concertina: the English, in which there

ABOVE: *The concertina is unusual in that it has 14 keys to the octave and is tuned to mean rather than equal temperament.*

is a uniform tone – the same note being sounded on both extension and contraction of the bellows – and the German, which sounds different notes on extension and compression.

Although it was played by people such as Giulio Regondi (1822–72), a guitarist and player of the *mélophone*, and Richard Blagrave (1826–95) whose playing was once described as a "first-rate workman on a miserable tool", the concertina was never a popular instrument and its use today is almost solely restricted to folk music, although composers such as Charles Ives (1874–1954) and Percy Grainger (1882–1961) did occasionally score for the instrument.

ABOVE: *South America has many accordion aficionados. This young man is playing at the Vallanato Festival in Colombia.*

Harmonium

It is astonishing what an effect the sound of some simple air played on an harmonium on a Sunday evening has on the loiterers in the streets.

MUSICAL OPINION, JUNE 1905

The harmonium, which resembles a small organ, was often used as a substitute for its big brother in small churches and chapels, as well as being popular as a household instrument. A distant relation of the mouth organ, it consists of a series of free reeds operated by a keyboard and activated by a wind supply from foot-operated compression bellows.

Early French harmonium

The harmonium evolved from Gabriel Grenié's *orgue expressif*, a free-reed keyboard instrument of about 1810. The register of Grenié's instrument was supplied by bellows

ABOVE: *The popularity of the harmonium in the 19th century was mainly due to its price. This New Cottage Harmonium cost seven guineas, a fraction of that of a piano.*

worked by two pedals. The "expression" was a stop that enabled direct contact between the bellows and the wind-reservoir by means of the pedals, thereby permitting dynamic gradations for the first time in the history of the organ.

In 1834 an improved version by the eminent French organ builder Aristide Cavaillé-Coll was exhibited at the Paris exposition. Built in the form of a small, square piano, Cavaillé-Coll's instrument, which was called the *poïkilorgue*, had a range of one and a half octaves. In 1843 Grenié's pupil Théodore-Achille Muller patented a portable model that could be folded up into a rectangular box.

Although the French were the leaders in making and perfecting

LEFT: *Built by the leading firm of Alexandre of Paris in 1859, this harmonium was widely used both in homes and churches.*

the harmonium, experiments were also being carried out in Bavaria. Here, in 1815, Bernhard Eschenbach devised a free-reed keyboard instrument that was capable of "expression", which he called an *Aoline*.

Improvements

The harmonium achieved its ultimate popularity in the form patented by the Parisian Alexandre-François Debain (1809–77) in 1842. Debain's harmonium incorporated a three-octave keyboard with sets of reeds of different thicknesses and widths. One of the new features was that each key controlled a valve that regulated the amount of wind produced by the compression bellows. This made possible, for the first time, the production of different tones. Further improvements, added by Debain in 1848, included the shifting keyboard, a device that permitted transposition by any interval, while playing the music as noted. In 1854 Victor Mustel added a divided expression stop worked by knee-levers.

Experimental harmoniums

Because of its ability to sustain a constant tone, the harmonium was well suited for acoustical experiments

and demonstrations of different tuning systems. The best known of these experimental harmoniums was that designed by Shohé Tanka and built by Johann Kewitsch of Berlin in 1889. Such was the accuracy of Tanka's instrument that it was tuned to pure intervals, with no less than 20 keys to the octave. This, however, was child's play compared with Banquet's experimental harmonium, which was constructed to produce 53 microtones to the octave.

India

The harmonium was introduced into India by missionaries around the mid 19th century to accompany hymn-singing. Since the 1920s small portable harmoniums have been made in India and Pakistan; Palitana in Gujarat Is the centre of manufacture of the reeds. Harmoniums are very popular, and many homes have one. They are widely used to accompany devotional music, to the dismay of aficionados of traditional Indian music, as their

fixed pitch is at odds with the flexible intonation of Indian vocal and instrumental music They have also led to the demise of indigenous instruments such as the *bajona sruti*, or Indian bagpipe.

As is common with Indian musicians, the harmonium player sits on the floor, playing the keyboard with one hand and operating the bellows with the other. Harmoniums are, however, now giving way in their turn to the ubiquitous electronic keyboard.

Indian harmoniums

LEFT, BELOW AND RIGHT: Small portable harmoniums have been very popular in India, with many homes owning one. The musician usually sits on the floor, playing the keyboard with one hand and operating the bellows with the other.

Mechanical Instruments

*A good melody is such a one as would grind
about the streets upon the organ.*

THOMAS ARNE (1710–78)

In the years before recording and broadcasting, instruments that played pre-set tunes became popular. When no musician was available, turning a handle could provide music, whether at home, for street entertainment, dancing, or for church services.

Barrel organ

The barrel organ made its appearance in Italy in the early 1700s. One of the first makers of the instrument was Giovanni Barbieri of Modena; his name was perpetuated by the French, who called the Italian's invention *orgue de Barbarie*. However, by 1774 many had obviously forgotten the Italian's pioneer work, for in that year an advertisement appeared offering for sale *"Un veritable orgue de barbarie fait par les sauvages."*

These early constructions were small enough to rest on the player's left hip

LEFT: This 19th-century English barrel organ has three barrels. Two play dance music and popular songs, while the third provides hymn tunes.

while the right hand turned the handle. The barrel organ's mechanism consisted of two or more ranks of organ pipes placed above a set of bellows in an enclosed cabinet, while the music was supplied by a pinned cylinder or barrel that was mounted on a metal spindle. Each pin raised a trigger-shaped key that opened a pallet, allowing wind to enter the required pipe. Each tune required one complete rotation of the barrel.

In the 19th century, with the demand for longer and more complicated music, barrel organs became larger and larger. In 1887 Michael Welte patented an instrument in which the barrels were pegged spirally and rotated 12 times during one piece of music, making it possible for quite long compositions to be played.

Street organ

In the early 19th century an Italian named Gavioli, who was established in Paris, started making portable organs in which the barrel was replaced by perforated cardboard strips, concertina-folded and based on the

THE STREET ORGAN.

LEFT: The organ grinder was once a familiar sight in the streets of most European towns, surrounded by children. The music made a welcome break in an otherwise monotonous day.

card patterns used by jacquard weavers. Gavioli's organs were often mounted on handcarts and wheeled about by "organ grinders", who were invariably accompanied by little monkeys. These organs were very successful and were seen on the streets of most European cities until well into the 20th century.

Church barrel organ

Until the introduction of the harmonium, many small churches and chapels used a "barrel and finger organ" as a substitute for a conventional organ. These were so-called because they had a conventional keyboard at the front and a barrel movement at the back. The barrels were pegged with hymns, chants, psalms and even voluntaries so that if no organist was available for a service, music could still be produced by turning the handle.

ABOVE: Early barrel pianos, operated by turning a handle, were quite small domestic instruments.

ABOVE: An orchestrion or "orchestral organ", showing the internal mechanisms, including the pipes and barrel.

Orchestrion

The main drawback of the barrel organ was its monotonous sound, and in an attempt to rectify this the orchestrion was invented. Intended for indoor use in wealthy households, the orchestrion was composed of ranks of organ pipes of differing timbres that were constructed to imitate the sounds of orchestral instruments. It was an elaborate assembly with refined cabinet work and had as many as eight ranks of pipes with a chromatic compass of over five octaves, plus percussion instruments such as cymbals, drums and triangles.

One of the first successful orchestrions was built in Holland in 1789. Said to be capable of imitating a whole orchestra, it was encased in a 3m/10ft cube and was complete with four manuals and a pedalboard for obtaining *crescendos* and *diminuendos*. The componium, a Dutch invention of 1821, could compose variations on a theme, using two movable barrels.

Apollonicon

In 1817, Flight & Robson of London exhibited their massive apollonicon, which had been constructed the previous year. No less than 7.2m/24ft in height and 6m/20ft wide and deep, it had nearly 2000 pipes, disposed in 46 registers. It had five manuals that could be played either mechanically or, when detached from the main body, manually by five performers, all facing the public. It was displayed and operated in the window of the company's London showroom for some years, but was not a financial success and was dismantled in 1840.

Music box

Small musical movements were first made in the late 18th century for snuff boxes. By the 1830s the music box was established in its standard form, with tuning combs that had as many as 250 teeth covering a range of about six octaves. Many of these boxes were finely decorated and embellished with marquetry and mother-of-pearl. The early combs were fitted to cylinders, but by the 1890s disc-operated boxes were appearing, with discs up to 85cm/34in in diameter. They were eclipsed by the arrival of the gramophone.

ABOVE: This internal view of a music box built in the last year of the 19th century in Sainte-Croix, Switzerland, shows the steel comb whose tuned tongues are plucked by pins on the clockwork-driven cylinder, as well as the bells and drum.

Electronic Keyboards and Computers

The synthesizer is no more inhuman than the piano.

MILTON BABBITT (BORN 1916)

One of the first electronic instruments was Thaddeus Cahill's keyboard-operated "dynamophone" or "telharmonium", the first full-size version of which was completed in 1906. It supplied current to telephone receivers fitted with cardboard horns, and was used for daily concerts. Although the aim of the instrument was "to generate music electrically with tones of good quality", Cahill's pioneer work was too far ahead of its time and his invention was eventually sold for scrap, but his ideas were the basis of later developments during the 1920s and '30s.

Theremin

The Russian scientist Lev Theremin invented the theremin in 1924. Its signals were produced by oscillators, and were modified by the position of the player's hands. Volume was controlled by the proximity of one hand to a metal loop, and pitch by moving the other hand towards or away from an antenna protruding vertically out of the instrument. Although some musicians were able to demonstrate its vocal qualities, it was very difficult to play and as such did not become widely used. The radical composer Edgard Varèse (1885–1965) used two theremins in *Ecuatorial* (1934) but later replaced them with the more reliable *ondes Martenot*.

LEFT: The electronic keyboard has become one of the most important instruments in many small bands. The sound of almost every instrument of the orchestra — and other sounds — can be achieved.

Ondes Martenot

The *ondes Martenot*, invented by the French musician and engineer Maurice Martenot (1896–1980), was produced in 1928. Although its oscillating valves are similar to those of the theremin, it is very much easier to control the pitch produced, as the player is guided by a five-octave keyboard. A substantial number of works have been written for it, and it produces haunting sounds.

Hammond organ

The American Laurens Hammond invented the Hammond organ in 1935, with the intention of replacing the pipe organ for both church and domestic use. Like the conventional organ, it has two small manuals and a pedalboard, but produces sounds electronically. This versatile organ became very popular in the 1960s,

RIGHT: The eponymous Hammond organ, with its ability to produce (albeit limited) special effects, was a forerunner of the modern electronic keyboard.

especially with rock musicians. Special stops and tabs control the manuals and produce effects such as "wah-wahs", *glissandos* and arpeggios.

Synthesizer

The first synthesizer of major importance was the RCA Mark II, which was acquired in 1959 by the Columbia-Princeton Electronic Music Center in New York. It had been developed at the Sarnoff Research Center, New Jersey, from the Mark I of 1955 by Harry Olsen and Herbert

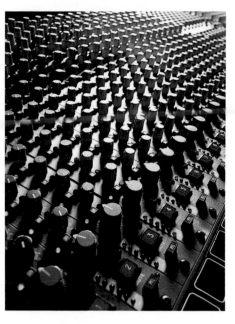

ABOVE: Composing music has come a long way from the quill pen of Purcell to the MIDI keyboard and computer of the modern composer.

ABOVE: A mixing desk is standard equipment in the modern recording studio.

Belar. Using transistors instead of valves, it was much smaller than the Mark I, a colossal machine that almost filled a room with controls for the multitude of oscillators, mixers, filters and amplifier.

Since 1966 much smaller synthesizers have been made available commercially, including the Moog Sonic Six and the Buchla. Originally developed for producing tapes for recordings, by the mid 1960s synthesizers had reached the concert platform as chordal instruments for live performances, and were especially popular with rock bands.

Although the synthesizer keyboard looks like that of a piano, it behaves in a different way: it controls not only the pitch of a note (which may not be the same as that on a piano), but also its length. Some keyboards are touch-sensitive so that, depending on the way the keys are depressed or released, different functions may be performed.

Some modern synthesizers, such as the Kawai CP150, have dummy keyboards to give the performer the feeling of playing a "real" piano. The Kawai CP150 has a unique weighted action with wooden keys that simulate a hammer action by using a dummy hammer within the mechanism. The effect is so natural that in time the action beds down and settles in, just like a real piano keyboard.

Digital revolution

Today almost every recording studio has an abundance of computer-related equipment. The music is digitally saved on to a hard disk and then edited on a mixing desk using sophisticated software before the final version is mastered on to digital audio tape. This Musical Instrument Digital Interface (MIDI) deals with all aspects of the performance, including pitch, velocity and duration. As well as the MIDI keyboard, there are conventional MIDI instruments that connect electronically with the mixing desk. Even acoustic instruments can have tiny microphones attached to convert analogue pitch into digital information. Such is modern technology that it is almost possible to play a flute concerto on a kazoo.

ABOVE: This mixing desk, a Virtua Digital Console, has eliminated the need for long rows of buttons and dials.

ABOVE: The computer combines all the functions of a mixing desk and multi-track tape machine to create a "virtual studio".

The Voice

The Human Instrument

Song is man's sweetest joy.

ARISTOTLE (384–322 BC)

The fundamental musical instrument is the human voice. Singing is the most natural and spontaneous mode of musical expression, and since it is almost always linked to a text it can unambiguously express thought as well as emotion. As the singer is his or her own instrument, the voice is never altogether distanced from the personality. However, a good voice does not make a singer unless it is combined with accurate rhythm, good sense of pitch and enunciation. As in other instruments, the sound of the voice is the result of amplified vibrations. The vibrations of the

ABOVE: *Boys' choirs have been a feature of Christian ritual for a thousand years. As women were banned from taking part in the service, when polytonal music developed it was the youthful soprano voices that sang the top line of the music, while men sang the alto and baritone lines.*

ABOVE: *Diana Ross was a founder member of the Supremes, one of the singing groups that emerged from Detroit in the 1960s.*

vocal cords resonate in the cavities of both the chest (in the lower register) and the head (in the upper register). The singer automatically adjusts the shapes and sizes of these cavities to produce the required notes.

Vocal ranges

When men and women sing together, men usually sing an octave lower: the normal range of women's voices is in the treble clef, and the men's is in the bass clef. Each voice has its own natural range of pitch. The highest woman's voice is the soprano, and the lowest the contralto, or alto, with the mezzo-soprano lying between the two extremes. These pitches are also within the range of boys' voices (known as trebles).

The lowest male voice is the bass and the highest is usually the tenor, with the baritone between them. Some male singers have a natural extension at the top of their range which allows them to sing in the alto, or countertenor, range.

Madrigals

The early church forbade women to participate in services, so treble parts were sung by boys and countertenors.

Until the 15th century most music was written for high voices, but with the expansion of polyphony, songs began to feature two parts below the tenor and the qualities of the bass voice became better appreciated.

By the 16th century all secular music used vocal ranges that were comfortable for male voices, with countertenor parts never going above *d"*. When women joined singing groups, madrigals with parts as high as *g"* appeared. Madrigal singers and composers became increasingly interested in secular music and the ornamentation – forbidden in church music – that could be added to it.

Opera

The birth of opera between 1575 and 1625 resulted in an entirely new kind of singer. The madrigal singer had a relatively limited range, rarely exceeding an octave and a half. Opera singers began to extend their range, both up and down, to accommodate the composers who were experimenting in new forms of vocal music, just as instrument makers were experimenting in the construction of musical instruments.

Voice production

Singing styles and techniques before the advent of sound recordings are even harder to study than instrumental playing styles, as once the singer has died their voice is forever lost. There is no surviving instrument to help with research into the lost sound.

Although styles of singing changed, the Italian method of voice production, known as *bel canto* ("beautiful singing"), remained the same from the time of Monteverdi to that of Rossini. The main characteristic of *bel canto* voice production is the forward-placing of the voice, with a concentration of resonance in the nasal cavities to give a light, florid effect.

ABOVE: The music of a cathedral choir is a joy to hear in a candlelit setting.

ABOVE: The British mezzo-soprano Anne Murray (born 1949) was especially praised for her Covent Garden performance of the title role in Handel's Xerxes *in 1985.*

In the 20th century there were two main developments in singing. One is the *verismo*, or realistic style, as perfected by Enrico Caruso (1872–1921). Operatic composers around 1900 – particularly Italians such as Pietro Mascagni (1863–1945) and Giacomo Puccini (1858–1924) – began to write operas with more contemporary, realistic plots, for which the artifice of the traditional *bel canto* vocal style was unsuitable.

The second development was due to the invention of electronic amplification. Until the 1920s there was little difference between classical and popular singing. However, as popular singers began to use microphones, new singing styles developed. There was now no need to project the voice as before. Because it was easier for sound engineers to amplify a soft voice, early radio performers who sang with light, intimate voices were preferred.

ABOVE: The London Philharmonic Choir in rehearsal.

Choirs

Let the pealing organ blow To the full-voiced quire below
In service high and anthems clear.

JOHN MILTON (1608—74)

Organized choral singing has been known for at least 3000 years, since it is mentioned in Homer's *Iliad*, composed in about 850 BC. The ancient Greek chorus, from which choirs derive, included dancers as well as singers, and participated as a group in religious festivals. Some of these groups were very large, and could comprise up to 600 people. In Greek drama, the chorus provided a moral commentary on the action. Tragedies had a chorus of between 12 and 15 people, while comedies had from 24—50.

Polyphony

Choral music, in the form of plainsong, was an essential component of services in the early church. Early medieval choirs were small: they usually consisted of from four to eight boys and from 10 to 18 men, women being absolutely excluded from church services. One of the largest choirs of the 12th and 13th centuries was that of Notre-Dame in Paris, which consisted of almost 30 singers.

As polyphonic composition gradually replaced unharmonized chant, the range of voices widened. The earliest surviving mass, by Guillaume de Machaut (c.1300—77) is written in four parts. Antiphonal music, which was developed at St Mark's in Venice by Andrea and Giovanni Gabrieli, involved a solo voice and a choir, or two or more contrasting choirs, who sang verses and responses from different parts of the church. The increasing richness and complexity

ABOVE: A 14th-century French church choir. These singers are sharing a single manuscript copy of their text and musical line.

Vienna Boys Choir

The Hofmusikkapelle, which evolved into the world-famous Wiener Sängerknaben (the Vienna Boys Choir), was founded in 1498 by the Holy Roman Emperor Maximilian I. Its original purpose was to provide musical training for the choir of the Hofburg in Vienna. Now, however, it is a private boarding school. The 150 boys are divided into four choirs, each of which tours Europe and the United States for three months of the year.

ABOVE: The world-famous Vienna Boys Choir.

ABOVE: *To say that the Welsh love singing is like saying that fish like swimming. Almost every village has its own choir, an institution that binds the communities together.*

century, choral singing has been an important focal activity of the *eisteddfod* since it was first introduced in 1825. For many years virtually the only songs the singers knew were hymns, but by the second half of the 19th century cantatas, oratorios and works by contemporary Welsh composers such as Joseph Parry (1841–1903) and David Jenkins (1849–1915) were added to the repertoire.

During the 20th century many outstanding choirs were formed, and choral festivals have included Harlech (1867–1934), Cardiff (1892–1910) and the Three Valleys Festival (1930–39). Since 1947 choral singers from all over the world have flocked to Llangollen for the annual International Eisteddfod.

ABOVE: *A girls' choir performing at a concert.*

of polyphony culminated in works by the Roman school, led by Giovanni Pierluigi da Palestrina (1525–94).

Church choir

The sung mass became one of the most important forms of church music. Composers of all periods have written settings of it, and choral singing has a central role in almost every religious service. Renaissance choirs sang in a minimum of four parts, often six, eight or more. The choirs grew larger, and were accompanied by instrumental groups. After the Reformation, Protestant choirs were modelled on the Catholic pattern, and women therefore continued to be excluded, preserving the tradition of using boys' voices. This tradition is only gradually being challenged.

Choral societies

The overwhelming popularity of Handel's oratorios in late 18th-century Britain – especially *The Messiah* (1742) – led to the formation of new choral

societies, which did include women, in almost every town. At first only religious music was sung, including, as well as Handel, Haydn's *Creation* (1799) and later Mendelssohn's *Elijah* (1846), but secular music eventually crept in, such as the popular songs of Gilbert and Sullivan's Savoy Operas.

Choral singing reached extraordinarily high standards in Germany, where choral societies grew up in the industrial towns, a movement that was fostered by numerous choral festivals, such as those held at Frankenhausen, Mannheim, Magdeburg and Halle. Excellent folk choirs still flourish today.

Male voice choir

One country synonymous with choral singing is Wales. Growing up with the enormous rise in the urban population in the early 19th

ABOVE: *The choir of St John's College Chapel, Cambridge.*

Soloists

Let but thy voice engender with the string
And angels will be born, while thou doest sing.

ROBERT HERRICK (1591–1674)

The earliest solo singers were poet-composers who sang their own songs, and few singers were famous as soloists before the mid 16th century. However, they acquired greater importance as secular music became more highly ornamented. At the same time, women began to perform as singers, and a preference for the soprano voice was established. The birth of opera, which drew its earliest performers from the ranks of popular court singers of madrigals, eventually led to the rise of the professional opera star. Although many singers restrict their singing to one medium, such as opera or recital work, some have made a name for themselves in both.

ABOVE: Adelina Patti was famous for her wealth and for never attending rehearsals, but was a great actress.

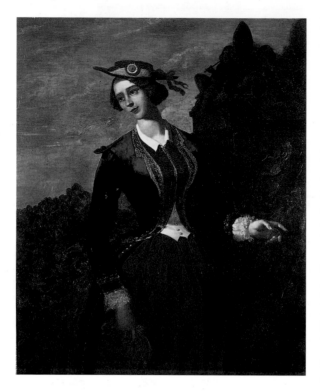

ABOVE: Jenny Lind, "The Swedish Nightingale", was the pop idol of the mid 19th century. She was in such demand that tickets for her concerts were usually sold out within hours of being put on sale.

Male voices

One of the best examples of operatic singers "going solo" is the outstanding success of Luciano Pavarotti (born 1935), José Carreras (born 1946) and Plácido Domingo (born 1941) – three men whose successes in opera have been equalled if not excelled by their appearance as "The Three Tenors" at concerts held in conjunction with the three football World Cup finals in Italy (1990), the United States (1994) and France (1998).

Without doubt the most popular tenor of his generation, Pavarotti, with his trademark white handkerchief in his left hand, has brought operatic arias to enormous audiences. His recording of *Nessun dorma*, an aria from Puccini's *Turandot* that was used as the theme song of Italia '90, hit the pop charts worldwide. Many people who had hitherto felt alienated from opera realized the beauties of the music they had so long resisted.

Some classically trained male singers have deliberately pursued a solo career rather than performing in opera. These include the Austrian Richard Tauber (1892–1948), the Irish singer Josef Locke (1917–99) and the German Ivan Rebroff, whose fantastic voice ranges from the ultra bass, which must be one of the deepest known, to a high falsetto.

Female voices

One of the most popular singers of the 19th century was Jenny Lind (1820–87), known as the "Swedish Nightingale", whose appearances often caused more excitement than a royal visit. On more than one occasion when Lind was singing in London the House of Commons was unable to continue business as there were not enough MPs present to constitute a quorum – they were all at her concert. Her singing was so pure that her audiences could hardly believe that such powers existed in the human voice. She was married to the conductor Otto Goldschmidt, who often accompanied her on the

piano. Another factor that endeared her to the public was her custom of donating part of her salary to a charitable institution in whichever town she performed.

Another 19th-century diva was the *coloratura* soprano Adelina Patti (1843–1919), who began her career as a child prodigy in the United States. Hearing her voice so affected Rossini that he rewrote the role of Rosina in *The Barber of Seville* for her. He once said to her: "Madam, I have cried twice in my life. Once when I dropped a wing of chicken into Lake Como, and once when for the first time I heard you sing."

Joan Sutherland (born 1926) is arguably the 20th century's finest *coloratura* soprano, and made many of the great roles of Delibes, Massenet, Rossini, Donizetti and Bellini her own. She conquered the world in 1959 with

her performance in Donizetti's *Lucia di Lammermoor*, her rich and agile voice making her one of the most popular singers of the time. She gave her

farewell performance on New Year's Eve 1990, in a guest appearance with the American mezzo-soprano Marilyn Horne and Luciano Pavarotti in the Covent Garden production of Johann Strauss's operetta *Die Fledermaus*.

Kiri Te Kanawa (born 1944) had begun her recording career by the time she was 20. One of the most famous sopranos of modern times, she made her debut as the Countess in *Le nozze di Figaro* at Covent Garden in 1971.

ABOVE: *One of the most remarkable "discoveries" of the 1990s was "The Three Tenors". The trio of Plácido Domingo, José Carreras and Luciano Pavarotti brought opera to enormous audiences worldwide, especially at the three football World Cup finals in Italy (1990), the United States (1994) and France (1998).*

ABOVE: *Kiri Te Kanawa has become one of the most famous sopranos in the world. She is seen here giving one of her popular solo concerts.*

Other Voices

God giveth speech to all, song to the few.

WALTER CHALMERS SMITH

Many composers, particularly in modern times, have sought to use the voice as an instrument in new and unusual ways, whether by extending its range outside the normal compass or by incorporating vocal sounds other than singing into their music. The style called *Sprechgesang* that Schoenberg used in *Pierrot Lunaire* (1912) falls between singing and speaking. Humming is a device that is often used in choral works, and sometimes in solos: Villa-Lobos's *Bachianas Brasileiras No. 5* uses a solo soprano voice humming a soaring tune, accompanied by cellos. Speech and shouting add new colours to choral writing, and the use of the microphone has opened up many new possibilities for vocal effects, in rock and pop as well as serious music.

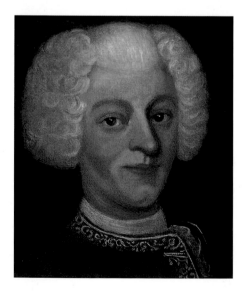

ABOVE: The castrato Carlo Broschi Farinelli (1705–82) sang all over Europe, including a three-year stay in London.

Castrati

The castrato, whose voice was prevented from breaking by castration in childhood, first appeared in church choirs to sing the high parts that women, who were banned from the church, supplied in secular music. In the late 16th and early 17th century castrati found a role in the new medium of opera, and opera composers began to write special parts for them.

Some castrati achieved great wealth. One of the most famous of the 18th century was the Italian Carlo Broschi Farinelli, whose voice, it was claimed, was able to reach and sustain seven or eight notes above any other singer of the period. Farinelli's artistry was such that when King Philip V of Spain heard him he was so impressed that he commissioned the Italian to sing him four arias a night for the rest of his life. When Philip died, his successor Ferdinand VI awarded Farinelli the rank of prince and a generous pension.

The barbaric practice of castration for artistic purposes eventually died out, and castrati were banned from the papal chapel in 1903. The last castrato, Alessandro Moreschi, who had been musical director of the Sistine Chapel, died in 1922, aged 66.

Jazz singing

An oratorical style of singing that exploits the contours and cadences of speech, jazz singing is concerned with emphasizing the text rather than the tone. Because jazz singers usually follow the dynamics of speech rather than of the melody, their voices tend to be low-pitched; soprano jazz singers are very rare.

In some jazz styles the interest lies in musical effect rather than emotional content, a prime example being scat singing. This is a wordless performance, usually improvised, that uses the voice like an instrument. Although many jazz singers include scat singing in their acts, not many are capable of keeping it up for more than 32 bars. Louis Armstrong's solos in the 1920s and '30s began a vogue for the style.

ABOVE: Jazz singing has arisen from the traditions of blues singing and popular songs. It usually involves improvisation to fit the lyrics to the music.

Human voice orchestra

In the 19th century there were various choral groups that sang not words but sounds. One such was Hoffmann's Organophonic Band or "human voice orchestra". Wearing military uniform, the 12 members, who imitated by voice alone a complete orchestra of instruments, were popular over most of Europe. This type of wordless singing was revived in the 1960s by the Swingle Singers.

Yodelling

Yodelling is the sudden change from chest voice to falsetto head voice and back again in rapid alternation. It originated in the Swiss mountains where it was, and still is, intended to be a joyful sound. In the 1930s yodelling entered American blues music where, instead of being a happy sound, it was turned into a lonesome and sad expression, first typified by Jimmy Rodgers and copied by many others since.

ABOVE: The French-Canadian singer Celine Dion (born 1967) made the transition from child star to French-language chanteuse to an internationally acclaimed ballad singer.

RIGHT: A Tyrolean yodelling party in national costume.

Composition
through
the Ages

A beautiful example of a medieval choirbook emanating from Germany, now in the State Library in Gdańsk, Poland. The pages illustrated show the beginning of the plainsong chant for the antiphon Rorate coeli, used in the liturgy for the Ascension season.

Music as a Language

We — are we not formed, as notes of music are,
For one another, though dissimilar?

<small>PERCY BYSSHE SHELLEY (1792–1822), "EPIPSYCHIDION"</small>

Musical composition is one of the most mysterious of all art forms. People who can easily come to terms with a work of literature or a painting are still often baffled by the process by which a piece of music – appearing in material form as notation – must then be translated back into sound through the medium of a third party – the performer. Unlike a painting, a musical composition cannot be owned (except by its creator); and although a score may be published, like a book, it may remain incomprehensible to the general public until it is performed. Although a piece may be played thousands of times, each repetition is entirely individual, and interpretations by different players may vary widely.

ABOVE: An early example of neumatic notation, from a German illustrated liturgical manuscript.

Origins of musical notation

The earliest musical compositions were circumscribed by the range of the human voice. People from all cultures have always sung, or used primitive instruments to make sounds. Notation, or the writing down of music, developed to enable performers to remember what they had improvised, to preserve what they had created, and to facilitate interaction between more than one performer. Musical notation, like language, has ancient origins, dating back to the Middle East in the third millennium BC. The ancient Greeks appear to have been the first to try to represent variations of musical pitch through the medium of the alphabet, and successive civilizations all over the world attempted to formulate similar systems of recognizable musical notation.

Neumatic notation

The earliest surviving Western European notational system was called "neumatic notation" – a system of symbols which attempted to portray the rise and fall of a melodic line. These date back to the 9th century AD, and were associated with the performance of sacred music – particularly plainsong – in monastic institutions. Several early manuscript

ABOVE: An early example of musical notation, a 3rd-century BC Greek song. The letters above the text indicate the notes.

ABOVE: *Guido d'Arezzo (c.977–1050), who devised the hexachord. His statue stands outside the Uffizi Gallery in Florence.*

sources contain sacred texts with accompanying notation, although there was no standard system. The first appearance of staff notation, in which pitch was indicated by noteheads on or between lines with a symbol called a clef at the beginning to fix the pitch of one note, was in the 9th-century French treatise *Musica enchiriadis*. At the same time, music for instruments (particularly organ and lute) was beginning to be written down in diagrammatic form known as tablature, which indicated the positions of the player's fingers.

Guido d'Arezzo

The 11th-century Italian monk Guido d'Arezzo invented the "solmization" system — the precursor of "tonic solfa" — in which various syllables were used to indicate pitches in a musical scale. He also invented the "Guidonian Hand", in which the tips and joints of the five fingers

were used as an aid to remembering the various notes. At the same time, attempts were being made to indicate rhythm in performance, by varying the length and angle of the tails of the neumes, and the earliest polyphony (the simultaneous performance of more than one melodic line) was being explored.

The modal system

From around 400 BC until AD 1500, European music was built on modes. In the 4th century BC, the Greek mathematician Pythagoras worked out a scale roughly corresponding to the (modern-day) white keys of the piano, and two centuries later this scale was being used by the Greeks in seven different ways. The early Christian church adopted four so-called "authentic" modes (corresponding to white-note scales beginning on D, E, F and G), and under the 6th-century Pope Gregory, four more modes were added for the performance of plainsong.

ABOVE: *Pope Gregory (c.540–604), who gave his name to "Gregorian" plainsong melodies for liturgical use.*

ABOVE: *The so-called "Guidonian Hand", Guido d'Arezzo's device for showing the notes of the scale.*

In 1547, the Swiss monk Henricus Glareanus postulated the theory of 12 modes, giving them somewhat inauthentic Greek names:

Dorian (range D–D)
HypoDorian (range A–A)
Phrygian (range E–E)
HypoPhrygian (range B–B)
Lydian (range F–F)
HypoLydian (range C–C)
Mixolydian (range G–G)
HypoMixolydian (range D–D)
Aeolian (range A–A)
HypoAeolian (range E–E)
Ionian (range C–C)
HypoIonian (range G–G)

Of these, the Aeolian and Ionian modes later became the basis of the minor and major scales respectively, which have since underpinned Western European music. The modes finally gave way to the keys we know today with the development of harmony in the late Renaissance period.

Emergence of Composers

Lovely forms do flow
From conceit divinely framed;
Heaven is music.

THOMAS CAMPION (1567–1620), "OBSERVATIONS IN THE ART OF ENGLISH POESIE"

Much medieval music survives in manuscript anthologies, some copied by monks for a particular monastery, others – often exquisitely illuminated – commissioned by an aristocratic patron. The earliest surviving ones date from the 10th century. Among the most famous manuscripts are two 15th-century English sources, the Old Hall Manuscript and the Eton College Choirbook. There are also two French sources dating from around 1470, the beautiful heart-shaped *Chansonnier cordiforme* and the *Mellon chansonnier*. Many pieces in these manuscripts are anonymous, but some were attributed to individual composers.

Ars antiqua

The Parisian composers Léonin and Pérotin were among the finest exponents of the style called *ars antiqua*, or "ancient style", a method of harmonizing plainsong melodies by adding between one and three secondary voices to the main vocal line, moving in parallel motion. This was known as *conductus*, and was an early form of polyphony – a compositional technique in which several melodic lines are combined, moving independently (as opposed to

ABOVE: An example of the ars antiqua *– a page from the* Jeu de Robin et Marion *by Adam de la Halle (1230–c.1288).*

homophony, in which the voices move together, forming blocks of harmony). European music was dominated by the polyphonic principle from the 13th to the 16th centuries.

By the 13th century, musical notation had become more sophisticated and standardized, with only the finer points of rhythmic

notation still open to interpretation. *Conductus* was gradually superseded by a new form known as the motet, a sacred Latin song, usually with a Biblical text, in which other voices moved in counterpoint to the main tune. The motet has remained a standard form of liturgical music.

Ars nova

At the same time, secular songs, such as those sung by French troubadours and *trouvères*, were being written down. Their flexibility and tunefulness led to the development of a new style (*ars nova*) in the 14th century, initiated by the theorist Philippe de Vitry. The music of the *ars nova*, which flourished particularly in France and Italy, had greater rhythmic vitality, and composers such as Guillaume de Machaut began to experiment with new techniques such as isorhythm, in which the same rhythmic pattern appears in successive repetitions of the melody, but not necessarily using notes of the same value. Many motets of the period were based on this technique, and on a *cantus firmus* – a familiar tune (either a plainsong melody or a folk song) which underpinned a polyphonic composition

increasing sophistication of musical instruments. This was the invention of "monody", a new style in which the old principle of equal voices moving in counterpoint gave way to a single vocal line accompanied by instruments. While the tenor line still carried the main tune of a composition, it was now underpinned by a "ground bass", or *basso continuo* – a strong bass line played on keyboard and reinforced by cello and other bass instruments, which provided a harmonic foundation. The new style – the basis of all Baroque music – originated in Florence, where the composer Giulio Caccini published a famous collection of monodies, *Nuove musiche*, in 1602. The invention of monody coincided with the birth of a new secular musical genre, opera. The concept of a drama set to music, performed by costumed singers with instrumental accompaniment, originated in Florence with early examples by Peri and Caccini. Its greatest early exponent was Claudio Monteverdi.

ABOVE: An example of ars nova *notation – an anonymous 14th-century French virelai (song). Note the increasing complexity of the notation.*

by appearing throughout, usually in the tenor line.

By 1500 the system of Western European musical notation had become largely standardized, and from then onwards it became increasingly sophisticated and refined. The 16th century (the High Renaissance) was dominated by the principle of polyphony, brought to a height of perfection by composers such as Palestrina in Italy, Lassus in Germany, Victoria in Spain, and William Byrd in England.

Radical change of style

Around 1600, a musical sea-change occurred, partly as a reaction against polyphony, partly as a result of the secularization of society, and the

ABOVE: An exquisitely illuminated page from the 15th-century Squarcialupi codex showing Francesco Landini (c.1325–97) with the score of his madrigal Musica son.

Baroque Forms

[Opera is] one of the most magnificent and expenseful diversions the wit of man can invent.

JOHN EVELYN (1620–1706), DIARY, 1645

Music in the Baroque era (c.1600–1750) was dominated by an insatiable demand for recreational art-forms. The great aristocratic and royal households, which could support their own orchestras, also employed composers to supply a constant need for new works. In 18th-century Europe, the growing size and wealth of the new middle classes led to a gradual democratization of musical appreciation and the advent of public performances in new concert halls and opera houses.

Music and drama

Opera became a favourite entertainment at the many princely courts which dotted Europe; the first public opera house opened in Venice in 1637, followed by others in major European cities. New musical forms were developed to suit the genre, including recitative and aria: the recitative allowed the singer (accompanied only by keyboard) to advance the story rapidly; while the aria, accompanied by the orchestra, allowed for expansive and lyrical reflection on a given situation or emotion.

The Baroque era was dominated by *opera seria*, based on plots drawn from ancient mythology, legend or history, with heroic characters fulfilling their destinies according to approved behavioural concepts. The most prolific 17th-century opera composers included

ABOVE: A sumptuous court entertainment of 1747 in the Teatro Argentina in Rome to celebrate the marriage of the son of Louis XV.

Alessandro Scarlatti and Antonio Vivaldi in Italy, Reinhard Keiser in Germany, and Jean-Baptiste Lully in France.

But by far the greatest exponent of Italian *opera seria* was Handel, who managed to make his characters express real human emotions. His operas have survived, while works by his contemporaries have been consigned to history. *Opera seria* lasted into Mozart's time, but by then audiences were demanding a lighter, more naturalistic type of drama, often dealing with comic subject-matter, which flowered in the hands of Gluck and especially Mozart.

Oratorio

Despite initial resistance, not even the church could remain unaffected by these new developments. A sacred – and normally unstaged – type of musical drama called oratorio, using the same musical forms as opera, but based on biblical stories, came into

being. Most opera composers (such as Scarlatti and Vivaldi) also wrote oratorios, but again it was Handel's fine examples which have survived to the present day. Bach's *St John* and *St Matthew Passions*, relating the story of Christ's death according to the Gospels, belong to this genre.

Instrumental forms

A growing demand for purely instrumental music led to the development of other new forms, such as the sonata. This was conceived both as a form suitable for church performance – the *sonata da chiesa*, which the Italian composer Corelli developed as a standard four-movement form – and its lighter counterpart the *sonata da camera*, which had an unspecified number of dance-like movements. Dance types – gavotte, minuet, courante, allemande, gigue – found their way into instrumental compositions, and their enormous variety formed the basis of the Baroque suite, perfected by Bach and Handel.

Another new form was the concerto, a genre pioneered by Giovanni Gabrieli in the late 1500s, in which a small group of instruments (later one solo instrument) is contrasted with the main body of the orchestra (the earlier form is known as a *concerto grosso*). While Renaissance music had exalted the principle of equality, Baroque music thrived on contrast.

Transition to Classicism

The still, sad music of humanity.

WILLIAM WORDSWORTH (1770–1850), "TINTERN ABBEY"

Baroque music reached its zenith in the works of Bach and Handel. Bach concentrated on sacred music, notably in his many cantatas – dramatic works for voices and instruments intended for church performance; Handel worked in both secular and sacred genres, writing Italian operas and English oratorios. The opening instrumental overtures, or "sinfonias", of such pieces gradually expanded into the 18th-century symphony, which eventually settled into a standard four-movement form with an opening fast movement, a lyrical slow movement, a short dance movement (usually a minuet and trio) and a fast finale. This was the form which Joseph Haydn perfected in over 100 examples, together with another new instrumental genre, the string quartet, written for two violins, viola and cello.

Sonata form

These works, together with the Classical sonata itself, were dominated by the structural principle of "sonata form", in which an opening exposition, usually presenting two main, contrasting themes, is succeeded by a central "development" section, in which the themes are subjected to a variety of treatments. Then comes

ABOVE: *A group of musicians playing stringed and keyboard instruments at the court of the Duke of Modena in the late 17th century, painted by Antonio Gabbiani (1652–1726).*

a "recapitulation", in which the opening themes are repeated (often in shortened or slightly varied form),

followed by a short "coda" to round off the movement.

Haydn's great Viennese contemporaries Mozart and Beethoven consolidated and developed the symphony and string quartet, as well as the solo concerto – which was now becoming primarily a vehicle for one virtuoso performer. As the 18th-century harpsichord gave way to the more powerful and reliable pianoforte, the piano concerto – and the solo piano sonata – became favoured forms from Mozart's time onwards.

ABOVE: *An 18th-century concert with wind, string and keyboard players held at a private Italian palazzo (probably in Venice).*

The Romantic Heyday

There is nothing stable in the world; uproar's your only music.

JOHN KEATS (1795–1821)

While Napoleon Bonaparte swept across Europe, toppling the decadent aristocratic rulers of the *ancien régime*, Beethoven's powerful musical vision heralded a new age of individualism. His massive *Eroica* Symphony (No. 3) pushed Classical symphonic form to its limits, while his Sixth (*Pastoral*) Symphony showed how music could be used to illustrate humanity's relationship with nature (a favourite concept of the Romantic era, as illustrated in the art and literature of the period). Meanwhile, as aristocratic patronage declined, the burgeoning middle classes began to demand music on a domestic scale for private enjoyment – a market filled by the music of

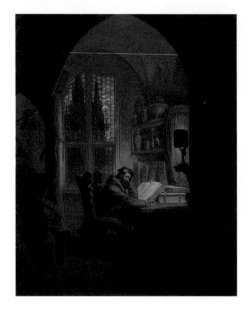

ABOVE: One of the seminal literary works of Romanticism – an artist's impression of Goethe's Faust in his study, painted in 1829.

Schubert, Schumann, Chopin, Mendelssohn and Brahms, who produced songs with piano accompaniment, chamber music (for combinations of string and wind instruments) and solo piano pieces.

The rapid expansion of the orchestra during this period, together with the invention of new instruments such as the clarinet and the improvement of existing ones, particularly woodwind and brass, led to the creation of much larger ensembles with increased power, colour and tonal range. These demanded new types of music on a vastly expanded scale. In line with the expansionist vision of the 19th century, the symphonic canvases of Schumann, Brahms, Bruckner and Mahler became

ABOVE: A typical Romantic seascape: Moonrise over the Sea, *by Caspar David Friedrich (1774–1840).*

ABOVE: *An impression of Wotan from Wagner's massive operatic cycle* Der Ring des Nibelungen *(1853–74).*

ABOVE: *The Russian composer Nikolay Rimsky-Korsakov was the most prominent member of "The Mighty Handful". His nationalistic works include* Voskresenaya *(Russian Easter Festival Overture) and the opera* Sadko, *a setting of Russian folk legends.*

ever more inflated; while Wagner's massive "music-dramas", culminating in the epic saga *Der Ring des Nibelungen*, first performed complete in 1876, pointed the way forward to the "music of the future".

Rise of nationalism

While Germany led the musical world in symphonic terms, composers such as Smetana and Dvořák in Bohemia, Glinka, Borodin and Rimsky-Korsakov in Russia, Grieg in Norway and Chopin in Poland were beginning to discover an individual musical culture by introducing the colourful inflections of their native folk music into standard musical genres. Liszt, the Hungarian composer and virtuoso pianist, tackled the symphony from a different angle, inventing the one-movement symphonic "tone-poem" (usually inspired by a poetic, artistic or literary idea); this form was later adopted by Richard Strauss.

For much of the 19th century, England languished as "the land without music" until it was rescued from oblivion on the one hand by the enchantingly witty "Savoy Operas" of Gilbert and Sullivan, and on the other by the genius of Edward Elgar, the first major British composer since Purcell. Italy, however, continued to consolidate its reputation as the operatic centre of the world, with masterpieces by Rossini, Donizetti, Bellini, Verdi and Puccini.

ABOVE: *A poster advertising three operas by Gilbert and Sullivan –* The Gondoliers, The Mikado *and* The Yeomen of the Guard *– produced by the D'Oyly Carte Opera Company.*

Lives and Works
of the Great
Composers

The Ride of the Valkyries, *inspired by an episode from Act III of* Die Walküre
by Richard Wagner, painted by William T. Maud (1865–1903).

Introduction

I would rather write 10,000 notes than one letter of the alphabet.

Ludwig van Beethoven (1770–1827)

For the past six centuries, Western classical music has been largely defined by the role of the composer, and this section presents a historical survey of the exceptional figures whose imagination and skill has shaped its development. The invention of notation meant that music could be preserved and musicians were no longer limited by the number of notes they could memorize. The music could become far more ambitious and complex in scope, and the act of composition became distinct from the performance of the work: the role of the composer began to evolve.

Improvisation, however, remained an important part of music. Until the 18th century, notation provided little more than the bare bones of a piece of music. Couperin wrote that "we write one thing and play another", and

ABOVE: *Vienna has been a major centre for composers and musicians since the Baroque era. This painting depicts a court banquet in the Great Antechamber of the Hofburg Palace.*

descants, ornaments, figured basses and cadenzas were extemporized by the performers. During the 19th century, written music became more prescriptive, but since the 1950s composers have returned to improvisatory techniques, using graphic notation to stimulate the creativity of the performer, and introducing elements of chance.

Composers may use improvisation themselves, as a way of finding their way into a piece of music. Even though Mozart was said to write his scores without revision, he liked to compose at a keyboard so that he could try out his ideas, while Tippett found it satisfying to feel his music coming through his fingers on to the keys before he committed it to paper. Haydn liked to "extemporize, sadly or joyously, gravely or playfully, as I happen to be feeling, until I lay hold of an idea."

Composition means "putting together", and various elements are involved: the composer's intrinsic talent, technical skill and the rules that have evolved to frame the music –

ABOVE: *This beautifully illustrated French manuscript dates from the 13th century, when composers such as Léonin and Pérotin were working at Notre-Dame in Paris.*

ABOVE: *Joseph Haydn spent his career in the service of a single aristocratic family. He practically invented the Classical forms of symphony, concerto, string quartet and sonata.*

ABOVE: Beethoven was a revolutionary composer who expanded musical forms and brought new levels of emotion into his compositions. This manuscript shows an excerpt from Egmont (1809–10), *Beethoven's music to Goethe's five-act play about the Count of Egmont.*

which are there not only to be followed but also to be broken or changed. Debussy's teacher, perplexed by his work, asked what rules of harmony he was following. "Mon plaisir," answered Debussy. And yet, as the old rules were stretched to their limit by the Expressionists of the early 20th century, Schoenberg sensed the need for a new musical framework, and developed the 12-note system.

As the stories of the great composers are told and put into context, the connections between them become clear: most were not isolated artists, but teachers and pupils, fathers and sons, friends or, indeed, enemies. Many were drawn to congregate in centres of excellence such as Paris and Vienna, while others – like Wagner – took an individual course.

Just as music is subject to external influences, from the expertise of performers and instrument makers to political upheaval, the prevailing religious climate and fashions in entertainment, it is also the product of personal experience. While a piece of great music has the power to move the listener regardless of the circumstances in which it was written, it is fascinating to learn more about its background. We might expect episodes of depression, bereavement or political oppression to result in sombre music, and happy romances to produce lyrical song-cycles, but even more interesting are the examples of composers who have been able to transmute their personal misery or disappointments into music of inspiring beauty.

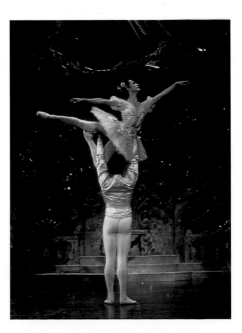

ABOVE: Tchaikovsky's ballet, The Nutcracker (1891–2). *Despite the death of his mother and an unhappy marriage, Tchaikovsky was able to write inspiring, romantic music.*

Lives and Works of the Great Composers **267**

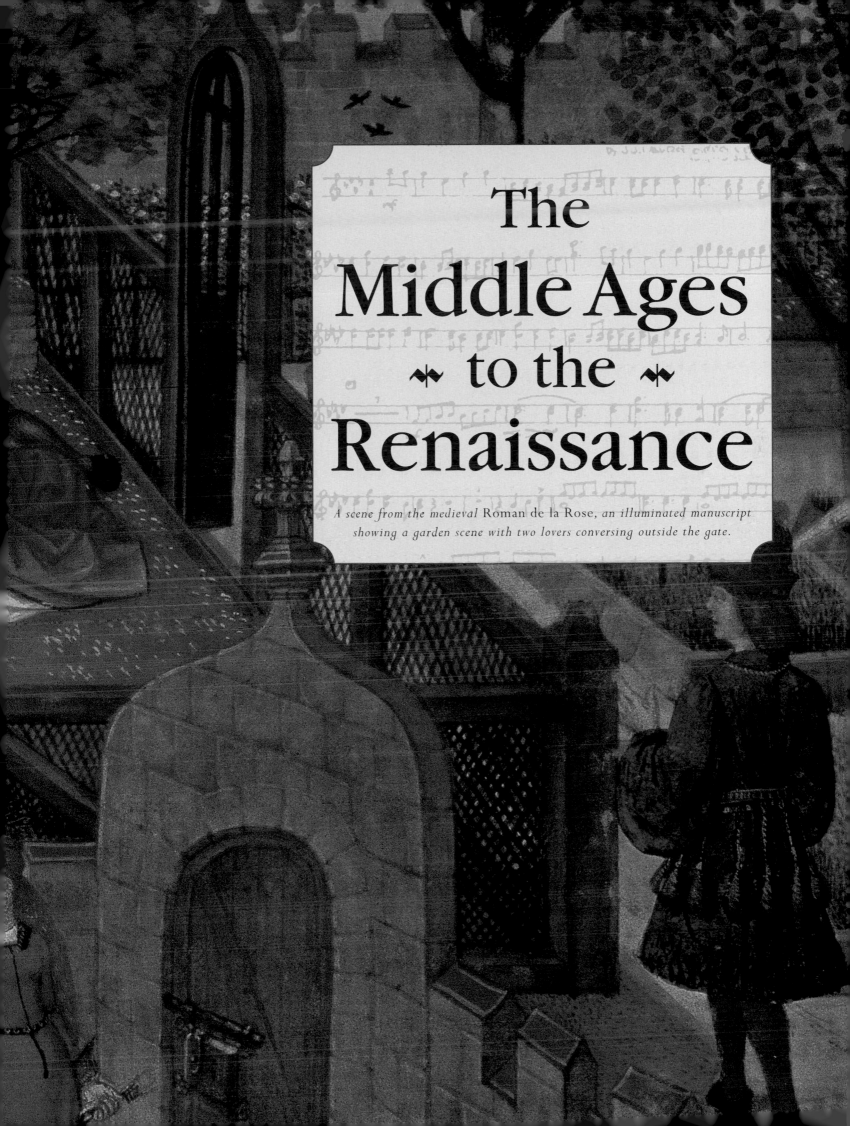

The Middle Ages
❧ to the ❧
Renaissance

A scene from the medieval Roman de la Rose, *an illuminated manuscript
showing a garden scene with two lovers conversing outside the gate.*

Medieval and Polyphonic Music

The sound of the cornet, flute, harp, sackbut, psaltery, dulcimer,
and all kinds of music.

DANIEL, 3:3

Until the 20th century, there was a general perception that the history of music began with Bach. Only with the huge growth in musical research and scholarship, together with the explosion of the "early music movement" in the later decades of the 20th century, did many lost masterpieces of the medieval and Renaissance periods come to light, prompting a re-evaluation of their composers' achievements.

Sacred music

Music in the Middle Ages was largely the preserve of the church. Surviving medieval sources were mostly produced by monastic scribes, and kept in monastery libraries. While secular music existed, much of it was improvised,

ABOVE: A page from an illuminated Flemish medieval psalter dating from c.1470.

so the earliest music to survive was generally intended for sacred use.

The names of individual composers become scarcer the further back into history we travel. Among the earliest musicians who may be singled out from the 12th and early 13th centuries are the French composers Léonin and Pérotin, who were associated with the newly built cathedral of Notre-Dame in Paris. A spate of enormously popular recordings has recently revealed the visionary music of the 12th-century nun Hildegard of Bingen, who not only has the distinction of being one of the

earliest known composers, but was also a woman working in a field where women have traditionally not been prominent. She is now something of a feminist icon. Performances and recordings by early music groups have also uncovered a wealth of music by unnamed composers derived from medieval manuscript sources, such as the 13th-century Spanish *Cantigas* of Alfonso X.

Polyphony

The French composer Guillaume de Machaut was the single most important musical figure of the 14th century. His many innovations included being the first to compose a complete setting of the Ordinary of the Mass, the first to write music in four parts (which became the

ABOVE: French church singers dating from the 14th century, the time of the innovative composer Guillaume de Machaut.

ABOVE: A heart-shaped score, in red and black ink, of a three-part French chanson Belle, bonne *by Baude Cordier (fl.1390s).*

such as Filippo Brunelleschi (1377–1446), evident in Florentine churches such as San Lorenzo and Santo Spirito, or the wonderful ducal palace at Urbino, found a musical counterpart in Renaissance polyphony. Music, too, acquired new depth and perspective. While three Flemish composers had dominated the 15th century, the polyphonic art of the High Renaissance was perfected by a trio of musicians – Palestrina from Italy, Lassus from Flanders, and Victoria from Spain – who all spent long periods in Italy.

The polyphonic principle continued to dominate 16th-century music, from the Masses and motets written for performance in the great Catholic churches of France, Italy, Spain and southern Germany, to the equivalent settings of both Catholic and Protestant liturgies by the English composers Tallis and Byrd, and the enchanting secular partsongs of the Elizabethan madrigal school. Meanwhile the plangent songs and solo lute music of Dowland looked forward to a new age of individualism.

ABOVE: An illumination from a 15th-century manuscript showing secular musicians playing a variety of instruments – crumhorn, fiddle, lute, bagpipes, nakers (drums) and triangle.

standard polyphonic combination), and one of the first to set the typical secular poetic forms of his day: *ballade, rondeau* and *virelay*.

For the next century, the musical centres of gravity remained the courts and churches of northern France and Flanders, which produced the sacred and secular works of the Flemish composers associated with the court of the dukes of Burgundy: Dufay, Ockeghem, Josquin des Prez and their contemporaries. However, many drew inspiration from prolonged visits to Italy, where musical activity flourished at important courts such as those of Ferrara and Mantua.

The harmonious exercises in perspective of Renaissance architects

ABOVE: The nave and choir of the church of Santo Spirito in Florence, designed by Filippo Brunelleschi in the mid 15th century. This church is a classic Renaissance masterpiece of perspective.

Hildegard of Bingen

A feather on the breath of God.

HILDEGARD

This remarkable woman was one of the earliest known composers. A contemporary of the famous medieval lovers Abélard and Héloïse, who also ended their lives in monastic institutions, Hildegard was born into a noble German family. As the tenth child she was considered a tithe and therefore due to the church, and was dedicated to religious service. When she was eight years old, she was sent as a novice to the Benedictine monastery of Disibodenberg.

In 1136 Hildegard became an abbess in her own right, and around the age of 50 she founded a nunnery near Bingen in the Rhine Valley. She died at the advanced age of 81, and her name was

ABOVE: A modern plaque in the German town of Bingen commemorating its famous Abbess, Hildegard of Bingen.

put forward by several popes as a candidate for canonization. Though never formally canonized, she is often referred to as a saint, and has a feast-day which is particularly celebrated in Germany.

Mysticism and music

Hildegard was a visionary, and soon gained a widespread reputation as a prophetess. Popes, emperors, monarchs, archbishops and clergymen of all kinds flocked to Bingen to consult this "Sybil of the Rhine". Between 1141 and 1170 she recorded her mystical experiences; she also wrote two important works on natural history and medicine, and a great deal

of lyric and dramatic poetry, collected together in a volume called *Symphonia armonie celestium revelationum*.

Most of her poetry is liturgical, including antiphons, sequences and hymns designed for performance on the feast-days of particular saints. Among her work is the earliest known surviving morality play, *Ordo virtutum*, which describes the 16 Virtues battling with the Devil for a human soul. This and many of her poems have music attached, written in German neumatic notation. Unlike much music of this period, Hildegard's melodies are not drawn from monastic plainsong, but are strikingly original, and sometimes highly complex and decorative.

Many of her works have been performed and recorded during the recent revival of interest in early music: the album released under the title *A Feather on the Breath of God* (1984) has enjoyed huge popularity.

ABOVE: An illustrated 13th-century manuscript depicting The Vision of St Hildegard, *compiled 50 years after her death in 1179.*

Life and works

NATIONALITY: German

BORN: Böckelheim, 1098;
DIED: Bingen, 1179

SPECIALIST GENRES: Plainsong settings of her own poetry.

MAJOR WORK: *Ordo virtutum*; *Symphonia armonie celestium revelationum*.

The Notre-Dame School

*Who could retain a grievance against the man
with whom he had joined in singing before God?*

ST AMBROSE (C.339–97)

Léonin and Pérotin –
sometimes referred to as
Master Leoninus and Master
Perotinus – were the best-known
of a group of composers who
worked in medieval Paris in the
late 12th and early 13th centuries.
This was the age of King Philippe-
Auguste (Philippe II), during
whose reign, from 1180 to 1223,
the medieval kingdom of France
was consolidated. Little is known of
the lives of Léonin and Pérotin,
but both are associated with the
cathedral of Notre-Dame de Paris,
whose foundations were laid in the
mid 1160s, and its high altar
consecrated in 1182.

Léonin

The major work attributed to Léonin
was the *Magnus liber* ("great book")
designed for use by the choir of the
new cathedral. He is mentioned by an
anonymous 13th-century theorist as
"the best composer of organum for the

*ABOVE: An initial letter from an illuminated
French psalter dating from the 13th century
– the time of Léonin and Pérotin.*

amplification of divine service",
suggesting that he wrote polyphonic
settings for two independent voices of
parts of the liturgy intended for
performance on the main feast-days of
the church's year. Léonin may also have
been among the first to indicate
rhythm as well as pitch in his musical
notation. His vocal writing was
imaginative, free-flowing and
improvisatory in style.

Pérotin

Some time after Léonin's death,
Pérotin, who may have been his pupil,
seems to have revised and shortened
the *Magnus liber*. Pérotin remains a
shadowy figure. He may have been
born around 1160, and died some
time between 1205 and 1225. Some

scholars have suggested that he
may have worked at the royal
parish church of St Germain-
l'Auxerrois, near the Tuileries Palace,
since there is no direct evidence
that he worked at Notre-Dame.

Pérotin was active in the creation of
the four-voice motet, an ecclesiastical
musical form which survives to the
present day. His contribution towards
the development of three- and four-
voice polyphony was one of the most
important steps forward in musical
history. Of his works, two
graduals in four voices for the
Christmas season survive, as do
about a dozen liturgical works in
three voices, and about 160 *clausulae* –
polyphonic passages written for
insertion into liturgical plainsong to
vary the texture.

*ABOVE: A view of medieval Paris showing
the cathedral of Notre-Dame, where Léonin
and Pérotin worked, from the 15th-century
Book of Hours of Etienne Chevalier.*

Lives and works

NATIONALITY: French

ACTIVE: Léonin, c.1163–90;
Pérotin, c.1200

SPECIALIST GENRES: Early
polyphonic sacred music.

MAJOR WORKS: *Magnus liber*,
motets and graduals.

The Baroque Era ❦

A concert given to the Procurators of Venice by the girls of an 18th-century Venetian orphanage. Vivaldi taught at such an institution.

Harmony and Ornament

Architecture in general is frozen music.

FRIEDRICH VON SCHELLING (1775–1854)

The term "Baroque", which is derived from *barroco*, the Portuguese word for a misshapen pearl, was originally used – in a pejorative sense – to describe the flamboyant, ornate architecture found in German, Austrian and Italian churches of the 17th century, which were designed as a reaction to the cool classicism of Renaissance architecture. One of the most prominent Baroque architects was the Italian sculptor Gianlorenzo Bernini (1598–1680), who worked principally in Rome. His work exhibits the fluid, dynamic shapes, theatricality and illusion that characterize the style.

In music, the Baroque period covers the years from c.1600–1750, during which Renaissance polyphony gave way to a new, highly ornamental style with a strong harmonic basis. Most Baroque music – from operatic arias to *concerti*

ABOVE: *Baroque flamboyance at its height – the interior of St Peter's Basilica in Rome in 1730.*

grossi for groups of instruments – was supported by a *basso continuo*, a firm bass line played on keyboard and reinforced on cello or bass, which provided a harmonic foundation.

Opera

The Baroque period saw the introduction of several new forms, mostly developed in Italy. In the late 16th century, a group of poets and musicians formed an association in Florence called the Camerata, and several of their members – the poet Ottavio Rinuccini (1562–1621) and the composers Jacopo Peri (1561–1633) and Giulio Caccini (c.1550–1618) – collaborated to produce

the earliest music-dramas, or operas. The new form was taken up and transformed by the genius of Claudio Monteverdi, whose three surviving operas are the earliest still to be regularly performed today.

Opera spread like wildfire, with demand coming not only from aristocratic patrons, but also from newly opened public opera houses. Monteverdi's pioneering work was carried on by composers such as Vivaldi and Alessandro Scarlatti in Italy, Hasse in Germany, Lully, Charpentier and Rameau in France, and the German-born Handel in England. Alongside secular operas (usually based on plots derived from ancient history or mythology), a similar sacred form – oratorio – developed, using the same forms and styles as opera, but based on biblical stories. Oratorio flourished both in the Catholic South and the

ABOVE: *An opera theatre in Munich, Germany, in 1665.*

ABOVE: A realistic depiction of an 18th-century private concert against an allegorical background, one of a set of four Fine Arts designs by Giuseppe Zocchi (1711–67).

Bach and Handel

In musical terms, the Baroque era reached its height in the works of Bach and Handel. Both were reared in the German Protestant tradition, but their careers took very different paths.

Bach concentrated on church music, whether for voices and instruments (in the form of the church cantata, a kind of unstaged mini-drama performed during the Sunday services), or for instruments alone (particularly solo organ). His Passion settings brought a German tradition to its peak, and his monumental Mass in B minor took the form to an unprecedented level.

Handel flourished in a more cosmopolitan environment, first in Italy and then in England, where he stepped neatly into the void left by the early death of Henry Purcell. Handel's many Italian operas, written for London theatres, have recently resumed their place in the repertoire, while his English oratorios have always been a well-loved feature of the British choral tradition.

Protestant North, where Heinrich Schütz pioneered it in Germany, paving the way for the great sacred works of J. S. Bach. It reached its apogee in the works of Handel, written in English, of which *Messiah* has been the most frequently performed.

Spanish courts, where he developed his own highly individual form of keyboard sonata.

Instrumental forms

The Baroque period also saw a huge demand for instrumental music, particularly concertos, *concerti grossi*, sonatas and suites, and almost all major composers worked in these new forms. Again, they flourished in Italy in the hands of Corelli, Vivaldi and Alessandro Scarlatti, but were equally popular in Germany. Bach's *Brandenburg Concertos* and Handel's sets of *concerti grossi* brought the genre to its peak, while the solo concerto and solo sonata underwent further metamorphosis in the Classical era. Meanwhile Alessandro Scarlatti's son Domenico, an exact contemporary of Bach and Handel, defied convention by removing to the Portuguese and

ABOVE: The Rehearsal, *with viols, flute, oboe and voice, by Etienne Jeaurat (1699–1789).*

Claudio Monteverdi

Claudio Monteverdi, in moving the affections...
becomes the most pleasant tyrant of human minds.

Aquilino Coppini, 1608

Monteverdi was a composer of enormous significance in the history of music. Like his contemporary Heinrich Schütz in Germany, he bridged the worlds of the High Renaissance and the Baroque era. He can also be compared to Stravinsky: during the course of long lives both men showed an endless capacity to re-invent and adapt their musical styles according to changing tastes.

Early years

Monteverdi began his career as a chorister at the cathedral in his birthplace, Cremona. By the age of 16 – already a fine instrumentalist – he had published a volume of three-part motets and a book of sacred madrigals. In 1587 he published his first volume of secular madrigals, followed by a second volume in 1590. Around that time he found a job as a string player at the ducal court in Mantua, and by the

ABOVE: *Claudio Monteverdi (1567–1643),*
painted around 1640 by Bernardo Strozzi.

time his third madrigal collection appeared in 1592 his fame as a composer was spreading rapidly. He married in 1599 and had three

children, of whom two sons survived: the elder became a musician, the younger a doctor.

Triumph and tragedy

In 1601 Monteverdi became *maestro di cappella* at the Mantuan court, where he published two more madrigal collections over the next four years. In 1607 he made his first foray into the new genre of opera with *L'Orfeo*, which was performed in Mantua in February. Seven months later his wife died after a long illness, leaving Monteverdi a grief-stricken widower with two small children.

He was obliged to pull himself together enough to finish his second opera, *L'Arianna*, which was performed in May 1608 to celebrate the marriage of the Gonzaga heir, Francesco, to Margaret of Savoy. (Only one aria from this opera has survived.) During rehearsals another tragedy struck when Caterina Martinelli, the young principal singer and a close friend of Monteverdi, died of smallpox. Monteverdi then suffered a complete collapse, although his glorious setting for voices and instruments of the *Vespro della beata vergine* (*Vespers of the Blessed Virgin*, 1610) dates from this unhappy period.

Venice

After making several attempts to leave the service of the Gonzagas, Monteverdi was finally dismissed in

ABOVE: *The interior of the Teatro Olimpico in Vicenza, designed by Andrea Palladio (1508–80).*

NATIONALITY: Italian

BORN: Cremona, 1567;
DIED: Venice, 1643

SPECIALIST GENRES: Opera,
madrigals, motets.

MAJOR WORKS: Nine
books of madrigals; *Vespro
della beata vergine* (1610);
La favola d'Orfeo (1607);
Il ritorno d'Ulisse in patria
(1640); *L'incoronazione di
Poppea* (1642).

ABOVE: A scene from a 1975 production of Monteverdi's L'incoronazione di Poppea *(1642), shortly after its re-introduction to modern audiences.*

1612, and in 1613 became *maestro di cappella* at St Mark's Cathedral in Venice, where he remained for the rest of his life. He also continued to write ballets and operas for the Mantuan court, but many of his scores were destroyed when Austrian troops sacked the palace in 1630. In the same year Venice was ravaged by plague, and shortly afterwards Monteverdi renounced the world and took holy orders.

In 1637, after the first public opera house opened in Venice, he was commissioned to write several operas. The two that survive – *Il ritorno d'Ulisse in patria* (*The Return of Ulysses*)

ABOVE: The sinfonia da guerra *(Battle Sinfonia) from the score of Monteverdi's* Il ritorno d'Ulisse in patria *(1640).*

and *L'incoronazione di Poppea* (*The Coronation of Poppea*) – are masterpieces of the genre in their superb characterization and instinctive feel for dramatic effect. The final scene of *L'incoronazione di Poppea*, despite celebrating the union of two ambitious and deeply unpleasant people, contains one of the most intensely passionate love duets in all opera.

The works of Monteverdi's Venetian years include three more madrigal collections. Book 8 of 1638, entitled *Madrigali guerrieri et amorosi* (*Songs of War and Love*), contains substantial dramatic works such as *Il ballo delle ingrate*, and the famous *Combattimento di Tancredi e Clorinda*, a graphic description of a duel between the Christian knight Tancred and the pagan Clorinda, who is disguised as a man. As a whole, the madrigal collections show Monteverdi moving with the times, from typically Renaissance polyphonic pieces in the earlier volumes (one of the most beautiful and frequently performed of these is the five-voice *Zefiro torna*, a setting of words by Petrarch), to highly expressive dramatic works for

solo voices with instrumental accompaniment in the later ones. All his music, early or late, is characterized by qualities of emotional intensity, depth of expression and understanding of human nature comparable with those that inform the works of Shakespeare.

ABOVE: The title page of a collection of poetical tributes in commemoration of Monteverdi's death, published in 1644.

Heinrich Schütz

The most spiritual musician the world has ever seen.

ALFRED EINSTEIN (1880–1952)

The achievements of J. S. Bach would not have been possible without the ground-breaking work of his illustrious predecessor, Heinrich Schütz. Born into a middle-class family of innkeepers in Saxony, Schütz became the most esteemed German composer of the 17th century. During two prolonged visits to Italy – the first, made while he was still a law student, enabling him to study in Venice with Giovanni Gabrieli – Schütz absorbed the Italian style, which he then amalgamated with the very different musical tradition of his native Germany.

Dresden *Kapellmeister*

On his return from Italy in 1613 after Gabrieli's death, Schütz became organist and then *Kapellmeister* at the electoral

ABOVE: *A portrait of Heinrich Schütz (1585–1672), by his contemporary Christoph Spetner.*

court in Dresden, the most important musical centre in Protestant Germany. He published his first important compositions in 1619. These were a collection of settings for voices (some with instrumental interludes in the Venetian style) of the Psalms of David, described as "various motets and concertos". In the same year he married Magdalena Wildeck, daughter of a court official. Their happy union, which produced two daughters, was tragically brief: Magdalena died in 1625, and the grief-stricken composer never remarried. He outlived both his children: the elder died at the age of 16, and the younger in 1655, aged 31.

Schütz's court duties included writing music for official events, such as weddings and funerals. For the wedding of the elector's daughter to the Landgrave of Hessen-Darmstadt in 1627, he wrote the first German opera, setting the same libretto (*Dafne*) which the Italian composer Jacopo Peri had set 30 years earlier. Unfortunately the music has not survived.

In 1628 Schütz paid a second visit to Italy, where he met Monteverdi. This contact with recent musical developments bore fruit in a second published collection of vocal and instrumental music, *Symphoniae sacrae*. But there were troubles at home: Germany had entered the Thirty Years

ABOVE: *Schütz's birthplace in Bad Köstritz, Germany. The building is now a museum devoted to the composer.*

War, and the Elector of Dresden found himself unable to pay his employees. Schütz escaped for two years to the court of the Crown Prince of Denmark, for whose wedding festivities he provided elaborate musical entertainments. But despite constant financial problems, he remained in the service of the Dresden court (apart from two more visits to Denmark) until 1657, when he was pensioned off. After his retirement he continued to write works for the electoral chapel until his death at the age of 87.

Schütz's music

Although Schütz was an enormously prolific composer, many of his manuscripts were destroyed by fire or the ravages of war. Even so, some 500 works survive. *Die Geburt unsers Herren Jesu Christi* (*The History of the Birth of Jesus Christ*), performed at Christmas Vespers at the Dresden court in 1660,

ABOVE: Gondolas moored near the Rialto Bridge in Venice, where Schütz studied with Giovanni Gabrieli.

is the earliest known German setting of the Nativity story in which the words of the Evangelist – or Narrator – are sung in recitative, rather than chanted as in earlier settings. His settings of the four Passions, together with innumerable psalm and motet settings and Italianate madrigals, influenced later composers such as Bach. Although Schütz's music fell out of fashion fairly rapidly, it was rediscovered in the 20th century, and championed by performers such as Roger Norrington in Britain, who founded first the amateur Heinrich Schütz Choir in 1962, and then the professional Schütz Choir of London.

Life and works

NATIONALITY: German

BORN: Köstritz, 1585; DIED: Dresden, 1672

SPECIALIST GENRES: Sacred vocal and instrumental music, including oratorios and Passions.

MAJOR WORKS: *Psalmen Davids* (1619); *Cantiones sacrae* (1625); opera *Dafne* (1627); *Symphoniae sacrae* (1629, 1647, 1650); *Sieben Worte Jesu Christi am Kreuz* (*Seven Words of Christ on the Cross*, 1645); Christmas Oratorio (1660); Passions according to Matthew, Mark, Luke and John (1664–6).

ABOVE: The title page of Schütz's Psalmen Davids, *settings of the Psalms for voices and instruments published in 1619.*

Jean-Baptiste Lully

The musician is to follow the poet's direction, only in my opinion, Lully is to be exempted,
who knows the passions and enters further into the heart of man than the authors themselves.

SEIGNEUR DE SAINT-EVREMOND (1610–1703)

The founder of French opera owed his success partly to his exceptional talent, and partly to his ruthless, ambitious nature – only Wagner has rivalled Lully in sheer single-mindedness of purpose and grandiose vision. His career mirrored that of his patron, the "Sun King" Louis XIV (1643–1715), perhaps the greatest European monarch of his age, who saw his own glory reflected in the sumptuous entertainments devised by his clever court composer.

King and composer enjoyed a close, symbiotic relationship: indeed Lully's death, in 1687 at the age of only 55, marked the zenith of the Sun King's reign. Thereafter it was a long, slow story of royal decline, marked by personal misfortunes and military defeats.

ABOVE: *Louis XIV's court composer, Jean-Baptiste Lully (1632–87).*

The ambitious page

The son of a humble Florentine miller, Lully's singing voice was spotted at the age of 13 and he was taken to Paris and employed as a pageboy to a distant member of the royal family. Having perfected his own talents for dancing and playing the violin, he applied himself to social climbing, and quickly got his first royal appointment. His job was to write music for the lavish court ballets, and to drill the orchestra which accompanied them, the *Vingt-quatre violons du roi*. He soon established himself as a strict disciplinarian with a quick temper – later in life, as director of the opera house in Paris, he allegedly punched his pregnant leading lady in the stomach, causing her to miscarry, rather than jeopardize his productions.

ABOVE: *The courtyard of Louis XIV's palace at Versailles, the envy of many other European monarchs. Many of Lully's court ballets and comedy-ballets were performed here.*

ABOVE: *A 17th-century engraving of Lully in his role as director of the royal orchestra.*

NATIONALITY: Italian

BORN: Florence, 1632;
DIED: Paris, 1687

SPECIALIST GENRES: Court ballets, comedy-ballets, opera.

MAJOR WORKS: 36 court ballets; 14 *comédies-ballets,* including *Les fâcheux* (1661) and *Le bourgeois gentilhomme* (1670); 16 *tragédies-lyriques,* including *Alceste* (1674), *Atys* (1676), *Amadis* (1684), *Roland* (1685) and *Armide* (1686).

ABOVE: *An original stage design by Jean Berain for Lully's* tragédie-lyrique, Armide, *first performed at the Académie Royale de Musique in Paris in 1686.*

Lully's ruthless nature suited his purposes well. He made an expedient marriage in order to disguise his homosexuality – a predilection which the king (a great lover of women) abhorred – and consolidated his position at court by choosing as his bride the daughter of the court composer, Michael Lambert. Meanwhile he cultivated the playwright Molière (1622–73), with whom he collaborated on several *comédies-ballets* (a hybrid form – half play, half ballet) for the entertainment of the court. The most famous of these was *Le bourgeois gentilhomme* (1670).

Opera at Versailles and Paris

Lully's next move, in 1672, was to take advantage of the bankruptcy of a fellow musician who had obtained a royal licence to import Italian opera. Lully seized the licence for himself, and while continuing to supply music for lavish court entertainments at the magnificent new palace of Versailles, he established a virtual monopoly over operatic productions, opening his own opera house in a disused tennis court

in Paris. The following year he turned his old friend Molière's troupe of actors out of their centrally sited theatre in the Palais Royal, and took it over, with the king's permission, rent-free.

Over the next 14 years, Lully and the poet Philippe Quinault (1635–88) produced a succession of brilliant operas in an entirely new and original style. These "lyric tragedies" were

ABOVE: *A costume design for a character in* Armide, *regarded as Lully's masterpiece.*

based on subjects drawn from mythology and legend (such as *Isis, Thésée, Phaëton* and *Armide*), worked into plots which subtly flattered Louis XIV – his victories, his devotion to duty and his personal concept of glory. Audiences of the time loved them – as did the king. Lully had struck gold, and made a huge fortune.

A bizarre end

Lully's court position required him to compose sacred music for the royal chapel, and while conducting a Te Deum written to celebrate Louis XIV's recovery from illness, he accidentally struck his foot with the heavy stick he used to mark the beat by banging it on the floor. Gangrene set in, but Lully refused to have the toe amputated.

As he lay dying, he was visited by a priest. In a final dramatic gesture to mark his penitence, Lully threw his last opera manuscript on to the fire, and received absolution. After the priest had gone, a horrified friend asked Lully why he had wantonly destroyed his last great work. "Don't worry," whispered the dying man, "I've got another copy!"

Arcangelo Corelli

I never met with any man that suffered his passions to hurry him away so much whilst he was playing on the violin as the famous Arcangelo Corelli, whose eyes will sometimes turn as red as fire.

FRANÇOIS RAGUENET (C.1660–1722)

While 17th-century German composers were bringing the art of organ-playing to a peak of perfection, Italy remained pre-eminent for nurturing the art of the violin. With the products of an unsurpassed school of instrument-makers – the Amati and Guarneri families, Stradivari, Gasparò da Salo and Maggini – at their disposal, Italian performers could hardly fail to establish a European reputation as masters of their art. One of the most influential of these – both in terms of violin technique and musical style – was Arcangelo Corelli.

Success as a performer

Corelli came from Fusignano, a town between Bologna and Ravenna. He took music lessons from a priest in nearby Faenza, and in 1666 arrived in Bologna, where he studied the violin

ABOVE: *Arcangelo Corelli, probably painted by the Flemish artist Jan Frans van Douven around 1700.*

with several fine players. By 1675 he had made his professional debut in Rome where, over the next few years, he established himself as a brilliant performer, taking part in the elaborate church performances commissioned by Rome's decadent but artistically inclined prelates, and in secular performances at the theatres. In 1679 he became chamber musician to the exiled Queen Christina of Sweden, to whom he dedicated his first compositions, a set of 12 *sonate da chiesa*.

Before long, the ambitious violinist had decided to replace his patron with a more influential one: Cardinal Pamphili, one of the richest men in Rome. From 1684 onwards Corelli began to play regularly at musical events organized by Pamphili, while introducing his own works – including a set of chamber trios

LEFT: *A highly romanticized impression (1913) of the violin maker Antonio Stradivari in his workshop at Cremona, by Edgar Bundy (1862–1922).*

RIGHT: *The* Hellier Stradivarius, *made in 1679.*

ABOVE: The title page of Corelli's Op. 1 trio sonatas, published in 1685 with a dedication to Queen Christina of Sweden.

dedicated to Pamphili — at the musical academies held on Sunday afternoons at the cardinal's sumptuous palazzo. His social climbing bore fruit, and in July 1687 he was formally engaged as the cardinal's music master, and given a suite of rooms in the palace.

Orchestral compositions

In 1690 Pamphili moved to Bologna, but Corelli declined to follow him. Instead, he was engaged by a rival cardinal, the young Pietro Ottoboni, nephew of Pope Alexander VIII, another ostentatious patron of the arts. Corelli and Ottoboni became good friends, and Corelli dedicated a second set of chamber trios to him in 1694. He also began to write orchestral works (sinfonias and concertos), which attracted much attention. He was described as "the famous violinist…the Orpheus of our time," whose works were "prized and esteemed".

In 1702, however, his self-esteem was shaken when he visited Naples to play in the opera orchestra, taking with

him two Roman players since he distrusted the abilities of the Neapolitans. To his surprise, he found that the despised southerners could actually play quite well, while he himself had embarrassing difficulty with a particular passage that his hosts managed fluently.

In 1707 Corelli met Handel (who was working in Rome), and played in a performance of an early Handel oratorio. Shortly afterwards he retired from playing to devote himself to composition. His health deteriorated, and he died early in 1713. He was buried in the Pantheon. His reputation both as performer and composer long outlived him: his compositions were reprinted many times and sold all over Europe. They were particularly popular in England and Germany, where they influenced many later composers, including Handel, Telemann and Bach.

Life and works

NATIONALITY: Italian

BORN: Fusignano, 1653; **DIED:** Rome, 1713

SPECIALIST GENRES: Violin music, sinfonias, concertos.

MAJOR WORKS: Four sets of 12 trio sonatas; 12 solo sonatas; 12 *concerti grossi*.

ABOVE: Queen Christina holding court. She is talking with the French philosopher René Descartes (painting by Dumesnil the Younger, 1698–1781).

Henry Purcell

*Mr Purcell, in whose person we have at length found
an Englishman equal with the best abroad.*

JOHN DRYDEN (1631–1700)

Unlike some European countries, which enjoyed a strong and continuing musical tradition from the Renaissance onwards, England – while strong on literature – has suffered from a distinctly patchy musical heritage. After the Elizabethan flowering, only a few distinctive figures emerged in the early 17th century – notably the Lawes brothers, Henry (1596–1662) and William (1602–45), and later John Blow (1649–1708); but England produced no composer of European stature until the brilliant but tragically short-lived Henry Purcell.

Occasional music

Purcell began his career as a chorister in the Chapel Royal; in 1679 he succeeded Blow as organist of Westminster Abbey. He seems to have married around 1680, and had several children, of whom a son and a daughter survived him. In 1682 he was appointed an organist of the Chapel Royal, and a year later became organ-maker and keeper of the king's instruments. His court appointments were renewed after Charles II's death, and he continued to produce many odes and welcome songs (cantata-like compositions) for occasions such as royal birthdays, marriages and New Year's Day. Most of these "occasional" works are now among the least known of his output, but the 1692 Ode for St Cecilia's Day, *Hail, Bright Cecilia*, is one of his best-loved works.

ABOVE:
*A 19th-century
lithograph of
Henry Purcell by
Alfred Lemoine
(1824–81).*

LEFT: *William III
(1650–1702)
and his wife
Mary II (1662–
94), who reigned
jointly as King
and Queen of
England from
1689.*

Life and works

NATIONALITY: English

BORN: London, 1659;
DIED: London, 1695

SPECIALIST GENRES: Opera
and incidental music for the
stage, odes, anthems,
instrumental music.

MAJOR WORKS: *Dido and Aeneas*
(1689); *King Arthur* (1691);
The Fairy Queen (1692); *Hail,
Bright Cecilia* (1692);
Come, Ye Sons of Art (1694);
Te Deum and Jubilate in D
(1694); Funeral music for
Queen Mary (1695).

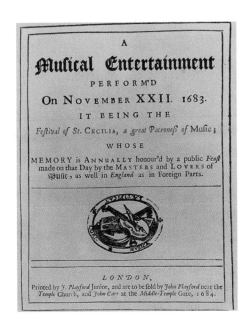

LEFT: The opening of Purcell's Golden Sonata *for two violins and* basso continuo.

RIGHT: The frontispiece to the text of Purcell's 1683 Ode to St Cecilia, Welcome to all the pleasures.

Stage works

During the last decade of his life, Purcell combined his court duties with writing music for the stage. Opera as such did not exist in England at the time, but between 1690 and 1695 Purcell provided incidental music for five major "semi-operas" put on at London theatres: Betterton's *Dioclesian, King Arthur* and *The Indian Queen* (with texts by John Dryden), *The Fairy Queen* and *The Tempest* (both loosely based on Shakespeare).

Purcell's most famous stage work, however, is the opera *Dido and Aeneas*, long thought to have been written around 1689 for a girls' school in Chelsea, but possibly dating from several years earlier. He also provided individual musical items for over 40 other plays by the most notable playwrights of the time. The Rondeau from his music for Aphra Behn's 1695 play *Abdelazer* was used by Benjamin Britten as the theme of his *Young Person's Guide to the Orchestra* (1946).

Purcell's legacy

Apart from his dramatic music, Purcell wrote many exquisite anthems, a Magnificat and a Te Deum, a vast number of solo songs and partsongs (some with extremely bawdy texts which have only recently been permitted to surface), instrumental music including fantasias for viol consort, a set of 12 trio sonatas for two violins and continuo, a set of 10 sonatas "in four parts", clearly influenced by Corelli, and some charming keyboard music, including eight suites. Among his last works was the moving Funeral Music for Queen Mary, written for the young and much-mourned queen: within a short

ABOVE: *The choir of Westminster Abbey, where Purcell was buried at the foot of the organ.*

while Purcell had followed her to the grave at the age of only 36. The music he had written for the queen was played at his own funeral.

Purcell's genius lay in his unique response to the setting of English words, whether sacred or secular, his gift for appealing melody, his assimilation of elements from both Italian and French music – notably Corelli's violin writing, and Lully's unusual effects (the "Frost Scene" from *King Arthur*, in which each note is sung with a shiver, was borrowed from a similar scene in Lully's opera *Isis*) – and his forward-looking treatment of the orchestra, particularly the strings.

Though regarded as a "one-off" genius, the end of a tradition rather than an initiator, Purcell is still held in high esteem. *Dido and Aeneas* is often performed, and in the last decade of the 20th century, particularly during the tercentenary celebration of his death, most of his music was made widely available through high-quality performances and recordings.

Antonio Vivaldi

He is an old man, who has a prodigious fury for composition. I heard him undertake to compose a concerto, with all the parts, with greater despatch than a copyist can copy it.

CHARLES DE BROSSES, 1739

For many people, the name Vivaldi is associated with just one piece of music – *Le quattro stagioni* (*The Four Seasons*) – which has been recorded countless times. But many other gems of Vivaldi's output are worth exploring: he was one of the most prolific and influential composers of his time, and without his contribution to the development of concerto form, the instrumental music of later composers such as Bach would have been the poorer.

The Red Priest
Vivaldi was born (during a minor earthquake) in Venice, to a baker turned professional violinist,

ABOVE: The violinist and composer Antonio Vivaldi (1678–1741), painted in 1723 by François Morellon La Cave.

and its reputation was such that many leading performers took part in its concerts. Vivaldi was required to teach and rehearse the students and to maintain the instruments. His initial appointment lasted six years, during which time he published a set of 12 trio *sonate da camera* and a set of solo violin sonatas. He had already begun to write concertos, which became his favourite medium.

Vivaldi's concertos
In all Vivaldi wrote well over 200 violin concertos, around 27 cello concertos, around a dozen for flute, three for

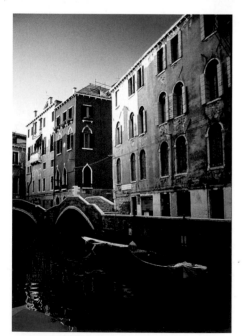

ABOVE: Vivaldi's family home on the Fondamenta del Dose in Venice.

with whom the young Antonio studied. In 1693 he began to train for the priesthood, while still living at home and continuing his violin studies. He was ordained in 1703, and his startling red hair earned him the nickname of *il prete rosso* (the Red Priest), but the ecclesiastical life did not entirely suit him, and several times he found himself at odds with the church authorities.

In the year of his ordination, Vivaldi was appointed violin teacher at the Conservatorio dell'Ospedale della Pietà, a Venetian orphanage which housed and educated young girls. Music was held in high esteem there,

ABOVE: A page from the cello part of Vivaldi's collection of concertos L'estro armonico.

piccolo, 20 for oboe, 37 for bassoon (an instrument for which few other composers have written concertos), and many more double and multiple concertos, of which the E minor concerto for four violins, Op. 3 No. 4, is very well known.

The fanciful titles of some of his concertos gave Vivaldi plenty of opportunity for descriptive writing. As well as the famous *Four Seasons*, programmatically depicting seasonal activities such as skating on the ice (winter), hunting (autumn), and listening to birdsong (spring), their titles include *La tempestà di mare* (Storm at Sea), *L'amoroso* (The Lover), *La caccia* (The Hunt) and *Il corneto di posta* (The Posthorn).

A set of 12 concertos for one, two or four solo violins was published in Amsterdam in 1711 under the title *L'estro armonico*, and instantly sold all over Europe (Bach made keyboard transcriptions of five of them). Another set of 12 *(La stravaganza)* appeared in 1714, and from then on Vivaldi's music was much in demand (the collection

ABOVE: *The title page of Vivaldi's* L'estro armonico, *published 1711 with a dedication to the Grand Duke of Tuscany.*

containing *The Four Seasons* was published in 1725). He also wrote around 60 *concerti grossi* for strings and bass.

In 1711 Vivaldi returned to the Pietà, where he took the opportunity to write sacred as well as instrumental music. His cheerful *Gloria* is still much

performed today. He was associated with the institution until his death, although his frequent absences were not popular. He also began to write operas (about 45 in all) for various Italian courts and opera houses, including Mantua, Venice and Rome. Several have recently been revived, although interest still tends to be academic.

Fall from grace

Vivaldi spent much of the last two decades of his life on the move. Around 1725 he became involved with his singing pupil, Anna Giraud. The church authorities cannot have been pleased with the whiff of scandal surrounding the "Red Priest" and in 1737 he was censured for unpriestly conduct. In 1741 Vivaldi undertook a mysterious journey to Vienna (perhaps connected with Anna's work as an opera singer). He arrived on 28 June, and a month later he was dead, apparently of unknown causes. His arrogance and egotism had made many enemies, but his posthumous influence was immense.

Life and works

NATIONALITY: Italian

BORN: Venice, 1678; **DIED:** Vienna, 1741

SPECIALIST GENRES: Instrumental music, especially violin concertos.

MAJOR WORKS: Over 400 concertos published in sets, including *L'estro armonico* (1711); *Il cimento dell'armonia e dell'inventione* (1725 – 12 concertos of which the first four are *Le quattro stagioni*).

ABOVE: *The Piazza San Marco in Venice, painted in 1723 during Vivaldi's lifetime by the Italian artist Canaletto.*

Johann Pachelbel

A perfect and rare virtuoso.

DANIEL EBERLIN (1647–C.1715)

Johann Pachelbel, an important predecessor of J. S. Bach, is remembered today chiefly for a single composition, known as "Pachelbel's Canon" (of which many versions – including rock – now exist). But in his day he was much admired for his contribution to German Protestant church music, particularly for the organ.

Born in Nuremberg, he began his career as organist at St Stephen's Cathedral in Vienna. In 1677 he became organist at Bach's birthplace, the Thuringian town of Eisenach, but a year later he moved a few miles east to Erfurt,

ABOVE: The title page of Pachelbel's Hexachordum Apollinis, *printed in Nuremberg in 1699, six "arias" for organ or harpsichord, with variations.*

where for the next 12 years he was organist at the Predigerkirche. There he came into contact with members of the Bach family (he was godfather to one of J. S. Bach's sisters, and taught his elder brother Johann Christoph, who in turn taught Johann Sebastian).

While at Erfurt, Pachelbel married, only to lose his wife and their baby son two years later in a plague epidemic. He remarried in 1684, and raised a family of seven children. He then spent two years as court organist at Stuttgart, and three as town organist at Gotha, before finally moving back to his own birthplace as organist of St Sebald's Church.

Pachelbel's music

The organ chorales composed by Pachelbel – complex polyphonic pieces based on Protestant hymn tunes – had

enormous influence on those of Bach. He was also a master of various other keyboard genres of the time, including toccatas, *ricercari*, fantasias, chaconnes and variations – his *Hexachordum Apollinis* (1699) is a group of six arias with variations for organ or harpsichord, each in one of five keys making up a perfect fifth.

Pachelbel also wrote six suites for two violins and keyboard, the masterly and justly famous Canon (a set of 28 canonic variations originally scored for three violins and bass), motets, sacred concertos and 11 fine settings of the Magnificat for chorus and instruments, intended for the Vesper services in Nuremberg.

ABOVE: A 1732 engraving of a concert with organ, strings, wind and brass instruments. Pachelbel specialized in organ church music.

🎼 Life and works

NATIONALITY: German

BORN: Nuremberg, 1653;
DIED: Nuremberg, 1706

SPECIALIST GENRES:
Organ music.

MAJOR WORKS: Canon
and Gigue in D major;
six suites for two violins;
organ chorales.

Dietrich Buxtehude

*I should place an organist who is master of his instrument
at the very head of all virtuosi.*

LUDWIG VAN BEETHOVEN (1770—1827)

The Danish organist and composer Dietrich Buxtehude was an almost exact contemporary of Pachelbel, and like him, proved a formative influence on J. S. Bach. Probably of German origin, he was born some time around 1637 in the duchy of Holstein, where his father was a school-master and organist. In 1668 Buxtehude himself became organist at St Mary's Church in Lübeck, in north Germany. This appointment was one of the most important and lucrative in Germany, and competition was fierce (even though one of the stranger conditions attached to it was that the successful

ABOVE: *A painting by Johannes Voorhout depicting the friendship between Dietrich Buxtehude and his colleague J. A. Reincken (at the harpsichord).*

candidate should marry a daughter of his predecessor). This Buxtehude did – although Handel apparently declined an offer of the post nearly 40 years later when confronted with the necessity of marrying Buxtehude's own ageing daughter.

Buxtehude remained at Lübeck for the rest of his life. His duties at St Mary's required him to play and compose music for the main services, but he also reinstated an old tradition of giving substantial concerts in the church on the five Sundays before Christmas, just after the afternoon service. These *Abendmusiken*, as they were called, became famous, as was Buxtehude's extraordinarily accomplished organ-playing. In the winter of 1705–6, the young J. S. Bach is reputed to have walked from Thuringia to Lübeck just to hear the great man play.

Buxtehude's music

Buxtehude left a substantial body of compositions, including cantatas, several oratorio-like works intended for the *Abendmusiken*, many organ works including chorale preludes, fantasias, fugues and variations based on chorale themes, as well as some lighter chamber and keyboard music. His organ works, which had enormous influence on Bach, exploit the characteristic range of tone-colour of north German organs of the period, and liberate the pedal from its traditional role as harmonic foundation – some of Buxtehude's pedal parts require virtuoso footwork in their own right.

ABOVE: *St Mary's Church in Lübeck, where Buxtehude was organist for nearly 40 years, and where Bach heard him play.*

Life and works

NATIONALITY: Danish

BORN: Oldesloe, c.1637;
DIED: Lübeck, 1707

SPECIALIST GENRES: Organ music, cantatas for the German Protestant liturgy.

MAJOR WORKS: 120 sacred cantatas and other vocal pieces; many organ works; chamber and keyboard music.

Johann Sebastian Bach

Johann Sebastian Bach has done everything completely,
he was a man through and through.

FRANZ SCHUBERT (1797–1828)

For many music-lovers, the music of J. S. Bach fulfils a profound spiritual need: it has a timeless, other-worldly quality which could only come from a composer who felt himself close to God. Just as Bach's birthplace was over-shadowed by the Wartburg mountain, topped by the fortress in which Martin Luther hammered out the fundamental principles of Protestant theology, so his life was dominated by his devotion to the Lutheran faith, and his music was dedicated to its service.

Early years

Unlike many of his more cosmopolitan contemporaries, Bach spent his entire career in Germany – mostly in the central regions of Thuringia and Saxony. He was born into a long dynasty of Thuringian organists and composers who worked as church organists and choir-masters, municipal musicians, and at the many small princely or ducal courts which flourished in the region. Bach's father, Ambrosius, was himself employed as a musician by the town council of Eisenach, where Johann Sebastian was born on 21 March 1685.

After losing both parents by the age of ten, Bach was sent to live at Ohrdruf with his married elder brother, Johann Christoph, who was organist there. It seems likely that Johann Christoph helped with his young brother's musical training, but once Johann Sebastian reached the age of 15, there was no longer room for him in the Ohrdruf household, and he obtained a free place at St Michael's

ABOVE: *The house where Bach is believed to have been born in the Rittergasse in Eisenach, Thuringia, now a Bach museum.*

ABOVE: *Johann Sebastian Bach, four years before his death, in a painting by E. G. Haussmann.*

RIGHT:
A room in Bach's probable birthplace, containing contemporary instruments.

School in Lüneburg, 320km (200 miles) away in north Germany. There he benefited from a solid musical education and sang in the choir, but his formal education came to an end in 1702.

Arnstadt and Mühlhausen

At the age of 17, Bach returned to his native Thuringia to look for a job. After a temporary spell as a violinist at the Weimar ducal court, he was appointed organist at the New Church in Arnstadt, not far from Weimar. There he started to compose in earnest, and in the winter of

1705–6 he made his legendary pilgrimage (allegedly on foot) to Lübeck, 420km (260 miles) to the north, to hear the celebrated organist Dietrich Buxtehude.

After his return to Arnstadt, Bach's relationship with the church council deteriorated (he had a stubborn and at times arrogant streak, which caused problems with all his employers), and in the summer of 1707 he left to take up a new post as organist at the imperial free city of Mühlhausen, some 58km (36 miles) to the north-west. His salary was now such that he felt able to marry his second cousin, Maria

Barbara Bach. But although his personal life had settled down, Bach quickly became dissatisfied with conditions at Mühlhausen, and in 1708 he moved again, this time to the ducal court at Weimar.

Life and works

NATIONALITY: German

BORN: Eisenach, 1685; **DIED:** Leipzig, 1750

SPECIALIST GENRES: Sacred music for the German Protestant liturgy, especially cantatas, instrumental and keyboard music.

MAJOR WORKS: *Brandenburg Concertos* (1721); 4 orchestral suites; 7 harpsichord concertos; 3 violin concertos; *Goldberg Variations* (1722); *The Well-Tempered Clavier* (1722–44); over 200 cantatas; *St John Passion* (1723); *St Matthew Passion* (1729); *Christmas Oratorio* (1734); *Italian Concerto* (1735); *The Musical Offering* (1747); Mass in B minor (1749); *The Art of Fugue* (1750).

ABOVE: Bach directing a concert in 1714 at the Court Chapel in Weimar, where he worked from 1708 until 1717.

Weimar

In the early 18th century Weimar was just another small, provincial town – its period of glory was to come some 80 years later, when its residents would include Goethe, Wieland and Schiller. Bach's job was as organist at the ducal chapel in the castle, but six of his children – including the future composers Wilhelm Friedemann (1710–84) and Carl Philipp Emmanuel (1714–88) – were christened at the City Church of St Peter and Paul during the Weimar years.

It was here that Bach began composing cantatas in earnest for performance at court, and he also provided instrumental music for the court orchestra. His early years at Weimar were happy and productive but, after 1713, relations with his employer, Duke Wilhelm Ernst, began to deteriorate and in 1717 Bach accepted

ABOVE: *A romanticized artist's impression of Bach's visit to Frederick the Great at the palace of Sans Souci in Potsdam, May 1747.*

with concertos for violin (including the famous Double Concerto in D minor), orchestral suites, sonatas for harpsichord, violin, and flute, the suites for solo cello and the sonatas and partitas for solo violin. These works show that Bach had thoroughly absorbed the Italian style, through intensive study of works by Corelli and Vivaldi.

Remarriage

In May 1720, while Bach was away at a spa with his employer, Maria Barbara died suddenly. Bach remarried the next year: his bride, Anna Magdalena Wilcken (1701–60), proved a great asset to her husband, both domestically and professionally (the daughter of a musician, she was a singer, harpsichordist and music copyist). She inherited Bach's four surviving

the job of *Kapellmeister* to the court of Prince Leopold of Anhalt-Cöthen. The duke was so reluctant to let him go that he placed him under house arrest for a month. Eventually, in December 1717, the Bach family was allowed to leave.

Cöthen

While most of Bach's compositions up to 1717 had been organ works and sacred cantatas, he now exploited the instrumental resources available to him at the Cöthen court. Most of his work there was secular, since the Calvinist Prince Leopold required little sacred music. Among the works he composed during this period were the six *Brandenburg Concertos* for various instrumental combinations, together

ABOVE: *Bach's eldest son, Wilhelm Friedemann (1710–84), painted around 1760. Like his father, he was a composer.*

ABOVE: *The trumpeter Gottfried Reiche (1667–1734), who played the high clarino parts in Bach's works in Leipzig.*

children, to whom she added another 13, including another future composer, Johann Christian (1735–82), later known as the "English Bach", since he spent much of his career there. Shortly after their marriage Bach began to compile two *Clavierbüchlein* (*Little Keyboard Books*) for his wife, which contain, among other works, the 15 Inventions and Sinfonias and several preludes and fugues, which were later assembled with others as *Das wohltemperierte Clavier* (*The Well-Tempered Clavier*).

In 1721 Prince Leopold of Anhalt-Cöthen married his cousin, and life changed irrevocably at the Cöthen court. The frivolous new princess was uninterested in music, and Bach soon felt obliged to move on – probably with some regret. In June 1722 the post of Kantor of the Thomasschule in Leipzig became vacant. The town council wanted Telemann, but he could not be released from his job at Hamburg, and so, after much deliberation, they appointed Bach. On 22 May 1723 he moved into his new quarters in the Thomasschule, where he stayed until his death 27 years later.

Leipzig

Bach's years at Leipzig, where he was required not only to teach, but to supply music for the town's two principal churches, St Thomas and St Nicholas, were relatively uneventful, but were punctuated by acrimonious disagreements with the council over pay and conditions. Nonetheless, they were amazingly fruitful. One of his principal jobs was to write, rehearse and direct cantatas for the Sunday services at the two churches, and his output included around 250 of these substantial works for voices, chorus

ABOVE: A page from the manuscript score of Bach's St Matthew Passion, *first performed in Leipzig on Good Friday in 1729.*

and orchestra, mostly based on well-known Protestant chorale tunes.

In addition, he produced two magnificent settings of the Passion story, according to St Matthew and St John, the Mass in B minor, the *Christmas Oratorio*, and other major sacred works, into which he poured all the resources of vocal and instrumental writing available to him. Towards the end of his life, several books of keyboard music were published, but Bach's fame remained local. Among his last major

works were the *Goldberg Variations* for harpsichord, allegedly written for an aristocratic insomniac; *Das musicalisches Opfer* (*The Musical Offering*, based on a fugue subject devised by Frederick the Great when Bach visited him at Potsdam in 1747), and the almost visionary *Kunst der Fuge* (*The Art of Fugue*), a complex series of canons on which Bach worked during the last years of his life, when his sight began to fail. He was almost totally blind when he died, leaving his widow in dire financial straits.

By the time of Bach's death, musical fashions were fast changing, and his music was perceived as antiquated. During his lifetime he had been more celebrated as an organist than as a composer. Unlike Mozart or Beethoven, he had little posthumous influence until Mendelssohn rediscovered his choral masterpieces in the 19th century, and his works began to be performed once more. He is now revered as one of the greatest of all composers.

ABOVE: A romanticized 19th-century impression of the Bach family at their morning prayers.

George Frideric Handel

Handel understands effect better than any of us –
when he chooses, he strikes like a thunderbolt.

WOLFGANG AMADEUS MOZART (1756–91)

ABOVE: George Frideric Handel (1685–1759). He never appeared in public without his voluminous wig.

Handel and Bach were born in the same year, in much the same area of central Germany – Halle, Handel's birthplace in Saxony, is about 160km (100 miles) north of Thuringia. Both men lived to a reasonable old age, and both had lost their sight when they died. But their respective careers could not have been more different.

Early years

While Bach was content to live and work within the musical tradition of his family, Handel had to struggle to make a career in music. His father wanted his son to study law, and tried to stifle the boy's interest in music. But Handel persisted, and was eventually allowed to study music as part of his general education. Only after his father's death did he take it up full-time and in 1703, aged 18, he set out for Hamburg in search of employment.

Hamburg

One of Hamburg's attractions was as a flourishing centre of opera. Germany's first commercial opera house had opened there in 1678, and had scraped along financially under a succession of entrepreneurial directors with flair but no money. Here Handel found an ideal proving-ground for his early attempts at the genre which would dominate his life. But he refused the offer of a permanent post, and instead departed for Italy – the birthplace of opera.

The Italian experience

Handel travelled to Italy under the patronage of Prince Ferdinando de'Medici, and in 1707 his first mature opera, *Rodrigo*, was produced at a Florentine theatre. It was a success, earning Handel the favours of the grand duke's mistress, the singer Vittoria Tarquini. Perhaps wisely, Handel quickly departed for Rome, where he found employment at the court of Cardinal Pietro Ottoboni, the immensely wealthy papal vice-chancellor. There he met celebrated musicians including Corelli and the Scarlattis, and tried his hand at music for the unfamiliar Catholic liturgy, including a setting of the Vespers. His first oratorio, a setting of the Resurrection story, was performed with great splendour on Easter Sunday 1708 at the Palazzo Bonelli.

From Rome Handel travelled on to Naples and then to Venice, where his opera *Agrippina* was performed during

ABOVE: An anonymous painting of Hamburg, one of the most important of the Hanseatic ports, in 1700.

ABOVE: *The square in front of St Peter's Basilica in Rome, painted in 1754 by G. P. Pannini.*

ABOVE: *A romantic impression depicting Handel making music at the keyboard with his friends.*

the 1710 carnival season. Then, ever eager for new experiences, he returned north to Hanover, to be appointed *Kapellmeister* to the elector at a good salary and with the promise of a year's sabbatical leave. He took it immediately, and promptly left with an invitation to London. His transformation from a German to an English composer had begun.

England

In Queen Anne's England, Handel stepped into a musical vacuum left by the deaths of John Blow and his gifted pupil Henry Purcell. He decided to fill it by satisfying the growing middle-class demand for opera. His opera *Rinaldo* scored a huge success at the Queen's Theatre in London, both musically and dramatically. Audiences were particularly intrigued by a dramatic masterstroke – the release of a flock of sparrows onstage to lend verisimilitude to the aria "Augelletti" ("Little Birds"). But Handel was under an obligation to return to Hanover, where he spent some 15 months

perfecting his instrumental compositions – overtures and *concerti grossi*.

In the autumn of 1712 Handel obtained another period of leave from the indulgent Elector of Hanover, and

Life and works

NATIONALITY: German

BORN: Halle, 1685;
DIED: London, 1759

SPECIALIST GENRES:
Italianate operas,
English oratorios.

MAJOR WORKS:
Water Music (1717);
Acis and Galatea (1718) and
45 other operas; *Chandos Anthems* (1717–20);
12 *concerti grossi* (1739);
Messiah (1742); 15 other oratorios; *Music for the Royal Fireworks* (1749).

returned to London, where his next opera, *Il pastor fido (The Faithful Shepherd)*, was put on at the Haymarket Theatre. This time the public was disappointed. As one critic put it: "The habits [costumes] were old. The opera short." Handel immediately hit back with a full-length, five-act opera, based on the Greek myth of Theseus. At the same time he began to fulfil royal commissions, supplying royal odes and a triumphantly received Te Deum and Jubilate to celebrate the Treaty of Utrecht, which ended the War of the Spanish Succession.

Life under a new king

Handel had absented himself from his duties in Hanover for two years when in 1714 he received a rude shock: Queen Anne died childless, and the English throne passed to his neglected former employer the Elector of Hanover, now George I of England. It is said that the famous *Water Music*, written to accompany the king's triumphal procession up the Thames, was composed as a peace-offering (although it was probably written three

ABOVE: Handel playing one of his organ concertos at the Covent Garden Theatre in London.

years after George's accession). In any case, Handel was quickly forgiven, and remained a favoured royal composer for the rest of his life. He also acquired a new patron, the Duke of Chandos, for whose magnificent estate in Edgware Handel wrote the 11 *Chandos Anthems*, a Te Deum, the masque *Acis and Galatea*, and his first attempt at an English oratorio, *Esther*.

The Royal Academy

In 1719 the grandly named Royal Academy of Music came into being. This institution, supported by a group of 62 royal and noble subscribers, aimed to establish a regular opera company in London, with Handel as its composer-in-residence. Over the next eight years he supplied some 14 Italian operas for the company, including

Radamisto, Rodelinda, Admeto, Giulio Cesare and *Tamerlano*, and engaged some of the finest European singers to perform them. These included the great castrato Senesino, a man possessed of a "powerful, clear, equal and sweet contralto voice", and the sopranos Francesca Cuzzoni and Faustina Bordoni, all engaged at astronomical salaries. Apart from the entertainment of the operas themselves, London society was soon treated to the diverting spectacle of the two rival divas fighting on stage while Senesino spent his time sulking in the background.

Change to oratorio

George I died in 1727. For his successor, George II's, coronation Handel provided four anthems (including *Zadok the Priest*, which has been sung at British coronations ever since). By this time the Academy was in deep financial trouble, and Handel's own financial losses – combined with waning public enthusiasm for this "exotic and irrational entertainment", the unexpected popularity of John Gay's satirical *Beggar's Opera* in 1728, and a complete breakdown in health – prompted a change of direction. He was already

LEFT: The aria "How beautiful are the feet" from Handel's autograph score of Messiah.

RIGHT: Handel's choir singing an oratorio by Willem de Fesch, as drawn by Hogarth in 1731.

writing instrumental music, especially organ concertos, for the London pleasure gardens, but although he continued to write Italian operas, including *Ariodante* and *Serse*, until 1740, he needed a new genre. He found it in the English oratorio, beginning with *Deborah*, *Athaliah*, *Saul* and *Israel in Egypt* in the 1730s, but reaching its apogee in *Messiah*, written for performance in Dublin in 1742.

In setting these Biblical stories, Handel adapted elements from Italian opera, particularly the recitative-aria format; but reduced the soloists' importance in order to give more prominence to the chorus and orchestra. This clever ploy ensured the survival of his oratorios as a mainstay of the repertoire of British choral societies. *Messiah* was followed by some 15 further oratorios, including *Samson* (1741–2), *Semele* (1743), which is more of an opera than an oratorio, *Judas Maccabaeus* (1746), *Alexander Balue* and *Joshua* (1747), *Solomon* (1748) and *Jephtha* (1751), all of which are still regularly performed.

ABOVE: *Handel's memorial in Westminster Abbey, London.*

Last years

Handel's fortunes were mixed in the last years of his life. He had amassed considerable wealth despite his losses, and used some of it to support philanthropic causes, such as the Foundling Hospital. In April 1749 he fulfilled his last royal commission: music to accompany a grand firework display in London's Green Park to mark the Peace of Aix-la-Chapelle — an occasion marred when the firework pavilion burnt to the ground. But Handel's *Music for the Royal Fireworks* ranks with the *Water Music* among his most popular instrumental compositions.

Two years later his sight was failing. A painful operation to cure cataracts proved useless, and for the last seven years of his life he was totally blind. But the people of his adopted land had taken him to their hearts, and while Bach's death went largely unremarked, Handel was buried with full honours in Westminster Abbey. His epitaph summed up his extraordinary achievement:

The most Excellent Musician
any Age ever produced:
Whose Compositions were
a Sentimental Language
rather than mere Sounds;
And surpassed the Power of Words
In Expressing the various Passions
of the Human Heart.

ABOVE: *A contemporary artist's view of the structure erected in Green Park for the 1749 firework display celebrating the Peace of Aix-la-Chapelle.*

ABOVE: *The Handel Centenary Commemoration concert (1785) in Westminster Abbey.*

Domenico Scarlatti

*Scarlatti frequently told M. L'Augier that he was sensible
he had broke through all the rules of composition...*

CHARLES BURNEY (1726–1814), "GENERAL HISTORY OF MUSIC"

The son of the composer Alessandro Scarlatti, Domenico probably began his musical training with his father. At the age of 16 he was appointed organist in the Neapolitan royal chapel, where his father was *maestro di cappella,* but in the spring of 1705 Alessandro ordered his son to seek his fortune in the northern Italian cities of Florence and Venice, describing him in a letter of recommendation as "a young eagle whose wings are grown: he must not remain idle in the nest, and I must not hinder his flight". In fact, Alessandro continued to interfere with his son's career until Domenico obtained legal independence in 1717, at the advanced age of 32.

In 1709 Domenico entered the service of the exiled Polish Queen Maria Casimira in Rome, where he encountered other up-and-coming musicians, including his contemporary,

Handel. After a spell as *maestro di cappella* at the Julian Chapel in the Vatican, he decided to leave Italy for Portugal, and from 1719 until 1728 he worked in Lisbon.

Keyboard sonatas

Scarlatti's duties in Lisbon included teaching the king's musical daughter Maria Barbara. When the princess married the Crown Prince of Spain and moved to Madrid in 1728, Scarlatti accompanied her. He remained in her service for the rest of his life, and it was for her that he wrote the 550 or so one-movement keyboard sonatas on which his fame rests.

These sonatas are unique in the keyboard repertoire. Apart from their unusual binary format, they explore new playing techniques, including hand-crossing and rapid note repetition. Each sonata, which Scarlatti himself described as "an ingenious jesting with art", focuses on a particular technical problem, and many incorporate special effects in imitation of Spanish idioms, such as the thrumming of guitars and the clicking of castanets.

ABOVE:
A contemporary portrait in oil of Domenico Scarlatti by Antonio de Velasco.

LEFT: The Harpsichordist, *by Edith Hipkins (1885), now in the Royal Academy of Music in London.*

Life and works

NATIONALITY: Italian

BORN: Naples, 1685;
DIED: Madrid, 1757

SPECIALIST GENRES:
Virtuoso harpsichord music.

MAJOR WORKS:
550 keyboard sonatas.

Jean-Philippe Rameau

*The expression of thought, of sentiment, of the passions,
must be the true aim of music.*

RAMEAU

The French composer Jean-Philippe Rameau is now chiefly remembered for his operas, but like Janáček, he was a late starter in the operatic field. Born two years before the great Bach-Handel-Scarlatti triumvirate, he spent the earlier part of his career working as an organist, moving between various major towns in central France and Paris, where he eventually settled in 1722. In that year he published a textbook on harmony, *Traité de l'harmonie*, which established him as one of the most innovative and controversial musical theorists of his age.

Over the next 25 years or so Rameau worked principally as a harpsichord teacher, and his volumes of enchanting "character" pieces for keyboard in the tradition of François Couperin became very popular. In 1730 he found a wealthy patron, the tax-collector Le Riche de

ABOVE: *Jean-Philippe Rameau with his violin, a famous portrait by Joseph Aved (1702–66).*

ABOVE: *Sophie Arnould (1740–1802), one of the most celebrated French opera singers of Rameau's time.*

la Pouplinière, who introduced him to the playwright Abbé Simon-Joseph Pellegrin. Rameau's first opera, *Hippolyte et Aricie,* to a libretto by Pellegrin, was produced at the Paris Opéra in October 1733. It established the composer as a worthy successor to Lully in the operatic field.

Rameau went on to write some 30 stage works – full-blown *tragédies-lyriques* in the Lullian mould such as *Castor et Pollux, Dardanus* and *Les boréades;* opera-ballets (operas with a substantial dance element, often written to celebrate royal victories or marriages), such as *La princesse de Navarre, Les fêtes de Polymnie* and *Zaïs;* and straightforward ballets such as *Pygmalion.* All are characterized by

sensitive handling of the text, whether comic, sentimental or tragic; colourful and innovative use of the orchestra (especially evident in the many brilliant and lively dances); and expressive and powerful choral writing.

War of the Buffoons

In the early 1750s Rameau (or rather his supporters) became embroiled in the celebrated *"Querelle des bouffons"* – a war of words between admirers of Rameau's traditional French style, and those of the newly imported Italian style of Pergolesi. In the long run, the Italians won, and Rameau's operas finally dropped out of fashion. They were resurrected some 200 years later by William Christie's *Les arts florissants* in France and the British conductors John Eliot Gardiner and Nicholas Kraemer.

Life and works

NATIONALITY: French

BORN: Dijon, 1683;
DIED: Paris, 1764

SPECIALIST GENRES: Opera and opera-ballets in the French style.

MAJOR WORKS: *Les Indes galantes (The Courtly Indies,* 1735); *Castor et Pollux* (1737); *Pièces de clavecin* (1741).

Other Composers of the Era

The Italian style and the French style have for long divided the Republic of Music in France.

FRANÇOIS COUPERIN (C.1626–61)

The Baroque era produced a plethora of minor composers, many of whom are remembered today only for a handful of works.

Italy

Among these was the Italian priest and singer Gregorio Allegri (1582–1652), who worked at the Sistine Chapel in Rome. His chief claim to fame is the nine-part Miserere which he wrote for the exclusive use of the chapel, and which was jealously guarded until the young prodigy Mozart wrote it out from memory after hearing it twice on a visit in 1770.

Giacomo Carissimi (1605–74), who worked in Rome as choir-master to Queen Christina of Sweden, adapted Monteverdi's operatic style to the sacred oratorio, of which he wrote

ABOVE: Gregorio Allegri (1582–1652), noted particularly for his nine-part Miserere.

over a dozen, together with many motets and cantatas. He was the last composer to use the ancient folk tune "L'homme armé" as the musical basis for a Mass setting.

Carissimi's pupil Alessandro Scarlatti (1660–1725) also worked for Queen Christina, and spent his life moving between Rome and Naples in the service of court and church. More than half of his 115 operas survive, but only a handful, including *La Griselda* (1721), have been revived. Scarlatti invented the *da capo* aria, with its long introduction and closing orchestral *ritornello*. He is credited with introducing recitative accompanied by orchestra rather than keyboard, and invented the "Italian overture", a two-part slow-fast orchestral introduction

to a dramatic work, which later developed into the symphony. He also wrote a large volume of sacred music, and around 700 chamber cantatas.

The Venetian composer Tomaso Albinoni (1671–1751) is now more famous for one work which he did not compose – the Adagio for organ and strings constructed from musical fragments by Remo Giazotto in 1945 – than for his genuine 81 operas, 99 sonatas, 59 concertos and nine sinfonias. His solo concertos for oboe (the earliest known) and trumpet, and some of his *concerti grossi*, are now back in the repertoire.

Giovanni Battista Pergolesi (1710–36) died of tuberculosis at the age of only 26. Many of his works were lost, but he is remembered for a brilliant comic opera, *La serva padrona*

ABOVE: Alessandro Scarlatti (1660–1725), father of Domenico, and a noted composer in his own right.

ABOVE: Giovanni Battista Pergolesi (1710–36), a highly talented composer who died young of tuberculosis.

ABOVE: *An atmospheric contemporary portrait of the great Italian violinist and composer Giuseppe Tartini (1692–1770).*

(*The Maid as Mistress*, 1733), a Stabat Mater (1736), and for tunes he probably did not write (but which were ascribed to him after his death because of his popularity) which Stravinsky recycled in his ballet *Pulcinella* (1920).

Like Corelli, Giuseppe Tartini (1692–1770) is remembered for his daringly original violin music. A brilliant virtuoso, he wrote 42 violin

ABOVE: *Johann Hasse (1699–1783), upon hearing the 15-year-old Mozart, remarked "This boy will cause us all to be forgotten."*

sonatas of immense technical difficulty (the most famous is the *Devil's Trill*, said to have been played to him in a dream by the Devil), 135 violin concertos, and many other instrumental pieces.

France

In France, the vacuum left by Lully's death in 1687 was filled by Marc-Antoine Charpentier (c.1645–1704), who began his career as music master and court singer to the Duchesse de Guise. From 1672 until 1686 he was also associated with Molière's troupe, writing music for the original production of *Le malade imaginaire*, among other works. He wrote a great deal of fine sacred music: 10 Magnificats, 37 antiphons, 84 psalms, over 200 motets and four Te Deums (one of which is now often performed) for Sainte-Chapelle on the Ile de Paris. Among his many fine stage works, *Les arts florissants* (1685–6) has lent its name to one of the foremost modern French ensembles playing music of the Baroque period.

Another French composer, François Couperin (c.1626–61), worked for the courts of Louis XIV and Louis XV. Born into a famous musical dynasty (his uncle Louis was a fine composer for organ and harpsichord), François became organist at the royal chapel. His harpsichord works (four published volumes contain around 230 pieces) are masterpieces of delicacy and musical description; many have enigmatic titles. He also wrote several instrumental suites in the fashionable style of Corelli.

Germany

The composer Johann Hasse (1699–1783) concentrated on opera, becoming director of the Dresden court opera. In 1763 he moved to Vienna, where he continued to write *opere serie* on texts by Metastasio, even though fashions were changing.

ABOVE: *François Couperin, known as "Le grand" ("the Great"), one of the finest composers of keyboard music of his time.*

Georg Philipp Telemann (1681–1767) spent most of his career as music director to the Hamburg churches. Probably the most prolific composer in the history of music (his output includes 600 overtures, 40 operas, 44 Passion settings and a huge quantity of instrumental music), he was in his day more highly regarded than Bach. His instrumental music is still popular today.

ABOVE: *Georg Philipp Telemann (1681–1767) holds the record as the most prolific composer of all time.*

The Classical ❧ Period ❧

A painting by J. F. Greipel (1720–98) of the 1765 performance of Gluck's
one-act "theatrical serenata" Il parnaso confuso (Parnassus in Confusion).

Music of the Enlightenment

*Dust as we are, the immortal spirit grows
Like harmony in music.*

<small>WILLIAM WORDSWORTH (1770–1850), "THE PRELUDE"</small>

By classical music, most people today mean serious music of any period, as opposed to jazz, pop, rock or other similar genres. But the term Classical is strictly applied to music written between about 1750–1830, corresponding to a period of classicism in art and architecture.

Classical style

During this period, the flamboyant, heavily ornate Baroque style of architecture (exemplified by the interior of the church of St Nicholas in Prague's Old Town, where Mozart played the organ on one of his visits) gave way to a cooler, more restrained style, based on the serene proportions of the ancient world. The 18th century was the age of the Grand Tour, when upper-class young men were despatched to Italy to study Greek and Roman architecture, as revealed through recent archaeological excavations.

Contemporary architects such as Robert Adam designed grand country houses with Classical façades, while the furniture designed by Sheraton and his colleagues took on a graceful, delicate look. In England, the fashion for the

ABOVE: The building which inspired much 17th- and 18th-century neo-classical architecture – the Parthenon (Temple of Athena) on the Acropolis in Athens, built between 447 and 422 BC.

ABOVE: A fine example of 18th-century neo-classical architecture – designs for Home House in Portman Square, London, by Robert Adam (1728–92).

ABOVE: Vienna in the 18th century – a view of one of its main streets, the Kohlmarkt. St Michael's Church can be seen on the right.

Classical look reached its height around the turn of the 19th century (the age of Jane Austen), continuing into the Regency period (1811–20). In France, particularly, there was a short period of transition between the Baroque and Classical styles known as Rococo, characterized by delicate but elaborate ornamentation, as seen in French furniture of the mid 18th century, and the paintings of artists such as Antoine Watteau (1684–1721) and François Boucher (1703–70).

Classical style in music

Musical tastes inevitably followed the decorative arts, and the florid, ornamental, technically intricate styles of late Baroque composers gave way to a new emphasis on clarity, order and balance, exemplified by the Classical symphony, string quartet and solo sonata. A few composers fitted the Rococo label, including C. P. E. Bach, François Couperin, the English composer William Boyce (1710–79), and Gluck and Rameau – both primarily opera composers – in some of their works. But generally speaking, the Classical period in musical history is dominated by four giants, all associated with Vienna, and sometimes collectively known as the First Viennese School. They were Haydn, Mozart, Beethoven and Schubert. Their works are still part of the core repertoire of classical music as a whole.

Music's place in society

The late 18th century was a period of great social upheaval. The breakdown of the old social order reached its culmination in the French Revolution (1789–99), and music ceased to be the exclusive preserve of pampered aristocrats or prelates. This radical social shift is reflected in the careers of the four great Classical composers.

Haydn, the oldest, spent his long career in the service of a single

ABOVE: *A charming example of 18th-century Rococo art –* The Dance *(c.1719) by Antoine Watteau (1684–1721), a favourite artist at the French court.*

aristocratic family, who regarded him as a valued servant. Mozart began his career in a similar way, in the employment of the Archbishop of Salzburg, but when more lucrative court appointments eluded him, he took the radical step of trying a freelance existence, which allowed

ABOVE: *Private music-making –* The Lost Chord *by Stephen Lewin (fl.1890–1910).*

him personal liberty, but failed to provide sufficient financial security.

Beethoven, in a similar situation, enjoyed the friendship and patronage of several wealthy noblemen, but he was not so fettered by 18th-century convention as Mozart. He understood his own worth as an individual, and his patrons played to his tune, not the other way round. Beethoven was one of the first composers to free himself from the idea of musician as servant, and to produce powerfully individualistic music which he himself promoted to an audience of the rising middle class.

Schubert, a native of Vienna, never tried to obtain a permanent job. A composer who stood on the threshold of the Romantic age, he wrote music out of personal choice, aimed at people like himself (he had a close circle of musically inclined friends). Much of his music – particularly his songs and chamber music – was intended for a domestic market, and none of his symphonies was professionally performed during his lifetime.

Christoph Willibald Gluck

*Hearing "Iphigénie" I forget that I am in an opera house
and think I am hearing a Greek tragedy.*

BARON GRIMM

ABOVE: *Christoph Willibald Gluck, painted by Duplessis in 1775, when Gluck was alternating between Vienna and Paris.*

Gluck's career overlapped with that of Rameau, his senior by over 30 years, and like Rameau, he worked during the transitional period between Baroque and Classical styles, often known as the Rococo age. Born into a German family of foresters who lived in Upper Bohemia, he escaped being coerced into the family profession by running away from home when he was about 13. He went to Prague, and then to Vienna, where he was attached to a nobleman's household. When the nobleman moved to Milan, Gluck went with him, and it was in Italy that he realized his true profession – that of opera composer.

By 1744 eight of his operas had been produced in Italy, many based on

libretti by the great Italian dramatist Pietro Metastasio. In 1745 Gluck went to London, where he found himself in competition with Handel (who is said to have remarked that "Gluck knows no more of counterpoint than my cook", though in fact he liked Gluck and arranged a concert with him). After leaving London, Gluck spent several peripatetic years travelling around Europe with an Italian opera company, before making an advantageous marriage and settling in Vienna. In 1754 the Empress Maria Theresa appointed him composer to the court theatre.

"Reform" operas

Over the next few years Gluck evolved the operatic style which would make him famous. It was clear that *opera seria*, and its French equivalent, the *tragédie-lyrique*, had run their course. Audiences were beginning to demand different types of entertainment, portraying real people in real-life situations rather than cardboard-cutout ancient heroes. To Gluck's mind, opera had been taken over by the often absurd demands of star singers, who felt able to dictate their wishes to librettists and composers, usually in defiance of dramatic reason. In collaboration with the poet Raniero de Calzabigi (1714–95), and with the active encouragement of the Intendant of

ABOVE: *Gluck at the keyboard, by the French artist Eugène Delacroix.*

ABOVE: *The opening of Act II of Gluck's "azione teatrale", Orfeo ed Euridice.*

320 *The Classical Period*

ABOVE: A design by V. D. Polenov (1844–1927) for Act I of Gluck's opera Orfeo ed
Euridice, *for a performance of the French version in Moscow, 1897.*

the court theatres, Count Giacomo Durazzo, Gluck set out to "reform" operatic convention.

He began by writing a series of comic operas in the French style, including *La fausse esclave* and *L'île de Merlin* (1758), but his first major collaboration with Calzabigi and the choreographer Gasparo Angiolini was the ballet *Don Juan* (1761), a work of great dramatic force which influenced Mozart's opera *Don Giovanni* (1787). It was followed in 1762 by the opera *Orfeo ed Euridice* – the most expressive setting of this tragic love story since Monteverdi. Orfeo's aria "Che farò senza Euridice" is one of the most affecting operatic laments, while the scenes in Hades and Elysium (especially the famous "Dance of the Blessed Spirits") gave Gluck ample opportunity for dramatic instrumental and vocal effects, backed up by innovative staging.

In 1767, Gluck and Calzabigi produced the second of their "reform" operas, *Alceste*. In a famous preface to the score, Gluck laid out the principles of this new type of opera, free of the

abuses "which have so long disfigured Italian opera and made of the most splendid and beautiful of spectacles the most ridiculous and wearisome". Gluck aimed to "restrict music to its true

ABOVE: The title page of the first edition of the score of
Orfeo ed Euridice, *published in Paris in 1764.*

office of serving the poetry by means of expression and by following the situations of the story", seeking "a beautiful simplicity", free of unnecessary vocal display at the whims of individual singers. He also tried to make the overture an integral part of the drama. These principles governed his next Viennese opera, *Paride ed Elena* (*Paris and Helen*, 1770).

In 1774 Gluck moved to Paris, where over the next six years he wrote three new operas (two based on the story of Iphigenia, and *Echo et Narcisse*), as well as revisions (in French) of *Orfeo* and *Alceste*. He also found himself drawn into competition with the Italian composer Niccolò Piccinni (1728–1800). After *Echo et Narcisse* failed to please, Gluck returned to Vienna, where he died of the last of a series of strokes incurred, it was said, after drinking an after-dinner liqueur in defiance of his doctor's instructions.

Joseph Haydn

So far as genius can exist in a man who is merely virtuous,
Haydn had it.

FRIEDRICH NIETZSCHE (1844–1900)

Joseph Haydn was the eldest and longest lived of the four great composers of the so-called "First Viennese School". Born when Bach and Handel were at the height of their fame, he outlived his friend Mozart by 18 years, and saw his former pupil Beethoven well established in his own career. It was Haydn who practically invented the Classical musical forms of symphony, concerto, string quartet and sonata. Mozart, Beethoven and Schubert all owed an incalculable debt to their genial, hard-working predecessor.

Haydn's life spanned a period of great social change. He was one of the last major musicians to work for a single aristocratic patron – in his case, the Hungarian Esterházy family, whose seat was the castle of Eisenstadt, some 80km (50 miles) from Vienna.

ABOVE: *Joseph Haydn at the keyboard (c.1795) with the score of his penultimate symphony – the* Drumroll *(No. 103).*

The arrangement worked quite well for Haydn – his employers treated him fairly – but in their eyes he was no better than a servant. His life-long desire for freedom was granted only towards the end of his long career, when he was effectively pensioned off and was able to travel and enjoy his spreading European reputation.

Early years

Haydn was one of 12 children born to the village wheelwright in Rohrau, about 50km (30 miles) south-east of Vienna. When he was only six, his budding musical talent was noticed by his family and neighbours, and a relative in Hainburg, who was a schoolmaster, offered to take the child as a boarder and begin his musical education. Shortly after his eighth birthday, Haydn was taken on as a choirboy at St Stephen's

LEFT:
Prince Nikolaus Esterházy ("the Magnificent"), Haydn's patron and employer from 1762–90.

RIGHT:
The courtyard of the Esterházy family palace at Eisenstadt, near Vienna, where Haydn worked.

ABOVE: A performance in 1775 of Haydn's opera L'incontro improviso (The Unforeseen Encounter), *in the theatre at Eszterháza. The composer is playing the harpsichord.*

Cathedral in Vienna, under the harsh regime of the choir-master Karl Georg Reutter. Haydn said later in life: "I never had a proper teacher. I started with the practical side…I listened more than I studied, and tried to turn to good account all the things that impressed me."

Haydn left the choir in 1749, and for the next decade he eked out a meagre living in Vienna as a music teacher. His major breakthrough came when Prince Paul Anton Esterházy happened to hear a symphony of Haydn's and immediately offered the young composer a job. Haydn accepted, but first he took the disastrous step of getting married. His first love had become a nun, and perhaps out of a mistaken sense of duty to her father, Haydn agreed to marry her elder sister, Maria Anna Keller. His wife turned out to be bad-tempered,

unattractive, and didn't care "whether her husband was a cobbler or an artist". She was also apparently unable to have children. During the years ahead Haydn found consolation with other women, but by the time his wife died in 1800 he was too old to think of remarriage.

ABOVE: The exquisite mirrored concert room at the summer palace of Eszterháza, built in the mid 1760s.

LEFT: A 19th-century edition of Haydn's Symphony No. 84 in E flat, first published as the fourth of the set of six Paris Symphonies.

RIGHT: A 19th-century artist's impression of Haydn and friends playing string quartets. Haydn was a good violinist.

Eisenstadt

In May 1761 Haydn took up his new post. His duties included training the choir and orchestra at Eisenstadt, maintaining all the instruments and music, and keeping discipline. He was also required to compose to order. Among the first works that Haydn wrote for his new patron were three symphonies called *Morning*, *Noon* and *Evening*, possibly intended to be played by the prince himself.

Less than a year later, Prince Paul Anton died. His successor, his brother Prince Nikolaus, was far more socially ambitious (he acquired the nickname "the Magnificent"), and soon Haydn found himself turning out a stream of music for his patron's entertainment: symphonies, concertos, string quartets, trios, and a vast quantity of chamber music for the prince's own instrument, the archaic, six-stringed baryton (similar to the viola d'amore).

Move to Eszterháza

In 1764 Nikolaus decided that Eisenstadt was no longer equal to his pretensions. He ordered the construction of a new summer palace – fit for a prince – on the shores of Lake Neusiedler. It had 126 lavishly decorated guest rooms, an art gallery, a concert hall, a ballroom and a 400-seat theatre. The Empress Maria Theresa attended a performance of one of Haydn's operas there in 1775, and declared: "If I want to hear a good opera, I go to Eszterháza." All in all, Haydn wrote some 25 operas for Eszterháza, including *L'infedeltà delusa* (*Infidelity Deluded*, 1773), *Il mondo della luna* (*The World on the Moon*, 1777) and *Armida* (1783).

While Haydn enjoyed the isolation of Eszterháza, where there was no one to bother him, and he was, as he said, "forced to become original", the other musicians hated it. Each year Prince Nikolaus found it harder to tear himself away from his fairy-tale palace, and he and his courtiers spent as little time at Eisenstadt as possible. But many of the court musicians had families in Vienna, and they begged Haydn to intercede with the prince.

ABOVE: A romantic impression of Haydn walking in the streets of Vienna carrying one of his scores under his arm.

His witty answer was the *Farewell* Symphony (No. 45), written in November 1772, in which one by one the musicians left the stage, packing up their instruments and blowing out their candles, until only two violins were left playing. The prince apparently took the hint.

The *Farewell* Symphony is one of a group of distinctive symphonies written during the 1770s in the fashionable, literary-influenced style known as *Sturm und Drang* ("storm and stress"). Many are in unusual keys, and exhibit a wide variety of moods. The same emotional style also influenced Haydn's other work of the period, including his highly original string quartets – of which he wrote 68 – and piano sonatas.

ABOVE: Haydn's last public appearance, at a performance of his oratorio The Creation *in the Great Hall of the University of Vienna on 27 March 1808, in honour of his 76th birthday.*

International fame

By the 1780s, Haydn's international reputation was spreading rapidly, and he managed to negotiate a new contract with his employer which

ABOVE: A romantic impression of Haydn crossing the English Channel in the 1790s.

allowed him to compose for other patrons, and to have his works published. In 1785 he became a Freemason, and around the same time he was commissioned to write several symphonies by a Parisian masonic lodge. The result was the "Paris" symphonies (Nos. 82–7) – several of which carry nicknames such as *The Bear*, *The Hen* and *The Queen* (a tribute to Marie Antoinette). Their success helped to consolidate his fame abroad.

After the death of Prince Nikolaus Esterházy in 1790, Haydn was free to travel for the first time. He was persuaded by the impresario Johann Peter Salomon to visit London, where he was – to his surprise – fêted by the court and high society. In July 1791 Oxford University honoured him with the degree of Doctor of Music. His twelve "London" symphonies (Nos. 93–104, some again with nicknames including *The Surprise*, *The Miracle*, *The Military* and *The Clock*) met with great public enthusiasm. Haydn made a further trip to England in 1794–5, but resisted King George III's invitation to stay permanently.

Last years

Haydn returned to Vienna as *Kapellmeister* to a new Esterházy prince, Nikolaus II, who in contrast to his predecessors required only sacred music for his newly austere court. Between 1796 and 1802 Haydn produced six fine masses, including the *Missa in tempore belli* (*Mass in Time of War*) and the *Missa in Angustiis* (*Nelson Mass*), both reflecting the political turmoil of the Napoleonic wars. He also wrote two Handelian oratorios, *Die Schöpfung* (*The Creation*, 1798) and *Die Jahreszeiten* (*The Seasons*, 1801). These, his last major works, teem with vibrant detail and an undimmed creative impulse.

The increasingly frail composer made his last public appearance at a performance of *The Creation* at Vienna University in honour of his 76th birthday, and died at the end of May 1809, during the Napoleonic occupation of Vienna. The whole art-loving world of Vienna attended his memorial service, which included a performance of Mozart's Requiem. Eleven years later his remains were reinterred in the chapel at Eisenstadt.

Wolfgang Amadeus Mozart

Mozart is sunshine.

Antonín Dvořák (1841–1904)

The works of Mozart and Beethoven stand at the heart of Western art music. Until the mid 20th century, Beethoven was perhaps the more revered as a heroic figure, battling against personal misfortune to produce his visionary and powerfully original music; while Mozart's music tended to be dismissed as "galant" and superficial. But over the past half-century, the re-evaluation of Mozart, together with the performance and recording of many of his lesser-known works, has revealed a composer of inestimable profundity and infinite variety, whose music has enriched the lives of performers and listeners alike.

ABOVE: Wolfgang Amadeus Mozart, painted nearly three decades after his death by Barbara Krafft.

Family background

The "miracle whom God let be born in Salzburg" made his appearance on 27 January 1756, the last of seven children born to Leopold Mozart and his wife Anna Maria, and one of only two to survive infancy. Leopold Mozart – a talented violinist, and the author of a successful treatise on violin technique – played in the court orchestra of the Archbishop of Salzburg, one of the most powerful prelates in Austria.

Mozart's relationship with his father was central to his life. Leopold Mozart has been vilified as the archetypal domineering father, dragging his prodigiously talented son around the courts of Europe at an early age, not only subjecting him to the rigours of prolonged travel, but forcing him to display his skills on the keyboard to any bored aristocrat who would pay money to listen; then hectoring him when he grew older, trying to obstruct him from leaving a miserable existence in Salzburg for the excitements of Vienna, and interfering in his personal life. In fact, there is no evidence to suggest that Leopold was motivated by anything other than love and solicitude for his son. The Mozart family was

LEFT: Mozart's birthplace on the Getreidegasse in Salzburg, where the family lived from 1747 until 1773.

RIGHT: Mozart's father Leopold (1719–87), painted in 1756 – the year of his son's birth.

ABOVE: Mozart at the age of six in court dress, painted by P. A. Lorenzoni.

Childhood

At the age of four, Wolfgang began to study keyboard and composition with his father. Wolfgang's elder sister Maria Anna (Nannerl) was also a talented pianist, though once she reached adulthood, the conventions of the time obliged her to confine her talents to the domestic sphere. Leopold saw it as his duty to exhibit his exceptional children to the world. When they were six and 11 respectively, he took them to perform before the Elector of Bavaria at Munich, and the Empress Maria Theresa in Vienna.

In 1763 the whole family undertook a trip to Paris and London, where Wolfgang played to both French and English monarchs. By this time he was already composing: four early keyboard sonatas were published in Paris, and he wrote his first symphonies in London. The family arrived back in Salzburg in November 1766. A further trip to Vienna failed to result in a hoped-for opera commission, but on returning home Mozart wrote one anyway, and *La finta semplice (The Pretend Simpleton)* was performed at the Archbishop's palace in May 1769.

very close, and their voluminous correspondence is full of protestations of affection. Leopold's only concern was for Wolfgang's well-being and success. He was one of the few people who fully recognized his son's unique gift, and he took every step to prevent it being squandered.

Life and works

NATIONALITY: Austrian

BORN: Salzburg, 1756; **DIED:** Vienna, 1791

SPECIALIST GENRES: Opera, symphonies, piano concertos, string quartets, church music.

MAJOR WORKS: *Le nozze di Figaro* (1786); *Don Giovanni* (1787); *Così fan tutte* (1790); *Die Zauberflöte* (1791); 21 piano concertos; five violin concertos; concertos for clarinet and other wind instruments; 41 symphonies; 24 string quartets and other chamber music; 17 Masses.

ABOVE: A concert given by the young Mozart in the Redoutensaal (ballroom) of the Schönbrunn Palace in Vienna.

ABOVE: Leopold Mozart and his two talented children, Maria Anna and Wolfgang, 1763.

ABOVE: The young Mozart (aged six) being presented by Joseph II to his wife, the Empress Maria Theresa, at Schönbrunn Palace on 13 October 1762.

Years of travel

In December 1769 Leopold took Wolfgang to Italy for the first time. After visits to Milan, Florence, Rome and Naples, Mozart received his first opera commission. *Mitridate, rè di ponto* was performed at Christmas 1770 at the Milanese court; but although both it and a further opera, *Lucio Silla*, were well received, Mozart's request for a job was turned down.

Back in Salzburg, Mozart settled down reluctantly as *Konzertmeister* to the court orchestra of a new (and less tolerant) Archbishop, and continued to compose. In January 1775 he and his father travelled together for the last time, to Munich, for the performance of Mozart's comic opera, *La finta giardiniera* (*The Pretend Gardener*). Two years later he asked for another period of leave, for an extended trip to Paris. The Archbishop promptly dismissed him, and Leopold, realizing that his own position was now in jeopardy, decided not to go. Mozart set out with his mother as chaperone.

The trip was a disaster. After a prolonged stay in Mannheim, where Wolfgang fell madly in love with a young singer called Aloysia Weber, he was peremptorily ordered by Leopold on to Paris. There he found the sophisticated French capital totally uninterested in an unknown provincial composer, now too old to be

ABOVE: A romantic artist's impression of Mozart composing, painted around 1880 by Josef Büche.

interesting as a prodigy. Although the Paris experience did produce some fine works – the *Paris* Symphony (No. 31) and a concerto for flute and harp (both fashionable French instruments) – there was no financial gain and a severe loss, when Mozart's mother died suddenly. Saddened and disillusioned, Mozart returned home.

Idomeneo

For the next 18 months he buried himself in his official court duties, writing sacred music for the Salzburg court, as well as symphonies, serenades, the Sinfonia Concertante for violin and viola (inspired by the French model) and a double piano concerto for himself and Nannerl. Then, in the summer of 1780, he was commissioned to write a new opera for Munich, on the subject of Idomeneus, king of Crete. *Idomeneo* is Mozart's first great opera – the first in which he demonstrated his extraordinary talent for bringing characters to life, allowing them to express real human emotions through the medium of music.

Vienna: early years

After being fêted in Munich, Mozart felt stifled by the petty humiliations of life in Salzburg. In March 1781 he was summoned to Vienna in the Archbishop's retinue, and took advantage of the rising antagonism between himself and his employer to engineer his own dismissal – albeit "with a box on the ear and a kick on the backside".

To Leopold's dismay, Mozart announced his intention of remaining in Vienna, where he would teach, compose, and give concerts. It was a bold idea, but ultimately an unsuccessful one. Austria was at war with the Turkish Empire, money was short, and fashions ephemeral, but for a few years, Mozart's novelty value paid dividends.

During his first year in Vienna he composed a group of three new piano concertos to play at his own subscription concerts, three magnificent wind serenades, and a new opera, *Die Entführung aus dem Serail* (*The Abduction from the Seraglio*), with a German text and spoken dialogue (a type known as a *Singspiel*). Its success

ABOVE: Mozart's first-floor apartment (with bay-window, second from right) in Vienna. He composed The Marriage of Figaro *there.*

was marred only by the laconic remark of the emperor that it seemed to have "too many notes".

Mozart also got married, much against his father's wishes. His bride, Constanze Weber, was the younger sister of his first love, Aloysia, who had turned him down. Constanze was an amateur singer: Mozart described her as "kind-natured…not ugly, but no beauty either". She has often been accused of ruining her husband's life by her bad housekeeping, but the accusation seems to have been unfounded, and the marriage – which produced two surviving sons (four other children died in infancy) – was very happy. When Leopold Mozart finally visited his son in 1785, he was much impressed with Wolfgang's fine apartment and high standard of living.

Vienna: middle years

For several years Mozart's new career proved successful. He had a busy teaching and concert programme, for which he turned out a string of piano concertos, raising the genre to new heights of virtuosity, passion and expression. Among these may be singled out the Concerto in D minor (K466), a highly emotional work in the *Sturm und Drang* ("storm and stress") style; and its companion in C major (K467), whose exquisite slow movement featured in the 1967 film *Elvira Madigan*.

ABOVE: Mozart's wife Constanze (1763–1842), painted by Hans Hansen in 1802, 11 years after Mozart's death. She remarried in 1809.

ABOVE: The final page from Mozart's own thematic catalogue of his works, which he kept from 1784 until his death. This page shows entries for the operas Die Zauberflöte *and* La clemenza di Tito, *the Clarinet Concerto and a Masonic cantata, finished in November 1791.*

ABOVE: *Stage set for* The Magic Flute, *designed by Simon Quadligo for a performance in Munich on 27 November 1818.*

Mozart's first love, however, was for opera – the genre which could make or break a composer – and in 1785 he began work on a daring new operatic venture, based on Pierre Beaumarchais's notorious French play *La folle journée, ou le mariage de Figaro*, which had been produced the previous year. This attack on aristocratic morals, disguised as a comedy, had already been banned in Vienna. Mozart's literary collaborator was the Italian adventurer, ex-priest and poet Lorenzo Da Ponte (1749–1838), with whom Mozart also worked on two later operas, *Don Giovanni* and *Così fan tutte*.

Le nozze di Figaro (*The Marriage of Figaro*) is one of the great monuments of Western art – a masterpiece of characterization, quicksilver wit and emotional depth. But Vienna failed to appreciate it. By this time, Mozart's arrogance had made him many enemies, including the powerful court composer, Antonio Salieri. Salieri and his friends were intensely jealous of

Mozart's abundant talent, and did all they could to sabotage the opera's production. (Salieri may not literally have poisoned Mozart, as some later claimed, but he certainly stifled his rival's career.) However, the music-lovers of Prague, where Figaro was

ABOVE: *A seduction scene from Mozart's opera* Don Giovanni *(1787).*

produced in 1787, took the opera to their hearts (the city went "Figaro-mad"), and immediately commissioned a new opera, *Don Giovanni*. Mozart's visit to Prague also produced a new symphony (No. 38), known as the *Prague*.

Vienna: last years

The final years of Mozart's brief life were a dismal catalogue of financial worry, constant moves to cheaper apartments, and failing health. He finally achieved his desire of a court appointment, but only as chamber composer, writing dance music for court balls, for a meagre salary. By June 1788 he was writing begging letters to his fellow Freemasons, asking for loans. *Don Giovanni* had been performed with even less success than *Figaro*.

In the summer of 1788, Mozart wrote his last three symphonies, including the *Jupiter* (No. 41), in the space of a few weeks; it is not known

ABOVE: A scene from Act II Scene 3 of the original 1791 production of The Magic Flute *at the Theater auf der Wieden in Vienna.*

if he ever heard them performed. A third opera written with Da Ponte, *Così fan tutte* (literally, "so do all women"), was premièred in the autumn of 1789, but the emperor died shortly afterwards and all theatres were closed. Two trips to Berlin and Frankfurt to give concerts failed to make any money, and by the end of 1790 Mozart was deeply depressed.

In the spring of 1791, he busied himself with dance music and pieces for mechanical organ and glass harmonica, several works for clarinet, including a fine concerto and quintet, and also with the serious and beautiful Piano Concerto in B flat (K595), a work tinged with melancholy. He also began work on another *Singspiel*, written for an actor-manager friend who ran a small suburban theatre. On the surface, *Die Zauberflöte* (*The Magic Flute*) appears to be an amusing pantomime with glorious music attached. But closer inspection reveals that the piece is infused with Masonic symbolism, including thinly disguised versions of Masonic rites and initiation ceremonies. Mozart was taking an

enormous risk, and it has been suggested – probably wrongly – that he paid for his presumption with his life.

While working on *The Magic Flute*, he received two more commissions, one for an *opera seria*, *La clemenza di Tito* (*The Clemency of Titus*), which was produced in Prague in September 1791 and was to be the last major work of this type, and another for a Requiem Mass. The latter was commissioned anonymously, via an emissary dressed in grey, by a Viennese nobleman whose young wife had died. Mozart's own health was failing by this time, and as he worked on the Requiem, he became obsessed by the idea that it would be his own, and that he was being poisoned. In fact he had advanced kidney disease. He died on the morning of 5 December in his wife's arms. Because he left little money, he was given the cheapest possible funeral in an unmarked grave. Few mourners accompanied the cortège. The unfinished Requiem was completed after his death by Franz Süssmayr, one of his pupils.

ABOVE: A 19th-century artist's impression of Mozart's last hours, by Henry O'Neil (1817–80). The composer died in his wife's arms, aged 35.

Ludwig van Beethoven

Nature would burst should she attempt to produce nothing save Beethovens.

ROBERT SCHUMANN (1810–56)

Mozart died in Vienna in the late autumn of 1791, a victim of the stifling class conventions of the *ancien régime*. A year later, a 20-year-old named Ludwig van Beethoven arrived in Vienna, keen to make his name as a musician. By this time, the face of European society was changing fast. The French Revolution was in full swing, and Austria – horrified at the treatment meted out to the French monarchs, particularly Queen Marie Antoinette, a former Austrian archduchess – had declared war on France. For more than two decades, Europe would be ripped apart by war. While Mozart's life had remained largely unaffected by international politics, Beethoven's revolutionary artistic vision was shaped by the ideology and volcanic social change of the turbulent times in which he lived.

ABOVE: *Ludwig van Beethoven (1770–1827), painted in 1823 by Ferdinand Georg Waldmüller.*

ABOVE: *Beethoven's birthplace in Bonn. He was born in the third-floor attic.*

Early years
Beethoven was born into a musical family. His grandfather had been music director to the Archbishop-Elector of Cologne, and his father was also employed at the electoral court, though in the lowlier position of singer and instrumentalist. As with the Mozart family, the majority of the seven children born to Johann van Beethoven and his wife died in infancy. Three boys survived: Ludwig, born on 16 or 17 December 1770, and two younger brothers, Caspar Carl and Nikolaus.

Johann van Beethoven, an alcoholic bully, was determined that his eldest son should follow in the young Mozart's footsteps as a child prodigy. But Johann lacked Leopold Mozart's abilities as a teacher, and forced his son to practise the keyboard constantly at the expense of his general education. From around 1780 Beethoven received more kindly and sympathetic instruction from the court composer and organist Christian Neefe, who organized the publication of his pupil's first compositions – a set of keyboard variations. In 1783 a set of three piano sonatas appeared in print with a dedication to the elector, whose successor appointed Beethoven second court organist the following year.

In 1787 Neefe suggested that Beethoven should travel to Vienna to take lessons from Mozart, who was much impressed with the young man's talent. But Beethoven's trip was curtailed by news of his mother's serious illness: she died of tuberculosis in the summer of that year, leaving him to cope with his father's violence and alcoholism. At the age of 18 Beethoven assumed responsibility for the family affairs, being granted half his father's court salary as well as his own. He also found an influential patron, Count Ferdinand Waldstein, who persuaded the elector to allow Beethoven leave to study with Haydn in Vienna. The

Life and works

NATIONALITY: German

BORN: Bonn, 1770;
DIED: Vienna, 1827

SPECIALIST GENRES:
Symphonies, piano
concertos, string quartets,
piano sonatas.

MAJOR WORKS: First period:
Symphonies No. 1 (1800) and 2
(1802); six string quartets; Piano
Sonatas No. 8 (*Pathétique*, 1799)
and No. 14 (*Moonlight*, 1801).

Second period: Symphonies No. 3
(*Eroica*, 1803) to No. 7; *Kreutzer*
Sonata for violin and piano
(1803); *Fidelio* (1805); Violin
Concerto (1806); *Razumovsky*
Quartets (1806); Piano
Concerto No. 5 (*Emperor*, 1809);
Archduke Trio (1811).

Third period: *Diabelli Variations*
(1823); last piano sonatas and
string quartets; *Missa solemnis*
(1823); Symphony No. 9
(*Choral*, 1824).

elector agreed, and in 1792 Beethoven
arrived in Vienna, the city which
became his permanent home.

Vienna

Beethoven found that his lessons with
Haydn were not a great success, but
he quickly began to make a name as a
pianist, with a formidable reputation
for improvisation. "He is greatly
admired for the velocity of his playing,
and astounds everybody by the way he
can master the greatest difficulties with
ease," a local paper reported. He also
found a new and powerful patron,
Prince Lichnowsky (in whose mansion

he had an apartment), and despite
his unprepossessing appearance –
stocky, swarthy, with an ugly, red,
pockmarked face – and rather boorish
manners, he found himself tolerated
by fashionable society.

He gave his first public concert,
playing a new piano concerto of his
own, at the Burgtheater on 29 March
1795, astonishing the audience with his
fiery virtuosity and establishing a
pattern which would continue for
several years. By 1796 he had
published a set of piano trios and three
piano sonatas (a genre he would
develop far beyond the Classical
"galant" style of Mozart and Haydn),
and had earned enough money to set
himself up in his own apartment.
Over the next four years he went
on occasional concert tours, gave
subscription concerts in Vienna, and
issued his chamber works in print –
sonatas for piano (including the
magnificent *Pathétique* Sonata No. 8 in
C minor), violin and cello, and the
Op. 16 Quintet for piano and wind.

All these works show Beethoven's
desire to push at the boundaries of
conventional compositional technique,
to expand sonata form, and to infuse
his work with unheard-of drama
and passion.

These principles were already
evident in the first of his nine
symphonies (written in 1800), which,
while conforming to the standard
Classical four-movement format,
relies not so much on lyrical themes
as on rhythmic dynamism and the
development of short melodic
fragments, or motifs. Clearly, the
old courtly "minuet and trio" which
traditionally constituted the third
movement of a symphony had outlived
its purpose: from the Second
Symphony onwards Beethoven
replaced it with a faster, more dynamic
and rhythmically propelled scherzo,
while retaining a tripartite structure
with a slower, more lyrical central
section. "There is something
revolutionary about that music,"
remarked the emperor.

ABOVE: *Beethoven, aged 17, playing to Mozart. Mozart declared that the young genius would
"soon astonish the world".*

ABOVE: *A view of rural Heiligenstadt, where Beethoven escaped from city life to compose and recuperate, and where he wrote the "Heiligenstadt Testament".*

The Heiligenstadt crisis

Around the turn of Beethoven's 30th year, just as his career seemed to be soaring, he was struck by an appalling personal crisis. He was forced to acknowledge the fact that he was going deaf. For several years he had tried to hide his hearing problems for both professional and social reasons, but it became clear that the affliction was incurable.

In the summer of 1802 he reached a nadir of despair, while staying at the country retreat of Heiligenstadt, just outside Vienna. He wrote a long letter (known as the "Heiligenstadt Testament") to his brothers, in which he described his utter misery: "For me there can be no pleasure in human society, no intelligent conversation, no mutual confidences. I must live like an outcast." But though he had contemplated suicide, Beethoven concluded that he must henceforth live for his art: "It seemed impossible to leave the world before I had accomplished all I was destined to do." The letter was never sent, and was found among his effects after his death.

Years of struggle

Beethoven's inner struggle is reflected in the titanic works of the next few years. These included the massive Eroica Symphony (No. 3), originally dedicated to Napoleon, nearly twice as long as a conventional symphony, with a powerful and tragic funeral march as its slow movement; the Triple Concerto for piano, violin and cello; two piano sonatas (No. 21, the *Waldstein* and No. 23, the *Appassionata*); and his only opera, *Fidelio*.

The opera's plot was based on a French Revolutionary tale of a wife's heroic efforts to save her imprisoned husband. (For political reasons, Beethoven was obliged to move the action to 18th-century Spain.) By the time of the opera's production, in 1805, Napoleon's army had occupied Vienna and *Fidelio* received only two performances. It remains a lone masterpiece of its kind in Beethoven's output, perhaps lacking the innate sense of theatre of Mozart's mature operas, but containing memorable dramatic moments such as Leonora's great "Abscheulicher" aria, the quartet "Mir ist so wunderbar" and the moving chorus when the prisoners are brought from their cells and greet the light of day.

ABOVE: *Napoleon Bonaparte (1769– 1821), the original dedicatee of Beethoven's Symphony No. 3 (the* Eroica*), but whom Beethoven despised when he proclaimed himself Emperor of France.*

ABOVE: *The "Heiligenstadt Testament", a letter written in 1802, in which Beethoven expressed his suicidal despair at his deafness.*

ABOVE: The première of Beethoven's opera Fidelio *at the Theater an der Wien in Vienna, 1805. The opera was not an immediate success, owing to the French occupation.*

Disillusioned after *Fidelio*'s failure, Beethoven concentrated on instrumental pieces, producing a set of three string quartets dedicated to the Russian ambassador to Austria, Count Andreas Razumovsky, the Fourth Symphony, the Violin Concerto (again a lone masterpiece), and his Fourth Piano Concerto. Just before Christmas 1808 the Fifth and Sixth Symphonies, both revolutionary in concept, were premièred at the same concert. The Fifth, with its progression from tragedy to hope, has been interpreted as representing Beethoven's own struggle against adversity, and is one of the first symphonic works to recycle thematic material between movements. The Sixth (the *Pastoral*) is a harbinger of Romanticism. One of the earliest symphonic examples of "tone-painting", it illustrates scenes of Austrian country life, including a realistic thunderstorm, birdsong and a village festival.

By this time, Beethoven was enjoying a measure of financial security through the support of several wealthy patrons, including the Archduke Rudolph (to whom Beethoven dedicated his Fifth Piano Concerto, known as *The Emperor*). When Napoleon's troops invaded Vienna in 1809, the imperial family fled to safety: Beethoven celebrated their return from exile in 1810 with the Piano Sonata No. 26, *Das Lebewohl* (*The Farewell*). Seven years later Rudolph also received the dedication of the *Hammerklavier* Sonata (No. 29).

Disappointment in love

Apart from his deafness, Beethoven's life was marred by his failure to find a partner: the objects of his affection were usually either married, or else above him in social station (such as Countess Giulietta Guicciardi, the dedicatee of the *Moonlight* Sonata). An unsent letter written in 1812 reveals a deep attachment to an unspecified

ABOVE: The triumphant entrance of Napoleon's army into Vienna in 1805. The French occupation caused hardship for Viennese citizens.

ABOVE: Countess Giulietta Guicciardi, to whom the Moonlight *Sonata was dedicated.*

woman, "the immortal beloved", who may possibly have been Antonie Brentano, the wife of a Frankfurt businessman. She and Beethoven never met in later life, but many years later he dedicated to her his last work for piano, the *Diabelli Variations*.

Beethoven seems to have despised women of a lower social class: an attitude which led to acrimonious rows with his brothers over their "unsuitable" choice of wives. In 1820, after a long legal battle begun after his brother's death in 1815, he became sole guardian of his nephew Karl, perhaps fulfilling his own frustrated desire for an heir. Their relationship, however, proved a stormy one, and overshadowed the later years of Beethoven's life.

Last years

In 1813 Beethoven celebrated Napoleon's defeat on the Iberian Peninsula with his *Battle Symphony*. Originally written for a mechanical instrument called the "panharmonicon", the piece is far inferior to the contemporary Seventh and Eighth

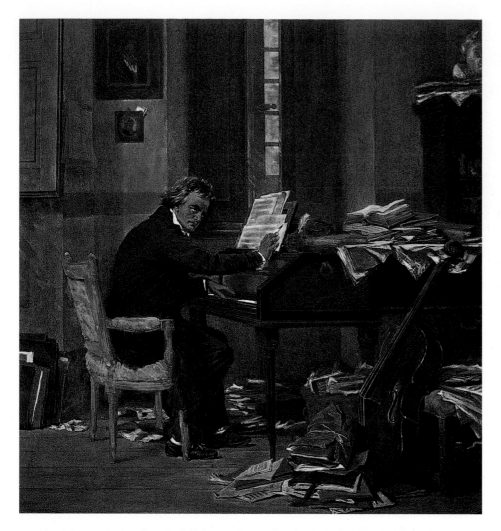

ABOVE: *A 19th-century artist's impression of Beethoven (in later life) composing in his Viennese apartment. He was notably untidy.*

ABOVE: *Beethoven's ear-trumpet lying on the manuscript of his* Eroica Symphony.

ABOVE: *The opening of the Theater in der Josefstadt in Vienna, 1822, for which Beethoven wrote the overture* The Consecration of the House.

ABOVE: *The Kärntnertor Theatre in Vienna, where the première of Beethoven's Ninth Symphony took place on 7 May 1824.*

Symphonies. By this time Beethoven had more or less abandoned public performance, and by 1818 he was stone deaf.

He became increasingly withdrawn and anti-social, but continued to compose. Sacred music had never figured largely in his output, but in 1822 he completed the *Missa solemnis*, originally intended to celebrate Archduke Rudolph's enthronement as Archbishop of Olmütz. This great work, written "from the heart to the heart", ranks with Bach's B minor Mass as one of the crowning achievements of its composer's career. Sections of it were performed in May 1824 at a concert which included the première of the Ninth Symphony, the result of Beethoven's desire to write a "choral symphony with voices". Within a traditional symphonic framework (except that the scherzo is placed second), Beethoven burst the bonds of convention by introducing into the finale a setting for solo voices and chorus of Schiller's *An die Freude* (*Ode to Joy*), with its ecstatic vision of an international brotherhood of man.

Beethoven's last instrumental compositions – the last three piano sonatas and the late string quartets (including the six-movement Op. 130, with its immense fugal finale) – have always been regarded as embodying Western musical art at a peak of perfection. They are introspective works, not intended to be "understood" or applauded in the conventional sense. They are the work of a man who had withdrawn into an inner life, which could only be expressed through the medium of pure, abstract music.

In 1826 Beethoven's nephew Karl attempted suicide. By this time the composer (a heavy drinker) was already mortally ill with liver disease. After months of suffering, Beethoven died on 26 March 1827. In contrast to Mozart's low-key burial, 10,000 people are estimated to have watched Beethoven's funeral procession. The poet Franz Grillparzer delivered the funeral oration, in honour of "the man who inherited and enriched the immortal fame of Handel and Bach, of Haydn and Mozart… Until his death he preserved a father's heart for mankind. Thus he was, thus he died, thus he will live to the end of time."

ABOVE: *A contemporary watercolour of Beethoven's funeral procession leaving the "House of the Black Spaniard", his last residence (to the right of the church).*

Franz Schubert

If you go to see him during the day, he says "Hello, how are you? — Good!"
and goes on working, whereupon you go away.

FRANZ VON SCHOBER (1798–1882)

On 29 March 1827, Beethoven was buried in the village cemetery of Währing, just outside Vienna. Among the torch-bearers in the funeral procession was a dark-haired, bespectacled young man of 30. His name was Franz Schubert, and he was paying homage to the member of his own profession he most revered. Less than two years later, Schubert's own body would be interred in the same cemetery, close to Beethoven's grave.

Unlike Beethoven, whose fame during his lifetime had spread all over Europe, Schubert's reputation was largely local. His composing career was short – a mere 15 years – and although he worked in the same genres as his three great predecessors, it was not his operas, or even his symphonies, but his more intimate works, particularly the songs and chamber music, which posthumously ensured his unique place in musical history.

By the time war in Europe ended with the Congress of Vienna (1815), European society had changed dramatically. A new generation of middle-class, independently minded citizens had sprung up, but conservative politicians, such as Prince Metternich in Vienna, attempted to maintain the status quo of the ruling classes and banish "subversive and revolutionary tendencies" by keeping the populace firmly under control through censorship and political repression.

ABOVE: Franz Schubert (1797–1828), aged about 28, painted by Wilhelm August Rieder around 1825.

People sought relief through social activity. Balls and parties became fashionable for the rich, while the less well-off built up a network of like-minded friends, meeting in private homes or at the local coffee houses. This was Schubert's social milieu.

Youth

Vienna was the centre of Schubert's universe. He was born on 31 January 1797 to a suburban schoolmaster, who taught all his children to play musical instruments. Franz learned the viola, and together with his father and brothers made up a string quartet. In 1808 he won a scholarship to the imperial seminary, where he had daily music lessons and played in the school orchestra. He also made several formative friendships, one with Joseph von Spaun, an ex-pupil and law student. By the time Schubert left school at the age of 16, he had already written a substantial quantity of music.

Schubert and Goethe

After his mother's death and his father's remarriage, Schubert spent some time as a teacher at his father's school. He also fell in love with a young singer named Therese

ABOVE: The great writer Johann Wolfgang von Goethe (1749–1832), the father of German Romanticism, painted c.1790.

Grob, who performed in his F major Mass in the autumn of 1814. Perhaps as a result of unrequited love, he began composing songs. His first efforts marked the beginning of a lifelong involvement with the poetry of Europe's most celebrated writer and the "father" of Romanticism, Johann Wolfgang von Goethe (1749–1832). Among these early songs was "Gretchen am Spinnrade" ("Gretchen at the Spinning Wheel"), from Goethe's *Faust*, a masterly characterization of the abandoned Margaret's distress.

The next year produced a huge crop of some 150 songs, many of them settings of Goethe's texts, such as the delicate ballad "Heidenröslein" ("Briar-rose"), and the stormy "Erlkönig" ("The Elf-king"), depicting a father's wild ride through the night to save his sick child from the grasp of Death. In spring 1816 Schubert's friend Spaun sent 28 Goethe settings to the poet, asking permission to dedicate them to him. Goethe, who loathed musical settings of his work, returned the volume without comment. Fortunately undeterred, Schubert went on to add another 100 songs – including the immortal settings of Goethe's "Nur wer die Sehnsucht kennt" ("Only he who knows yearning") and "Kennst du das Land" ("Do you know the country where lemon trees blossom?") – to his canon before the end of the year. In his 20th year he completed his Fourth and Fifth Symphonies, both very much in the Classical mould, for private performance by amateur orchestras.

Maturity

Schubert finally left the family home in December 1816, at the prompting of another close friend, Franz von Schober. A wealthy law student, Schober persuaded Schubert to abandon the drudgery of teaching and concentrate on composition (the song "An die Musik" – "To Music" – is a setting

ABOVE: *The autograph manuscript of Schubert's setting of Goethe's poem "Heidenröslein" ("Briar-rose"), one of his best-known early songs.*

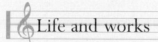

Life and works

NATIONALITY: Austrian

BORN: Vienna, 1797;
DIED: Vienna, 1828

SPECIALIST GENRES: Songs, piano music, symphonies, chamber music.

MAJOR WORKS: Symphonies No. 8 (*Unfinished*, 1822) and No. 9 (*The Great*, 1828); String Quintet in C (1828); Piano Quintet in A (*The Trout*, 1819); Octet in F (1824); String Quartet No. 14 in D minor (*Death and the Maiden*, 1824); Fantasy in C major for piano (*The Wanderer*, 1822); Fantasy in F minor for piano duet (1828); over 600 songs; song-cycles *Die schöne Müllerin* (1823) and *Winterreise* (1827).

of a Schober poem). He also introduced Schubert to the singer Johann Michael Vogl, who became the leading interpreter of his songs. These continued to pour out throughout 1817, together with seven piano sonatas, heavily influenced by Beethoven.

ABOVE: *A view of a Viennese square in Schubert's time. Schubert spent all of his short life in Vienna.*

ABOVE: An idealized portrait of the composer on his balcony, painted in 1917.

In 1818 Schubert's Sixth Symphony – a substantial work which shows Beethoven's influence – was performed (again by an amateur orchestra), and he spent five happy months on a Hungarian aristocratic estate as music teacher to the daughters of Count Esterházy of Galanta, concentrating on piano music for his young pupils. "I live and compose like a god", he told a friend.

Life in Vienna

The change of scene encouraged Schubert to broaden his horizons, and the next summer he and Vogl took a holiday in Steyr, where Schubert completed another piano sonata and the *Trout* Quintet, based on his own song "Die Forelle". From then onwards, Schubert's life took a regular shape. In Vienna, he was the focus of a close-knit group of talented young people – writers, poets and students – who enjoyed a happy and carefree existence, meeting at cafés, at parties in each other's homes or, in the summer, at a country estate owned by Schober's uncle. These informal gatherings, with games of charades, poetry readings and performances of Schubert's music, became known as "Schubertiaden". In the summers, Schubert and Vogl went on long walking tours of Upper Austria, where Schubert drew inspiration from the dramatic landscape.

The early 1820s brought mixed fortune. Vogl's performance of "Der Erlkönig" at a concert in the Burgtheater in 1821 brought public recognition for the as yet unpublished composer, but he had no experience of

ABOVE: Schubert playing the piano during an evening at Joseph von Spaun's.

business matters, and when demand for his work rose, he rashly sold the copyrights of ten volumes of songs to the publisher Diabelli. And by 1823 it was clear that Schubert's operatic ambitions would never be realized. Of his 17 stage works, none achieved success, and only the charming and popular incidental music to *Rosamunde* has survived.

Tragedy

The same year – 1823 – brought disaster. Schubert's hedonistic existence had left him suffering from syphilis, then a potentially fatal disease. At the height of his illness, he composed the two-movement *Unfinished* Symphony, restless and tragic in mood, as well as the great *Wanderer* Fantasy and the A minor Sonata, both for piano. He also composed his first song-cycle, a new genre consisting of a set of thematically linked songs based on a sequence of poems, telling a story. *Die schöne Müllerin* (*The Fair Maid of the Mill*) is a quintessentially Romantic tale of rejected love and death by drowning.

The last four years of Schubert's life were a constant struggle against

ABOVE: An excursion of the "Schubertians" from Atzenbrugg to Aumuhl, painted by Schubert's friend Leopold Kupelwieser. Schubert (wearing a top-hat) is walking behind the carriage.

ABOVE: A "Schubertiad" (Schubert evening) in a Viennese salon. Schubert at the piano is accompanying the singer Johann Michael Vogl.

depression and illness, interspersed with frantic creative activity. As well as the Ninth Symphony (a work of Beethovenian proportions and unstoppable rhythmic impulse, which a Viennese orchestra declared "unplayable"), the works of these years included a great deal of chamber music: the Octet for wind and strings, string quartets in A minor and D minor (*Death and the Maiden*), two massive piano trios, and the three last piano sonatas (which Schumann memorably described as "purely and simply thunderstorms breaking forth with Romantic rainbows over slumbering worlds").

Last months

Schubert continued to compose songs until the end of his life. Some, such as the radiant "Ständchen" ("Serenade"),

express a passionate delight in life; others – such as the bleak song-cycle *Winterreise* (*Winter Journey*), based on

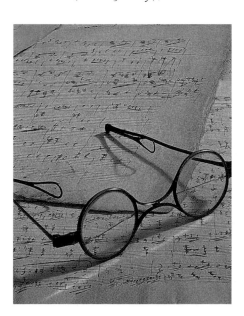

ABOVE: Schubert's spectacles lying on the manuscripts of some of his last works.

poems by Wilhelm Müller – plumb the depths of despair. Among the last was "Der Doppelgänger" – a terrifying setting of a poem by Heinrich Heine in which a young man sees his "double", foretelling his own death. It was a prophetic vision.

By September 1828, Schubert's health had worsened, and he moved in with his brother. That month he completed the sublime String Quintet in C major, followed in October by his last major work, *Der Hirt auf dem Felsen* (*The Shepherd on the Rock*), for soprano and piano with clarinet obbligato. He died of typhus on 19 November, aged 31, leaving only an unsurpassed musical legacy. His tombstone in the Währing cemetery carries the telling epitaph by Grillparzer: "The art of music has buried here a rich possession, but still fairer hopes."

Other Composers of the Era

Classicism is health, romanticism is sickness.

JOHANN WOLFGANG VON GOETHE (1749–1832)

Two sons of J. S. Bach bridged the gap between the Baroque and the Classical eras. Carl Philipp Emmanuel Bach (1714–88), born in Weimar, decided to follow a musical career, and in 1738 became keyboard player to the future Frederick the Great of Prussia. He remained in Berlin until 1767, when he succeeded Telemann as director of music at Hamburg. He is chiefly remembered for his inventive keyboard sonatas (of which he wrote over 200, for both "connoisseurs and amateurs"), which played a major role in the development of sonata form. His sinfonias, concertos and flute sonatas are also still performed today.

C. P. E. Bach taught the harpsichord to his younger brother Johann Christian Bach (1735–82). Bach's

ABOVE: Thomas Augustine Arne (1710–78), the composer of "Rule, Britannia!"

youngest son continued his studies in Italy, where he began a career as an opera composer, but moved to London in 1762 and remained there until his death, becoming known as "the English Bach". He was initially composer to the King's Theatre in London, and was later appointed music master to Queen Charlotte. His later operas were not very successful, but his instrumental works – particularly his skilfully crafted sinfonias and 40 or so piano concertos – had great influence on Haydn, Beethoven, and particularly Mozart, who met Bach when he visited London at the age of eight.

While British music in the 18th century was largely dominated by European imports, Thomas Arne (1710–78) was a notable home-grown

exception. Arne's output was largely theatrical, including masques and operas (his 1740 masque *Alfred* contained the song "Rule, Britannia!"), but he also wrote some charming symphonies, keyboard concertos and sonatas, and songs, including "The British Grenadiers".

Muzio Clementi (1752–1832) was born in Rome, but lived mostly in England. A brilliant pianist, who later went into publishing and piano-making, he toured Europe as a virtuoso from 1781–83, but then settled in London, where he became a much sought-after teacher (his pupils included John Field). Clementi's own compositions, which include sonatas, sonatinas and studies for piano, are still used as teaching pieces.

ABOVE: Carl Philipp Emmanuel Bach (1714–88), J. S. Bach's third son, who was an influential composer.

ABOVE: J. S. Bach's youngest son, Johann Christian Bach (1735–82), "the English Bach", who worked mostly in London.

ABOVE: *Luigi Boccherini (1743–1805), who worked in Vienna and Madrid. He was a fine cellist.*

Muzio Clementi's German contemporary, Johann Nepomuk Hummel (1778–1837), studied the piano with Mozart, and also worked for Haydn's employer Prince Esterházy. From 1819–37 he was

ABOVE: *The Italian Domenico Cimarosa (1749–1801), court composer in St Petersburg and Vienna, playing the clavichord.*

Kapellmeister to the Weimar court. His fluent, tuneful works were very popular: his Trumpet Concerto (1803) is still much performed, as are his *Septet militaire* (1829) and a Piano Quintet of 1802. His piano concertos and sonatas influenced Chopin.

While the Classical period was dominated by the four Viennese giants, Italy continued to produce its fair share of talented composers. Among them was Luigi Boccherini (1743–1805), whose music is similar in style to Haydn's. He worked in Vienna from 1757–64, but in 1769 moved to Madrid as composer to the Spanish court. An enormously prolific composer, Boccherini left a vast output of chamber music, including 91 string quartets, 154 quintets and 60 trios, as well as symphonies, concertos and church music. His famous Minuet (featured in the 1955 British film *The Ladykillers*) comes from his String Quintet in E, Op. 13, No. 5.

Mozart's rival Antonio Salieri (1750–1825) worked principally in Vienna, where he was first an opera composer, and then court conductor. His operas, unlike Mozart's, have not survived, but he was an influential teacher; Beethoven, Schubert and Liszt were among his pupils.

Domenico Cimarosa (1749–1801) spent some time in St Petersburg as court composer to Catherine the Great of Russia, before succeeding Salieri as court *Kapellmeister* in Vienna. After 1792 he returned to his native Naples. Most of his 65 operas have been forgotten, with the single exception of the comic opera *Il matrimonio segreto* (*The Secret Marriage*, 1792). He also wrote an oboe concerto, around 30 keyboard sonatas, and other instrumental works.

His rival and contemporary Giovanni Paisiello (1740–1816) also worked in St Petersburg and Naples, producing

ABOVE: *The title page of a comic opera by Antonio Salieri, produced a few months after Mozart's* Marriage of Figaro, *in 1785.*

over 100 operas as well as symphonies and piano concertos. His 1782 opera *Il barbiere di Siviglia* (*The Barber of Seville*), written when he was court composer to Catherine the Great, was at first more popular than Rossini's later version.

ABOVE: *Giovanni Paisiello (1740–1816), one of the most successful opera composers of his time, painted by Elisabeth Vigée-Lebrun.*

The Romantic ❧ Era ❧

Dancers at a court ball at the Hofburg Palace in Vienna in the late 19th century, painted by Wilhelm Gause.

Drama and Poetry in Music

Music, moody food
Of us that trade in love.

WILLIAM SHAKESPEARE (1564–1616), "ANTONY AND CLEOPATRA"

Schubert represented a turning-point in musical history. He inherited the Classical forms of his predecessors, but while his own musical style was essentially Classical, his inspiration looked forward to the age of Romanticism. One of the key features of Romantic music is its strong association with other art-forms, particularly literature or painting. Schubert responded instinctively to the poetry and drama of the great literary figures of his time: Goethe, Friedrich Schiller, Friedrich Rückert, Friedrich Klopstock, and Ludwig Hölty. Their writings, even when dealing with historical figures or events, expressed ordinary human emotions – love, happiness, sorrow –

and the beauty of the natural world. One of the most potent examples of literary Romanticism was Goethe's epistolatory novel *Die Leiden des jungen Werthers* (*The Sorrows of Young Werther*), published in 1774. It was inspired by Goethe's own unrequited love for a friend's fiancée, and the news of another friend's suicide as a result of disappointed love. *Werthers* had an enormous influence on European youth, and the theme of frustrated passion became a common one in the literature of the period.

Untamed nature

The other great Romantic theme was a response to nature, especially in its wilder aspects. Earlier generations had

sought to tame and cultivate the landscape; but in the late 18th century artists and writers – spurred on by Jean-Jacques Rousseau (1712–78) and his rejection of rationalism – reacted against the artificial moral code of Classical writers and philosophers, who believed in a neatly ordered world. Artists such as Théodore Géricault, J. M. W. Turner and Caspar David Friedrich began to depict the puny, helpless nature of human beings when pitted against terrifying natural phenomena such as avalanches or storms; while writers such as Lord Byron, William Wordsworth, Percy Bysshe Shelley and Sir Walter Scott identified human emotions with the turbulent moods of nature, and drew

ABOVE: This dramatic snow-capped landscape entitled Near Chamonix *was painted by James Stormont in the 19th century. Views such as this inspired many Romantic composers to write music that celebrated the beauty and ruggedness of nature.*

ABOVE: *A caricature by Gustave Doré of Berlioz conducting at the Jardin d'Hiver (Winter Garden) in Paris, 1850.*

orchestral masterpiece, the *Symphonie fantastique*, in which a young opium addict dreams he has killed his beloved and is led to the guillotine; while Mendelssohn's orchestral music records his vivid impressions of visits to Italy and Scotland. Much of Schumann's music was inspired by literary models; like Schubert, he had an immediate and passionate response to literature. At the same time, Liszt's newly invented "tone-poem" proved an ideal vehicle for musical responses to literature or art.

Virtuoso performers

The other hallmark of musical Romanticism was its emphasis on the individual – either the composer, fighting a lonely battle against incomprehension and intolerance, or the performer. The 19th century saw the rise of the star performer, and with it a division between creator and executant which became progressively more marked in the 20th century. Many 19th-century composers

ABOVE: *A poster advertising Massenet's opera* Werther *(1887), based on Goethe's novel* The Sorrows of Young Werther.

(Chopin, Liszt, Brahms, Paganini) carried on the tradition followed by Mozart and Beethoven in writing music for themselves to perform, but they also began to write for other virtuoso executants, such as the pianists Clara Schumann (1819–96), Eugen d'Albert (1864–1932) and his wife Teresa Carreño (1853–1917); the violinists Joseph Joachim (1831–1907), dedicatee of concertos by Brahms and Bruch, Ferdinand David (1810–73), for whom Mendelssohn wrote his concerto, and Pablo de Sarasate (1844–1908), for whom Lalo, Bruch and Saint-Saëns wrote concertos; and the clarinettist Richard Mühlfeld (1856–1907), for whom Brahms wrote his great chamber works for that instrument.

inspiration from the rugged landscapes of northern Europe, especially Scotland, or from the remoter, brigand-infested parts of Italy and Greece.

Portrayal of emotion

This was the climate which produced the great musical masterpieces of early Romanticism. Among these are Schubert's song-cycles *Die schöne Müllerin*, in which the brook (represented in the piano accompaniment) becomes an equal partner in a drama of rejection and suicide; and *Winterreise* (*Winter Journey*), in which both singer and accompanist paint a vivid picture of wintry desolation, mirroring the bleak emptiness in the betrayed protagonist's soul.

Berlioz left no listeners in any doubt about the "programme" behind his

ABOVE: *A painting by Edgar Degas (1876) of the divertissement in Meyerbeer's 1831 opera* Robert le diable, *seen from the viewpoint of the orchestra.*

Gioacchino Rossini

Rossini, in music, is the genius of sheer animal spirits.

LEIGH HUNT (1784–1859)

Towards the end of the 18th century, Italy was producing many composers of entertaining, accomplished, but undeniably ephemeral operas. Composers such as Giovanni Paisiello and Domenico Cimarosa wrote dozens of stage works, but very few survived for more than a season, and none could match the Italian masterpieces of Mozart. Opera in Italy had become stereotypical, subject to the tyrannical demands of audiences for a constant stream of hurriedly composed new works, and of singers for arias to show off their vocal technique, in defiance of dramatic exigencies. Italy needed an outstanding opera composer, and found one in the person of Gioacchino Rossini.

Rossini was the son of a horn player and a singer, and began to compose as a child. In 1806 he went to study at the Liceo Musicale in Bologna, and at the age of 15 was commissioned to write his first opera, *Demetrio e Polibio*. Further commissions followed, including several from the Teatro San Moïse in Venice for a series of one-act *farse* including *La scala di seta* (*The Silken Ladder*, 1811) and *Il Signor Bruschino* (1813).

Productive years

Rossini was able to work at high speed, and between 1810 and 1822 he turned out a steady flow of works, both comic and serious, for production in Venice, Milan, Naples and Rome, none of which took him more than a few weeks to write.

ABOVE:

A portrait of Gioacchino Rossini (1792– 1868), now in the Liceo Musicale in Bologna where he studied.

LEFT:

The interior of the Teatro San Carlo in Naples, where several of Rossini's operas were first performed.

Life and works

NATIONALITY: Italian

BORN: Pesaro, 1792; **DIED:** Paris, 1868

SPECIALIST GENRES: Opera (both "serious" and comic).

MAJOR WORKS: *Il barbiere di Siviglia* (1816); *La cenerentola* (1817); *Semiramide* (1823); *Guillaume Tell* (1829); Stabat Mater (1832–41); *Petite messe solennelle* (1863).

Among them were the serious operas *Tancredi*, *Elisabetta*, *Regina d'Inghilterra* and *Otello* (based on Shakespeare's play), and the comic operas *L'italiana in Algeri* (*The Italian Girl in Algiers*), *Il barbiere di Siviglia* (*The Barber of Seville* — Rossini's comic masterpiece), *La cenerentola* (*Cinderella*), and *La gazza ladra* (*The Thieving Magpie*). Of these, *The Barber of Seville* (based on Beaumarchais's prequel to *The Marriage of Figaro*) was a disappointing failure at its Roman première in 1816, thanks to a catalogue of onstage disasters, though by its third performance it had recovered from its initial setback. In one version of a famous story about Rossini, who was a notorious gourmet, he was asked by a journalist whether it was true that he had cried in public only twice in his life — the first time after the première of *The Barber*, and

ABOVE: A set for an 1830 production of Rossini's opera Le siège de Corinthe *(The Siege of Corinth) at the Berlin State Opera.*

the second when a particularly delicious piece of turkey stuffed with truffles had fallen in the river during a picnic. Rossini pondered, and then answered: "No, only once, and that was when the turkey fell in the river."

Rossini's greatest *opere serie* were written for the Teatro San Carlo in Naples between 1817 and 1823: they included *Mosè in Egitto* (*Moses in Egypt*), *La donna del lago* (based on Walter Scott's *The Lady of the Lake*), *Maometto II*, and *Semiramide*, the last of his Italian operas. In 1822 he married the singer Isabella Colbran, who had created the soprano roles in many of his operas, and after trips to Vienna and London, he settled in Paris as director of the Théâtre-Italien. He was still only 31 years old, rich and famous, with 34 operas to his credit.

Later life

Over the next six years he wrote several more operas for Paris, but after *Guillaume Tell* (*William Tell*), arguably his finest work, he effectively retired. In 1836 he returned to Italy, where he suffered prolonged periods of ill-health, but finally settled in Paris again with his second wife Olympe Pélissier, devoting himself to entertaining friends and eating (he invented, among other dishes, *tournedos Rossini*). The

only musical products of his later life are the delightful series of salon pieces which he called "the sins of my old age", and two sacred works, a Stabat Mater and the *Petite messe solennelle*.

Rossini's music

In the operatic field, Rossini's innovations included the replacement of keyboard-accompanied recitative by orchestral accompaniment, the expansion of the chorus and its dramatic integration, the development of the coloratura aria, and the revitalization of *opera buffa*; his characters, such as Figaro and the delightful Rosina, are real people with whom audiences of all ages can identify. His brilliant opera overtures (characterized by their famous, whipped-up *crescendo* endings) are still often performed in the concert repertoire today.

ABOVE: The title page of the fifth edition of the vocal score of Rossini's last opera, Guillaume Tell, *published in Paris.*

ABOVE: An 1829 cartoon by A. E. Chalon of the character of Figaro, the hero of Rossini's Il barbiere di Siviglia.

Gaetano Donizetti

I wallowed in rapture.

MIKHAIL GLINKA (1804–57), ON HEARING "ANNA BOLENA"

ABOVE: *A portrait of Gaetano Donizetti, now in the Liceo Musicale in Bologna.*

Italian opera in the early 19th century was dominated by three composers: Rossini, who gave up composing in 1829; Bellini, who died at the early age of 33 in 1835; and Donizetti. These three laid the foundations for the work of Giuseppe Verdi.

Donizetti was born to a poor Bergamo family, but was fortunate to be able to attend a free music school in Bergamo founded and run by the opera composer and local *maestro di cappella* Johann Mayr (1763–1845). After two years of further study in Bologna, he began composing with astonishing speed and fluency. In 1822 he wrote a successful opera for production at the Teatro Argentina in Rome, and then moved to Naples, where over the next few years he turned out up to five operas

a year. In 1828 he married Virginia Vasselli, a lawyer's daughter who died during a cholera epidemic nine years later – a tragedy from which Donizetti never recovered.

Maturity

In 1830 Donizetti achieved his first major international success with *Anna Bolena*. From then on he wrote for other operatic centres, including Milan, where he composed the enchanting comedy *L'elisir d'amore* (*The Love Philtre*), and the tragedy *Lucrezia Borgia*, performed at La Scala in December 1833. It was followed two years later by *Maria Stuarda*, based on Schiller's play about the Queen of Scots. Scotland also provided the

impetus for Donizetti's greatest success, *Lucia di Lammermoor*, based on Walter Scott's tragic novel, which opened at the Teatro San Carlo, Naples, in 1835. (The heroine's famous "mad" scene was parodied over 50 years later by Gilbert and Sullivan in *Ruddigore*.)

In 1838 Donizetti moved to Paris, where his new works – including *La fille du régiment*, *Les martyrs* and *La favorite* – were hugely successful. But he was suffering from syphilis, and both his physical and mental faculties were in decline. In 1842 he was appointed *Kapellmeister* to the Austrian court, but his last operatic masterpiece, *Don Pasquale*, was produced at the Théâtre-Italien in Paris in 1843. He was eventually committed to a lunatic asylum, before being taken home to die in Bergamo.

ABOVE: *The "Swedish Nightingale" Jenny Lind as Marie, the heroine of Donizetti's* La fille du régiment, *in an 1847 production.*

Life and works

NATIONALITY: Italian

BORN: Bergamo, 1797;
DIED: Bergamo, 1848

SPECIALIST GENRES:
Bel canto opera.

MAJOR WORKS:
L'elisir d'amore (1832);
Lucrezia Borgia (1833);
Lucia di Lammermoor (1835);
La fille du régiment
(1840); *Don Pasquale*
(1843).

Vincenzo Bellini

Long, long melodies, such as no one has ever written before.

GIUSEPPE VERDI (1813–1901)

Vincenzo Bellini was the youngest member of the trio of early Romantic Italian opera composers. He was taught from an early age by his father and grandfather, both musicians, and at 18 went to study at the Royal Music Conservatory in Naples. The first of his ten operas was performed there in 1825, leading to further opera commissions from Naples and Milan.

Bellini achieved more or less instant success with *Il pirata*, produced at La Scala in 1827. It was written in collaboration with the librettist Felice Romani, who went on to supply the texts for six more Bellini operas, including *I Capuleti ed i Montecchi* (*The Capulets and the Montagues*, Venice, 1830), *La sonnambula* (*The Sleepwalker*) and *Norma* (both Milan, 1831), and *Beatrice di Tenda* (Venice, 1833). The failure of this last opera coincided with a rift with Romani, and the termination of a long-standing love affair with a married woman.

In the spring of 1833 Bellini visited London and Paris, where he was fêted, and made many valuable social contacts. The Théâtre-Italien in Paris commissioned his last opera, *I puritani* (*The Puritans*, based on Walter Scott's *Old Mortality*), which was performed with huge success in January 1835. Eight months later the composer was dead, after a violent attack of gastro-enteritis, less than two months short of his 34th birthday.

Coloratura

The hallmarks of Bellini's mellifluous, essentially lyrical art are expressive declamation and the close relationship of music and words. "Bellini's music comes from the heart and it is intimately bound up with the text," said Wagner. His operas, like those of Rossini and Donizetti, were written for the great voices of his time. They fell out of favour after the art of *bel canto* declined in the late 19th century, but enjoyed a revival in the 20th century with the emergence of a new breed of coloratura sopranos, such as Maria Callas (1923–77) and Joan Sutherland (born 1926). The aria "Casta diva" from *Norma* became one of Callas's showpieces.

ABOVE:
Vincenzo Bellini (1801–35), a portrait now in the library of La Scala, Milan.

LEFT:
The interior of La Scala (1819), where Bellini's Il pirata was produced in 1827.

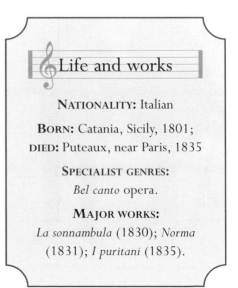

Life and works

NATIONALITY: Italian

BORN: Catania, Sicily, 1801;
DIED: Puteaux, near Paris, 1835

SPECIALIST GENRES:
Bel canto opera.

MAJOR WORKS:
La sonnambula (1830); *Norma* (1831); *I puritani* (1835).

Carl Maria von Weber

Weber, who seems to whisper in my ear like a familiar spirit,
inhabiting a happy sphere where he awaits to console me.

HECTOR BERLIOZ (1803–69)

Carl Maria von Weber, a leading pioneer of the German Romantic and nationalist movement, is chiefly remembered today for his opera *Der Freischütz* (*The Free Shooter*), the sparkling piano piece *Aufforderung zum Tanz* (*Invitation to the Dance*) which was orchestrated by Berlioz, the *Konzertstück* for piano and orchestra, and his brilliant works for clarinet.

Weber was born into a musical family in northern Germany, the son of a theatrical impresario and a singer. He took music lessons as a boy with Joseph Haydn's brother Michael in Salzburg, and by the age of 14 had already written his first opera. He completed his musical education in Vienna, and then spent over a

ABOVE: *A portrait of Carl Maria von Weber (1786–1826) by Caroline Bardua.*

ABOVE: *Costume designs for villains Samiel and Caspar in* Der Freischütz *(1821).*

decade working at various courts and municipal theatres in Germany (during which time he wrote many of his instrumental pieces) before being appointed director at the Prague Opera in 1813. During his tenure there he fell in love with the singer Caroline Brandt, but their tempestuous courtship lasted for four years before they were married.

A new German opera

On Christmas Day 1816 Weber was appointed to the prestigious post of *Kapellmeister* at the Dresden court. His brief was to establish a national German opera to rival the current dominance of the Italians, and throughout his time at Dresden he had to contend with the overt hostility of the royal *Kapellmeister* (an Italian), as well as with the early symptoms of tuberculosis. Nevertheless he persevered with building up his opera company, and with the composition of his German opera *Der Freischütz*.

The première of *Der Freischütz* in Berlin on 18 June 1821 was

Life and works

NATIONALITY: German

BORN: Eutin, near Lübeck, 1786; **DIED:** London, 1826

SPECIALIST GENRES: German Romantic opera, works for clarinet.

MAJOR WORKS: Two clarinet concertos; Clarinet Quintet (1814); *Grand Duo Concertant* (1816); *Aufforderung zum Tanz* (1819); *Konzertstück* in F minor (1821); *Der Freischütz* (1821); *Euryanthe* (1823); *Oberon* (1826).

ABOVE: Berlin in Weber's time — a view of the Brandenburg Gate and the Pariser Platz.

a triumph. Compared with the stuffy court operas of the period, it was entirely fresh and riveting, based on a story drawn from German folklore, and with music strongly influenced by German folk song idioms — the music of the people. It is based on the tale of a young forester who tries to win the hand of his beloved by selling his soul to the Devil in return for seven magic bullets which cannot fail to hit their targets. This gave Weber the opportunity for a marvellous supernatural scene in the "Wolf's Glen", a gift to designers and producers, with spine-chilling music to match.

Although *Der Freischütz* went on to take Europe by storm, Weber's next two operas were less successful. Both *Euryanthe* and *Oberon*, while containing marvellous individual numbers (the overture to *Oberon* is a masterpiece), suffered from muddled, incomprehensible plots and little sense of drama. *Euryanthe* opened in Vienna in 1823, but was given only 20 performances.

Last performances

Oberon, commissioned by the manager of the Covent Garden Theatre in London, was scheduled for performance in the spring of 1826. By the end of 1825 Weber knew that he was dying. Athough his wife and friends tried to dissuade him from travelling to London to conduct the opera, Weber was so worried about making financial provision for his young family that he insisted on making the journey.

He managed to conduct the première of *Oberon* on 12 April 1826, also undertaking many other concert engagements, but he was failing fast. He died at his lodgings in Great Portland Street in London on 5 June, aged only 39. Eighteen years later, Wagner, whose own early operas in the German Romantic style owed an enormous debt to Weber's pioneering work, had his predecessor's remains taken back to Dresden.

ABOVE: The "Wolf's Glen" scene from Der Freischütz — *the 1982 production of Weber's famous opera performed at the Royal Opera House in Covent Garden, London.*

Giacomo Meyerbeer

Meyerbeer feels as Michelangelo felt.

GEORGES BIZET (1838–75)

While the operas of Rossini, Donizetti, Bellini and Weber have all to some extent held their place in the repertoire, those of Giacomo Meyerbeer have been revived only occasionally over the past century. In his own time, however, Meyerbeer was one of the most successful opera composers and one of the richest men in Europe. This inevitably provoked envious sniping from his less fortunate colleagues – particularly Wagner, who launched a vitriolic attack on Meyerbeer in his anti-Semitic pamphlet *Das Judenthum in der Musik* (1850).

Child prodigy

Meyerbeer was a truly cosmopolitan figure. Born in Berlin, into the same affluent, cultured, Jewish milieu as his younger contemporary Mendelssohn, Jakob Liebmann Beer (as he was originally called) showed early promise

ABOVE: *Giacomo Meyerbeer (1791–1864), creator of French "grand opera". He and Berlioz shared a taste for the "monumental".*

as a pianist, appearing as soloist in a performance of a Mozart concerto at the age of 11. He began writing German operas while still in his teens.

From 1816 he spent nine years in Italy, where he wrote six operas in the style of Rossini. The last of these, *Il crociato in Egitto* (*The Crusader in Egypt*, 1824), was subsequently staged with equal success in London and Paris, where Meyerbeer met the librettist Eugène Scribe (1791–1861). From then onwards, Paris became the focus of Meyerbeer's activities, although he never lived there permanently. In the 1840s he was appointed *Generalmusikdirektor* in Berlin, where he wrote a *Singspiel* for the Swedish soprano Jenny Lind (1820–87).

Grand opera

Meyerbeer's reputation rests on the "grand operas" he created for the Paris Opéra in collaboration with Scribe, beginning with *Robert le diable* (*Robert the Devil*) in 1831, continuing with *Les Huguenots* and *Le prophète*, and ending with *L'Africaine* (premièred posthumously in 1865). All were staged with spectacular and innovative effects, such as storms, ships sinking on stage and massive crowd scenes.

Unlike Rossini, Meyerbeer was not a fast worker, and his productions were eagerly awaited. He wrote with specific voices in mind, and was always searching for new vocal and orchestral timbres.

ABOVE: *Costume for the role of Marguerite de Navarre, worn at the première of* Les Huguenots *in Paris on 29 February 1836.*

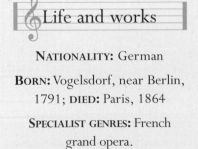

Life and works

NATIONALITY: German

BORN: Vogelsdorf, near Berlin, 1791; **DIED:** Paris, 1864

SPECIALIST GENRES: French grand opera.

MAJOR WORKS: *Robert le diable* (1831); *Les Huguenots* (1836); *Le prophète* (1849); *L'Africaine* (1865).

Niccolò Paganini

Paganini is the turning-point in the history of virtuosity.

ROBERT SCHUMANN (1810–56)

The Italian violinist and composer Niccolò Paganini is still revered as the greatest virtuoso of all — a true "wizard of the violin" whose technical mastery has never been equalled. His brilliant Twenty-four Caprices for solo violin have spawned many imitations, and his concertos and variations are still part of the violin repertoire.

Born into a poor Genoese family, he was forced as a small child to practise the violin constantly by his bullying father. In 1795 he spent a year studying in Parma, and at 18 was appointed leader of the orchestra (and then solo violinist to the court) in Lucca. At one of his court concerts he improvised a musical "love scene" using only

ABOVE: *The legendary violinist Niccolò Paganini inspired composers and performers, including Schumann, Liszt and Chopin.*

two strings of the violin, and he also wrote and performed a sonata entirely on the G string, demanding outstanding dexterity and accuracy.

From 1810 onwards, Paganini travelled Europe as a freelance virtuoso. After his 1813 debut concert at La Scala, Milan, a critic wrote: "He is without question the foremost and greatest violinist in the world. His playing is truly inconceivable. He performs certain passage-work, leaps, and double stops that have never been heard from any violinist…"

Pact with the Devil

The astonishing virtuosity of Paganini's playing, combined with his bizarre appearance — he was lean and gaunt, with a shock of long black hair, and very long, thin fingers — caused rumours that he was in league with the Devil. He never married, but a four-year relationship with a singer, Antonia Bianchi, produced one son, Achille, to whom he was devoted.

Between 1828 and 1834 Paganini's career as a touring virtuoso was at its height: he was acclaimed in Vienna, Berlin, Warsaw, Paris and London, but deteriorating health precipitated his retirement to Italy in 1834. Six years later he died of cancer of the larynx, but the church, having denounced him as a heretic, refused to allow his burial in consecrated ground. In 1845 his remains were transferred from the French Riviera to a private burial-ground in Parma, and were re-interred in Parma Cemetery in 1876. His Guarneri violin is preserved in the municipal museum in Genoa.

Paganini had enormous influence, both on composers (including Schumann), and performers: not only violinists, but also pianists. Both Liszt and Chopin were encouraged by his example to extend the frontiers of keyboard technique. Liszt's *Transcendental Studies* were directly inspired by Paganini's Caprices.

Life and works

NATIONALITY: Italian

BORN: Genoa, 1782;
DIED: Nice, 1840

SPECIALIST GENRES:
Virtuoso violin music.

MAJOR WORKS:
24 Caprices for unaccompanied violin (1820); violin concertos and shorter works, including *Le streghe* (*Witches' Dance*) and *Moto perpetuo* (*Perpetual Motion*).

Hector Berlioz

Berlioz composes by splashing his pen over the manuscript
and leaving the issue to chance.

FRÉDÉRIC CHOPIN (1810–49)

Like Schumann and Chopin, Berlioz is regarded as an archetypal "Romantic" artist, both for the nature of his work and for the colourful events of his life, which are documented in his entertaining *Memoirs*.

The son of a provincial French doctor, he intended to pursue a medical career, but the grisly scenes of carnage he encountered at medical school in Paris put him off. Instead he began music lessons, first privately and then at the Paris Conservatoire.

ABOVE: Hector Berlioz composing his opera Les Troyens *(The Trojans).*

Scaffold", the artist dreams that he has murdered his beloved and is being led to the guillotine; in the last, a grotesque witches' sabbath, the beloved has been transformed into a hag, her theme obscenely distorted.

In 1832 Berlioz finally persuaded Harriet Smithson to marry him. But proximity to the Beloved proved less appealing than worship from afar. Although he never divorced Harriet (who died of alcoholism in 1854), he formed a liaison from 1841 onwards with the

ABOVE: A cartoon of Berlioz conducting, surrounded by some of the bizarre instruments he deployed – including a cannon!

Sensitive, passionate and impulsive by nature, Berlioz was prone to violent emotions. In 1827 he saw an English theatre company performing *Hamlet* at the Odéon Theatre, and was immediately stricken with wild admiration, both for Shakespeare and for Harriet Smithson, the attractive Irish actress who played Ophelia. His unrequited passion found an outlet in 1830 in the extraordinary, programmatic *Symphonie fantastique*, subtitled "Episodes in the life of an artist". In the first three of its five movements, "the beloved" appears in various transformations as a melodic motif (which Berlioz called the *idée fixe*), whether in "passions and dreams", at a ball, or during a pastoral idyll (which owes much to Beethoven). In the fourth movement, "March to the

ABOVE: Harriet Smithson as Ophelia. Berlioz became obsessed with her and eventually married her, with disastrous consequences.

Life and works

NATIONALITY: French

BORN: La-Côte-Saint-André,
near Grenoble, 1803;
DIED: Paris, 1869

SPECIALIST GENRES: Romantic
orchestral and choral works,
large-scale opera.

MAJOR WORKS: *Symphonie
fantastique* (1830); *Harold
en Italie* (1834); *Grande
messe des morts* (1837);
Roméo et Juliette (1838–9);
overtures *Le corsaire*
(1831) and *Le carnaval
romain* (1844); *La damnation
de Faust* (1846); *Te Deum*
(1849); *Les Troyens* (1856–8).

singer Marie Recio, who later became
his second wife.

During the 1830s Berlioz produced
some of his finest works, including the
symphony with obbligato viola, *Harold
en Italie*. This work was commissioned
by Paganini, who paid the struggling
composer 20,000 francs for the piece,
although he never played the solo part
because he said it did not adequately
display his talents as a virtuoso.

Large-scale works

Berlioz's predilection for the
monumental led him to compose
enormous scores for huge orchestral
forces (although he himself played only
the guitar, he was a master of
orchestration and wrote an influential
treatise on the subject). His colossal
works for chorus and orchestra
included a Requiem (1837), the
dramatic symphony *Roméo et Juliette*
(1838–9), the *Grande symphonie
funèbre et triomphale* (1840), and the

operas *Benvenuto Cellini* (1834–7),
and *Les Troyens* (*The Trojans*, 1856–8).

Berlioz never had enough money.
He was forced to supplement his
income by working as a music critic,
and by touring Europe as a conductor.
In 1846 *La damnation de Faust*, a
"dramatic cantata" based on the play
by Goethe – whom Berlioz declared,
together with Shakespeare, the guiding
influence of his life – failed to attract
attention in Paris, though it scored a
great success in Russia. But his oratorio
L'enfance du Christ (*The Childhood of
Christ*) achieved a modest success in
1854, and the exquisite "Shepherds'
Farewell" scene has always remained
a popular favourite.

Les Troyens finally reached the stage
in 1863, when the second part only,
Les Troyens à Carthage, was performed
in Paris. Its failure broke Berlioz's
heart, and his last years were clouded
by depression and ill-health. (The
opera was not staged in its entirety in
French until 1969.) In the early 1860s
he completed his last work, the

sparkling Shakespearean opera *Béatrice
et Bénédict*, but thereafter wrote little
until his death.

Re-evaluation

While his large-scale works are still
performed relatively infrequently
because they are so expensive to
mount, the *Symphonie fantastique* and
the concert overtures (especially *Les
francs-juges*, the Byronic *Le corsaire* and
Le carnaval romain) have remained
popular, as has the delicately scored
orchestral song-cycle, *Les nuits d'été*
(*Summer Nights*, 1841), based on a
series of poems by Théophile Gautier.

Berlioz is still perceived as an
"oddball" composer, and his originality
has been derided as incompetence. But
the persuasive advocacy of writers such
as David Cairns and conductors such as
Colin Davis and Roger Norrington
have restored some previously
neglected masterpieces, such as *Les
Troyens*, to the repertoire, and affirmed
Berlioz's importance as one of the
foremost 19th-century composers.

ABOVE: Caricature of Berlioz conducting, by Georges Tiret-Bognet (born 1855).

Felix Mendelssohn

A romantic who felt at ease within the mould of classicism.

PABLO CASALS (1876–1973)

Felix Mendelssohn was born into a wealthy and cultured Jewish family. His grandfather Moses was a liberal philosopher, and his father, Abraham, a prominent banker who fled from Hamburg (where Felix and his sister Fanny were born) to Berlin, to escape Napoleon's marauding troops. The Mendelssohn family enjoyed a privileged middle-class existence in Berlin, where the children (two girls and two boys) were baptized as Christians, and their father became a town councillor.

At the family home, the young Felix encountered many well-known philosophers, actors, artists, writers and musicians, and showed precocious talent in music, drawing and poetry. By the age of 13 he was already an accomplished composer, and in 1821 he was introduced by his teacher Karl Zelter to Goethe. A strong friendship

ABOVE: Felix Mendelssohn (1809–47), painted by Gustav Zerner.

based on shared interests developed between the literary giant (then aged 70) and the talented boy. Mendelssohn dedicated his Third Piano Quartet to Goethe, who greatly appreciated the young man's frequent visits to his home in Weimar.

Musical impressions

Mendelssohn travelled a great deal as a young man, visiting Switzerland, Italy and Britain. He responded passionately both to literature and to impressions of people and landscapes encountered on his travels, both of which influenced his essays in the Classical musical forms of his day – symphony, overture, concerto, sonata and quartet. At the age of 16 he composed the brilliant Octet for strings, whose scherzo was inspired by the "Witches' Sabbath" scene in Goethe's *Faust*; two early overtures were inspired

LEFT: The Leipzig Conservatory of Music, founded by Mendelssohn in 1843.

RIGHT: The autograph score of the first of Mendelssohn's six Songs Without Words *for piano (1829).*

NATIONALITY: German

BORN: Hamburg, 1809;
DIED: Leipzig, 1847

SPECIALIST GENRES:
Symphonies, overtures,
concertos, piano pieces, songs.

MAJOR WORKS: Five
symphonies; incidental music
to *A Midsummer Night's Dream*
(1826–42); Octet for strings
(1825); *Hebrides* overture
(1830); Violin Concerto
(1844); two piano concertos;
eight books of *Lieder ohne Worte*
(*Songs Without Words*) for piano
(1829–45); *Elijah* (1846).

respectively by Shakespeare (*A Midsummer Night's Dream*) and Goethe (*Calm Sea and Prosperous Voyage*). Two of his five mature symphonies – the *Scottish* (No. 3, dedicated to Queen Victoria) and the *Italian* (No. 4) – reflect his impressions of landscapes. His 1829 tour of Scotland also inspired the famous *Hebrides* overture, written after a visit to Fingal's Cave on the Isle of Staffa.

Classical style

In Mendelssohn's two piano concertos, the much-loved Violin Concerto and the *Scottish* Symphony, he made original experiments in form, such as the recycling of thematic material and the linking of movements, which later became a feature of much Romantic music. Yet, for all his Romantic traits, he was a worthy successor to Beethoven and Schubert in his fluent handling of musical material. Schumann called him "the Mozart of the 19th century – the one who sees

most clearly through the contradictions of the period and for the first time reconciles them".

Mendelssohn's musical legacy

Through his tireless work as adminstrator and conductor, especially of the Lower Rhine Music Festival in Düsseldorf and the Leipzig Gewandhaus Orchestra, Mendelssohn was responsible for resurrecting buried treasures such as Bach's Passions and B minor Mass, and Handel's oratorios (on which he modelled his own *St Paul* and *Elijah*). He also helped to establish the role of the conductor, and raise standards of choral and orchestral performance.

In addition, Mendelssohn promoted the careers of other composers and performers, including Robert and Clara Schumann, Berlioz, the violinists Joseph Joachim, Ferdinand David (1810–73) and Henri Vieuxtemps (1820–81), and the pianist and composer Anton Rubinstein (1829–94). Many of his protégés were invited by Mendelssohn to join the staff of the newly opened Leipzig Conservatory (inaugurated in 1843), which under his direction became one of the most respected musical institutions in Europe.

ABOVE: An Art Deco programme cover for a dramatized pageant performance in London in 1936 of the oratorio Elijah *by Mendelssohn.*

In 1837 he married Cécile Jeanrenaud, daughter of a Lutheran pastor. They had five children and their marriage was happy but all too short: Mendelssohn died of overwork and grief in November 1847, aged only 38, shortly after hearing of the death of his beloved sister Fanny.

ABOVE: An annotated drawing made by Mendelssohn during his 1829 tour of Scotland.

Frédéric Chopin

*After playing Chopin, I feel as if I had been weeping over sins that I had never committed,
and mourning over tragedies that were not my own.*

OSCAR WILDE (1854–1900), "THE CRITIC AS ARTIST"

Chopin epitomizes the figure of the "Romantic artist": withdrawn, temperamental, talented and doomed to a premature death from tuberculosis. Like Paganini, he was both composer and performer (although his concert-giving was actually very limited), but his music established the piano as the 19th century's most popular instrument. He was also an important figure in the early nationalist movement, drawing inspiration from the folk idioms of his native Poland.

Born of mixed French and Polish parentage, Chopin began to compose before he was seven, and made his first public appearances as a pianist. On leaving school at 16 he enrolled at the Warsaw Conservatory, where he began to compose in earnest, and on graduating three years later he decided to seek his fortune abroad. In August

ABOVE: *Frédéric Chopin (1810–49), painted by Albert Graefle.*

1829 he made his debut in Vienna, playing two of his own piano works, including the set of Variations, Op. 2, whose publication Robert Schumann greeted with the immortal words, "Hats off, gentlemen, a genius!"

Polish themes

Chopin then returned to Warsaw, intending to leave soon afterwards on a European concert tour, but the tour was postponed owing to the volatile political situation and, meanwhile, Chopin fell in love. While he dallied in Warsaw, unwilling to leave, he worked simultaneously on two piano concertos. From his early youth he had been fascinated by the rhythms and melodic vitality of Polish folk music, and the finales of both concertos are strongly influenced by Polish dances – particularly the mazurka. After giving their premières with great success,

LEFT: *An artist's impression of Chopin at the piano, composing his Preludes.*

RIGHT: *The monastery of Valldemosa on the island of Majorca, where Chopin and George Sand took refuge in 1838.*

Chopin left Poland for Paris. On the way, he composed the great *Revolutionary* Study, in response to the devastating news that the Russians had captured Warsaw.

Paris

Chopin gave his first concert in Paris in February 1832. Although he was not a great success with the public, he was introduced to Parisian *salon* society, where his music was a triumph. From then onwards – although he rarely played in public – he became an instant celebrity. He was a sought-after teacher, consorted with the wealthy and powerful, and enjoyed the friendship of fellow composers (Liszt, Berlioz, Bellini and Meyerbeer), writers such as Heinrich Heine and Honoré de Balzac, and artists such as Eugène Delacroix.

Chopin also found lovers in this talented milieu – first the aristocratic singer Delfina Potocka, and then the writer Aurore Dudevant (George Sand), whom he met in 1836 at the home of Liszt's mistress. Their intense relationship lasted for nine years. They

ABOVE: *Chopin playing the piano in Prince Radziwill's salon in Paris, painted in 1887 by Hendrik Siemiradzki.*

ABOVE: *The writer Aurore Dudevant, alias George Sand (1804–76), Chopin's lover during the 1840s.*

spent the winter of 1838 in Majorca, hoping to reap the benefits of peace and a warm climate; but inclement weather and local hostility forced them to take refuge in the derelict monastery of Valldemosa. There Chopin finished his Twenty-four Preludes and other works, including the C sharp minor Scherzo. From then on he spent the winters in Paris and the summers at George Sand's country estate, but the affair finally fizzled out in 1847. By this time Chopin was seriously ill with consumption.

In 1848, Chopin was persuaded to visit England, where he played privately for fashionable social occasions. His last public appearance was at a charity concert for the benefit of Polish refugees. He died at his Paris home on 17 October 1849.

Chopin's music

Apart from the concertos and a handful of pieces for cello and flute, Chopin's output is all for solo piano. He borrowed the Irish composer John Field's new form, the nocturne, and raised it to fresh heights of subtle expression. His *études*, preludes, waltzes, impromptus and mazurkas were written to exploit and develop

piano technique; while the later polonaises, the *fantaisies*, the scherzos, ballades, the Barcarolle and the two sonatas, were all virtuoso works.

Contemporaries praised the "exquisite delicacy and liquid mellowness" of his tone, and the "pearly roundness of his passages of rapid articulation". These are still the hallmarks of great Chopin interpretation.

 Life and works

NATIONALITY: Polish

BORN: Zelazowa Wola, near Warsaw, 1810; **DIED:** Paris, 1849

SPECIALIST GENRES: Solo piano music.

MAJOR WORKS: Two piano concertos; three sonatas; four scherzos; 25 preludes; 27 *études*; 19 nocturnes; 44 waltzes; ten polonaises; 56 mazurkas; four ballades.

Robert Schumann

To me, Schumann's memory is holy.
The noble, pure artist forever remains my ideal.

JOHANNES BRAHMS (1833–97)

Just as Mozart and Beethoven dominated the musical scene in the late 18th and early 19th centuries, Mendelssohn and Schumann were the standard-bearers until 1850. Schumann's personality and career exemplify musical Romanticism: his moody nature, fluctuating between exuberance and deep depression; his prolonged struggle to win the hand of his adored Clara; his receptiveness to literary stimuli, his obsession with numerology and secret ciphers, and finally his collapse into madness and early death, possibly as a result of syphilis (which, together with tuberculosis, put a premature end to many a flourishing Romantic talent).

Literary influences

Schumann was the youngest child of a bookseller, whose interest in literature

ABOVE: *Robert Schumann (1810–56), painted by Gustav Zerner.*

he clearly inherited. While still a schoolboy he began to compose music, and also to write articles and drama. He formed a society for the study of German literature, and in the novels of Jean Paul (pseudonym of Johann Paul Richter, 1763–1825) he found a role model for the two conflicting sides of his own personality, which he later characterized as Florestan (extrovert and impetuous) and Eusebius (dreamy, melancholic, introverted).

While studying law in Leipzig he began to take piano lessons with Friedrich Wieck, whose nine-year-old daughter Clara was showing extraordinarily precocious talent as a pianist. By now Schumann had decided to follow a career in music, but a hand injury (possibly a result of muscular weakness caused by mercury treatment

ABOVE: *The market-place at Zwickau, where Schumann was born.*

ABOVE: *Schumann's study at his home in Zwickau.*

for syphilis) put paid to his hopes of becoming a concert pianist. Instead, he decided to concentrate on composition and criticism.

Early works

By 1832 Schumann had published two major piano pieces: the *Abegg* Variations, based on a waltz theme derived from the name of a girl who had taken his fancy, and *Papillons* (*Butterflies*), a set of pieces linked by events at a masked ball described in a novel by Jean Paul. He also began work on a symphony.

In 1834 he founded the influential music periodical *Neue Leipziger Zeitschrift für Musik*, which he used to promote new musical talent, including Brahms and Chopin. He also used its pages to fight artistic philistinism by way of an imaginary society, the Davidsbund, or "League of David" (named after the vanquisher of

ABOVE: *A romantic lithograph of Schumann composing his song-cycle* Dichterliebe (*A Poet's Love*).

Goliath), whose members were given fanciful names: Schumann himself was either Florestan or Eusebius; Clara Wieck was Chiara or Chiarina; her father was Master Raro, and Mendelssohn was Felix Meritis. These names appeared in Schumann's set of 18 "characteristic pieces" for piano, *Davidsbündlertanze* (*Dances of the League of David*, 1837).

Marriage to Clara

In 1834 Schumann fell in love with Ernestine von Fricken, to whom he became secretly engaged (and for whom he wrote the set of piano pieces later titled *Carnaval*). When he discovered that she was only the illegitimate daughter of a Baron, he broke off the engagement and

RIGHT: *Schumann composing at his piano. He had hoped to be a pianist, but was overshadowed by his more accomplished wife, Clara.*

ABOVE: *Clara and Robert Schumann. Their marriage in 1840 marked the beginning of a partnership that was rare for its time.*

which overshadowed his own reputation as a composer), Clara stimulated her husband's creative imagination, acting as muse, confidant and critic.

Productive years

From 1840 onwards, almost in regular annual cycles, Schumann poured out song-cycles – including *Myrthen* (*Bridal Wreath*), his wedding present to Clara, *Liederkreis* ("song-cycle"), *Frauenliebe und -leben* (*Woman's Love and Life*), and *Dichterliebe* (*A Poet's Love*) – chamber music (including a piano quartet and quintet, and three piano trios), and a body of piano music unsurpassed by any other contemporary composer. It was Clara who encouraged Robert to try his hand at larger-scale works. These included concertos for piano (the popular A minor Concerto was written for her), violin and cello; four symphonies, and other symphonic works including the exuberant *Konzertstück* for four horns and orchestra and the *Manfred* overture, inspired by Byron.

Schumann's orchestral music has been criticized for heavy-handed orchestration (partly the result of his

ABOVE: *Clara Schumann (1819–96), photographed in middle age. She outlived her husband by 40 years.*

transferred his affections to Clara Wieck, by now a delicate, dark-haired beauty of 15. Clara's father, who guarded his daughter jealously, was furious, and forbade Schumann to contact Clara. Then began an acrimonious six-year battle between Wieck – who made outrageous allegations against Schumann's character – and the lovers. Finally, in 1840, a court ruling paved the way for Schumann's marriage to Clara, which took place on 12 September.

Thus began one of the most remarkable musical marriages –

a partnership far ahead of its time – in which both husband and wife tried to combine family life with successful, independent careers. Clara Schumann (1819–96) was one of the most extraordinary women of her time. Her fragile appearance belied a steely inner strength, which enabled her to continue her demanding schedule of concert appearances all over Europe (she was one of the finest pianists of her age) while also coping with repeated pregnancies and child-rearing. While the marriage was not without its strains (Schumann resented his wife's success,

ABOVE: An illustration to "Du bist wie eine Blume" ("You are Like a Flower") from Myrthen, *Schumann's wedding present to Clara.*

own ineptitude as a conductor), but any defects are amply compensated for by its melodic charm and ingenious construction. Schumann's innovations include the recurring use of motto themes and other cyclical devices: in the D minor Symphony (No. 4), he directed that the thematically linked movements should be played without a break.

His large-scale vocal works include the secular oratorio *Das Paradies und die Peri* (1843), one opera, *Genoveva* (1850) and choral music including *Scenes from Goethe's "Faust"* (1853). As a composer of songs and piano music, he proved himself a worthy successor to Schubert. His piano music encapsulates an enigmatic private world, full of literary and musical allusions, autobiographical references and cryptograms: many of the piano pieces are built around references to Clara, such as the musical equivalents of the letters of her name. His songs include settings of Goethe, Adelbert von Chamisso (1781–1838), Eduard

Mörike (1804–75) and Joseph von Eichendorff (1788–1857), but his settings of Heinrich Heine (1797–1856), particularly the *Dichterliebe* cycle and some of the *Romanzen und Balladen*, are unsurpassed for their subtlety and lyricism.

Final years

In 1843 the Schumanns were reconciled with Friedrich Wieck, no doubt anxious to see his first grandchild. After a concert tour of Russia the following year they moved from Leipzig to Dresden. Schumann had always been prone to fits of deep depression and ill-health, and in 1846 he was so beset by nerves and chronic illness that he composed very little. By 1849 (when a revolutionary insurrection forced the family temporarily to flee Dresden), Schumann was becoming disillusioned by his failure to find a real job, and in 1850 he accepted an offer to become municipal music director in Düsseldorf.

His years in Düsseldorf were marked by failing health and mental instability, which adversely affected his abilities as

ABOVE: A page from the autograph manuscript of Schumann's Piano Sonata No. 3 in F minor, Op. 14, signed by the composer.

ABOVE: An illustration to Schumann's song "Der Nussbaum" ("The Walnut Tree"), No. 3 in the song-cycle Myrthen.

a conductor and caused increasing problems with his employers. He became obsessed with phenomena such as table-turning, and suffered aural and cerebral disturbances. Among the highlights of his later years were his meetings with the young Johannes Brahms, whom Schumann hailed in his magazine as a musician of the future, and the violinist Joachim, for whom Schumann wrote his Fantaisie for violin and orchestra and the Violin Concerto. Among his last compositions were the charming *Phantasiestücke* (*Fairy-tales*, 1849) for clarinet, viola and piano, and five Romances (1853) for cello and piano.

Schumann's mental faculties finally gave way completely in February 1854, and he began to experience hallucinations. After a failed suicide attempt, he was committed to an asylum. During the two and a half years in which he was incarcerated there, he was not allowed to see Clara. She was finally summoned to his bedside two days before his death on 29 July 1856.

Franz Liszt

I have not seen any musician in whom musical feeling ran, as in Liszt,
into the very tips of the fingers and there streamed out immediately.

FELIX MENDELSSOHN (1809–47)

As a composer, Liszt tends to stand on the sidelines of music history, partly because he does not fall neatly into the German symphonic tradition, stretching from Beethoven and Schubert, through Schumann and Mendelssohn, to Brahms and Bruckner. But his influence on 19th-century music was enormous: he was a superlative performer (the pianistic equivalent of Paganini), an outstanding teacher, and a dedicated champion of the "music of the future", expressed both in his own innovative and highly individual work, and in his promotion of Wagner.

Liszt was the son of an official at the Hungarian court of Haydn's employer, Prince Nikolaus Esterházy. He showed prodigious talent as a pianist, giving his first piano recital at the age of nine, and Prince Nikolaus funded his education in Vienna, where he moved from an early age in aristocratic circles.

ABOVE: *A portrait of Franz Liszt in old age, when he styled himself the "abbé Liszt" (Liszt the abbot).*

Paris

In the 1820s the flamboyant young virtuoso began to cause a sensation in Paris (where his family moved) and London, where he played for King George IV. Back in Paris in the early 1830s he met Berlioz and Paganini, and made piano transcriptions of some of their works, including Paganini's Caprices, which in Liszt's version became the *Grandes études de Paganini*. He was also greatly influenced by Chopin's Romantic style.

In 1834 he began a liaison with the Countess Marie d'Agoult, which produced three children (their second daughter Cosima later married Wagner). They began a peripatetic existence in Switzerland and Italy, during which time Liszt compiled his *Années de pèlerinage* (*Years of Pilgrimage*) for piano, and the *Album d'un voyageur*.

LEFT: *Liszt's summer residence on the corner of the Ilm Park in Weimar.*

RIGHT: *Title page of the score of Liszt's* Hungarian Rhapsody *No. 11.*

By 1839 the relationship was under strain, and Liszt resumed his touring career as a virtuoso. He and the countess finally separated in 1844, and Liszt began a period of wild womanizing, which contrasted oddly with his secret desire to become a priest. In 1848 he became music director to the ducal court at Weimar, where he eventually settled with his new companion, Princess Carolyne Sayn-Wittgenstein (who was trying to obtain a divorce from her husband). She shared Liszt's interest in religion and mysticism, and encouraged him to write his most ambitious works.

Weimar

The Weimar years (1848–59) represent the zenith of Liszt's composing career. Most of his major works date from this period. They include two pieces inspired by the Faust legend – the *Faust* Symphony (based on Goethe) and

ABOVE: *Liszt playing at a Parisian salon in 1840, painted by Joseph Danhauser. Listening (from left to right) are Alexandre Dumas, Victor Hugo, George Sand, Niccolò Paganini, Gioacchino Rossini and Countess Marie d'Agoult, Liszt's mistress.*

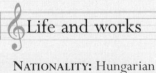

Life and works

NATIONALITY: Hungarian

BORN: Raiding, 1811; DIED: Bayreuth, 1886

SPECIALIST GENRES: Tone-poems, programme symphonies, piano works.

MAJOR WORKS: *Années de pèlerinage* (1836–77); 19 *Hungarian Rhapsodies* (1846–85); piano concertos; *Funérailles* for solo piano (1849); tone-poems *Mazeppa, Tasso, Les préludes* and *Orpheus* (1851–4); Piano Sonata in B minor (1853); *Dante* Symphony (1856); *Faust* Symphony (1857); *Mephisto Waltz* No. 1 (1861).

Episodes from Lenau's "Faust" – the *Dante* Symphony; over a dozen symphonic poems inspired by literary or pictorial models, including *Tasso, Les préludes* (after a poem by Alphonse de Lamartine), *Mazeppa, Hamlet* and *Hunnenschlacht* (*The Battle of the Huns*); the E flat Piano Concerto, the *Totentanz* (*Dance of Death*) for piano and orchestra, and piano works including the Transcendental Studies, the B minor Sonata, many of the Hungarian Rhapsodies, and the *Harmonies poétiques et religieuses*. In addition, Liszt championed works by other up-and-coming composers, giving the premières of operas by Wagner, Schumann, Berlioz, Verdi and Donizetti, among others. During his tenure, Weimar became known as the haven of the "New German School".

Holy orders

By 1860, however, Liszt had fallen out with conservative Weimar society (which disapproved of his open affair with Carolyne Sayn-Wittgenstein, and his promotion of "avant-garde" music).

He spent most of his later life in Rome, separated from the princess (who was never granted her divorce), and in 1865 he took minor holy orders.

A historian who saw him at the time described him as "Mephistopheles disguised as an abbé": his "diabolical" qualities, like Paganini's, were enhanced by his excessively tall, thin appearance, with long hair, originally blond, now white. He was still much sought-after as a teacher.

Liszt's later compositions are mostly sacred, and include the oratorios *Die Legende von der heilige Elisabeth* (*Legend of St Elisabeth*, 1857–62) and *Christus* (1862–7). However, they also include the Second and Third *Mephisto Waltzes*, one for orchestra (1880) and one for piano (1883). Among his last works – which became increasingly impressionistic in style – was *La lugubre gondola*, inspired by a premonition of his son-in-law Richard Wagner's death in Venice in 1882. Liszt himself died of pneumonia four years later in Bayreuth, having travelled there to attend the music festival.

Charles Gounod

*A man has only a certain number of virtues, and all of Gounod's
are concentrated on his art.*

GEORGES BIZET (1838–75)

Gounod is remembered today chiefly for his opera *Faust*, based on Goethe's drama; and for the song "Ave Maria", an arrangement of his Meditation for violin on Bach's Prelude No. 1 in C. In fact, he was a prolific composer whose music was influential in both France and England.

Gounod's father was a painter and his mother a pianist. Like Berlioz, he studied at the Paris Conservatoire, winning the Prix de Rome in 1839. In Italy he fell under the spell of 16th-century polyphonic music, and began to write sacred music of his own (he also seriously considered becoming a priest). But he also met two influential women – the singer Pauline Viardot-Garcia (1821–1910), who introduced Gounod to the theatrical world, and Fanny Hensel (1805–47), who introduced him to her brother Felix Mendelssohn.

ABOVE: Charles Gounod (1818–93). His operas influenced Bizet and Tchaikovsky.

In 1843 Gounod visited the Mendelssohns in Leipzig, where he heard the famous Gewandhaus Orchestra, and music by Bach (then rarely performed).

Opera

On returning to Paris Gounod began to write grand operas in the currently fashionable style of Meyerbeer, together with elaborate masses and other church music. His opera *Faust* was performed at the Théâtre-Lyrique in 1859, and was an instant success: Gounod's gift for memorable tunes (such as the "Soldier's Chorus" and Marguerite's "Jewel Song"), and his subtle musical characterization of the doomed lovers, appealed to a Parisian audience growing weary of Meyerbeerian bombast. None of his other operas (even *Roméo et Juliette*, 1867) was ever quite as successful.

England

Between 1870 and 1875 Gounod took refuge from the Franco-Prussian War in England, where his music appealed to Victorian sentimentality. Here, he acquired a ferocious English mistress, Georgina Weldon (he was chronically unfaithful), and founded the Gounod Choir, which eventually became the Royal Choral Society. In the 1880s he was preoccupied with composing oratorios (two of which were written for the Birmingham and Norwich festivals). Apart from the popular *Petite symphonie* for 10 wind instruments (1885), few of his later works have survived the test of time.

ABOVE: A scene from Goethe's Faust *– Faust tempted by Mephistopheles, painted in the mid 1820s by Eugène Delacroix.*

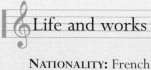

Life and works

NATIONALITY: French

BORN: Paris, 1818;
DIED: Paris, 1893

SPECIALIST GENRES: French grand opera, oratorios.

MAJOR WORKS: *Faust* (1859); *Roméo et Juliette* (1867); *La rédemption* (1881); *Mors et vita* (1884).

Georges Bizet

I am not made for the symphony; I need the theatre,
I can do nothing without it.

BIZET

Bizet's fame rests largely on just one work – the opera *Carmen* – but although his output was primarily operatic, several of his instrumental works, particularly the early Symphony in C, the suite *Jeux d'enfants* (*Children's Games*) and the incidental music to Alphonse Daudet's play *L'Arlésienne* (*The Girl from Arles*), have found a regular place in the repertoire.

Bizet studied at the Paris Conservatoire, winning many prizes, including the coveted Prix de Rome in 1857. Among his teachers was the opera composer Jacques Halévy, whose daughter he later married. The coolly classical Symphony in C was written at the age of 17, and in 1857 Bizet's one-act opera *Le docteur miracle* won joint first prize in a composition competition. He spent the years 1858–60 in Rome, where he picked up the chronic throat complaint which eventually killed him.

ABOVE: *Georges Bizet (1838–75), composer of the highly popular opera* Carmen, *the tragic story of the life, loves and death of a gypsy. Bizet wrote* Carmen *towards the end of his short life.*

Early set-backs

In 1863 Bizet's first important opera, *Les pêcheurs de perles* (*The Pearl-fishers*), was put on at the Théâtre-Lyrique in Paris. It failed, although the famous duet from Act 1, "Au fond du temple saint", has always been a popular favourite. Afterwards Bizet was obliged to take up hack work from publishers in order to survive financially. Meanwhile he worked on several more operatic projects, none of which achieved success. The colourful Provençal background of Daudet's play *L'Arlésienne*, for which Bizet provided incidental music in 1872, inspired him to find his true métier, and it was the similarly exotic setting and tragic story of Prosper Mérimée's *Carmen* which finally fired his imagination.

Carmen

Bizet's great opera was produced at the Opéra-Comique on 3 March 1875. It met with initial hostility, but within the next four years critics and audiences had come to appreciate the subtlety, power and originality of this vibrant score, and it was being performed all over Europe and in America. Bizet did not live to see its success. He died of a heart attack brought on by rheumatic fever on the night of its 33rd performance, just after the singer playing Carmen had fainted during the famous card-scene in which the gypsy heroine foretells her own death.

ABOVE: *Célestine Galli-Marié, the first* Carmen, *who fainted on stage in the fortune-telling scene on the night Bizet died.*

Life and works

NATIONALITY: French

BORN: Paris, 1838;
DIED: Bougival, 1875

SPECIALIST GENRES: Opera.

MAJOR WORKS: Symphony in C (1855); *Les pêcheurs de perles* (1863); *Jeux d'enfants* (1871); *Carmen* (1874).

Other Composers of the Era

Sounds overflow the listener's brain
So sweet, that joy is almost pain.

PERCY BYSSHE SHELLEY (1792–1822)

Although the main focus of early Romantic opera lay in Italy, France did not lag far behind. One of the most influential figures was Luigi Cherubini (1760–1842), who straddled the transitional period between Classicism and Romanticism. He began his career in his native Italy, where several of his early operas were produced, and then settled in Paris just before the Revolution. During the early Napoleonic era, Cherubini produced his most influential operas in Paris, including *Médée* (*Medea*, 1797), *Les deux journées* (*The Two Days*, also known as *The Water-carrier*, 1800) and *Anacréon* (1803). He then fell out with Napoleon, and in 1805 went to Vienna, where he met Haydn and Beethoven

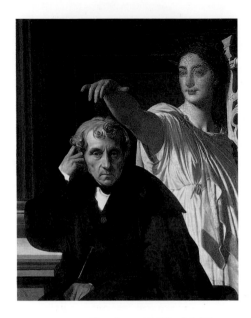

ABOVE: *Luigi Cherubini (1760–1842), in front of an Italian painting. This portrait was done in the year of his death by Ingres.*

ABOVE: *Daniel-François-Esprit Auber (1782–1871), a pupil of Cherubini and a successful opera composer.*

(whose *Fidelio* owes much to *The Water-carrier*). In 1816 Cherubini became a professor (later, from 1822, director) of the Paris Conservatoire, where his influence as a teacher was far-reaching.

Among Cherubini's pupils was Daniel Auber (1782–1871), who in 1842 succeeded his teacher as director of the Paris Conservatoire. He wrote nearly 50 operas, many in collaboration with the dramatist Eugène Scribe, of which the most famous are *La muette de Portici* (*The Dumb Girl of Portici*, 1828, which ends with a dramatic earthquake), *Fra diavolo* (*Brother Devil*, 1830), *Le domino noir* (*The Black Mask*, 1837) and *Manon Lescaut* (1856, a subject later tackled by Massenet and Puccini).

Bizet's teacher, Jacques Halévy (1799–1862), was another pupil of

ABOVE: *Costume designs for an 1827 German production of Daniel Auber's opera* Le maçon (The Mason)*, a musical drama written in the style of French* opéra comique.

ABOVE: *The Irish composer John Field (1782–1837), who invented the nocturne.*

Cherubini and also taught at the Paris Conservatoire from 1827 onwards. He was the principal singing coach at the Paris Opéra, 1829–45. Of his 30 or so operas, only *La Juive* (*The Jewess*, 1835) is occasionally revived.

Opera in Germany

Several German contemporaries of Weber advanced the cause of German Romantic opera, including Albert Lortzing (1801–51), one of the few composers who actually starved to death (he needed money so badly that he sold the valuable copyrights in his successful operas for a pittance). These included *Zar und Zimmermann* (*Tsar and Carpenter*, 1837), *Der Wildschütz* (*The Poacher*, 1842) and *Undine* (1845), based on Friedrich la Motte Fouqué's Romantic fairy-tale of 1811. This story had previously been adapted by the composer and writer Ernst Theodore Amadeus Hoffmann (1776–1822) for his 1816 opera of the same name.

Heinrich August Marschner (1795–1861), Weber's co-conductor at Dresden in the 1820s, was also influenced by the Romanticism of Hoffmann. He fared better than Lortzing, although his earlier operas – including the Gothic horror opera *Der Vampyr* (Leipzig, 1828), *Der Templar und die Jüdin* (*The Templar and the Jewess*, based on Scott's *Ivanhoe*, 1828) and *Hans Heiling* (Berlin, 1833) – achieved far greater success than his later works. He stands midway between Weber and Wagner as a pioneer of German Romantic opera.

Instrumental music

In the instrumental field, the violinist, conductor and composer Louis Spohr (1784–1859) scored great success in Germany, Vienna (where he led the orchestra at the Theater an der Wien) and London, where there was a considerable vogue for his work. From 1822 he was court conductor and later music director at the German court of Hesse-Kassel. He was one of the first conductors to use a baton. Spohr's operas have not survived, but his instrumental pieces are still played. They include 10 symphonies, 18 violin

ABOVE: *The Frenchman Jacques Fromenthal Halévy (1799–1862) taught Bizet.*

ABOVE: *The Swedish violinist and composer Franz Berwald (1796–1868).*

concertos, 4 clarinet concertos, and a quantity of chamber music, including string quartets and quintets, an octet for strings and wind, a fine nonet for strings and wind, and a quintet for piano and wind.

His Swedish contemporary Franz Berwald (1796–1868) was an amateur composer. He ran an orthopaedic institute in Berlin, and then managed a glassworks in Sweden, before being appointed Professor of Composition at the Swedish Royal Academy of Music shortly before his death. Berwald is now remembered for his *Symphonie singulière* (No. 3, 1845), and for his charming *Grand septet* in B flat for wind and strings.

The Irish composer John Field (1782–1837) studied with Clementi in London, and went on to enjoy a successful European career as a virtuoso pianist, from his base in St Petersburg. He invented the short piano piece known as the "nocturne", a form and style borrowed by Chopin. Field's 19 examples are still in the solo piano repertoire.

The Rise
❧ of ❧
Nationalism

A traditional Catalan festival held on Ash Wednesday to celebrate the beginning of Lent, painted in 1907 by Xavier Nogues (1873–1940).

The Nationalist Movement

The art of music above all other arts is the expression of the soul of a nation.

RALPH VAUGHAN WILLIAMS (1872–1958)

Up to the 19th century, music had been perceived as a common international language. Italian opera held sway in all European countries, as popular in Vienna, Stockholm, Madrid or London as in Venice or Rome; while the German symphonic style of Haydn, Mozart and Beethoven was adopted and copied by all European composers of their time. Only towards the middle of the 19th century did composers start to become aware of cultural differences between nations, an awareness prompted partly by political events, and partly through the Romantic cult of individualism, celebrating the unique qualities of both individuals and nations.

Revolutions of 1848

The nationalist movement took root in central Europe, where in the 1830s a wave of nationalist sentiment swept through Germany, Poland, Belgium and northern Italy (at that time ruled

ABOVE: A Bohemian Landscape with Shepherds, *painted in 1841 by Ludwig Richter.*

by Austria). Over the next decade, the desire of autonomous states for political independence from the mighty empires that ruled them coincided with the democratic urge to replace monarchies with republican governments more in tune with the needs of ordinary citizens. This

unstoppable force flared into violence in the year 1848, when patriotic sentiment and revolutionary fervour spread across France, Italy, Germany and central Europe. Although the revolutions failed, and autocratic rule tottered on in some countries until World War I, a new spirit of

LEFT: The Old Market-place in Prague, painted in 1865.

RIGHT: Mlle Eglantine's Dancing Girls — *a poster of the Belle Epoque in Paris, by Henri de Toulouse-Lautrec (1864–1901).*

nationalistic patriotism informed European politics from this time onwards, spreading into culture and the arts.

Folk music

In music, this patriotic fervour encouraged composers to seek inspiration in their national roots, particularly folk culture (often viciously suppressed by the ruling authorities). In beleaguered Poland, carved up by neighbouring powers after the Congress of Vienna, Chopin indicated his revolutionary sympathies by his use of Polish folk dances, especially the polonaise and the mazurka.

The nationalist movement was particularly strong in Russia (where Italian music – and Italian composers – had long reigned supreme at the cosmopolitan court in St Petersburg). Glinka was the first composer to draw inspiration from the distinctive melodic patterns and rhythms of Russian folk songs and dances, and his example was taken up with proselytizing zeal by Balakirev and his disciples, known as "The Mighty Handful", or "The Five". They in turn influenced Tchaikovsky, whose music, while not consciously "nationalistic", is still recognizably Russian in inspiration, drawing on folk legends and idioms, and epic tales from Russian history.

Landscape and people

The central European areas of Bohemia, Slovakia and Hungary, whose native culture had been suppressed by centuries of foreign domination, were particularly receptive to the new spirit of nationalism. The Bohemian composer Smetana was the first to celebrate the rich history and characteristic landscape of his native land in a series of tone-poems entitled *Má vlast* (*My Homeland*), and in a series

ABOVE: Spanish gypsy flamenco dancers, painted in 1898 by Ricardo Canals y Llambi (1876–1931).

of operas based on Czech subjects, from historical or mythical figures such as Libuše, to contemporary peasant life in *The Bartered Bride*. He in turn

ABOVE: The colourful costumes of 19th-century Russian ballet dancers.

influenced his pupil Dvořák, who effortlessly incorporated Czech song and dance idioms into European symphonic structures.

Nationalism was by no means confined to central Europe. Edvard Grieg, Norway's greatest composer, was trained in the German musical tradition, but his music draws plentifully on the folk idioms which he picked up on walking excursions into the Norwegian mountains.

In Spain, Albéniz and Granados exploited the colourful characteristics of Moorish-derived flamenco in their piano and orchestral works; in Austria, the talented Strauss family turned Vienna into the waltz capital of the world, and in England, then languishing under a dearth of native talent, the quintessentially "English" Savoy Operas of W. S. Gilbert and Arthur Sullivan exploited a rich vein of satirical English humour.

Mikhail Glinka

*I should like to unite in legitimate bonds the Russian popular song
with the good old Western fugue.*

GLINKA

Mikhail Glinka is regarded as the founding father of Russian nationalism in music. A contemporary of the Romantic poet Alexander Pushkin (1799–1837), he spent his early childhood with his grandmother, in whose care he first came into contact with the real music of Russia – the folk songs, pealing bells and ecclesiastical chants which would later inform his own music.

Glinka encountered Western music for the first time in his early teens, after he was sent to school in St Petersburg, where he studied violin and piano (including some lessons with John Field). On leaving school he became a minor civil servant, a job

ABOVE: *Mikhail Glinka (1804–57) working on his opera* Ruslan and Lyudmila, *painted by Ilya Repin.*

which left him plenty of time to indulge his passion for music as an enthusiastic amateur singer and pianist.

Opera

He began to compose songs and chamber music in the 1820s, but a prolonged trip to Italy in the early 1830s left him with a passionate interest in opera. His own first opera, *A Life for the Tsar* – based on the patriotic story of a heroic Russian peasant who saves the tsar's life at the cost of his own – was written after his return to Russia, and proved hugely successful on its première in 1836.

Glinka found himself acclaimed as Russia's leading composer (although, to be fair, there was little competition), and encouraged by his success he immediately embarked on his next

opera, *Ruslan and Lyudmila*. Unlike his earlier work, *Ruslan* was not well received. Its plot, based on Pushkin's fairy-tale (and involving such staging nightmares as a gigantic talking head), was cumbersome and ill-suited to the stage, and Glinka composed the score piecemeal. But its musical content – an appealing blend of elements drawn from Russian folk music, exotic orientalism and touches of "grotesquerie" – proved a rich legacy for all later Russian composers, as did his enthusiasm for the music of Spain (evinced in his two Spanish Overtures). Although Glinka died relatively young, his influence stretched far into the 20th century.

ABOVE: *A cartoon of Mikhail Glinka by V. Samoilov (1853).*

Life and works

NATIONALITY: Russian

BORN: Smolensk, 1804;
DIED: Berlin, 1857

SPECIALIST GENRES: Opera and orchestral works in Russian nationalist style.

MAJOR WORKS: *Ivan Susanin* (*A Life for the Tsar*, 1836); *Ruslan and Lyudmila* (1842); Spanish overtures *Jota Aragonesa* (1845) and *Night in Madrid* (1848).

"The Mighty Handful"

Show me a people who have more songs!

NIKOLAY GOGOL (1809–52), "THE CONTEMPORARY"

This curious crowd of dedicated drinkers, who were largely amateur composers, was given its nickname ("moguchaya kuchka") by the critic Vladimir Stasov in 1867. Their self-styled leader was Balakirev, while Borodin worked as a chemist, Rimsky-Korsakov was a naval officer and César Cui was a military engineer, and the most gifted, Mussorgsky, was a civil servant whom the rest regarded with a certain contempt. Nevertheless, their influence on Russian music in the late 19th century was immense.

Mily Balakirev

Balakirev began piano lessons with his mother as a young child and

ABOVE:
Mily Balakirev (1837–1910), the driving force behind Russian musical nationalism.

RIGHT: The statue of Peter the Great in front of the Cathedral in St Petersburg (1844).

became a proficient pianist. While still quite young he came into contact with the music of Mikhail Glinka – one of his own earliest compositions was a piano fantasy on Glinka's opera *A Life for the Tsar*. Glinka imbued Balakirev with a strong sense of the importance of Russian nationalism, especially in music.

In the early 1860s Balakirev began to assemble a small band of like-minded disciples around him, and also played a major role in founding the Free School of Music in St Petersburg (he became its director in 1868). From this period date the beginnings of Balakirev's twin obsessions – collecting Russian folk music from far-flung regions and editing the works of other composers.

Balakirev was prone to fits of chronic illness and depression, and he was never a prolific composer. His single most frequently performed work is the ferociously difficult "oriental fantasy" for piano, *Islamey*. His main reputation was as an uncompromising critic of other composers' works. Tchaikovsky, among others, fell victim to Balakirev's stinging criticisms.

Of Balakirev's disciples, César Cui (1835–1918) was the least important. He wrote some 15 operas and other stage works, all of which have now disappeared from the repertoire.

Life and works

NATIONALITY: Russian

BORN: Nizny-Novgorod, 1837;
DIED: St Petersburg, 1910

SPECIALIST GENRES:
Romantic orchestral and piano works using Russian idioms.

MAJOR WORKS: *Overtures on Russian Themes* (1858, 1864); two symphonies; *Islamey* (1869); many other works for piano; symphonic poem *Tamara* (1882).

Alexander Borodin

Borodin wrote only one opera, but music from it is still a concert favourite. The illegitimate son of an elderly Russian prince, Borodin was brought up by his gentle, cultured mother, and showed an early interest in music. But his chief love was science, and he became a distinguished professor of chemistry, founding a School of Medicine for Women.

In 1862 Borodin met Balakirev, and immediately began work on a symphony. It was performed in 1867 with great success, and he started work on his second. Shortly afterwards, in 1870, he began work on the opera *Prince Igor*, whose composition dragged on over the next 17 years, and remained unfinished at his death. Although it was subsequently completed by Rimsky-Korsakov, it is rarely performed, but the exotic "Polovtsian Dances" which end Act II (in Rimsky-Korsakov's orchestration) have always been highly popular, as have the Second Symphony in B minor

ABOVE: *Alexander Borodin (1833–87), the composer of* Prince Igor, *one of the most colourful Russian nationalist operas.*

and the languorous Nocturne from the Second String Quartet. Many of Borodin's most famous tunes formed the basis of the 1953 musical *Kismet*.

Modest Mussorgsky

Arguably the most original composer of "The Five", Mussorgsky was bedevilled by mental instability, exacerbated by his heavy drinking. He showed an early talent for music, becoming a proficient pianist, but was destined for an army career. He completed his training and enlisted in the élite Preobrazhensky Regiment, but resigned his commission within two years. By then he had met Balakirev, with whom he began to study music seriously.

Financial difficulties then forced him to take a job in the civil service, while he continued to struggle with his first opera, *Salammbô*, based on Flaubert's novel. Although he started various projects with great enthusiasm, he finished few of them, and his three great operas — *Boris Godunov*, *Khovanshchina* (*The Khovansky Affair*) and *Sorochintskaya yarmarka* (*Sorochintsy Fair*) — were all left incomplete at his death (from alcoholic epilepsy), just after his 42nd birthday. He is also remembered

Life and works

NATIONALITY: Russian

BORN: St Petersburg, 1833;
DIED: St Petersburg, 1887

SPECIALIST GENRES:
Opera and orchestral works influenced by Russian and oriental idioms.

MAJOR WORKS: Symphony No. 2 in B minor (1877); *V srednei Azii* (*In the Steppes of Central Asia*, 1880); String Quartet No. 2 (1885); *Kniaz Igor* (*Prince Igor*, 1887).

ABOVE: *Russian folk dancers. All five composers in "The Mighty Handful" drew inspiration from their native folk music.*

Life and works

NATIONALITY: Russian

BORN: Karevo, 1839;
DIED: St Petersburg, 1881

SPECIALIST GENRES:
Opera in nationalistic idiom, piano works, songs.

MAJOR WORKS:
Boris Godunov (1872); *Khovanshchina* (1872–5); *Kartinki s vistavki* (*Pictures at an Exhibition*) for piano (1874); *Night on the Bare Mountain* (1877); songs; song-cycles.

ABOVE: *Modest Petrovich Mussorgsky (1839–81), painted in the year of his death by Ilya Repin.*

for his orchestral piece *Ivanova noch na Lisoi gore* (*Night on the Bare Mountain*), inspired by a witches' sabbath, the famous *Kartinki s vistavki* (*Pictures at an Exhibition*) for piano, later orchestrated by Ravel, and his affecting song-cycles *Detskaya* (*The Nursery*, 1870), *Bez solntsa* (*Sunless*, 1874) and *Piesni i plyaski smerti* (*Songs and Dances of Death*, 1875–7).

Nikolay Rimsky-Korsakov

The most active and prominent of "The Mighty Handful" (and the youngest), Rimsky-Korsakov was born into a well-to-do naval and military family. He managed to combine a career as a naval officer with a productive sideline in composition. In 1871 he became professor of composition and instrumentation at the St Petersburg Conservatory.

Like his musical colleagues, he was deeply influenced by the nationalist work of Glinka, and he too fell under Balakirev's spell. Orchestration was Rimsky-Korsakov's great strength,

and his talent for orchestral colour, combined with exotic, oriental-sounding harmonies, produced many rich and glowing works including the *Capriccio espagnol* (*Spanish Caprice*), the symphonic suite *Sheherazade*, inspired by tales from the *Thousand and One Nights*, and the *Voskresenaya* (*Russian Easter Festival Overture*). This heady blend of Russian folk material and orientalism also informed the scores of many of his 15 operas. Rimsky-Korsakov devoted as much time to his friends' work as to his own. He was responsible for orchestrating and completing, among others, Borodin's *Prince Igor*, and several works by Mussorgsky, including *Night on the Bare Mountain* and the operas *Boris Godunov* and *Khovanshchina*. Naturally he applied his own ripe orchestral palette to these works, and the modern trend in performance is to return as far as possible to the originals.

ABOVE: *Sheherazade and the Sultan — a scene from the Russian Ballet version of Rimsky-Korsakov's* Sheherazade.

ABOVE: *Nikolay Rimsky-Korsakov (1844–1908), one of the most popular Russian composers of his day.*

Life and works

NATIONALITY: Russian

BORN: Tikhvin, near Novgorod, 1844; **DIED:** Liubensk, near St Petersburg, 1908

SPECIALIST GENRES: Operas based on Russian fairy-tales.

MAJOR WORKS: *Snegurochka* (*The Snow Maiden*, 1881); *Capriccio espagnol* (1887); *Sheherazade* Suite (1888); *Voskresenaya* Overture (1888); *Sadko* (1898); *Tsar Saltan* (1900); *Skazkanie o nevidimom gradie Kitezhe* (*The Tale of the Invisible City of Kitezh*, 1903–4); *Zolotoy Petushok* (*The Golden Cockerel*, 1906–7).

Pyotr Ilyich Tchaikovsky

Music is not illusion, but revelation.

Tchaikovsky could claim to be the world's most popular "classical" composer. His music has always held a special appeal, for its passion, lyricism, extravagant emotionalism, and glowing orchestral colour. It reflects the extremes of temperament of its composer — a moody, melancholy character, prone to fits of depression, but also of heightened optimism.

Throughout his life, Tchaikovsky was torn between his desire for a "normal" family life, and his homosexual nature. This constant, unhappy struggle was reflected in his music, particularly the later symphonies. Although associated with "The Mighty Handful", Tchaikovsky was never a member of that nationalist group. Much of his own work, however, draws on a rich vein of Russian folk culture, which he successfully fused with the Western symphonic tradition. He wrote: "As far as the Russian element in my music is concerned, this is because I grew up in the provinces, imbued from earliest childhood with the indescribable beauty of the characteristic features of Russian folk music."

Early life

Tchaikovsky was the son of a mining engineer, and was born near the Urals. From his delicate, epileptic, French mother he inherited his hypersensitive nature and a tendency to hypochondria. When he was eight, the family moved to St Petersburg, where Tchaikovsky enrolled in the junior department of the School of Jurisprudence, a training-ground for the civil service. By this time, he had acquired twin younger brothers, Anatoly and Modest. He was exceptionally close to his mother, and her shocking death in a cholera epidemic when Tchaikovsky was 14 was a trauma from which he never really recovered.

ABOVE: Pyotr Ilyich Tchaikovsky (1840–93), arguably the greatest and most popular Russian composer of the 19th century.

LEFT: Tchaikovsky's father, Ilya Petrovich, with his twin sons Anatoly and Modest.

RIGHT: The square in front of the Mariinsky Theatre in St Petersburg in 1812.

Tchaikovsky graduated from the School of Jurisprudence in 1859, but found life in the civil service uncongenial. When a new music conservatory opened in St Petersburg in 1862, he enrolled as a student. He graduated in 1866, and found a job as a harmony teacher at the Moscow Conservatory, which had just been established by his mentor, the pianist and composer Nikolay Rubinstein (1835–81). The successful performance of an early overture in March 1866 encouraged him to start work on a symphony, entitled *Winter Daydreams*, which was performed under Rubinstein's baton in 1868. Modelled on Mendelssohn's *Italian* and *Scottish* Symphonies, it uses melodies influenced by Russian folk tunes.

Music for the stage

Meanwhile Tchaikovsky was working on his first opera, *Voyevoda*, which was performed at the Bolshoy Theatre in Moscow in February 1869. Shortly afterwards Tchaikovsky met Balakirev, who recognized a major new talent and

ABOVE: A page from the autograph piano reduction of Tchaikovsky's ballet Swan Lake *(1877). The score is a masterpiece and the ballet is a major part of the dance repertoire.*

encouraged Tchaikovsky to tackle the tone-poem *Romeo and Juliet*. Its subject-matter, dealing with the favourite Russian themes of love and death, fired the composer's imagination, and it quickly became one of his most popular works.

In May 1872, while staying at the country estate of his beloved sister Alexandra and her family, Tchaikovsky wrote his Second Symphony, known as the *Little Russian*, which incorporates genuine Ukrainian folk tunes into its musical fabric. It was well received, but he still wanted to achieve operatic success. This eluded him until after his first venture into the world of ballet, with *Lebedino ozero* (*Swan Lake*), written for the Imperial Ballet in Moscow. Though its first production in 1877 was a disaster, it was the first of his three great ballet scores – the others are *Spyashchaya krasavitsa* (*The Sleeping Beauty*) and *Shchelkunchik* (*The Nutcracker*) – which are still the cornerstones of the classical ballet repertoire.

In 1874 Tchaikovsky's confidence received another severe dent when Nikolay Rubinstein contemptuously

rejected his First Piano Concerto as "worthless and unplayable". Tchaikovsky rightly ignored the criticism, and refused to alter the score. After Hans von Bülow gave its première in Boston, USA, the following year with great success, Rubinstein was forced to admit his

ABOVE: The Swan Princess *by M. A. Vrubel (1867–1910), inspired by the heroine of* Swan Lake.

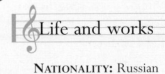

Life and works

NATIONALITY: Russian

BORN: Kamsko-Votkinsk, 1840; **DIED:** St Petersburg, 1893

SPECIALIST GENRES: Symphonies, ballets, opera.

MAJOR WORKS: Symphonies No. 1–6; Piano Concerto No. 1; *Swan Lake* (1877); Violin Concerto (1878); *Eugene Onegin* (1879); *Manfred* Symphony (1886); *The Sleeping Beauty* (1889); *The Queen of Spades* (1890); *The Nutcracker* (1891–2).

Bedřich Smetana

Here is a composer with a genuine Czech heart,
an artist by the Grace of God!

FRANZ LISZT (1811–86)

Nationalist feeling was particularly strong in 19th-century Bohemia, where Czech customs, culture, and even language were suppressed by its German-speaking Austrian rulers. Smetana was the first Czech composer openly to draw inspiration from national legends, history and landscape, and to incorporate the melodic patterns and rhythms of folk music into his work.

The son of a German-speaking master brewer, Smetana showed early promise as a pianist, and having studied in Prague and Plzen despite parental opposition, he decided to make music his career. He began by making a precarious living as a concert pianist and teacher, during which time he met the Schumanns and Liszt. In 1848 he took an active role in the unsuccessful Prague Revolution, helping to man the street barricades, and the following year he married a fellow pianist, Kateřina Kolářová.

ABOVE: *Bedřich Smetana, influential in the central European nationalist movement.*

Of their four daughters, three died in childhood, followed by the consumptive Kateřina herself in 1858. The family had spent much of the previous two years in Göteborg, Sweden, where Smetana had opened a music school, and where he had begun to compose symphonic tone-poems modelled on the works of Liszt, including *Richard III* and *Wallensteins Lager*, based on Schiller's play.

Czech nationalism

A few months after his wife's death, Smetana became engaged to his brother's sister-in-law, whom he married in 1860. He returned to Sweden that year, but events in his homeland were changing fast. The Austrians had suffered heavy defeats at the hands of Napoleon III's armies, and the time was ripe for a resurgence of Czech national feeling.

Smetana returned home early in 1861, hoping to become conductor

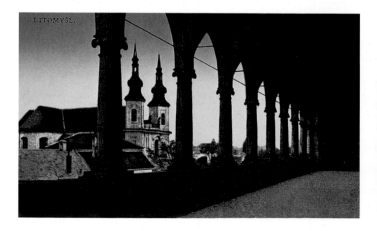

ABOVE: *The Bohemian town of Litomyšl, where Smetana was born in 1824. Bohemia was part of the Austrian Empire at this time.*

ABOVE: *A view of Prague, showing the banks of the river Vltava, the inspiration for one of the movements in Má vlast (My Homeland).*

of the new Prague Provisional Theatre, which had just opened for the performance of opera and drama, but having been raised as a German-speaker it took time to convince the authorities of his ambitions for Czech music. His first opera, *Braniboři v Čechách* (*The Brandenburgers in Bohemia*), with a libretto by the nationalist poet Karel Sabina, was produced there in January 1866 to great enthusiasm. It was quickly followed by *Prodaná nevěsta* (*The Bartered Bride*), which, with its appealing blend of rustic lyricism and the skilful incorporation of Czech dances, became Smetana's most popular opera.

Prague Provisional Theatre

In the autumn of 1866 Smetana was finally appointed conductor to the Provisional Theatre, where he introduced many major works to the repertoire, among them his own *Dalibor* (1868), based on a legendary Czech hero, and *Dvě vdovy* (*The Two Widows*, 1874). His most overtly patriotic work, *Libuše* (dealing with the legendary founder of the Czech ruling dynasty), was composed

ABOVE: Smetana at his piano, composing the opera The Bartered Bride *(1866).*

between 1869 and 1872, but had to wait until June 1881 for its première, at the triumphant opening of the National Theatre.

During the composition of *Libuše*, Smetana also worked on his great cycle of symphonic poems celebrating Czech history, legend and topography, entitled *Má vlast* (*My Homeland*). The most popular individual item has always been *Vltava*, a portrait of the river that runs through Prague.

Deafness and disability

In the early 1870s Smetana became aware that his health was deteriorating: he complained of giddiness and hearing problems (the result of syphilis). In October 1874 he went completely deaf in one ear. He was also suffering from financial problems, but nevertheless managed to complete a new opera, *Hubička* (*The Kiss*), in 1876. At the same time he wrote his E minor String Quartet, subtitled "From My Life",

whose last movement is dominated in the coda by a sustained high note representing the shrill whistling sound which Smetana suffered permanently as a result of his deafness.

Like Beethoven, Smetana continued to compose in spite of his disability. A seventh opera, *Tajemství* (*The Secret*, 1878), was followed by two new patriotic symphonic poems, *Tábor* (1878) and *Blaník* (1879), both inspired by episodes from Czech history. (*Tábor* is built around an early 15th-century Hussite chorale, effectively the Czech national anthem.)

Smetana's last opera, *Čertova stěna* (*The Devil's Wall*, 1882), took three years to write, during which time he complained of feeling as if he were standing "under a huge waterfall". He completed his Second String Quartet in March 1883, but his condition deteriorated and a year later he was taken to the Prague lunatic asylum, where he died on 12 May 1884.

Life and works

NATIONALITY: Czech

BORN: Litomyšl, 1824; **DIED:** Prague, 1884

SPECIALIST GENRES: Nationalistic Czech operatic and orchestral music.

MAJOR WORKS: *The Bartered Bride* (1866); *Má vlast* (1872–9); String Quartet No. 1 in E minor *From My Life* (1876); *The Kiss* (1876).

Antonín Dvořák

I should be glad if something occurred to me
as a main idea that occurs to Dvořák only by the way.

JOHANNES BRAHMS (1833–97)

Dvořák stands at the heart of the Czech nationalist musical movement. Like his contemporary Tchaikovsky, he succeeded in fusing folk idioms (the inflections of folk melodies and the characteristic rhythms of Czech dances such as the "furiant") with the symphonic techniques of his predecessors Beethoven and Brahms. His symphonies (particularly the three later ones), tone-poems, chamber and piano music are all part of the mainstream repertoire, and his operas (especially *Rusalka*, 1900) are becoming more widely known through frequent revivals.

Dvořák's father was the village butcher, and wanted his son to follow the same trade, but Antonín began to learn the violin at an early age and was eventually allowed to study music. He attended the Prague Organ School, and began his career as principal viola in the orchestra of the Provisional Theatre. He also began to compose and teach. He fell in love with a pupil, Josefina Čermáková, but when she rejected him he married her younger sister, Anna, in 1873.

By 1874 Dvořák had already completed four symphonies and two operas. That year he achieved his first real breakthrough when he entered several compositions in a competition intended to help struggling young artists. The jury included Brahms, who recognized Dvořák's talent, awarded him first prize, and took a fatherly interest in promoting his career.

ABOVE: *Antonín Dvořák, the most famous Czech composer of his time. He was equally popular in England and the USA.*

Brahms recommended Dvořák to his own publisher, who in 1878 commissioned a set of eight orchestral *Slavonic Dances* and within a year had published them, together with three *Slavonic Rhapsodies*, a Serenade for wind instruments, a String Sextet and Quartet, songs and piano duets. The infectiously tuneful *Slavonic Dances* in particular were a huge success, and assured Dvořák's international reputation.

England

From then on, Dvořák's works were performed as far afield as London and New York. In 1882 August Manns conducted the Sixth Symphony at the Crystal Palace in London, and the Stabat Mater was performed with great success in London the following year.

In 1884 Dvořák visited England for the first time, conducting some of his own works, including the Sixth Symphony and the *Scherzo capriccioso* for orchestra. He was immediately invited to write a new symphony (the Seventh, in D minor) for the Royal Philharmonic Society, and two large-scale choral works for the Birmingham and Leeds Festivals: the dramatic cantata *The Spectre's Bride* for Birmingham, and the oratorio *St Ludmila* for Leeds.

Life and works

NATIONALITY: Czech

BORN: Nelahozeves, 1841;
DIED: Prague, 1904

SPECIALIST GENRES: Opera, symphonies, tone-poems, chamber music.

MAJOR WORKS: Nine symphonies, including No. 9 *From the New World* (1893); Serenade for strings (1875); Stabat Mater (1877); *Slavonic Dances* (1878 and 1886); Requiem (1890); Cello Concerto in B minor (1895); operas; chamber music; piano music; songs.

London also saw the performance in 1887 of the *Symphonic Variations*, conducted by Hans Richter, and, in 1890, of the Eighth Symphony – often known as the *English*, although it is a thoroughly "Bohemian" work. The next year Dvořák received an honorary doctorate from Cambridge University.

America

In 1891 he was invited to become director of the new National Conservatory of Music in New York, at a very attractive salary. Dvořák spent five months touring Bohemia with several new works – including the Dumky Piano Trio and a cycle of three overtures, *V přírodě* (*In Nature's Realm*), *Carnaval* and *Othello* – before sailing for New York in spring 1892.

He spent three years there, teaching, conducting and composing. The Ninth Symphony (*From the New World*), the *American* String Quartet and Quintet, the Cello Concerto (whose coda reflects Dvořák's grief at hearing of the death of his sister-in-law Josefina), and the charming Violin Sonatina (dedicated to his six children) were all composed there. Several of these works show the influence of American folk music, especially the negro spiritual.

ABOVE: The National Theatre in Prague, opened on 18 November 1883. Dvořák's opera The Jacobin *was premièred there six years later.*

Return to Prague

The lure of his native Bohemia eventually proved too strong, and after 1895 Dvořák decided not to return to America. Instead he resumed teaching at the Prague Conservatory, and spent time with his family. The last decade of his life produced many new works, including two string quartets, four symphonic poems based on Czech folk tales – *Vodník* (*The Water Goblin*), *Zlatý kolovrat* (*The Golden Spinning-wheel*), *Polednice* (*The Noonday Witch*) and *Holoubek* (*The Wild Dove*), 1896–7 – and his two best-known operas, *Čert a Káča* (*Kate and the Devil*, 1899) and *Rusalka* (1900), both based on fairy-tales. He died on 1 May 1904, and had a state funeral.

LEFT: Dvořák with his wife and children, photographed shortly after their arrival in New York, 1892.

RIGHT: Dvořák conducting at the Chicago World Fair in 1893. The programme included the Eighth Symphony and three of the Slavonic Dances.

The ❦ Later ❦ Romantics

Patrons arriving at the Bayreuth Festspielhaus, 1892. Wagner's music-dramas are still performed in this opera house at an annual festival directed by his descendants.

mother's death in January 1865, was a bitter blow (Brahms commemorated her death in the slow movement of his powerful Horn Trio).

In 1868 Brahms decided to settle permanently in Vienna, but continued playing his own works on frequent concert tours. In 1872 he became conductor of the Vienna Gesellschaftskonzerte, but held the post for only three years. A new breed of professional virtuoso conductors such as Hans Richter (1843–1916), Hans von Bülow (1830–94), and Hermann Levi (1839–1900) had arrived on the scene, and Brahms wisely realized his own limitations. In 1869 he had already had a taste of critical vitriol when Wagner (fearing a new and talented rival) had viciously

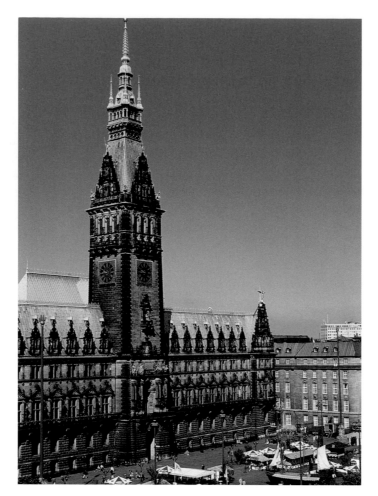

ABOVE: *The Town Hall in Hamburg, the city where Brahms was born in 1833.*

attacked him in an article entitled "On Conducting". From then onwards, Brahms devoted himself to composition.

After many years of work, in 1868, Brahms had completed *Ein Deutsches Requiem* (*A German Requiem*) for soloists, chorus and orchestra – a deeply felt response to biblical passages on the subject of death, mourning and consolation – and during the Franco-Prussian War he was hailed as a "patriot", having used material from the Lutheran Bible rather than the traditional Latin text of the Catholic liturgy. He responded by composing the *Triumphlied* (*Song of Triumph*) in the summer of 1871 to celebrate Germany's victory. By 1873, when he finished his popular *St Anthony Variations* (*Variations on a*

Theme of Haydn) for orchestra, he was earning enough to be able to live on the income from his concerts and publications, and felt sufficiently secure to turn down a lifelong contract offered by the publisher Fritz Simrock (he also rejected an honorary doctorate offered by Cambridge University).

Symphonic success

Three years later, with Clara Schumann's constant encouragement, Brahms finally completed his First Symphony in C minor, begun over 20 years earlier. Its long gestation had been haunted by the ghost of Beethoven, and by Brahms's fear that the work would be rejected because it was not "programmatic". But the Viennese public received it with enthusiasm, and

ABOVE: *The opening page of the autograph score of Brahms's Double Concerto for violin and cello (1887).*

ABOVE: *Brahms (centre) on the day of Clara Schumann's funeral, 20 May 1896. He had loved her ever since their first meeting.*

Brahms immediately began work on a second symphony.

In the late 1870s he adopted the habit of spending the summers in the Austrian countryside, at Pörtschach on Lake Wörther in Carinthia. There he completed the Second Symphony in D, the brilliant Violin Concerto (whose gypsy finale pays homage to Joachim, its Hungarian dedicatee), the G major Violin Sonata, the two Rhapsodies, Op. 79, and the eight Piano Pieces, Op. 76. From 1880 onwards he found another summer refuge at Bad Ischl, where he wrote the Piano Trio in C, the Quintets in F and G, the Three Motets, Op. 110, and many of his late chamber and vocal works.

In 1881 Brahms conducted his satirical *Akademische Festouvertüre* (*Academic Festival Overture*), based on students' songs, in Breslau, where the University had awarded him a doctorate. He did not care for honours, and failed to attend the degree ceremony. That year he completed the Second Piano Concerto in B flat – a *tour de force* of power and vitality, and a milestone of pianistic virtuosity. He also had a major disagreement with Joachim, who was intending to divorce his wife. Brahms took Frau Joachim's side, and the violinist broke off all relations with Brahms. (They were eventually reconciled in 1887, when Brahms wrote the Double Concerto for Joachim and the cellist Robert Hausmann.)

Also from 1881, the conductor Hans von Bülow – a great admirer of Brahms – offered the composer the use of the Meiningen court orchestra to try out his new works. These included the Third and Fourth Symphonies. The Third, in F,

ABOVE: *Brahms at the piano – a posthumous sketch by Beckerath, 1899. Brahms had always been a fine pianist, having played since the age of seven.*

was written in Wiesbaden in 1883, and the Fourth, in E minor, during two summer holidays in southern Austria, and performed on a European tour with the Meiningen

Orchestra in the autumn of 1885. In its *passacaglia* finale, Brahms paid homage to another lifelong influence, that of J. S. Bach.

Last works

Brahms spent the following three summers at Hofstetten on Lake Thun, where he wrote his Second Cello Sonata in F major, two more violin sonatas, and the C minor Trio. By 1890 he had resolved to stop composing, but broke his resolution to write four clarinet works inspired by the brilliant playing of Richard Mühlfeld (1856–1907), principal clarinettist with the Meiningen Orchestra: the Clarinet Trio and Quintet and two clarinet sonatas. Clara Schumann's death in May 1896 prompted one final work – the *Vier ernste Gesänge* (*Four Serious Songs*) – but by then Brahms himself was mortally ill from liver cancer. He died on 3 April 1897, and was buried in Vienna's central cemetery.

ABOVE: *The sixth book of Brahms's* Collected Songs.

Anton Bruckner

Bruckner! He is my man!

RICHARD WAGNER (1813–83)

Bruckner's name is often coupled with Mahler's – but for no other reason than that both were Austrian and both wrote important, large-scale symphonies. In all other respects they were very different.

Bruckner's father was the village schoolmaster and organist at Ansfelden in central Austria. Anton, the eldest of five surviving children, was taught by his father, and by the age of ten was already a proficient organist. He also came into contact with the Catholic musical tradition at the nearby monastery of St Florian, where he enrolled as a chorister at the age of 13, after his father's death. St Florian was to remain the focus of Bruckner's life, and he chose to be buried there, beneath the organ.

Bruckner began his career as an ordinary schoolmaster in two provincial villages. Eventually, in 1845, he returned as a teacher and then as organist to St Florian. His first important compositions, including a Requiem Mass and the *Missa solemnis* in B flat, date from his early years there.

By 1855 Bruckner had decided he wanted to become a professional musician. While working as organist at Linz Cathedral, he enrolled on a correspondence course in harmony and counterpoint at the Vienna Conservatory. He graduated in 1861 at the advanced age of 37, with glowing references. But he still felt he lacked musical knowledge, and sought further tuition in symphonic form and orchestration with the principal cellist and conductor at the Linz municipal theatre, who engaged him in a thorough study of Beethoven and Mendelssohn.

ABOVE: The Austrian composer Anton Bruckner – a portrait by H. Kaulback.

LEFT: A page from Bruckner's Ninth Symphony, left unfinished at his death.

RIGHT: The organ at the Abbey Church of St Florian. Bruckner was a chorister and then organist there, and is buried beneath the organ.

NATIONALITY: Austrian

BORN: Ansfelden, 1824; **DIED:** Vienna, 1896

SPECIALIST GENRES: Symphonies, church music.

MAJOR WORKS: Nine symphonies, including No. 4 (*The Romantic*, 1874–81), No. 7 (1883), No. 8 (1885–90) and No. 9 (unfinished, 1896); Te Deum (1884).

ABOVE: The Graben, one of the principal streets in Vienna, in Bruckner's time. Bruckner lived in Vienna from 1868 until his death.

The impact of Wagner

Up to this point, Bruckner had been competent but characterless as a composer. Then, in 1863, he heard Wagner's *Tannhäuser*, and the experience changed his life. Overwhelmed by Wagner's genius, Bruckner immediately began to try his own hand at symphonic composition. During the mid 1860s he attended many performances of Wagner's music, and even met the great man, while his budding confidence led to the composition of three masses and the Symphony No. 1 in C minor (1865–6).

After suffering a nervous breakdown brought on by intense overwork, Bruckner was eventually persuaded to apply for a professorship at the Vienna Conservatory, to which he was appointed in 1868. He also became organist at the Imperial Chapel in Vienna, and received a government grant to allow him to compose. He lived in Vienna until his death, leaving for occasional visits to Paris and London, where his organ recitals were greeted with huge acclaim.

In Vienna (where he was appointed a lecturer at the University in 1875) he devoted much of his energy to composing symphonies. Between 1871 and his death, he turned out eight more (No. 9 remained unfinished).

Despite Bruckner's growing fame, he encountered enormous opposition and hostility from two anti-Wagnerite sources. The Vienna Philharmonic Orchestra either rejected his symphonies as "unplayable" or deliberately sabotaged their performances, and the influential critic Eduard Hanslick – a supporter of

ABOVE: The beginning of the Gloria from Bruckner's Mass in D minor (1864), a page from the autograph score.

Brahms – took every opportunity to denounce Bruckner's symphonies, especially the Third (which Bruckner, in an enthusiastic fit of hero-worship, had unwisely dubbed his *Wagner Symphony*). Diffident by nature and fatally lacking in self-esteem, Bruckner also suffered from the interference of well-meaning but misguided "friends" who persuaded him to make cuts and alterations to the scores of his symphonies, in the interests of "accessibility". Many still exist in various hybrid versions.

Bruckner's first real success came at the age of 60, with the Leipzig première of his Seventh Symphony in 1884. He had finally found critical acceptance, although he continued to revise his scores obsessively. Official honours came his way during the last decade of his life. A simple, pious, old-fashioned man, he never married, although he proposed to a succession of astonished young women. He had a morbid obsession with dead bodies, and left instructions that his own should be embalmed.

Giuseppe Verdi

It may be a good thing to copy reality;
but to invent reality is much, much better.

VERDI, 1876

Verdi was the greatest Italian opera composer of the 19th century. Unlike Wagner, who strove to create a new type of music-drama, Verdi worked within the Italian tradition of his predecessors, but throughout his long career his technique became ever more fluent, his characterizations more rounded and expressive, and his response to the text increasingly refined.

His masterpieces are the Shakespearean operas *Otello* (1887) and *Falstaff* (1893), written when he was in his 70s, but works from all periods of his life form the backbone of the present-day operatic repertoire.

ABOVE: *Giuseppe Verdi (1813–1901), the greatest Italian opera composer of the 19th century.*

son moved to Milan, where the opera had been accepted for production at La Scala. It was premièred in November 1839, a few weeks after his son's death, and in June 1840 Verdi's wife also died. During this sad period, Verdi was working on a new opera, the comedy *Un giorno di regno* (*King for a Day*), which failed utterly at its première at La Scala in September 1840.

Verdi was so discouraged that he almost gave up composing, but a friend persuaded him to begin work on *Nabucco*, based on the biblical story of Nebuchadnezzar. This – his earliest well-known work, famous for its chorus of Hebrew slaves "Va, pensiero" – was a triumphant

ABOVE: *The French dramatic soprano Rose Caron as Desdemona in Verdi's* Otello. *She created the role in 1894.*

Early years

Verdi was born in Lombardy, at a small village in the vicinity of Parma. He began to play the keyboard when he was three, and at ten he was sent to study in Busseto. In 1831 he became the protégé of a music-loving merchant, Antonio Barezzi, who financed his further musical education privately in Milan, Verdi having been rejected by the Milan Conservatory. Verdi then returned to Busseto as the town's music director. In 1836, aged 22, he married Barezzi's daughter Margherita. They had two children, who both died in infancy.

In 1838 Verdi began work on his first opera, *Oberto*. He, his wife and baby

ABOVE: *Arturo Toscanini, one of the great Verdi interpreters, conducting the orchestra of La Scala Opera House in May 1946.*

ABOVE: A set design (c.1862) by Carlo Ferrario for Verdi's grand opera La forza del destino *(The Force of Destiny).*

ABOVE: A scene from a performance of Verdi's Aida *at the 1991 Savonlinna Opera Festival in Finland.*

success, and was soon being performed all over Europe. Before long, Verdi's name was being linked with the emerging nationalist movement in Italy, as choruses such as "Va, pensiero" and the Scottish exiles' lament from *Macbeth* (1847) were interpreted as coded rallying-cries for the oppressed Italian nation.

Galley years

With *Ernani* (1844), Verdi entered on a period he later called his "galley years", producing a string of operas for Rome, Milan, Naples, Venice, Florence, Trieste, and even London (*I masnadieri – The Brigands*, 1847). His early operas, up to *La battaglia di Legnano* (*The Battle of Legnano*, 1849), were still influenced by Rossini, and generally dealt with historical subjects (including the Shakespearean opera *Macbeth*).

Luisa Miller (1849) was the first of a series of works in which the subject-matter became more personal and intimate. The finest operas of this period are *Rigoletto* – the tragic tale of a hunchbacked court jester who seeks to avenge his daughter's seduction but inadvertently causes her death; *Il trovatore* (*The Troubadour*), another tragedy with the motif of revenge at its heart; and *La traviata* (*The Woman Gone Astray*), Verdi's version of *La dame aux camélias* by Alexandre Dumas. The

story of the courtesan who finds true love, sacrifices it for her lover's honour, and dies of consumption, is one of the most popular operas ever written.

Grand opera

Verdi's third period began with *Les vêpres siciliennes* (*The Sicilian Vespers*, Paris, 1855), and includes *Simon Boccanegra*, *Un ballo in maschera* (*A Masked Ball*), *La forza del destino* (*The Force of Destiny*, produced in

St Petersburg in 1862), *Don Carlos* (Paris) and *Aida* (Cairo). During this period he spent much time on the country estate he had bought near his birthplace, with his second wife, the soprano Giuseppina Strepponi (1815–97).

In 1861, after the Italian War of Independence, Verdi was elected to the new Italian parliament, and for the next four years mixed politics with composition. After *Aida*, he wrote little except his dramatic Requiem commemorating the death of the Italian nationalist poet Alessandro Manzoni (1785–1873).

Last works

The huge success of the Requiem prompted Verdi's publisher, Ricordi, to suggest a collaboration with the composer-librettist Arrigo Boito (1842–1918), on an opera based on Shakespeare's *Othello*. It took Verdi another decade to begin work on *Otello*, which with *Falstaff* marked the culmination of his career. His last work, in 1898, was a set of *Quatro pezzi sacri* (*Four Sacred Pieces*), including a Te Deum and Stabat Mater. By then Verdi had lost his beloved second wife, he was over 80 and worn out. He died in Milan in January 1901, leaving his fortune to a home for aged musicians which he had built in Milan, and which he regarded as "his greatest work".

🎼 Life and works

NATIONALITY: Italian

BORN: La Roncola, near Busseto, 1813;
DIED: Milan, 1901

SPECIALIST GENRES: Italian grand opera.

MAJOR WORKS: *Nabucco* (1842); *Rigoletto* (1851); *Il trovatore* (1853); *La traviata* (1853); *Simon Boccanegra* (1857); *Un ballo in maschera* (1859); *La forza del destino* (1862); *Don Carlos* (1867); *Aida* (1871); *Requiem* (1874); *Otello* (1887); *Falstaff* (1893).

Richard Wagner

Wagner's opera style recognizes only superlatives.

EDUARD HANSLICK (1825–1904)

The figure of Richard Wagner straddles the 19th century like a colossus. Composer, critic, polemicist, his abundant energy allowed him to a pursue a vision with a ruthless single-mindedness beyond the comprehension of ordinary mortals.

His operas, rooted in the German Romantic tradition, remain (like Verdi's) the cornerstones of the modern repertoire, but they require performers of extraordinary power and stamina. There are still few sopranos and tenors able to do justice to roles such as Siegfried, Brünnhilde, Tristan and Isolde, and many singers have burnt out their voices in the attempt.

interested in the theatre, and in 1832 he began work on his first, abortive, opera. He realized from the start that he would only ever be able to work with his own librettos.

He began his theatrical career as a chorus-master in Würzburg, where he completed his first opera *Die Feen* (*The Fairies*). It remained unperformed, but already Wagner was showing a dogged determination to succeed. He began work on a third opera, *Das Liebesverbot* (*Love's Interdict*), based on Shakespeare's *Measure for Measure*, and joined a travelling theatre company as music director. *Das Liebesverbot* had a single performance in Magdeburg in 1836, before the company went bankrupt.

ABOVE: *A costume design by Franz Gaul for the 1873 production of Wagner's early opera* Rienzi *at the State Theatre in Brunswick.*

ABOVE: *An evocative portrait of Richard Wagner (1813–83), by Lenbach. Wagner was much given to striking romantic poses.*

Early years

Friedrich Wagner died of typhus soon after his son Richard was born, and his mother Johanna married Ludwig Meyer, who introduced his stepson to the world of the theatre and music. The family moved to Dresden, where the young Wagner came into contact with Weber, then conductor at the Royal Theatre. According to Wagner, it was Weber who instilled in him "a passion for music". After his stepfather's death the family returned to Wagner's birthplace, Leipzig, where he completed his education at school and university. By now he was passionately

ABOVE: *Senta leaps to her death — an Art Nouveau illustration of the final scene of* The Flying Dutchman.

ABOVE: A domestic vision of Wagner at home with his second wife Cosima, daughter of Franz Liszt.

ABOVE: A scene from the last act of Rienzi, *premièred at the Dresden Hoftheater on 20 October 1842.*

By this time Wagner had fallen in love with the actress Minna Planer, whom he married on 24 November. Six months later Minna ran off with another man, but was reconciled with her husband in October 1837. Their relationship remained stormy.

Paris

Wagner was working at Riga (now in Latvia) when he began *Rienzi*. By March 1839, when his contract ended, he was heavily in debt (a *Leitmotif* of his career). He, Minna and their huge dog were obliged to flee from his creditors by ship to London.

In September they arrived in Paris, where Wagner hoped to establish himself as a composer. Instead he found himself trying to make ends meet from journalism, while financial problems landed him in a debtors' prison. He did, however, come into contact with a great deal of new music, and with literature, especially the Germanic legends of Tannhäuser and Lohengrin. His Paris period thus laid the foundations of several future operas, including *Der fliegende Holländer* (*The Flying Dutchman*), which he finished in 1841. The famous, storm-tossed overture to this dramatic tale,

of a restless ghost who is finally redeemed by faithful love, was inspired by Wagner's own experiences on the ship from Riga.

Dresden

In 1842 *Rienzi* was finally performed, with considerable success, at the Dresden court theatre, which agreed to mount *The Flying Dutchman* in January 1843. Although Wagner was

disappointed with the latter's reception, his career was finally launched, and he was offered the post of conductor in Dresden. In April 1843 he completed *Tannhäuser*, based on the legend of the knight – seduced from his duties by the pleasures of Venus – who is redeemed by a divine miracle. *Tannhäuser* was premièred in Dresden in October 1845.

Wagner began work on *Lohengrin*, which was finished in 1848, the year of revolution in Europe. Wagner's pro-revolutionary sympathies implicated him (by default) in the Dresden uprising of May 1849, and in fear of his life he escaped to Switzerland. He settled in Zurich, where he worked on his creative manifesto, *Opera and Drama*, and also began work on the texts of a new project, based on the ancient Nordic saga of the Nibelungs. *Lohengrin* could not now be produced in Dresden, so Wagner sent the score to Liszt, who had sufficient confidence in it to risk censure by mounting a production in Weimar in August 1850. It eventually became an outstanding success, although Wagner himself was unable to attend a performance until 1861.

ABOVE: A Romantic impression of Wagner composing his epic saga Der Ring des Nibelungen, *a cycle of four operas completed in 1874.*

Music of the future

Lohengrin – another legendary tale of knightly chivalry with a strong magical element – marked the end of Wagner's involvement with conventional German Romantic opera. In *Opera and Drama* he set out his visionary ideal of the "music of the future", in which music and drama became indivisible. The last 30 years of his life were dedicated to realizing this ideal.

By 1852 Wagner was again chronically in debt. He was helped by the merchant Otto Wesendonk, with whose wife, Mathilde, he fell in love. Their affair inspired the opera *Tristan und Isolde*, which Wagner began in 1857. This passionate portrayal of an adulterous love which can find fulfilment only in death is one of the supreme achievements of Western art. In it, Wagner pushed chromatic harmony to its limits, from the unresolved, "yearning" motif of the Prelude to the ecstatic dignity of Isolde's "Liebestod" ("love-death")

in which she is finally united with Tristan as the strained "Tristan chord" achieves its radiant resolution.

Munich

Wagner's personal troubles continued. His wife discovered his liaison with Mathilde Wesendonk, and Wagner fled to Venice. With the police at his heels he moved on to Lucerne (where he finished *Tristan*) and then to Paris, where performances of *Tannhäuser* in 1861 were disrupted by an organized and noisy claque.

A political amnesty of 1860 allowed Wagner to return to Germany, but he spent the next three years travelling from city to city dodging his creditors, until a knight in shining armour appeared in the person of the "mad" King Ludwig II of Bavaria. Ludwig paid off Wagner's debts and offered him sanctuary in Munich, where *Tristan und Isolde* was first performed on 10 June 1865, under the baton of Hans von Bülow. Wagner repaid Bülow by beginning an affair with his wife Cosima (daughter of Liszt and the Countess Marie d'Agoult), who bore him two daughters, Isolde and Eva.

Wagner now had to leave Germany again in the face of Bavarian opposition to his powerful influence over the king and the vast sums of money that were being lavished on him from the public purse. Minna Wagner having died in 1866, Cosima von Bülow moved in with Wagner at his new home – financed by Ludwig – at Tribschen, outside Lucerne, where their son Siegfried was born in 1869. (This event inspired Wagner to compose the *Siegfried Idyll*, rehearsed in secret and played as a surprise for Cosima on Christmas morning.) After Cosima's divorce from Bülow, she and Wagner were married in 1870.

ABOVE: The Festspielhaus at Bayreuth, built to Wagner's specifications by Gottfried Semper between 1871 and 1876 for the performance of Wagnerian music-dramas.

Cosima – a formidable woman – kept Wagner on a short leash throughout their marriage, but protected his interests, and enabled him to compose in peace.

Bayreuth

In June 1868 *Die Meistersinger von Nürnberg* – a blend of comedy, philosophy, radiant young love and wisdom as embodied in the person of Hans Sachs the cobbler – had been premièred in Munich. At the same time, Wagner continued working on his *Ring* cycle, but realized that no existing theatre was suitable for such a large project. With King Ludwig's help, he raised the money to build a dedicated "Festival Theatre" at Bayreuth, where his operas are still performed at an annual festival directed by members of the Wagner family. The new theatre was inaugurated in August 1876 with three complete performances of the *Ring* cycle of four works – *Das Rheingold,*

ABOVE: *A 1914 stage set for the "Garden of Enchantment" in* Parsifal, *designed by Thomas Edwin Mostyn (1864–1930).*

Die Walküre, Siegfried and *Götterdämmerung* (*The Twilight of the Gods*).

Der Ring des Nibelungen – which contains over 12 hours of music – is held together by a complex system of musical references called *Leitmotifs*, in which characters and situations are identified by individual musical motifs, such as the joyous horn call associated with the hero Siegfried. By now Wagner's musical language had

succeeded in merging voices and orchestra into one continuous texture, at the opposite end of the spectrum from the Italianate concept of opera as separate arias, ensembles and choruses. This complex, endlessly evolving web of sound proved an ideal vehicle for the grandiose Nibelung drama, which reaches its shattering conclusion as Valhalla burns and the world ends.

In 1882 Wagner finished his last opera, *Parsifal*, based on the quasi-religious myth of the quest for the Holy Grail, with its miraculous powers of healing. It was performed at Bayreuth in the summer of 1882, conducted by Hermann Levi. Wagner himself conducted the last scene of the final performance. Two weeks later, suffering from a heart condition, he took his family to Venice, where he died of a heart attack on 13 February 1883.

LEFT: *Brünnhilde, from Arthur Rackham's 1910 watercolour illustrations to* The Rhinegold *and* The Valkyrie.

RIGHT: *The "Good Friday" scene from a 1950s Bayreuth production of* Parsifal, *produced by Wagner's grandson Wieland.*

Gustav Mahler

To write a symphony is, for me, to construct a world.

MAHLER

Mahler was a transitional figure. A contemporary of Sigmund Freud and the painter Gustav Klimt, his massive orchestral works are rooted in the 19th-century Austro-German symphonic tradition and speak in a rich, late-Romantic idiom inflected with folk idioms, yet look forward to 20th-century preoccupations such as neurosis and mysticism. His most important works are his ten symphonies and his songs with orchestral accompaniment, which influenced them. Four of the symphonies – Nos. 2, 3, 4 and 8 – have substantial vocal and choral parts, which has tended to limit their performance potential, and for almost five decades after Mahler's death his works were largely neglected, admired

He showed musical promise as a child, and studied at the Vienna Conservatory from 1875–8, where he wrote the cantata *Das klagende Lied* (*The Song of Sorrow*). From 1880 onwards he made his living as a conductor at provincial theatres in Upper Austria, Slovenia, Bohemia, and then at Kassel in Germany, where he composed the song-cycle *Lieder eines fahrenden Gesellen* (*Songs of a Wayfarer*), and started his First Symphony.

In 1885 Mahler spent a year in Prague, and then moved to Leipzig. There he met the Weber family, who introduced him to the folk poetry collection *Des Knaben Wunderhorn* (*The Youth's Magic Horn*, published in 1805–8). From 1887 onwards he began to set some of the

ABOVE: *Gustav Mahler in the loggia of the Vienna Court Opera House, where he was conductor from 1897 until 1907.*

only by a small band of devotees, until the advocacy of conductors such as Bruno Walter, Georg Solti and Rafael Kubelík in Europe, Leonard Bernstein in America and Norman del Mar in Britain, restored them to the repertoire.

Conducting

Mahler was born into a Jewish family and, although he later converted to Catholicism, his career was to some extent blighted by the anti-Semitic attitude of the Austrian establishment.

ABOVE: *A page from the autograph score of Mahler's Sixth Symphony (1903–6).*

ABOVE: *Mahler's wife Alma with their daughters Maria and Anna, c.1906–7.*

ABOVE: Mahler rehearsing his Eighth Symphony (Symphony of a Thousand). The huge choir extends all around the auditorium.

Wunderhorn poems, which were reworked in his earlier symphonies. Between 1888 and 1891 he worked as conductor of the Royal Opera in Budapest, before moving to the Stadttheater in Hamburg, where he conducted Wagner's *Tristan* in May 1891. By 1892 he had completed his First Symphony (first performed at Weimar in 1894), and had begun work on a second (the *Resurrection*). By then he had established a working pattern of conducting during the winter seasons, and retreating to the mountains to compose in the summer. The Third Symphony was finished in this way at Steinbach in the Salzkammergut.

Vienna

In 1897 Mahler was appointed conductor at the Vienna State Opera (one of his first productions there was Wagner's *Ring* cycle). He remained at Vienna for ten years, as one of the Opera's most distinguished music directors. In 1901 he found a new lakeside retreat at Maiernigg in Carinthia, where over the next few summers he composed the Fourth, Fifth,

Sixth and Seventh Symphonies, the *Rückert-Lieder*, the *Kindertotenlieder* (*Songs on the Death of Children*) and other works. The glorious *Adagietto* of the Fifth Symphony was an expression of his love for Alma Schindler, stepdaughter of the Viennese artist Carl Moll, whom Mahler married in 1902. Contrary to popular belief, the deeply affecting *Kindertotenlieder* pre-dated the death from scarlet fever of the couple's elder daughter Maria in 1907, although Alma believed that the cycle had "tempted providence".

ABOVE: The Metropolitan Opera House, New York, in the early 20th century. Mahler was appointed conductor there in 1908.

Mahler's Eighth Symphony (*Symphony of a Thousand*) dates from 1906–7. It was based on the text of a medieval hymn and the closing scene of Goethe's *Faust*, Part II. Mahler thought it "the greatest work I have yet composed". At the end of 1907, the victim of a vicious press campaign, he was obliged to resign his Vienna post, and also discovered that he had a potentially fatal heart condition. He was appointed conductor at the Metropolitan Opera House, New York, from January 1908, but continued to spend the summers in Europe, where he composed *Das Lied von der Erde* (*The Song of the Earth*), based on Chinese poems about the transience of life. He also completed his Ninth Symphony and began a Tenth.

In February 1911 Mahler became seriously ill, and died in Austria, aged 50. *Das Lied von der Erde* and the Ninth Symphony were given posthumous performances; the Tenth was completed in the 1960s by the British scholar Deryck Cooke.

Edward Elgar

Look out for this man's music;
he has something to say and knows how to say it.

HUBERT PARRY (1848–1918)

Like Arthur Sullivan (another composer knighted for his services to British music), Edward Elgar transcended the class barriers of his age, rising from humble origins to epitomize – in musical terms – Britain at the height of her Imperial glory.

Early life

He was born within sight of the Malvern Hills near Worcester, where his father ran a music shop and was organist at St George's Catholic Church. Edward's first job on leaving school was to help his father in both capacities, and he also began to play the violin in local orchestras and chamber groups. In the early 1880s he began to make a living as a freelance

ABOVE: *Edward Elgar revived British music almost single-handedly.*

player, teacher, conductor and self-taught composer with instrumental groups in the Malvern area. His composing ambitions were stimulated by his marriage in 1889 to his piano pupil Alice Roberts, daughter of a retired major-general. Alice, who was 40 when she married the 31-year-old Elgar, had social pretensions, and she persuaded her husband to move to London, where their only daughter, Carice, was born in September 1890.

Success as a composer at first eluded Elgar, and the following year the family moved back to Malvern, where he resumed his teaching activities and strove to overcome a sense of social inferiority. His persistence paid off when his overture *Froissart* was published.

Creative period

By the mid 1890s Elgar was becoming known for the cantatas he had composed for provincial festivals, including *The Black Knight* (1893) and *King Olaf* (1896), and in 1897 he finally achieved a breakthrough in London with the *Imperial March* for Queen Victoria's Diamond Jubilee.

In 1899 his first truly original composition, the orchestral *Enigma Variations*, was performed at St James's Hall in London. The Variations – each a

ABOVE: *Elgar conducting in the studio in 1919, the year he wrote his Cello Concerto.*

Life and works

NATIONALITY: English

BORN: Broadheath, near Worcester, 1857;
DIED: Worcester, 1934

SPECIALIST GENRES: Orchestral music, oratorios.

MAJOR WORKS: Symphonies No. 1 and 2; *Enigma Variations* (1899); *Sea Pictures* (1899); *Pomp and Circumstance* Marches (1901–30); *The Dream of Gerontius* (1900); Introduction and Allegro for string orchestra (1905); Violin Concerto (1910); *Falstaff* (1913); Cello Concerto (1919).

thinly disguised character portrait of a friend (including Elgar himself and his wife) – were recognized as a work of genius, while the underlying "enigma" – an unnamed tune which Elgar said "goes through and over the whole set" – has never been positively identified. The Variations encapsulate Elgar's musical style: noble, expansive, but tinged with plangent nostalgia for the English countryside.

In the autumn of 1899 the contralto Clara Butt sang Elgar's orchestral song-cycle *Sea Pictures* at the Norwich Festival, and he was commissioned to write an oratorio for the 1900 Birmingham Festival. The result was *The Dream of Gerontius*, based on a metaphysical Catholic text by Cardinal Henry Newman. Elgar was bitterly disappointed by the initial failure of this great work (which has since been recognized as a masterpiece), but the same year he was awarded an honorary doctorate by Cambridge University. His orchestral works were becoming popular, including the overture *Cockaigne*, inspired by London, and the first two *Pomp and Circumstance* Marches, of which the trio section from the first was later allied to the words of the verse "Land of Hope and Glory" written by A. C. Benson for the coronation of Edward VII. In 1904 Elgar was knighted.

The same year, the Elgars moved to a large house in Hereford, where over the next few years he wrote another oratorio (*The Kingdom*), the Introduction and Allegro for string orchestra (1905), and two symphonies. In 1910 Fritz Kreisler gave the première of Elgar's Violin Concerto,

ABOVE: The programme for a gala performance at the Royal Opera House, 1902, in the presence of the new King Edward VII and Queen Alexandra, at which Elgar's Coronation Ode *was performed.*

an eloquent work which bears an enigmatic dedication in Spanish: "Herein is enshrined the soul of…" This soul may have been that of John Everett Millais's daughter, Alice Stuart-Wortley, to whom Elgar seems to have been deeply attached.

In 1912 Elgar returned to London, to a grand house in Hampstead, where he wrote the cantata *The Music Makers* (1912) and the symphonic poem *Falstaff* (1913). He was greatly distressed by World War I, which he saw destroying the society in which his works were rooted, and his personal response was the elegiac Cello Concerto and three chamber works – a violin sonata, a string quartet and a piano quintet (all 1919). These were to be his last major works.

Post-war years

After Lady Elgar's death in 1920, Elgar wrote little more. He was created Master of the King's Music in 1924, and in 1932, the year the young Yehudi Menuhin made his historic recording of the Violin Concerto, the BBC commissioned a third symphony. Elgar was still working on it when he died of cancer on 23 February 1934. His wish that no one should "tinker" with it was respected for over 60 years, until it was completed by Anthony Payne (born 1936) and performed in 1997.

ABOVE: Yehudi Menuhin (aged 16) recording Elgar's Violin Concerto in 1932, with the composer conducting.

Jean Sibelius

Give me the loneliness either of the Finnish forest or of a big city.

SIBELIUS

The careers of Jean Sibelius and Edward Elgar have many parallels, although Sibelius, eight years Elgar's junior, outlived the English composer by more than 20 years. Each was responsible for a musical renaissance in his native land, and each developed a highly distinctive idiom, inspired to a certain extent by the musical characteristics of his native culture. Both composers lapsed into creative silence after middle age.

Sibelius was born into a Swedish-speaking family. His father, a doctor, died of cholera when Jean – who gallicized his given name, Johan – was still an infant, and the boy was brought up by his mother and grandmother. He was a promising violinist (he hoped to become a soloist), and was composing by the age of ten. From an early age he was much influenced by the *Kalevala*, the Finnish national epic, which – allied to an intense response to landscape and nature – was to provide the impetus for his own work.

ABOVE: *A coloured drawing from 1904 of the Finnish composer Jean Sibelius (1865–1957) by Albert Edelfelt.*

After leaving school Sibelius originally intended to study law, but gave it up in favour of music. In the 1880s he studied first in Helsinki, and then in Berlin and Vienna, where he made many influential contacts, but also began the heavy drinking and financial irresponsibility which were to mar his later life.

Nationalism

Sibelius returned to Finland in 1891, where he worked on *Kullervo*, a symphonic poem for soprano, baritone, chorus and orchestra based on the *Kalevala*. Its immediate success established him as Finland's leading composer. In June 1892 he married the daughter of a Finnish nationalist general, thereby cementing his own identification with the nationalist movement (Finland was at that time part of the Russian Empire).

Although Sibelius never used actual folk tunes, his works of the 1890s are all distinctively Finnish. They include the four tone-poems based on the exploits of the legendary hero Lemminkäinen, of which the third is *Tuonelan joutsen* (*The Swan of Tuonela*); two more tone-poems –

ABOVE: *A panoramic photograph of Helsinki, the capital of Finland, c.1910. Sibelius studied music at Helsinki's Conservatoire from 1886–8, where he became friends with the Italian/German composer Ferruccio Busoni (1866–1924) who was a member of the teaching staff.*

ABOVE: A photograph of Sibelius taken when he was a student in Vienna in his early 20s.

En saga and *Skogsrået* (*The Wood-nymph*) – and the incidental music to *Karelia* (from which Sibelius made an orchestral suite). All these show the characteristic features of Sibelius's musical style, especially his liking for short motifs which are spun out symphonically, his use of *ostinato* patterns, and his effective handling of orchestration, with woodwind highlighted against an atmospheric string background, giving the impression of wind-blown open spaces.

Symphonies

In 1897 Sibelius – who was constantly in debt – was awarded a state pension which allowed him to concentrate on composing. Two years later he completed the tone-poem *Finlandia* and his First Symphony, clearly influenced by Tchaikovsky. It was followed

by six more symphonies, written between 1902 and 1924, each of which is highly individual. The Second (1902) and the Fifth (1915) are perhaps the most popular (like Beethoven's, the Fifth is a "heroic" work); while the Fourth (1911) is compact and austere in tone, the Sixth more pastoral, and the short Seventh (originally called *Fantasia sinfonica*) is in a single movement. An Eighth Symphony was written, but immediately destroyed.

During the early years of the 20th century, Sibelius travelled extensively, visiting England, Bohemia and Italy. The Violin Concerto dates from 1903, a period in which Sibelius's drinking and debt put his marriage under strain. In 1904 he built himself a villa outside Helsinki, where he lived for the rest of his life. The tone-poems *Pohjolan tytär* (*Pohjola's Daughter*) and *Oinen ratsastus ja auringonnousu* (*Night-ride and Sunrise*) date from this period, as does the

ABOVE: An impressionistic illustration of Sibelius's tone-poem The Swan of Tuonela (1893–7) by I. J. Belmont.

incidental music to Maurice Maeterlinck's *Pelléas et Mélisande* (a play which Debussy used as the basis for his opera) and *Belsazars gästabud* (*Belshazzar's Feast*, a Biblical episode later set by William Walton).

Silence

In 1908 Sibelius underwent an operation for suspected throat cancer, and his later works have an intensified bleakness. He continued to travel throughout Europe and to America to conduct his works until the outbreak of World War I, an event which virtually ended his creative life. After the war he wrote only four more major pieces, including incidental music for Shakespeare's *The Tempest* (1925), and his last symphonic poem, *Tapiola* (1926). For the remaining 31 years of his life, he composed nothing, disliked talking about his music and became increasingly reclusive.

Life and works

NATIONALITY: Finnish

BORN: Hämeenlinna, 1865;
DIED: Järvanpää, 1957

SPECIALIST GENRES: Symphonies.

MAJOR WORKS: Seven symphonies; *En saga* (1892–1902); *Lemminkäinen Legends* (1893–7); *Karelia* Suite (1893); *Finlandia* (1899); Violin Concerto (1903–5).

Camille Saint-Saëns

There is nothing more difficult than talking about music.

SAINT-SAËNS

The French composer Camille Saint-Saëns was, like Mozart and Mendelssohn, a child prodigy. His father died just after he was born, and he was brought up by his mother and an aunt who began to teach him the piano when he was two. He was composing by the age of three, and played concertos by Mozart and Beethoven when he was ten. He also showed a keen interest in other intellectual pursuits, particularly archaeology, geology, astronomy and philosophy.

Saint-Saëns studied at the Paris Conservatoire, and was organist at the Madeleine church in Paris from 1857–76. After hearing him improvise, Liszt declared him the greatest organist in the world. In return, Saint-Saëns acknowledged Liszt's influence on his own symphonic poems of the 1870s: *Le rouet d'Omphale* (*Omphale's Spinning Wheel*), *Phaëton*, the enormously

ABOVE: Camille Saint-Saëns (1835–1921). He was an amazingly prolific composer — "I compose music as a tree produces apples", he said.

popular *Danse macabre*, and *La jeunesse d'Hercule* (*Hercules' Youth*). In 1871 he was a founder-member of the Société Nationale de Musique, set up to promote performances of works by younger French composers.

Saint-Saëns was much attached to his mother but, much to her disapproval, when he was 40 he married a girl half his age. Their two young sons died tragically within six weeks of each other, and after just six years of marriage, Saint-Saëns walked out on his wife. After his mother's death in 1888 he spent much time abroad, especially in North Africa, and many of his works, such as the Fifth Piano Concerto, make use of exotic harmonies.

His most famous and enduring works include the opera *Samson et Dalila*, the First Cello Concerto, the Introduction and Rondo Capriccioso for violin and orchestra, the five piano concertos, the Organ Symphony (No. 3), and *Le carnaval des animaux* (*The Carnival of the Animals*), written as a private joke for performance by friends.

LEFT: The entrance to the Paris Conservatoire de Musique et de Déclamation in the rue Bergère, where Saint-Saëns studied.

Life and works

NATIONALITY: French

BORN: Paris, 1835; **DIED:** Algiers, 1921

SPECIALIST GENRES: Tone-poems, piano concertos.

MAJOR WORKS: Piano Concerto No. 2 (1868); Cello Concerto No. 1 (1873); *Danse macabre* (1874); *Samson et Dalila* (1877); Symphony No. 3 (1886); *Le carnaval des animaux* (1886).

Gabriel Fauré

For me…music exists to elevate us as far as possible above everyday existence.

Fauré was Saint-Saëns' favourite pupil at the Ecole Niedermeyer in Paris. Like his teacher, he was a gifted pianist and organist, and began his career as an organist in Rennes. In 1871 he became organist at Ste Sulpice in Paris, and was also active in the foundation of the Société Nationale de Musique, where many of his own works were given their premières.

Fauré's engagement to Marianne Viardot (the daughter of a famous singer) produced three fine chamber works: the First Violin Sonata, the First Piano Quartet, and the Ballade for piano. In 1882, five years after Marianne broke off the engagement, he married Marie Fremiet, the daughter of a sculptor. The marriage, which produced two sons, was unhappy, and Fauré found consolation with other women, including Emma Bardac (the

ABOVE: Gabriel Fauré (1845–1924), aged 18. He studied with Saint-Saëns, and later taught at the Paris Conservatoire.

second Mme Debussy), for whom he wrote the tender song-cycle *La bonne chanson*, and for whose daughter Hélène (nicknamed Dolly) he wrote the *Dolly* Suite for piano duet.

Fauré continued to earn a living as organist, choir-master and teacher, and was able to compose only in his spare time. He was happiest with small-scale genres such as songs, piano and chamber music: many of his delicate, elusive songs are settings of texts by the Symbolist poet Paul Verlaine. His famous Requiem – probably his best-known work – took over 20 years to finish. In the late 1890s he was appointed principal organist of the Madeleine church in Paris, and also

became a professor of composition at the Paris Conservatoire, where his pupils included Ravel. He became director of the Conservatoire in 1905.

By the age of 50 Fauré was well-known in Parisian society (his friends included Marcel Proust). By this time he was attempting larger-scale works, including the incidental music to Maeterlinck's play *Pelléas et Mélisande* (which also inspired Debussy and Sibelius), the orchestral suite in 18th-century style *Masques et bergamasques* (1919) and the stage works *Prométhée* and *Pénélope*.

He retired from the Conservatoire in 1920, and was finally able to devote himself to composition, although by this time he was losing his hearing. His late works were mostly for chamber combinations, including a Piano Trio and Piano Quintet.

ABOVE: Fauré playing the organ at the Church of the Madeleine in Paris, where he was principal organist for many years.

Life and works

NATIONALITY: French

BORN: Pamiers, Ariège, 1845; **DIED:** Paris, 1924

SPECIALIST GENRES: Songs, piano and chamber music.

MAJOR WORKS: Songs and song-cycles; piano music, including *Dolly* Suite (1897); *Pavane* (1887); Requiem (1888); *Pelléas et Mélisande* (1892); *Pénélope* (1913).

Giacomo Puccini

*I shall feel it [the story of Manon] as an Italian,
with desperate passion.*

PUCCINI

Puccini was the last great exponent of Italian Romantic opera. His operas have always held a special place in the affections of audiences, and rival Verdi's in popularity. He was born into a dynasty of musicians who since the 18th century had been organists at the church of San Martino in Lucca. It had been intended that Puccini should follow the family tradition, but seeing a performance of Verdi's *Aida* at Pisa made him decide to become an opera composer.

Milan

In 1880 a scholarship enabled Puccini to enrol at the Milan Conservatory. He graduated in the summer of 1883, having entered a one-act opera, *Le villi (The Witches)*, in a competition sponsored by a music publisher. It came nowhere, but the next year Puccini played it through at a party attended by Verdi's publisher Ricordi. *Le villi* was staged in 1884, and

ABOVE: *A portrait of Giacomo Puccini (1858–1924) painted in Paris in 1899, three years after he wrote his highly popular opera* La Bohème.

Ricordi immediately commissioned another opera, *Edgar*, from the young composer, and signed him up.

Edgar was performed at La Scala in Milan in 1889, but was not well received (the composer himself described it as a "mistake"). But his next opera, *Manon Lescaut* (based, like Massenet's opera *Manon*, on the novel by Abbé Prévost), was a huge success at its Turin première in 1893. Puccini had found a winning formula: that of the young, doomed heroine whose flawed character leads to an affecting early death. He repeated it with *La Bohème (The Bohemian Girl)*, first performed at Turin in 1896 under Toscanini; but it took some time for this romantic drama of love and death in a Montmartre garret – now one of the world's most popular operas – to catch the public's imagination.

Puccini's next opera, *Tosca*, performed in Rome in 1900, was an excursion into the brutal world of *verismo*. Its

ABOVE: *Puccini at home in the music-room of his villa at Torre del Lago, near Lucca.*

ABOVE: *A stage set for Act I of Puccini's* Tosca, *set in the Roman church of S Andrea delle Valle.*

"body count" – an attempted rape, a murder, a faked execution by firing squad which turns out to be real, and a final, dramatic suicide – has rarely been surpassed. Critics have always been snooty about *Tosca* (one described it memorably as "a shabby little shocker"), but Puccini's marvellous melodic gift and innate sense of drama save it from mere sensationalism.

Based on a real-life incident, as related in David Belasco's play, *Madama Butterfly* (La Scala, 1904) returned to the "weepie" genre. The tragic tale of a Japanese geisha, betrayed and abandoned by the American naval lieutenant she believes to be her husband, took the operatic world by storm after Puccini revised it into three acts. Another Belasco play, *The Girl of the Golden West*, provided the subject-matter for Puccini's next opera, *La fanciulla del West*, premièred at the New York Metropolitan Opera in December 1910 with Enrico Caruso and Emmy Destinn in the leading roles.

Puccini made a political mistake with his next opera, accepting a commission from the directors of a Viennese theatre instead of an Italian one,

ABOVE: A poster for the original 1904 production of Madama Butterfly. *Butterfly is shown bidding farewell to her child before killing herself.*

drawing accusations of treachery. The little-known *La rondine* (*The Swallow*) was first performed during World War I, though in Monte Carlo rather than Vienna. Puccini worked simultaneously on a "Grand Guignol" triptych of one-act operas: the horrific *Il tabarro* (*The Cloak*), the sentimental tragedy *Suor Angelica* and his one comedy, *Gianni Schicchi*, the most successful of the three. The triptych was premièred in New York in December 1918.

"Nessun dorma"

Puccini had lived since 1891 at his villa at Torre del Lago outside Lucca, with his wife Elvira (his married mistress until 1904). In 1909 their servant girl committed suicide when unjustly accused by the jealous Elvira of having an affair with Puccini. This tragedy may have inspired the character of Liù, the gentle, lovable slave girl in Puccini's last opera *Turandot*, based on an oriental fairy-tale. The work includes the aria "Nessun dorma", popularized by the "Three Tenors" at a concert staged in conjunction with the 1990

football World Cup in Italy. *Turandot* was destined to have a happy ending, when the cruel princess Turandot is outwitted by Prince Calaf and finally succumbs to love. But Puccini died of a heart attack during treatment for throat cancer in November 1924, leaving the final love duet unfinished.

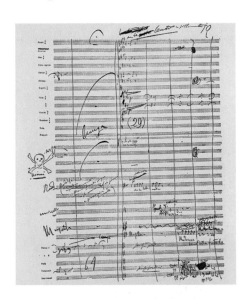

ABOVE: A page from the manuscript score of La Bohème *(1896). Puccini has indicated Mimi's death with a skull and crossbones in the margin.*

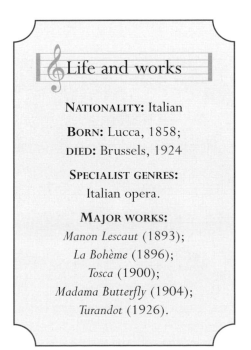

🎼 Life and works

NATIONALITY: Italian

BORN: Lucca, 1858;
DIED: Brussels, 1924

SPECIALIST GENRES: Italian opera.

MAJOR WORKS:
Manon Lescaut (1893);
La Bohème (1896);
Tosca (1900);
Madama Butterfly (1904);
Turandot (1926).

Richard Strauss

From time to time the cruellest discords are succeeded by exquisite suavities,
that caress the ear with delight.

CAMILLE SAINT-SAËNS (1835–1921), OF "SALOME"

Richard Strauss, like Rachmaninov, was a composer who outlived his era. Elgar and Sibelius stopped composing shortly after World War I, perhaps realizing that the spirit of the age contradicted their personal artistic visions; but their contemporaries Strauss and Rachmaninov enjoyed a late Romantic Indian summer, oblivious to stylistic change.

Strauss was born in 1864, the son of the principal horn player in the Munich court orchestra. His father Franz played horn solos in the premières of Wagner's *Tristan und Isolde* (1865) and *Die Meistersinger von Nürnberg* (1868), but the young Richard first encountered Wagner's operas a few years later. A precociously gifted child, he had learnt the piano from the age of four and the violin from eight.

Strauss's first important work, the *Serenade* for wind instruments, was performed in Berlin in 1882 by

ABOVE: *A portrait of the young Richard Strauss (1864–1949), probably dating from the 1890s.*

members of the famous Meiningen Orchestra, whose conductor Hans von Bülow commissioned the young composer's Suite in B flat. During this period Strauss also wrote his First Horn Concerto, a cello sonata, a symphony (No. 2, premièred in New York), and several song settings. In the summer of 1885 Strauss became von Bülow's assistant at Meiningen, and took over from von Bülow a month later. From then on, his career was divided between conducting and composing.

Tone-poems

In 1886 Strauss moved on to the Munich court opera, where he became interested in the theories of Wagner and Arthur Schopenhauer, and in Liszt's tone-poems. His own first venture into this genre, *Aus Italien*, dates from 1886. Between 1889,

LEFT: *Strauss directing an opera from the pit, 1929, by Wilhelm Viktor Krausz.*

RIGHT: *The frontispiece to the original piano score of* Elektra *(1909), designed by Louis Corinth.*

when he moved to Weimar as assistant conductor to the court opera, and 1898, when he became chief conductor of the Royal Opera in Berlin, he wrote a sequence of seven magnificent tone-poems: *Don Juan*, *Macbeth*, *Tod und Verklärung* (*Death and Transfiguration*), *Till Eulenspiegels lustige Streiche* (*Till Eulenspiegel's Merry Pranks*), *Also sprach Zarathustra* (*Thus Spake Zarathustra*), *Don Quixote* and *Ein Heldenleben* (*A Hero's Life*). Together with the *Symphonia domestica* (1902–4) and *Ein Alpensinfonie* (1911–15), they represent Strauss's most important orchestral works.

Opera

However, it was in the field of opera that Strauss achieved fame. Inspired by his marriage in 1893 to the soprano Pauline de Ahna, he began his long love affair with the voice – especially the female voice. His first opera, *Guntram*

ABOVE: The Dresden Court Opera House, where many of Strauss's operas were performed.

Life and works

NATIONALITY: German

BORN: Munich, 1864; **DIED:** Garmisch, 1949

SPECIALIST GENRES: Late Romantic tone-poems, Wagnerian-style opera.

MAJOR WORKS: Tone-poems *Macbeth* (1886–8), *Don Juan* (1888–9), *Tod und Verklärung* (1888–9), *Till Eulenspiegels lustige Streiche* (1894–5), *Also sprach Zarathustra* (1895–6), *Don Quixote* (1896–7) and *Ein Heldenleben* (1897–8); operas *Salome* (1905), *Elektra* (1909), *Der Rosenkavalier* (1911) and *Ariadne auf Naxos* (1911–12); *Capriccio* (1940–1); *Four Last Songs* (1948).

(1894), was a failure, and his second, *Feuersnot* (*Fire Famine*, 1901), is rarely performed; but from *Salome* (1905) onwards he created a series of magnificent and individual works which are rarely out of the repertoire. *Salome* (based on Oscar Wilde's scandalous play) and *Elektra* (based on Sophocles' drama) caused international sensations owing to Strauss's explicit treatment of their subjects. Musically, both owe much to Wagner; *Salome* in particular is a masterpiece of sensuous, overblown late Romanticism. The royalties from *Salome* alone enabled Strauss to build himself a luxurious villa at Garmisch.

The librettist of *Elektra*, Hugo von Hofmannsthal (1874–1929), worked with Strauss over the next two decades: their most successful collaboration was the Mozartian comedy *Der Rosenkavalier*. With Hofmannsthal, Strauss went on to create *Ariadne auf Naxos*, *Die Frau ohne Schatten* (*The Woman without a Shadow*, 1914–17), *Die ägyptische Helena* (*The Egyptian Helen*, 1923–7) and *Arabella* (1929–32), completed after Hofmannsthal's death. Strauss's librettist for his next opera, *Die*

schweigsame Frau (*The Silent Woman*, 1933–4) was the Jewish Stefan Zweig, but the prevailing political climate in Germany required Strauss to choose an Austrian librettist, Joseph Gregor, for his subsequent operas: *Friedenstag* (*Peace Day*, 1935–6), *Daphne* (1936–7) and *Die Liebe der Danaë* (*Danaë's Love*, 1938–40).

Strauss's political naivety led to his exploitation by the Nazi Reichsmusik-kammer, which appointed him its president in 1933 but removed him two years later (his daughter-in-law was Jewish). He spent the war years in Vienna (where he wrote his last opera, *Capriccio,* in 1940–1), but afterwards moved to Switzerland while he was investigated – and eventually cleared of Nazi affiliations – by the denazification tribunal.

Strauss's last works are mainly instrumental: they include *Metamorphosen* for 23 solo strings (1945, a lament for the devastation of Germany), the Second Horn Concerto, the Oboe Concerto, sonatinas for wind instruments, and the radiant *Vier letzte Lieder* (*Four Last Songs*, 1948) for voice and orchestra. He died at his home in Garmisch, aged 85.

Sergei Rachmaninov

I feel like a ghost wandering in a world grown alien.
I cannot cast out the old way of writing and I cannot acquire the new.

RACHMANINOV

Rachmaninov was the last of a tradition of great pianist-composers, and the last of the Russian Romantics. The dramatic sweep of his music, combined with a haunting Russian melancholy, holds a powerful appeal. His three symphonies and four piano concertos are much loved.

He had his earliest piano lessons from his mother, a trained pianist. In 1882 his family moved to St Petersburg, where Rachmaninov entered the Conservatory. But when his parents separated, he transferred to Moscow, where he studied with the strict teacher Nikolay Zverev, and from 1888 onwards, with Alexander Ziloti (1863–1945) for piano and Anton Arensky (1861–1906) for composition. He graduated from the piano class of the Moscow Conservatory in the summer of 1891, completing his First Piano Concerto at the same time. The next year, his one-

ABOVE: *Sergei Rachmaninov, painted in 1925 while he was living in the USA, by Konstantin Andreyevich Somov.*

act opera *Aleko* won him the Conservatory's highest award for composition and, shortly after graduating, he wrote one of his most popular pieces, the Prelude in C sharp minor for piano.

In 1897, Rachmaninov's good luck changed when his First Symphony, in D minor, was performed at a Russian Symphony Concert, conducted by Alexander Glazunov. The performance was a disaster (Glazunov was rumoured to be drunk), and the critic César Cui described the piece as "a programme symphony on the Seven Plagues of Egypt". It was not

performed again until 1945. Rachmaninov suffered a nervous breakdown, and could not compose anything for three years. In due course he underwent a successful course of hypnotic treatment with a Dr Nikolay Dahl, which restored his confidence and enabled him to start work on the Second Piano Concerto, the theme of whose slow movement was used to memorable effect in David Lean's 1945 film *Brief Encounter*.

Rachmaninov gave the première of his new concerto, dedicated to Dr Dahl, on 9 November 1901, and a few months later, after finishing his cantata *Spring*, he married his cousin Natalya Satina. Over the next few years he occupied himself with opera composition, until the illness of his daughter Irina obliged the family to move to Dresden in 1906. There he completed his Second Symphony (the

ABOVE: *Rachmaninov had unusually large hands, able to cope with big stretches — an advantage for a virtuoso pianist.*

ABOVE: *Alexander Glazunov is reputed to have ruined the première of Rachmaninov's First Symphony by conducting while drunk.*

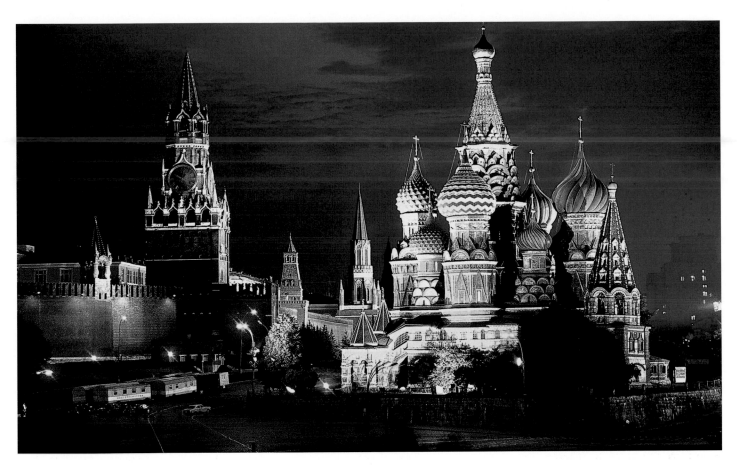

ABOVE: Red Square in Moscow, with St Basil's Cathedral illuminated. Rachmaninov drew inspiration from the Russian Orthodox liturgy, and wrote some fine sacred vocal music.

slow movement with its long-breathed clarinet solo is a masterly piece of writing), the First Piano Sonata, and the symphonic poem *The Isle of the Dead*, inspired by a painting by the Swiss artist Arnold Böcklin.

In 1909 Rachmaninov made his first visit to America, where he toured with a new work, the Third Piano Concerto. Over the next few years he spent the summers on his country estate, where he wrote the 13 Preludes for piano, Op. 13 (1910), the Liturgy of St John Chrysostom (1910), the *Etudes-tableaux* for piano, Op. 33 (1911), the 14 Songs, Op. 34, and the Second Piano Sonata (1913). During the winters he toured as a pianist, a routine that continued until the outbreak of World War I. His other major compositions of this period include the choral symphony *The Bells* (1913) and the *All-night Vigil* for unaccompanied choir (1915).

America

In 1917, the dangerous political situation in Russia forced Rachmaninov and his family into exile, first in Sweden, and then in America, where he remained for the rest of his life. From 1918 onwards he wrote little, spending most of his time performing. The Fourth Piano Concerto was written in 1926, but when it failed to achieve the success of its predecessors Rachmaninov was forced to revise and shorten it.

In 1931 he composed his last solo piano work, the *Variations on a Theme of Corelli*, followed by the brilliant *Rhapsody on a Theme of Paganini* for piano and orchestra (1934), the Third Symphony (1935–8), and the Symphonic Dances, his last work (1940). By early 1943 he was exhausted and ill, but he continued to tour. He died of cancer at his home in Beverly Hills on 28 March 1943, four days before his 70th birthday.

Life and works

NATIONALITY: Russian

BORN: Semyonovo, 1873;
DIED: Beverly Hills, 1943

SPECIALIST GENRES:
Piano concertos, solo
piano music.

MAJOR WORKS: Four
piano concertos; three
symphonies; 24 Preludes
for piano (1892–1910);
*Rhapsody on a Theme of
Paganini* (1934).

Other Composers of the Era

...some world far from ours
Where music and moonlight and feeling
Are one.

PERCY BYSSHE SHELLEY (1792–1822)

Like Rachmaninov, Alexander Glazunov (1865–1936) was among the late Russian Romantic composers. A pupil of Rimsky-Korsakov, he wrote his First Symphony at the age of only 16, and became a protégé of Balakirev. From the 1880s onwards he travelled widely, meeting Liszt in Weimar, and conducting in Paris and London. In 1905 he became director of the St Petersburg Conservatory. He suffered great hardship during the Russian Revolution, and in 1928 left Russia altogether, eventually settling in Paris. His works, which are more cosmopolitan than nationalist, include nine symphonies, two piano concertos, a popular Violin Concerto, a late Saxophone Concerto (1931), seven string quartets, and a ballet, *The Seasons* (1899).

ABOVE: *The Polish composer Karol Szymanowski (1882–1937), director of the Warsaw Conservatory.*

The Polish composer Karol Szymanowski (1882–1937) spent much of his early life in the Ukraine, but between 1905 and 1908 he lived in Berlin, where he wrote his first symphony. His Russian home was destroyed during the Revolution, and in 1920 he moved to Warsaw, where he became director of the Conservatory (later the Academy). He died of tuberculosis. His piano music was championed by Polish pianists including Artur Rubinstein, while his two violin concertos were premièred by the Polish violinist Paul Kochansky. His Stabat Mater (1925–6) is highly regarded.

Mahler's exact contemporary Hugo Wolf (1860–1903) was also his fellow pupil at the Vienna Conservatory. An enthusiastic Wagnerite, he antagonized many people with his critical attacks on Brahms. He is remembered for his exquisite songs – the worthy

successors of Schubert and Schumann. They include 53 settings of poems by Mörike, 20 by Eichendorff, 51 by Goethe, 44 songs in the *Spanisches Liederbuch* (*Spanish Songbook*, 1891), a total of 46 in the two volumes of the *Italienisches Liederbuch* (*Italian Songbook*, 1892–6) and three poems by Michelangelo (1898). Apart from songs, his best-known work is the *Italian Serenade* (1892) for string orchestra (originally for quartet). In 1897, a victim of syphilis, he went mad and was confined to an asylum.

The German composer Max Bruch (1838–1920) worked as a conductor in Berlin, Bonn, Liverpool, Breslau and Scotland, and became a professor of composition at the Berlin Hochschule. An enormously prolific composer, he is remembered today chiefly for three

ABOVE: *Alexander Glazunov (1865–1936). Like Rachmaninov, Stravinsky and Prokofiev he left Russia after the Revolution.*

ABOVE: *The Austrian composer Hugo Wolf (1860–1903). A brilliant composer of Lieder, he contracted syphilis and died insane.*

ABOVE: *Max Bruch (1838–1920) never quite lived up to his early promise, but his* Violin Concerto in G minor *is much played.*

ABOVE: *Vincent d'Indy (1851–1931), who founded the Schola Cantorum in Paris in the 1890s.*

ABOVE: *Paul Dukas (1865–1935). A contemporary of Debussy, he is remembered chiefly for* The Sorcerer's Apprentice.

works, the G minor Violin Concerto (1868), the *Scottish Fantasy* for violin and orchestra (1880), and *Kol Nidrei* (1881), an *adagio* on a Hebrew melody for cello and orchestra.

France

The Belgian born César Franck (1822–90) became organ professor at the Paris Conservatoire in 1872. An outstanding organist, he wrote a great deal of sacred music, but is chiefly

ABOVE: *Sir Hubert Parry (1848–1918), chiefly remembered for his setting of Blake's* Jerusalem *and for the six* Songs of Farewell.

remembered for his Organ Symphony in D minor (1886–8), the Symphonic Variations for piano and orchestra (1885), the Piano Quintet (1878–9), the Violin Sonata (1886) and *Panis angelicus* (1872, for tenor, organ, harp, cello and double bass).

His pupil Vincent D'Indy (1851–1931), an admirer of Wagner like his teacher, was a founder of the Schola Cantorum in Paris in 1894, originally for the study of church music but, from 1900 onwards, a general music school. He wrote several operas, but his best-known work is probably the *Symphonie sur un chant montagnard français* (Symphony on a French Mountaineer's Song, 1886).

Wagner also influenced the works of Paul Dukas (1865–1935), whose first major success, *L'apprenti sorcier* (*The Sorcerer's Apprentice*, 1897, based on a story by Goethe), is still much performed. Dukas wrote a fine opera based on a play by Maeterlinck, *Ariane et Barbe-bleue* (*Ariadne and Bluebeard*, 1907), similar in atmosphere to Debussy's *Pelléas et Mélisande*, but his strict self-criticism meant that he published only a few of his compositions and destroyed much of his work before he died.

Britain

In late Victorian England, Hubert Parry (1848–1918) and Charles Villiers Stanford (1852–1924) – both professors at the Royal College of Music, London – had enormous influence on a younger generation of British composers, whom they numbered among their many pupils. Parry taught at Oxford University; Stanford, the composer of seven symphonies, taught at Cambridge.

ABOVE: *Sir Charles Villiers Stanford (1852–1924) portrayed in a 1905* Vanity Fair *cartoon.*

The Early Twentieth Century

An example of post-impressionist art — Woman with a Yellow Jacket (1913) by the German artist August Macke (1887–1914).

Music in a New Framework

*Musical innovation is full of danger to the state, for when modes of music change,
the laws of the state always change with them.*

PLATO (C.428–347 BC)

By the closing years of the 19th century, it was clear that Romanticism had run its course. New trends were apparent in literature and art: in the Symbolist poems of Paul Verlaine, Charles Baudelaire and Stéphane Mallarmé and the plays of Maurice Maeterlinck; in the impressionist paintings of Claude Monet, Camille Pissarro and Edouard Manet, in which representational art gave way to blurred outlines and emphasis on the shifting play of light.

As the 20th century dawned, Impressionism was succeeded by post-Impressionism, and by a bewildering array of new artistic movements: the Fauves, with their bold outlines and brash colours, the Expressionist art of Edvard Munch and Wasily Kandinsky, the cubism of Pablo Picasso, the stark lines of Bauhaus art and architecture. Music, as ever, followed behind, when the focus of new trends moved decisively from central Europe to Paris.

ABOVE: Around the Piano *(1885) by Henri Fantin-Latour (1836–1904).*

ABOVE: An Allegory of Happiness *by Julio Romero de Torres (1880–1930).*

Impressionism in music

In musical terms, composers realized that they need no longer be subject to the tyranny of traditional tonality – a system which had lasted for 400 years. One of the pioneers of the "music of the future" was the Frenchman Claude Debussy, whose fluid structures, built out of the repetition of tiny motifs with colouristic instrumental effects, were likened to impressionist techniques in painting. Little of Debussy's mature music could be said to be in a "key"; instead, its gravitational centre constantly shifts as a result of his use of chromatic harmony.

Atonality

Meanwhile, the Austrian composer Arnold Schoenberg began writing in a lush, late-Romantic style, but in the first decade of the 20th century he pushed chromatic harmony to its limits, experimenting first with atonality, in which the 12 notes of the chromatic scale are treated equally, and then with an original method of musical organization called the "12-note system". This method – in which musical building-blocks are created from "tone-rows" consisting of all 12 notes of the scale – influenced many succeeding composers, including Berg

and Webern (who were Schoenberg's pupils), Stravinsky, Messaien, Boulez and Stockhausen. They used it in various ingenious ways and adapted it to their own particular ends.

Nationalism

Meanwhile, musical nationalism continued to flourish: in England in the works of Ralph Vaughan Williams, Frederick Delius and Gustav Holst; in Denmark in the works of Carl Nielsen; in central Europe in the works of the Hungarians Béla Bartók and Zoltán Kodály and the Czech composer Leoš Janáček, the spiritual descendant of Dvořák. All these composers were ardent collectors of their national folk songs, first by transcribing them manually, and then, when phonographic equipment became available, recording them.

The USA – still a relatively young nation – acquired its first major composer in the form of the highly original Charles Ives, quickly followed

ABOVE: Dancing in Vienna shown in a post-World War I painting entitled Once upon a Time.

by others: Samuel Barber, George Gershwin (a populist master), and Aaron Copland, who deliberately set out to create distinctively "American" music.

Music and politics

The political upheavals of the 20th century, particularly the two world wars, had a profound effect on music, as on other art forms. During the economic depression which followed World War I, composers were forced to pare down their musical resources. Works that had required huge and expensive symphony orchestras gave way to small chamber ensembles, evident in the post-war works of Igor Stravinsky and the eclectic group of mainly French composers known as "Les Six".

Another noticeable influence during the 1920s and '30s was that of jazz, exported to Europe from the USA, and taken up with enthusiasm in England, France and Germany (especially in the works of Kurt Weill).

The rise of Nazi Germany in the 1930s struck a grievous blow. The works of "decadent" composers such as Weill were banned, and central Europe was emptied of Jewish musicians, both composers and performers, and of "non-conformist" Aryans. Some – including Schoenberg, Hindemith and Weill – fled to Britain and the USA (where they greatly enriched the musical lives of their adopted nations), while others were murdered. Apart from the aged Richard Strauss, Germany lost most of its finest composers: perhaps the best-known composer who stayed was Carl Orff, remembered only for his popular cantata *Carmina burana*, and for an influential teaching method.

Similarly, in Soviet Russia, Stalin's purges struck fear into all serious composers. The two finest Russian composers of the 20th century, Prokofiev and Shostakovich, both survived, but suffered severely under a tyrannical regime driven by political dogma and opposed to artistic innovation.

ABOVE: L'homme au violon (The Man with the Violin)*, painted in 1918 by the Spanish artist Juan Gris (1887–1927).*

NEWS AND VIEWS OF ALL THE PLAYS.

The
THEATRE WORLD
and Illustrated Stage Review.

No. 4.　　　MAY, 1925.　　　SIXPENCE

ABOVE: This drawing on the cover of The Theatre World *review journal shows Spanish dancers in the 1920s.*

Claude Debussy

It's music on the points of needles.

CÉSAR FRANCK (1822–90)

From the late Baroque period to around 1890, mainstream Western music was firmly rooted in Germany and Austria. Not until the late 19th and early 20th centuries did the line of succession stretching from Bach to Mahler begin to branch out, with major composers emerging from Russia, Bohemia, England, Scandinavia and the USA. It was a Frenchman, Claude Debussy, who broke the German monopoly, revitalizing French music with his uniquely subtle art, and opening up a new sound-world for the 20th century. His music explored "the mysterious relationship between Nature and Imagination".

Debussy's life centred on Paris, which was fast becoming the hub of European culture. He was born on 22 August 1862 in the suburb of St Germain-en-Laye, where his parents ran a china shop. The young Claude

ABOVE: Claude Achille Debussy (1862–1918). His unique sound-world opened the door to a new century.

Achille and his siblings were often packed off to their Aunt Clémentine in Cannes, where Debussy began to learn the piano with a former pupil of Chopin. At the age of ten he entered the Paris Conservatoire, where he unnerved his teachers with experimental harmonic improvisations at the keyboard.

Despite his unorthodox tendencies, he won the coveted Prix de Rome in 1884 with his cantata *L'enfant prodigue*, but his sojourn in Rome was not a happy one, and he returned to Paris — where he had been conducting a love affair with a married woman — in the spring of 1887. The same year he became intoxicated with Wagner's music and in 1888 visited Bayreuth. Although Debussy later described Wagner's music as "a beautiful sunset that was mistaken for a dawn", it held a life-long fascination for him. He even began work on a Wagnerian opera, but

LEFT: Entrance to the Exposition Universelle (1889) by Jean Beraud (1849–1936).

RIGHT: Debussy with his daughter Chou-Chou. He was already gravely ill with cancer when this photograph was taken in 1916.

ABOVE: A drawing by René Bull illustrating Debussy's Prélude à "L'après-midi d'un faune" *dating from 1913, the year after Nijinsky's scandalous choreographic version for the Ballets Russes.*

abandoned it when he realized that his own music needed to be "flexible and adaptable to fantasies and dreams".

Impressionism

Debussy had already found inspiration in the elusive works of the Symbolist poets, including Verlaine, whose verses he had begun to match with delicate, ethereal settings. At the same time he began to experiment with new piano sonorities, and with a scale based on whole tones, without a firm key centre. Among his early piano works are a pair of Arabesques and the *Petite suite* for piano duet.

The Javanese gamelan music Debussy heard at the 1889 Paris Exposition left a lasting impression, when he realized that economy of means – a single, shrill clarinet or a gong – could

Life and works

NATIONALITY: French

BORN: St Germain-en-Laye, 1862; **DIED:** Paris, 1918

SPECIALIST GENRES: Orchestral and piano music.

MAJOR WORKS: *Prélude à "L'après-midi d'un faune"* (1892–4); *Pelléas et Mélisande* (1893–1902); *Nocturnes* (1899); *La mer* (1905); *Images* (1905–7); Preludes for piano (1910, 1913); *Jeux* (1913).

ABOVE: The Great Wave of Kanagawa *(1831) by the Japanese artist Katsushika Hokusai (1760–1849). This print inspired Debussy's symphonic seascape* La mer.

ABOVE: A piece of 17th-century Chinese embroidery. Debussy loved Oriental art, and drew inspiration from it for some of his piano pieces.

be just as effective as a full-blown symphony orchestra. The influence of Art Nouveau, then all the rage in Paris, resulted in his cantata *La damoiselle élue* (*The Blessed Damozel*, 1888), based on a poem by the Pre-Raphaelite artist and writer Dante Gabriel Rossetti.

In the early 1890s Debussy found a tiny apartment in Montmartre, then the centre of artistic "bohemian" life. Surrounded by the artists, writers, fellow musicians, laundresses and prostitutes who constituted the district's lively residents, he set up house with his girlfriend Gabrielle Dupont and embarked on a period of penniless squalor but artistic creativity. During this period he developed his characteristic style, capturing in subtle, shifting harmonies and fragments of melody the essence of a breath of wind, the rustle of leaves, or a shaft of moonlight.

Sometimes his inspiration came from an antique dream-world peopled by masked Harlequins and Columbines playing mandolins and dancing sarabands. These visions sprang to life in the *Suite bergamasque* (1890) for

piano, of which the third piece is the haunting "Clair de lune", the suite *Pour le piano* (1894–1901), and in the Verlaine settings called *Fêtes galantes* (1891 and 1904). From the same period dates the String Quartet

ABOVE: The Scottish soprano Mary Garden (1874–1967) as Mélisande, the heroine of Debussy's Pelléas et Mélisande. *She created the role at the Paris Opera in 1902.*

(1893), and his most famous orchestral piece, the *Prélude à "L'après-midi d'un faune"* (*Prelude to "The Afternoon of a Faun"*, 1894). Based on an erotic monologue by Mallarmé about a faun lying in the grass one hot summer's afternoon in ancient Greece, dreaming of making love to two beautiful but elusive nymphs, the piece – turned into a scandalous ballet in 1912 by the dancer Nijinsky – was a triumphant success. According to the conductor and composer Pierre Boulez, from the first languid notes of the faun's flute, "music began to beat with a new pulse".

In the mid 1890s Debussy worked on the opera *Pelléas et Mélisande*, based on a Symbolist drama by the Belgian writer Maurice Maeterlinck. His infinitely subtle music, economically scored, and using silence as "perhaps the only way of throwing the emotional weight of a phrase into relief", perfectly complemented Maeterlinck's perplexing play, in which the characters seem to lack normal motivation. It took nine years for *Pelléas* to reach the stage, when it was greeted with incomprehension and hostility. It is now recognized as a masterpiece.

During this period, Debussy had lived off a small annual allowance from a publisher. Constant lack of money caused friction between him and Gaby, and the couple finally separated in 1898, just as Debussy finished another orchestral work, the three *Nocturnes*. These poetic evocations of a cloudy day over the river Seine, a Parisian carnival complete with brass band, and a delicate seascape with mermaids singing, are among his most "impressionistic" pieces, as are the contemporary set of *Estampes* (*Prints*) for piano, consisting of the pseudo-oriental *Pagodes*, *Soirée dans Grenade* (*Evening in Granada*, a languid Spanish habanera), and the virtuosic *Jardins sous la pluie* (*Gardens in the rain*).

ABOVE: *A page from the autograph score of Act I of* Pelléas et Mélisande.

Marriage

In 1899 Debussy – whose dark, Mephistophelean looks made him immensely attractive to women – replaced Gaby with a pretty bottle-blonde model called Lilly Texier. Ill-educated and tubercular, Lilly proved an entirely unsuitable wife. In 1903 Debussy met Emma Bardac, Fauré's ex-mistress, now the wife of a banker. They fell passionately in love and eloped to Jersey (where he wrote the piano piece *L'île joyeuse*). Lilly Debussy tried to shoot herself and Debussy was ostracized by his friends, but he and Emma set up house together in the fashionable Avenue du Bois de Boulogne, where their adored daughter Claude-Emma (Chou-Chou) was born in 1905. For the rest of his life Debussy attempted to keep Emma in the style to which she had become accustomed, often with great difficulty, and their ten-year marriage was frequently under strain, especially when he was obliged to leave on long conducting tours.

In 1905 Debussy completed his symphonic seascape *La mer*, a vivid example of his ability to create, through a mosaic of melody and delicate touches of instrumentation, an impression of the interplay between light and water. Over the next few years he also completed two sets of *Images* for piano, the delightful *Children's Corner* (1906–8) for his daughter, two books of piano Preludes, and a set of orchestral *Images*: *Rondes de printemps* (*Dances of Spring*), *Iberia* and *Gigues*. In 1911 he tried his hand at ballet music in *Khamma*, written for the Canadian dancer Maud Allan, and in 1913, in the masterly score *Jeux* (*Games*), written for Diaghilev's Ballets Russes and choreographed by Nijinsky.

Last works

By 1914 Debussy knew that he was mortally ill with cancer of the colon. Deeply distressed by the carnage of World War I, he worked feverishly to finish two sets of piano studies, inspired by Chopin's, and three pieces for two pianos, *En blanc et noir* (1915), each dedicated to a friend killed in action. His last works were three out of a projected set of six sonatas – abstract music in a new, austere style

ABOVE: *The Russian impresario Sergei Diaghilev, the driving force behind the Ballets Russes. He commissioned Debussy's* Jeux.

– for cello and piano, violin and piano, and flute, viola and harp. He did not live to write the other three, dying during a German bombardment on 25 March 1918. His sonatas were published with the simple inscription: "Claude Debussy: musicien français".

ABOVE: *An impressionist seascape –* Storm at Agay, *1895, by Jean Baptiste Guillaumin (1841–1927).*

Béla Bartók

Bartók's name…stands for the principle and the demand for regeneration stemming from the people, both in art and in politics.

ZOLTÁN KODÁLY (1882–1967)

Bartók was the greatest Hungarian composer since Liszt. He and Kodály put Hungary on the international musical map.

Both Bartók's parents were musical, and he was taught the piano by his mother. He began to compose at the age of nine, and made his pianistic debut at 11. In 1903 he emerged from his studies at the Budapest Academy as a virtuoso pianist and a promising composer.

From the start, Bartók immersed himself in the idioms of Hungarian folk music. His first folk song collection was published in 1906, and in 1907 he became a piano professor at the Budapest Academy, a post which enabled him to pursue systematic research into folk music from Hungary, Romania, Slovakia and Transylvania. From this time onwards he began to publish folk song anthologies for voice and piano, and arrangements of

ABOVE: *An evocative portrait by Roboz of the Hungarian pianist and composer Béla Bartók (1881–1945).*

folk songs, such as *For Children* (1908–9). The Ten Easy Pieces, the 14 Bagatelles (both 1908) and the ferocious *Allegro barbaro* for piano (1911) are also strongly Hungarian in idiom. Another new influence, the atmospheric music of Debussy, informed Bartók's works from the First String Quartet (1908).

Works for the stage

In 1909 Bartók married his pupil Márta Ziegler, who gave birth to a son in 1910. The next year Bartók completed his one-act opera *A kékszakállú herceg vára* (*Duke Bluebeard's Castle*). This masterly score, based on a psychological interpretation of the Bluebeard legend, was not performed until 1918, after his ballet *A fából faragott királyfi* (*The Wooden Prince*) had been successfully staged in Budapest. Up to that point, Bartók's compositions had been largely neglected in his own country, but growing recognition of his talent prompted a second ballet, *A csodálatos mandarin* (*The Miraculous Mandarin*, 1918–19), whose sordid subject-matter caused outrage at its Cologne première in 1926. (The mandarin is lured into a robbers' den by a prostitute, but though stabbed and hanged by the men he refuses to die until he has had sex with her.)

During the post-war years Bartók began to tour widely as a pianist. In 1923 – when his Dance Suite, celebrating the 50th anniversary of the union of Buda and Pest, was premièred – he divorced Márta and married another young piano pupil, Ditta

ABOVE: *The opening manuscript page of Bartók's Hungarian folk song arrangements* Székely dalok *(Székely Songs) for six male voices (1932).*

ABOVE: *Bartók listening to his folk song recordings on a phonogram in 1915. He was one of the major folk song collectors.*

ABOVE: *Bartók giving a piano concerto performance in Budapest in 1938. His second wife, Ditta Pásztory, is sitting behind him.*

Pásztory. A second son was born in 1924.

Meanwhile, Bartók continued his dual career as pianist and composer. Many of his piano works – such as the First and Second Concertos (1926 and 1930–1), the Sonata, the Suite *Out of Doors*, and the Nine Little Pieces (all 1926) – were written for himself to play. His Third and Fourth String Quartets date from the late 1920s, as do the two Rhapsodies for violin and piano, both written for Hungarian virtuosi. The *Cantata profana* (1930) – a paean to the brotherhood of nations – was premièred in London in 1934, the year Bartók finally relinquished his teaching duties at the Budapest Academy to concentrate on his ethnomusicological work.

New musical structures

The late '30s – a period during which Bartók was preoccupied with musical structure, especially arch forms and constructions based on mathematical rules – produced some of his finest compositions, including the Fifth and Sixth String Quartets. He was equally concerned with timbre, exploiting the innovative sounds produced on conventional instruments, in works such as the *Music for Strings, Percussion and Celesta* and the 1939 Divertimento for strings. The Sonata for two pianos and percussion (1937) was premièred by Bartók and his wife; the Second Violin Concerto (1937–8) was written for Zoltán Székely and *Contrasts* for the violinist Joseph Szigeti and the clarinettist Benny Goodman. During the 1930s Bartók also published *Microkosmos*, six books of piano teaching pieces.

America

In 1940, alarmed by the threat of fascism, the Bartóks left for America, where they settled in New York.

The last five years of Bartók's life were clouded by public neglect, financial worries and declining health. In 1943 he was diagnosed as suffering from a rare form of cancer. He completed his most popular work, the Concerto for Orchestra (premièred by Serge Koussevitsky and the Boston Symphony Orchestra), in the summer of 1943, and the solo Violin Sonata, written for Yehudi Menuhin, the following March. His last works were the Third Piano Concerto (1945), written for his wife, and the Viola Concerto for the Scottish-born player William Primrose, which was left unfinished at his death in September 1945.

ABOVE: *The anti-hero of* Duke Bluebeard's Castle, *portrayed by Janos Kass.*

🎼 Life and works

NATIONALITY: Hungarian

BORN: Nagyszentmiklos (now in Romania), 1881;
DIED: New York, 1945

SPECIALIST GENRES: Orchestral and piano music influenced by central European folk idioms.

MAJOR WORKS: Six string quartets (1908–39); *Duke Bluebeard's Castle* (1911–18); *The Miraculous Mandarin* (1919); *Microkosmos* (1926–39); three piano concertos (1926–45); *Music for Strings, Percussion and Celesta* (1936); *Contrasts* (1938); Concerto for Orchestra (1943).

Zoltán Kodály

Some day the ringing tower of Hungarian music is going to stand.

KODÁLY, 1932

Like his friend and collaborator Bartók, Kodály raised the international profile of Hungarian music by fertilizing Western styles with Magyar folk idioms. An authority on folk music, he was also an important teacher, producing a vast body of musical educational material.

The son of a stationmaster, he spent his childhood and youth in the countryside, before enrolling at Budapest University to read languages. He simultaneously began to study composition at the Budapest Academy, where he was awarded a doctorate for his study of Hungarian folk song. From 1905 onwards he began to collect and record folk songs, often collaborating with Bartók, with whom he shared a vision of "an educated Hungary, reborn from the people". Like Bartók, Kodály devoted much of his life to the

ABOVE: Zoltán Kodály, photographed towards the end of his long life.

publication of folk song anthologies and arrangements.

In 1906 he received a travelling scholarship to study in Berlin and Paris, where he came into contact with Debussy's music. On his return he was appointed a professor at the Budapest Academy, becoming its deputy director in 1919. But his tenure of that post was abruptly curtailed by political intrigue, and his career was only rescued after the triumphant 1923 première of his oratorio *Psalmus hungaricus*, written — like Bartók's Dance Suite — to celebrate the 50th anniversary of the union of Buda and Pest. A performance in Zurich in 1926 marked the beginning of his international fame.

The same year (1926), Kodály's opera *Háry János* was performed in Budapest, and world-famous

conductors such as Arturo Toscanini, Rudolf Mengelberg and Wilhelm Furtwängler began to include the orchestral suite taken from it (which includes a prominent part for the cimbalom, a Hungarian dulcimer) in their repertoires. It was followed by other major orchestral works: the *Dances of Marosszek* (1930), the *Dances of Galánta* (1933), the *Peacock* Variations, based on a Hungarian folk tune (1939, written for the Amsterdam Concertgebouw Orchestra), and the Concerto for Orchestra (1939–40, for the Chicago Symphony). Like Bartók, Kodály opposed fascism, but he remained in Hungary when it came under Nazi rule. After the war he supervised the publication of the folk material he had collected, and continued to write educational works. In later life he was showered with honours.

ABOVE: The Liszt Academy of Music in Budapest, where Kodály studied composition, and where he later became deputy director.

Life and works

NATIONALITY: Hungarian

BORN: Kecskemét, 1882; **DIED:** Budapest, 1967

SPECIALIST GENRES: Orchestral and choral music influenced by folk music.

MAJOR WORKS: *Psalmus hungaricus* (1923); *Háry János* (1925–6); *Dances of Galánta* (1933); Concerto for Orchestra (1939–40).

Carl Nielsen

Music is life, and, like it, inextinguishable.

NIELSEN, MOTTO OF THE FOURTH SYMPHONY (1916)

Nielsen was the Danish equivalent of Grieg or Sibelius. Born into an impoverished family (his father was a painter), he began to scrape out melodies as a child on an instrument made from firewood. He started learning the violin at six and began playing in his father's folk band. In the mid 1880s he studied at the Copenhagen Conservatory, and first achieved success with his Little Suite for strings, performed at Tivoli in 1888.

The next year Nielsen became a violinist in the royal chapel, where he was able to broaden his musical outlook. During a trip to Paris in 1891 he met and married a sculptress, and on his return finished the first of a sequence of six symphonies, on which his reputation largely rests. No. 1 is an early example of "progressive tonality", beginning in one key and ending in another, while No. 2 (*The Four Temperaments*, 1901–2) uses the technique of thematic variation.

At much the same time Nielsen completed his first opera, *Saul og David*, followed a few years later by the comic opera *Maskarade*.

From 1908 until 1914 Nielsen combined composing with a position at the Royal Theatre, and then with teaching at the Copenhagen Conservatory, whose director he became in 1931, just before his death. He consolidated his foremost position in Danish musical life with three more symphonies (No. 3, *Sinfonia espansiva*, 1910–11; No. 4, *The Inextinguishable*, 1914–16; and No. 5, 1921–2), the Violin Concerto (1911), piano works including the Chaconne and the Theme and Variations, the tone-poem *Pan and Syrinx* (1917–18) and the exotic, colourfully scored incidental music to the play *Aladdin* (1918–19). His Fourth and Fifth Symphonies are imaginatively constructed, with innovative use of percussion (in a passage in the Fifth, the side-drum is instructed to improvise "in order to try to destroy the music").

Between 1914 and 1925 Nielsen published many volumes of Danish folk song arrangements, and his later works are mostly for chamber combinations or smaller orchestra. He died of heart disease in 1931.

Life and works

NATIONALITY: Danish

BORN: Nørre-Lyndelse, near Odense, 1865; **DIED:** Copenhagen, 1931

SPECIALIST GENRES: Symphonies.

MAJOR WORKS: Six symphonies; *Saul og David* (1898– 1901); *Maskarade* (1904–6).

ABOVE: The Danish composer Carl Nielsen (1865–1931), photographed as a young man.

RIGHT: The Royal Theatre in Copenhagen, where Nielsen's operas were performed, and where he worked from 1908–14.

Percy Grainger

I object to jazz and vaudeville having all the best instruments.

GRAINGER, 1930

The Australian composer and pianist Percy Grainger was brought up by his mother (to whom he was devoted) in Melbourne. In 1895 he left Australia for Europe, where he entered the Conservatory in Frankfurt; and in 1901 he settled in London to begin his career as a concert pianist, using it as a base for concert tours throughout Europe. He often visited Scandinavia, where he became a close friend of Grieg and a notable interpreter of his Piano Concerto; he was also a friend of Delius from 1907 onwards (Delius's orchestral rhapsody *Brigg Fair* is based on a Lincolnshire folk tune collected by Grainger).

In 1905 Grainger joined the English Folk Song Society, becoming an ardent folk song collector in company with

ABOVE: The Australian-born pianist and composer Percy Grainger (1882–1961).

Cecil Sharp, Holst and Vaughan Williams. Folk song infused much of his work, from piano arrangements such as the ever-popular *Country Gardens*, *Green Bushes*, *Molly on the Shore* and *Shepherds' Hey*, to arrangements for wind band, and original orchestral works such as *Mock Morris*. Much of his vocal music is now out of fashion, since he often set jingoistic verses by Kipling and other colonial writers. His original large-scale works, which include *The Warriors* for three pianos, orchestra and tuned percussion, have also fallen out of favour, with the exception of *Handel in the Strand* (1932) for strings, based

on Handel's *Harmonious Blacksmith* Variations treated in music-hall style.

In 1914 Grainger moved to the USA, where he became a US citizen, and settled in White Plains, New York State. His mother committed suicide in 1922, and over the next six years Grainger spent much time in Denmark, collecting Danish folk songs, and returned twice to Australia. In 1928 he married a Swedish artist, who was presumably willing to put up with his sado-masochistic sexual practices and other eccentricities – their wedding took place before a huge audience in the Hollywood Bowl. The rest of his life was a long creative decline, although he spent his last years experimenting with "free music", dispensing with the conventions of harmony, form and instrumentation.

ABOVE: Grainger at the piano with his adored (and domineering) mother, Rose, in the music room of their American home in 1921.

Life and works

NATIONALITY: Australian

BORN: Melbourne, 1882; **DIED:** White Plains, New York, 1961

SPECIALIST GENRES: Folk song settings and original works using ingenious instrumental combinations.

MAJOR WORKS: *The Warriors* (1912–16); *Handel in the Strand* (1932); Suite *A Lincolnshire Posy* (1940).

Charles Ives

*This fascinating composer…was exploring the 1960s during
the heyday of Strauss and Debussy.*

IGOR STRAVINSKY (1882–1971)

Charles Ives, one of the most innovative figures in music history, was America's first major composer. His father was a town bandmaster with a most original musical mind. His experiments with acoustics and pitch, using quarter-tones, polytonality, tone clusters and simultaneously playing pieces in different keys, intrigued his young son. Ives later incorporated the unusual sounds of his childhood experiences into his own music.

In 1894 Charles went to Yale University, where he studied composition and wrote the first of his four symphonies. After graduating he moved to New York, where he worked in insurance, and by 1906 he and his partner, Julian Myrick, had set up their own very successful insurance agency

ABOVE: Charles Ives (1874–1954), an essentially amateur composer who gave American music an individual identity.

which made them millionaires. Ives married Harmony Twichell in a union of lasting happiness, but long hours of work combined with spare-time composing undermined his health, and in 1918 he had a heart attack. During a year's convalescence he embarked on the publication of his music. He retired from the insurance business in 1930.

Most of Ives's major compositions were written before 1920. Many were inspired by "American" landscapes, festivals, traditions, or historical events. They include four numbered symphonies (the Fourth introduces a chorus into the finale); the *Holidays Symphony* (1904–13), in which the movements are "Washington's Birthday", "Decoration Day", "Fourth of July" and "Thanksgiving Day"; *Central Park in the Dark* (1906); and three Sets for

orchestra, of which No. 1 is entitled *Three Places in New England*. He also wrote several psalm settings for various vocal combinations and organ or orchestra; over 20 Studies for piano, of which several describe stages of a baseball game; the huge *Concord* Sonata for piano, with optional parts for viola and flute; the epigrammatic three-page Sonata (1905) and the early *Variations on "America"* for organ.

Ives was a Satie-like figure, who often used punning titles (such as *Five Take-offs* or *Six Protests*). In *The Unanswered Question* (1906) for chamber ensemble, a solo trumpet asks "the question", to which a woodwind choir frantically attempts to find an answer. His innovative musical style had enormous influence on later American composers.

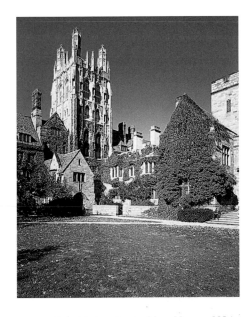

ABOVE: Yale University in New Haven, USA, where Ives studied in the 1890s. He was an enthusiastic member of the baseball team.

Life and works

NATIONALITY: American

BORN: Danbury, Connecticut, 1874; **DIED:** New York, 1954

SPECIALIST GENRES: Orchestral and piano music, often on American themes.

MAJOR WORKS: Five symphonies; *Variations on "America"* (1891); *Three Places in New England* (1904); Piano Sonata No. 2 *Concord* (1910–15); 114 songs.

George Gershwin

*I don't think there has been such an inspired melodist on this earth since Tchaikovsky...
but if you want to speak of a composer, that's another matter.*

LEONARD BERNSTEIN (1918–90)

Gershwin was one of the most popular composers of the 20th century, and one of history's greatest songwriters. From 1916 until his untimely death from a brain tumour at the age of only 39, he turned out a stream of great melodies which became instant classics. Songs such as "Swanee", "'S Wonderful", "Someone to Watch Over Me", "Embraceable You", "He Loves and She Loves", "I Got Rhythm" (and dozens more) rank with the best of Irving Berlin, Cole Porter and Jerome Kern, but were also much admired by "serious" musicians.

The son of a Russian Jewish immigrant family, Gershwin studied piano, theory and harmony as a child with several distinguished musicians, although he was never good at reading music. In 1914 he went to work for a Tin Pan Alley music publisher and began to write songs for other people's shows. From 1919 onwards he wrote his own Broadway musicals, many in collaboration with his brother Ira

(1896–1983). They included *Lady be Good* (1924), *Oh, Kay!* (1926), *Strike Up the Band* (1927), *Funny Face* (1927), *Girl Crazy* (1930) and *Of Thee I Sing* (1931). From 1931 onwards he also wrote film scores (the songs "Let's Call the Whole Thing Off", "Shall We Dance?" and "They Can't Take That Away From Me"

were written for the 1937 film *Shall We Dance?*).

In 1924 the bandleader Paul Whiteman commissioned Gershwin's famous *Rhapsody in Blue* for piano and jazz ensemble. The story goes that Gershwin did not know he was supposed to write it until he saw an advertisement for Whiteman's forthcoming "Experiment in Modern Music" concert in a newspaper. Ira Gershwin suggested the title, after a painting by Whistler. Its triumphant success led to commissions for the Piano Concerto, the orchestral tone-poem *An American in Paris*, and ultimately to the opera *Porgy and Bess*, set among the black community of the Deep South and using its folk music and rhythms. It is still the only American opera to be performed internationally on a regular basis.

ABOVE: George Gershwin, painted by himself a year before his death from a brain tumour.

LEFT: A poster advertising the 1959 film version of Porgy and Bess.

Life and works

NATIONALITY: American

BORN: Brooklyn, 1898;
DIED: Beverly Hills, 1937

SPECIALIST GENRES:
Popular songs.

MAJOR WORKS: *Rhapsody in Blue* (1924); Piano Concerto in F (1925); Preludes for piano (1926); *An American in Paris* (1928); *Porgy and Bess* (1935).

Samuel Barber

As to what happens when I compose,
I really haven't the faintest idea.

BARBER

Samuel Barber's style eschewed the idiomatic "Americanisms" of Copland and looked back to the late-Romantic European tradition. He began to learn the piano at the age of six, and began composing at seven. At 14 he became one of the first students at the Curtis Institute in Philadelphia, where he studied piano, composition, conducting and singing. He nearly became a professional baritone.

Barber's student years at the Curtis Institute produced his first mature compositions, including the popular *Dover Beach* (a setting of a poem by Matthew Arnold for baritone voice and string quartet which Barber himself recorded in 1935), the Serenade for string quartet, and the

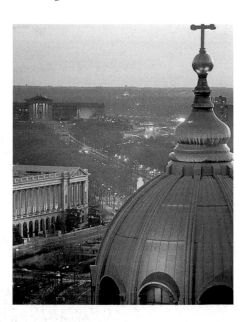

ABOVE: The American composer Samuel Barber (1910–81).

Cello Sonata, all of which gave him scope to develop his characteristic lyrical, expressive style. In 1928 he won a travelling scholarship with his Violin Sonata, and another in 1933 for his overture *The School for Scandal*. In the mid 1930s further scholarships, including the American Prix de Rome, enabled him to spend time in Italy. His compositions there included the First Symphony and a String Quartet, the slow movement of which, transcribed for orchestra, became the famous Adagio for strings (first recorded by Toscanini).

From 1939 until 1942 Barber taught at the Curtis Institute, and from 1943

until 1974 he lived in New York State with the Italian composer Gian Carlo Menotti (born 1911), who wrote the libretto for Barber's first opera, *Vanessa*. His Second Symphony (later withdrawn) was written during war service. His post-war works included a fine Cello Concerto (1945), the ballet *Medea* (1946), the Piano Sonata, *Summer Music* for wind quintet (1955), the vocal works *Knoxville: Summer of 1915* (1947), *Hermit Songs* (1952–3), and *Prayers of Kierkegaard* (1954), and three operas, of which *Antony and Cleopatra* (1965–6), based on Franco Zeffirelli's reworking of Shakespeare, was an expensive failure. A post-Romantic, Barber shunned innovation, and continued, as he said, to "go on doing his thing" until the end of his life.

Life and works

NATIONALITY: American

BORN: West Chester, Pennsylvania, 1910;
DIED: New York, 1981

SPECIALIST GENRES: Orchestral, chamber and operatic works, in neo-Romantic idiom.

MAJOR WORKS: *Dover Beach* (1931); *The School for Scandal* Overture (1933); Adagio for strings (1938); Piano Sonata (1949); opera *Vanessa* (1958); Piano Concerto (1962).

ABOVE: Philadelphia, Pennsylvania, at dusk. Barber studied there at the world-famous Curtis Institute.

Igor Stravinsky

Bach on the wrong notes.

SERGEI PROKOFIEV (1891–1953)

Stravinsky was arguably the greatest – and certainly the most versatile – composer of the 20th century. He was keenly receptive to new trends – from neo-classicism to 12-note music – and perceived the advantages of a protean approach to composition. He also shed his personal skin several times throughout his long life, acquiring two wives and three changes of nationality.

Russian period

The son of an opera singer, Stravinsky went to school in St Petersburg, and began piano lessons when he was nine. On a summer vacation in the country he met Rimsky-Korsakov, who became his teacher and mentor. His early Piano Sonata in F sharp minor was performed at Rimsky-Korsakov's house, and a Symphony in E flat and the orchestral fantasy *Feu d'artifice* (*Fireworks*, strongly influenced

ABOVE: *Igor Stravinsky, photographed by Tappe in 1965, while he was writing the* Requiem Canticles, *his last major work.*

ABOVE: *A portrait of Stravinsky conducting, by the artist Milein Cosman. Stravinsky conducted recordings of his entire output.*

by Debussy) were largely written under the elder composer's tuition. Stravinsky had no other formal musical education; during this time he spent a couple of years reading law at university, but found it uncongenial. He left in 1905 and the following year he married his cousin Katerina Nossenko, who bore him four children.

Diaghilev's Ballets Russes

In 1909 the *Scherzo fantastique* and *Feu d'artifice* were performed in St Petersburg. In the audience was the impresario Sergei Diaghilev (1872–1929), whose celebrated Ballets Russes employed the dancer Mikhail Fokine and the designers Léon Bakst and Alexandre Benois. Diaghilev lacked a composer for his 1910 Paris season, and he decided to try out the young Stravinsky with a commission for *L'oiseau de feu* (*The Firebird*), based on a Russian folk legend. Stravinsky's brilliant and colourful score – strongly influenced by his Russian forebears including Balakirev, Tchaikovsky and Rimsky-Korsakov – was a huge success.

His next score for Diaghilev began life as a concert piece for piano and orchestra, but then turned into *Petrushka*, based on a grotesque tale of lust and murder in a Russian puppeteer's booth. Another huge success at its Paris première in June 1911, *Petrushka* conjures up a vanishing world of Russian peasant life, complete

with exotic and exhilarating dances for Cossacks, coachmen, wet-nurses and a host of other characters.

During 1912 Stravinsky worked on his third Diaghilev ballet, *Le sacre du printemps* (*The Rite of Spring*). Its première at the Théâtre des Champs-Elysées on 29 May 1913 caused a riot among its outraged audience. Even now, the primitive violence of Stravinsky's score – especially when coupled with Nijinsky's explicit choreography (the ballet concerns an ancient fertility rite in which a young virgin is selected for ritual sacrifice) – still packs an electrifying punch.

In 1914 Stravinsky's first opera, *Le rossignol* (*The Nightingale*, based on Hans Christian Andersen's fairy-story), was produced under the aegis of the Ballets Russes at the Paris Opéra. (Five years later Stravinsky arranged the music as a symphonic poem, *Le chant du rossignol*, which was choreographed

ABOVE: *Stravinsky in his study in later life – a photographic portrait by Karsh of Ottawa.*

as a ballet by Leonid Massine with designs by Henri Matisse.)

When war broke out the composer and his family took refuge in Switzerland, where he worked on a new ballet score, *Les noces* (*The Wedding*), scored for four-part chorus,

four soloists, four pianos and percussion ensemble. Stravinsky's researches into Russian folk music for this project also inspired several secondary works, including the burlesque *Renard* (1915–16).

By 1918 Stravinsky had already abandoned the lush orchestral resources of his pre-war ballets in favour of more sparsely scored, chamber-orientated works. These included *L'histoire du soldat* (*The Soldier's Tale*, for three actors, dancer, and small instrumental ensemble) and the ballet *Pulcinella*, based on a *commedia dell'arte* theme with music "arranged" from fragments attributed to Pergolesi, at the suggestion of Diaghilev. *Pulcinella* – which ushered in Stravinsky's absorption in neo-classicism – was first performed at the Paris Opéra on 15 May 1920, with décor and costumes by Picasso. Stravinsky later arranged the music as suites for cello and piano and for violin and piano.

ABOVE: *The Moor, the Ballerina and Petrushka – a 1913 illustration by René Bull of the three main characters in Stravinsky's ballet* Petrushka.

Life and works

NATIONALITY: Russian

BORN: Oranienbaum, near St Petersburg, 1882; DIED: New York, 1971

SPECIALIST GENRES: Stage works (ballet, opera, oratorios), sacred music.

MAJOR WORKS: *L'oiseau de feu* (1910); *Petrushka* (1911); *Le sacre du printemps* (1912); *L'histoire du soldat* (1918); *Les noces* (1914–23); *Oedipus rex* (1926–7); *Symphony of Psalms* (1930); *Dumbarton Oaks* (1938); *Symphony in Three Movements* (1942–5); *The Rake's Progress* (1948–51).

ABOVE: *Cynthia Harvey and Anthony Dowell as the Firebird and the Prince in the Royal Ballet's production of* The Firebird, *Stravinsky's first ballet score for Diaghilev.*

ABOVE: *A scene from Stravinsky's third Diaghilev ballet,* The Rite of Spring.

French period

After the war, Stravinsky decided to make France his home, settling in Paris and Biarritz. The early 1920s saw the composition of several purely instrumental works, including the *Symphonies of Wind Instruments* (1921), dedicated to Debussy's memory, and the Concerto for Piano and Wind (1923–4). He also worked on *Mavra*: a one-act *opera buffa* based on Pushkin, and completed the orchestration of *Les noces*. These two works marked the

end of his "Russian" period. At the same time, he began an affair with a married actress, Vera Soudeikine, to whom he dedicated the Octet for wind instruments (1922–3). To his wife Katarina he dedicated the Serenade in A (1925), one of many piano works written in the 1920s which also included the Capriccio for piano and orchestra (1928–9) and the Sonata (1924).

In 1927 Stravinsky celebrated the 20th anniversary of Diaghilev's first

Paris season with the opera-oratorio *Oedipus rex*, based on a Latin version of the tragic myth by the poet Jean Cocteau. Neither Diaghilev nor the audience really appreciated this strange hybrid, which is now recognized as a masterpiece. Stravinsky had already begun to cut loose from Diaghilev. His next ballet score, *Apollon musagète* (a title later abbreviated to *Apollo*), was written to a commission from the American patroness Elizabeth Sprague Coolidge, and was the first of Stravinsky's ballets to be choreographed by George Balanchine (1904–83). It was followed by *Le baiser de la fée* (*The Fairy's Kiss*), a Tchaikovskian pastiche, for Ida Rubinstein's rival troupe. Diaghilev had little time to complain: he died in Venice in August 1929. The following year, Stravinsky was commissioned by Serge Koussevitzsky (1876–1951) to celebrate the 50th anniversary of the Boston Symphony Orchestra with the *Symphony of Psalms*; and in 1931 he began an association with the violinist Samuel Dushkin, for whom he wrote the Violin Concerto and the Duo Concertante for violin and piano.

In 1934 Stravinsky became a naturalized French citizen. The same year he collaborated with André Gide

ABOVE: *Stravinsky (right), photographed in 1921 with the impressario Sergei Diaghilev, founder of the Ballets Russes.*

ABOVE: *Stravinsky conducting in later life. He moved to the USA in 1939 and remained there for the rest of his life.*

ABOVE: Stravinsky rehearsing the orchestra of La Scala, Milan, in preparation for the première of his opera The Rake's Progress.

(1869–1951) on the musical melodrama *Perséphone*, again for Rubinstein, which was coolly received. But by the mid 1930s his main commissions were coming from the other side of the Atlantic. They included the ballet *Jeu de cartes* (*The Card Game*, choreographed by Balanchine in 1937 for the American Ballet), the pseudo-Baroque chamber concerto *Dumbarton Oaks*, and the Symphony in C for the Chicago Symphony Orchestra (1940).

American period

The imminent outbreak of World War II, combined with the deaths of his elder daughter, his wife and his mother, drove Stravinsky to seek sanctuary in the USA. On 9 March 1940 he married Vera Soudeikine, then settled in Hollywood and applied for US citizenship. The early works of his American years include the Symphony in Three Movements, the *Circus Polka* (1942) for dancing elephants in the Barnum and Bailey Circus, *Scènes de ballet* (1944) for a Broadway revue, the *Danses concertantes* (1941–2), and the *Ebony Concerto* for the jazz clarinettist

Woody Herman (1913–87). Stravinsky's last neo-classical work was the opera *The Rake's Progress* (1948–51), inspired by William Hogarth's famous series of etchings, to a libretto by W. H. Auden (1907–73) and Chester Kallman (1921–75). It was premièred in Venice in September 1951.

Last works

After *The Rake's Progress* Stravinsky's style underwent a major change. His meeting in 1948 with the conductor Robert Craft (born 1923), an admirer of Schoenberg, introduced Stravinsky to the music of the Second Viennese School. The first fruit of his own experiments with serial technique was the *Canticum sacrum* (1955), designed for performance in St Mark's, Venice. Two further stage works date from his later years: the ballet *Agon* (1953–4), and the musical play *The Flood*

(1961–2), based on the York and Chester mystery plays and first produced on American television.

Many of Stravinsky's later works, from the 1948 Mass onwards, sprang from religious impulses. They include *Threni* (*Lamentations of the Prophet Jeremiah*) for solo voices, chorus and orchestra (1957–8), the cantata *A Sermon, a Narrative and a Prayer* (1960–1), the "sacred ballad" *Abraham and Isaac* for baritone and chamber orchestra (1962–3), *Introitus* for men's voices and ensemble (1965), and his last major work, the *Requiem Canticles* for soloists, chorus and orchestra (1965–6). One of his last works was the charming setting for voice and piano of Edward Lear's poem "The Owl and the Pussy-Cat" (1966).

In 1969 Stravinsky and his wife moved to New York, where he died two years later. He was buried near Diaghilev in Venice.

ABOVE: The Rake's Progress *is a quasi-Mozartian full-length opera based on an English libretto. This photograh shows a 1952 performance at the Berlin State Opera.*

Music
❧ since ❧
World War II

A recording studio in Hollywood. Electronic studios were first used by post-war composers such as Edgard Varèse, Luciano Berio and Karlheinz Stockhausen.

The serial idea is based on a universe that finds itself in perpetual expansion.

PIERRE BOULEZ (BORN 1925)

From the late 20th century, music has become more fragmentary than at any previous historical period. There are no longer "schools" of composition: each composer now strives to find an original and entirely individual voice. If they draw inspiration from other music, it is from the works of individual predecessors rather than from general trends.

Both Shostakovich and Benjamin Britten came into their own after 1945, the year that Britten revitalized British opera with *Peter Grimes*. While Britten's principal importance lies in vocal music, especially his fine sequence of operas, Shostakovich was primarily an instrumental composer. Both were inspired by the playing of the Russian cellist Mstislav Rostropovich, for whom Shostakovich wrote his cello concertos and Britten his Cello Symphony and three solo suites. Both composers worked in an essentially tonal medium, unaffected by avant-garde developments.

Britain has maintained a strong operatic tradition since 1945, in the works of Britten, Michael Tippett, Harrison Birtwistle, Peter Maxwell Davies, and now a younger generation of composers, including Mark-Anthony Turnage and Thomas Adès. In America, Leonard Bernstein revitalized the American musical, especially with his brilliant *West Side Story* (1957), but has proved perhaps more influential as a conductor than as a composer. Meanwhile, Copland (though active up until his death) ceded the mantle of senior American composer to Elliott

ABOVE: VE Day, 8 May 1945. Crowds in Whitehall, London, cheering Prime Minister Winston Churchill and members of the Cabinet after the announcement of Germany's surrender.

ABOVE: The first landing on the Moon — the Apollo 11 mission, 1969.

Carter, whose orchestral and chamber music is characterized by the most rigorous intellectual discipline and formal perfection.

Minimalism

The experiments of John Cage proved a blind alley in themselves (the notorious *4' 33"* took music to its furthest extreme — complete silence), but Cage's ideas have taken root, most obviously in the American minimalist school of Steve Reich, Terry Riley, Philip Glass and John Adams, whose music relies on repetitive rhythmic and melodic *ostinati* for its hypnotic effect. The fact that such music has connections with the harmonic and rhythmic clichés of pop and rock music, as well as with Indian and African music (popular in the West since the 1960s), has contributed to its popularity. The British composer Michael Nyman (born 1944) uses similar techniques in his film scores.

Electronic music

Cage's use of aleatory, or chance, techniques (derived from the Chinese *I-Ching*, or *The Book of Changes*) has been independently adopted and developed to a limited extent by the Polish composer Witold Lutoslawski, and in a more intensely focused way by the Greek composer Iannis Xenakis, many of whose works use electronic tape. The use of electronic instruments, amplification and sampling has become widespread in "serious" music over the last 50 years. Composers who have

ABOVE: The American composer Philip Glass (born 1937) rehearsing with musicians in Los Angeles, March 1977.

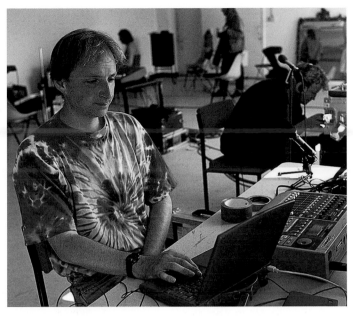

ABOVE: Students using computers on the Electro-Acoustic Composition Course at Dartington, 1999.

made use of such techniques include the early Franco-American experimenter Edgard Varèse, the Italians Luciano Berio and Bruno Maderna, the British composer Jonathan Harvey, and the German Karlheinz Stockhausen, one of the leaders of the European avant-garde in the 1960s and '70s.

French music in the later 20th century was dominated by two composers. The idiosyncratic style of Olivier Messiaen was influenced by Eastern music, birdsong, the serial technique of Webern – which he refined still further – and his profound Catholic faith. His pupil Pierre Boulez, who founded the major European research centre into modern composing techniques, is a central figure in 20th–21st-century European music. Equally well-known as a conductor, he has helped to co-ordinate the work of composers from many different countries, as well as producing an important and highly original body of work rooted in the French tradition, but cross-fertilized by European avant-garde techniques.

Female composers

One encouraging feature of music in recent years has been the emergence of women composers, and the rediscovery, after centuries of neglect, of the music of talented women of the past, such as Fanny Mendelssohn (1805–47) and Amy Beach (1867–1944). Composers such as Judith Weir (born 1954), Sofia Gubaidulina (born 1931), Elena Firsova (born 1950) and Roxanna Panufnik (born 1968) are now beginning to challenge the traditional male hegemony in composition, as in many other fields, and are proving particularly adept in the developing fields of television and film music.

ABOVE: Kurt Masur conducting the New York Philharmonic in the Avery Fisher Hall, New York, 1998.

Dmitri Shostakovich

*The music [Symphony No. 11] to me was self-evidently about
Shostakovich's own experiences in the catastrophe of his life.*

MICHAEL TIPPETT (1905–98)

Together with Stravinsky and Prokofiev, Shostakovich was one of the greatest Russian composers of the 20th century. His 15 symphonies and 15 string quartets are among the finest 20th-century works in those media.

Shostakovich began to learn the piano with his mother, a professional pianist. In 1919, aged only 13, he entered the St Petersburg Conservatory to study piano and composition: his teachers there included Glazunov. A phenomenally gifted student, his First Symphony (written as a diploma exercise) won international acclaim after its premières in Leningrad (1926), Berlin (under Bruno Walter), and Philadelphia (under Leopold Stokowski); a year later Shostakovich received an honourable mention as an entrant in the International Chopin Piano Competition.

During the 1920s Shostakovich – a firm adherent to Socialist ideals – concentrated on stage and film music. An opera, *Nos* (*The Nose*), and two

ABOVE: Dmitri Shostakovich (1906–75), photographed at the Moscow Conservatory in the early 1960s.

ballets, *Zolotoy vek* (*The Golden Age*, 1927–30) and *Bolt* (1930–1), showed him developing a brittle, witty and satirical style which owed much to current European avant-garde

influences, and for several years he was regarded as the "great white hope" of Soviet music.

Denunciation

Then came catastrophe. His opera *Lady Macbeth of the Mtsensk District*, a savage tale of adultery, murder and retribution, was produced in Moscow in 1934. At first it won critical acceptance both within Russia and abroad. But Stalin went to see it and was shocked by its graphic portrayal of sex and violence, and by its "advanced" musical idiom. On his orders, Shostakovich was savagely attacked in the press in 1936, in an article entitled "Chaos instead of Music".

Denounced also by his fellow composers, Shostakovich hurriedly withdrew the score of his Fourth Symphony, then in rehearsal, and responded with the more "accessible" Fifth Symphony (1937), which he described as "A Soviet artist's response to just criticism". For a while he

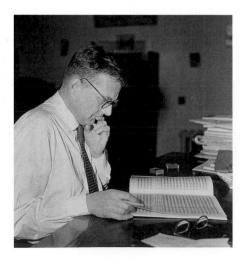

*LEFT:
Shostakovich
composing at
his Moscow flat.*

*RIGHT:
A view of the
Admiralty in St
Petersburg, where
Shostakovich
was born and
where he
studied.*

appeared to have been forgiven: the Fifth Symphony proved popular, his 1940 Piano Quintet received the Stalin Prize, and his Seventh Symphony, written during the German siege of Leningrad in 1941, became an international symbol of heroic resistance (even though its repetitive "invasion" theme was cruelly parodied by Bartók in his Concerto for Orchestra, written in America in 1943).

Shostakovich's next two symphonies were also inspired by the war: the Eighth (1943) by its savagery, and the Ninth (1945) in a spirit of rejoicing at its end. But in 1948 he was once again officially denounced (together with Prokofiev and others), accused of "formalist perversions" and "anti-democratic tendencies in music". Such denunciations, during the Stalinist purges of the late 1940s, were tantamount to a death sentence, and if Shostakovich's posthumously published *Memoirs* are to be believed, from then until Stalin's death in 1953 he lived in fear for his life. He kept his private artistic credo alive with intimate chamber works, while publicly he concentrated on "safe" works based on nationalistic themes.

ABOVE, FROM LEFT TO RIGHT: *The great Russian cellist Mstislav Rostropovich (for whom Shostakovich wrote his cello concertos), Shostakovich, Rostropovich's wife — the soprano Galina Vishnevskaya — and the violinist David Oistrakh.*

The post-Stalin era

After Stalin's death, Shostakovich returned to symphonic writing with the Tenth, Eleventh (*The Year 1905*) and Twelfth (*The Year 1917*) Symphonies. The late 1950s also produced the satirical musical comedy *Cheryomuschki* (*The Cherry Trees Estate*, 1958), a suite, *The Gadfly*, from his film score of 1955, the Second Piano Concerto (written in 1957 for his son Maxim, who became a well-known conductor), the First Cello Concerto (written in 1959 for Rostropovich), and the Seventh and Eighth String Quartets (1960).

In 1962 *Lady Macbeth* was restored to the Russian repertoire (under the new title *Katerina Ismailova*) and hailed as a masterpiece. Shostakovich then produced another controversial work, the Thirteenth Symphony (*Babi Yar*), based on poems by the Jewish writer Yevgeny Yevtushenko (born 1933). Its two successors, particularly the anguished Fourteenth Symphony of 1969 (settings of 11 poems by European writers), are preoccupied with death: the Fifteenth Symphony (1971), with its ironic references to other composers, seems to sum up

Shostakovich's own career. The last decade of his life produced seven more string quartets, sonatas for violin and viola, and a further concerto each for violin and cello.

Towards the end of his life, Shostakovich was allowed to visit the West. He became a friend of Benjamin Britten, to whom the Fourteenth Symphony is dedicated. Like Britten, he died of heart failure in his 60s.

ABOVE: *A programme for the first London concert performance of Shostakovich's opera* Lady Macbeth of Mtsensk, *in 1935.*

Life and works

NATIONALITY: Russian

BORN: St Petersburg, 1906; **DIED:** Moscow, 1975

SPECIALIST GENRES: Symphonies, concertos, string quartets, operas.

MAJOR WORKS: 15 symphonies; concertos for piano, violin and cello; chamber music, including 15 string quartets; operas *The Nose* (1927–8) and *Lady Macbeth of the Mtsensk District* (1934).

Benjamin Britten

If wind and water could write music, it would sound like Ben's.

Yehudi Menuhin (1916–99)

Together with Michael Tippett, Britten dominated the British musical scene from the 1930s onwards. His roots lay in the music of Mozart and Verdi, and he never abandoned tonality, but he developed a distinctive style with wide appeal. Much of his music was inspired by specific performers, particularly the tenor voice of his lifelong companion, Peter Pears (1910–86).

Britten was born on St Cecilia's Day, 22 November 1913. He went to boarding school, but studied composition privately with Frank Bridge (1879–1941) in school holidays. In 1930 he entered the Royal College of Music in London, where he studied composition with John Ireland and honed his already formidable skills as a pianist. He wanted to continue his studies in Vienna with Alban Berg,

ABOVE: Benjamin Britten, one of the major British composers of the 20th century.

having heard Berg's opera *Wozzeck* in 1934, but was discouraged by his parents and teachers.

Early works

In 1935, by which time several early works including a Sinfonietta and an Oboe Quartet had already been performed, Britten began to work for the documentary film unit of the General Post Office, where he met the poet W. H. Auden. They shared left-wing political sympathies and collaborated on several works, including the orchestral song-cycle *Our Hunting Fathers* (1936) and the choral work *Ballad of Heroes* (1939). In that year Britten and Peter Pears followed Auden to the USA. By this time Britten's natural predilection for vocal music had already been confirmed with the Rimbaud song-cycle *Les illuminations* (1939), but the

Seven Sonnets of Michelangelo of 1940 was the first of many works which Britten wrote expressly for Pears. Instrumental works of the late 1930s and early '40s included the charming Rossini pastiche *Soirées musicales* (1936), the brilliant *Variations on a Theme of Frank Bridge* for strings (1937), concertos for piano (1938) and violin (1940), and the *Sinfonia da requiem* (1940). From then onwards, Britten wrote few specifically orchestral works. Exceptions were the *Young Person's Guide to the Orchestra* (1946) and the exquisite Serenade for tenor, horn and strings (1943, written

ABOVE: Britten (left) with his lifelong companion Peter Pears in the garden of their house at Aldeburgh, Suffolk. This was one of the last photographs of Britten.

Life and works

NATIONALITY: English

BORN: Lowestoft, 1913;
DIED: Aldeburgh, 1976

SPECIALIST GENRES: Opera and other stage works, vocal music.

MAJOR WORKS: Operas *Peter Grimes* (1944–5), *Billy Budd* (1951), *The Turn of the Screw* (1954), *A Midsummer Night's Dream* (1960) and *Death in Venice* (1973); *War Requiem* (1962); three "church parables"; chamber music and songs, including song-cycles and folk song arrangements.

for Pears and the horn player Dennis Brain), two of his most popular works; the Cello Symphony for Rostropovich (1963); and two "occasional" works written to celebrate the respective openings of the Snape Maltings concert hall and the Queen Elizabeth Hall in London.

Aldeburgh Festival

Britten decided to return home from America in 1942, having by chance read George Crabbe's 19th-century poem *The Borough*, an unflattering portrait of the Suffolk fishing village of Aldeburgh, which inspired his first major opera, *Peter Grimes*. Its première at Sadler's Wells on 7 June 1945 marked a milestone in British music, and in the history of opera. Britten and Pears settled first at Snape, a few miles inland, and then in Aldeburgh itself, where in 1947 they established the annual Aldeburgh Festival. Twenty years later, the festival's main venue moved from Aldeburgh's tiny Jubilee Hall to a converted malthouse at Snape.

Opera and choral works

Three original chamber operas followed *Peter Grimes*: *The Rape of Lucretia* (1946), the comedy *Albert Herring* (1947), both performed at Glyndebourne, and *The Little Sweep* (1949). In 1951, *Billy Budd* (based on Herman Melville's nautical tragedy) was performed at Covent Garden, followed two years later by Britten's one failure, *Gloriana* (intended to celebrate Elizabeth II's accession in 1953): later productions have led to its reassessment. *The Turn of the Screw*, based on Henry James's ghost story, was premièred in Venice, the city which inspired Britten's operatic swansong (and the most direct expression of his love for Pears), *Death in Venice*, based on Thomas Mann's novella. Many people

ABOVE: The Maltings at Snape, converted by Britten's efforts from an abandoned malthouse to a fine concert hall, the major venue for the Aldeburgh Festival.

consider his operatic masterpiece to be the Shakespearean *A Midsummer Night's Dream*.

During the 1960s Britten temporarily eschewed conventional operas in favour of three "church parables" written for performance in Orford Church in Suffolk: *Curlew River* (1964, inspired by Japanese Noh drama), *The Burning Fiery Furnace* (1966) and *The Prodigal Son* (1968). His next opera, *Owen Wingrave*, was written for television in 1970, though it subsequently transferred successfully to the stage. In 1962

his *War Requiem* was performed at the newly opened Coventry Cathedral, with an international cast of soloists, in a spirit of post-war reconciliation. The Requiem text is interwoven with the poetry of Wilfred Owen (1893–1918), and the work is a powerful expression of Britten's pacifism.

Besides composing, Britten was a fine conductor and pianist, and often toured in recital with Pears. In 1973 he had heart surgery, which curtailed his activities, and shortly before his death in 1976 he became the first British composer to be made a life peer.

ABOVE: A scene from the 1995 Covent Garden production of Peter Grimes, *with Bryn Terfel as Captain Balstrode, and Ben Heppner as the fisherman Grimes.*

Michael Tippett

*I like to think of composing as a physical business. I compose at the piano
and like to feel involved in my work with my hands.*

TIPPETT

Like his younger contemporary Benjamin Britten, the English composer Michael Tippett grew up in Suffolk, and studied at the Royal College of Music in London. He left in 1928 and became a schoolteacher and part-time composer. His first mature works were the First String Quartet (1935), the First Piano Sonata (1936–7), and the Concerto for Double String Orchestra (1938–9), which belongs to the early 20th-century British tradition of works for string ensemble.

During the 1930s Tippett became involved in radical politics, organizing the "South London Orchestra of Unemployed Musicians". His passionate antipathy towards the horrors of war, initially aroused by the plight of European Jews, found expression in his deeply moving oratorio based on the true story of a Jewish boy who killed

ABOVE: For the last two decades of Michael Tippett's life he was the undisputed "Grand Old Man" of British music.

a Nazi diplomat, *A Child of Our Time* (1939–41), which articulates Tippett's lifelong belief in the opposing "dark" and "light" sides of human nature, present in everyone. The oratorio is influenced by Bach's Passions, with negro spirituals replacing Protestant chorales. Tippett was briefly imprisoned for his pacifist beliefs in 1943.

From 1940–51 Tippett was director of music at Morley College in South London. He subsequently became a full-time composer. His first opera, *The Midsummer Marriage*, was produced in 1952, and like each of its successors – *King Priam* (1961), *The Knot Garden* (1970), *The Ice Break* (1976), *New Year* (1989) – it spawned instrumental and

vocal works, including an important series of five string quartets, four symphonies, four piano sonatas and the *Songs for Dov* (1969–70) for tenor and chamber orchestra.

In 1995, the year of his 90th birthday, a Tippett Festival at the Barbican in London included the première of his last major work, *The Rose Lake*, a "song without words for orchestra". His last work was "Caliban's Song", part of a *Tempest Suite* commissioned by the BBC to mark the tercentenary of Purcell's death. Renaissance and Baroque music had been a major influence on Tippett's earlier works, including the *Fantasia Concertante on a Theme of Corelli* for strings (1953).

ABOVE: Tippett composing at the piano in 1992. His sight failed in the last years of his life.

Life and works

NATIONALITY: English

BORN: London, 1905;
DIED: London, 1998

SPECIALIST GENRES: Opera, symphonies, string quartets.

MAJOR WORKS: Concerto for Double String Orchestra (1938–9); *A Child of Our Time* (1939–41); five operas, including *The Midsummer Marriage* (1952); Piano Concerto (1953–5); *The Vision of St Augustine* (1965); *The Mask of Time* (1980–2); four symphonies; five string quartets.

John Cage

It is better to make a piece of music than to perform one.

CAGE, "SILENCE" (1961)

The American composer John Cage was one of the most interesting experimental artists of his time. He studied with Henry Cowell (1897–1965, himself a noted pioneer of innovative techniques) and with Schoenberg, who called him "an inventor – of genius". From 1937 onwards he developed a strong interest in dance and percussion techniques, and in 1942 he moved from the West Coast to New York, where he began a long association with Merce Cunningham's dance company.

In 1938 he invented the "prepared piano" by inserting small domestic objects such as paperclips and rubber bands between the strings. This instrument, capable of producing extraordinary timbres, was used in Cage's early pieces such as *Sonatas and*

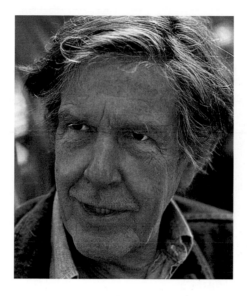

ABOVE: Experimental composer John Cage, more a "musical philosopher" than a composer.

Interludes (1946–8), and *Music for Marcel Duchamp* (1947). *The Wonderful Widow of Eighteen Springs* (1942) is a setting of a poem by James Joyce for voice and closed piano. A devotee of Zen Buddhism (before it became fashionable) and the *I-Ching*, Cage introduced aleatory (chance) techniques into his music, for instance in *Music of Changes* for piano (1951), in which the performance depends on the toss of a coin, and *Cheap Imitation* (1969), an alteration of Satie's *Socrate*, worked out using the *I-Ching*. With these works, he changed the nature of music by removing the necessity of intention from composition.

In 1952, with *Imaginary Landscape V*, Cage began to use electronic tape in his works. In the same year he "wrote" his notorious *4' 33"*, in which the performer sits at a silent piano and is required only to indicate the division

of the work into three movements: the attention of the audience is directed to life (including the chance sounds of the environment) rather than art. Also from 1952 dates *Theater Piece* for Merce Cunningham, the first "musical happening", combining theatre, art and music. From then on Cage used a wide range of electronic media in his works, which are often scored for bizarre combinations. For example, *Imaginary Landscape IV* (1951) is for 12 radios and 24 players, *Speech* (1955) for five radios and newsreader, *HPSCHD* (1967–9) for seven harpsichord soloists and 51 tape machines, and *Postcard from Heaven* (1983) for between one and 20 harpsichords.

Cage was a musical philosopher. He believed that art was whatever the artist said it was: "I have nothing to say, I am saying it, and that is poetry." An avowed anarchist, he followed a strict macrobiotic diet, was a brilliant chess player and an expert on mushrooms.

ABOVE: One of the "instruments" used in the performance by Ensemble Bash of The Art of Concealment *for percussion ensemble.*

Life and works

NATIONALITY: American

BORN: Los Angeles, 1912;
DIED: New York, 1992

SPECIALIST GENRES:
Experimental works for
bizarre combinations.

MAJOR WORKS: Numerous
works for percussion
ensemble, prepared piano
and various combinations
of instruments and
electronic media.

Leonard Bernstein

Any composer's writing is the sum of himself, of all his roots and influences.

BERNSTEIN, "THE JOY OF MUSIC" (1960)

Bernstein was one of the most flamboyant figures of 20th-century music. A talented pianist, composer of both "serious" works and extremely popular Broadway musicals and one of the finest conductors of his age, he excelled in every field he tackled (one of his fellow students remarked that he was "doomed to success").

He studied composition at Harvard University with Walter Piston (1894–1976), and conducting with Fritz Reiner (1888–1963) at the Curtis Institute in Philadelphia; in the early 1940s he attended summer schools at Tanglewood, Massachusetts, where he became Serge Koussevitzky's assistant. He was then invited to become assistant conductor of the New York Philharmonic Orchestra, and his big break came in November 1943, when he took over a concert at short notice from the indisposed Bruno Walter. This triumphant performance launched his career, helped by his striking good looks and charismatic personality.

From 1946 onwards Bernstein began to conduct opera, beginning with the US première of Britten's *Peter Grimes* at Tanglewood. In 1953 he became the first American to conduct at La Scala in Milan. He made his debut at the Metropolitan Opera House in 1964, and from 1958–69 he was principal conductor of the New York Philharmonic. He also guest-conducted many of the world's great orchestras.

Bernstein's parallel career as a composer began in 1944 with his ballet *Fancy Free* and his musical *On the Town*, which ran for 463 performances on Broadway. An adaptation of Voltaire's *Candide* (1954–6) had a disappointing reception and was later revised, but *West Side Story* (1957) made Bernstein's name. Written in collaboration with Stephen Sondheim (born 1930) and the choreographer Jerome Robbins (born 1918), this brilliant adaptation of the *Romeo and Juliet* story to a modern New York slum setting captured the spirit of the age.

The bisexual Bernstein was married to the Chilean actress Felicia Montealegre Cohn in 1951, and had three children.

ABOVE: Leonard Bernstein, photographed in the late 1960s.

LEFT: The ensemble song "America" from West Side Story, *as performed at the Prince Edward Theatre in London in 1998.*

Life and works

NATIONALITY: American

BORN: Lawrence, Massachusetts, 1918; **DIED:** New York, 1990

SPECIALIST GENRES: Populist stage works (ballets and musicals).

MAJOR WORKS: *On the Town* (1944); *Prelude, Fugue and Riffs* for clarinet and jazz ensemble (1949); *Candide* (1956); *West Side Story* (1957); *Chichester Psalms* (1965); *1600 Pennsylvania Avenue* (1976); three symphonies.

Elliott Carter

I am a radical, having a nature that leads me to perpetual revolt.

CARTER, C.1939

After Copland's death in 1990, Elliott Carter assumed the mantle of "Grand Old Man of American Music". But although he too studied with Nadia Boulanger in Paris in the early 1930s, his musical approach (apart from early works such as the First Symphony and the *Holiday Overture*) is very different from Copland's.

On returning to the USA after his Paris studies Carter became a musical director of Ballet Caravan (1936–40), and then began a long and distinguished teaching career in many major American universities and institutions. He has also spent long periods abroad, including fellowships of the American Academy in Rome, where he composed his Variations for Orchestra (1954–5). The Concerto for

Orchestra and the Third String Quartet (1971) were also written in Italy.

Carter's output includes choral music, songs (including "Warble for Lilac Time", 1943, "A Mirror on Which to Dwell", 1975, and "In Sleep, In Thunder", 1981) and incidental music (including the 1937–9 ballet *Pocahontas*). But his most significant works are for orchestra or chamber groups, particularly the five string quartets, which are regarded

as the most important since Bartók's. He is fascinated by the rhythmic and harmonic possibilities inherent in combining ensembles, as in the Symphony of Three Orchestras, the *Penthode* for five instrumental quartets (1984–5), and the Triple Duo (1982–3). The impact of experimental, radical influences on his underlying classical training has resulted in music of apparent complexity, underpinned by an inexorable musical logic of profound simplicity. The fusion of slow-moving formal structures with ebullient momentum gives Carter's work great dramatic power. His later works include an Oboe Concerto (1986–7) and Violin Concerto (1990), *Three Occasions* for orchestra (the third celebrated his own 50th wedding anniversary in 1989); and works for solo instruments, including *Changes* for guitar (1983), *Trilogy* (1992) for oboe and harp, and *Gra* (1993) for clarinet. A quintet for piano and wind, one of his finest later works, dates from 1992.

Life and works

NATIONALITY: American

BORN: New York, 1908

SPECIALIST GENRES: Complex polyrhythmic works.

MAJOR WORKS: Ballets *Pocahontas* (1937–9) and *The Minotaur* (1947); Piano Sonata (1946); Double Concerto for harpsichord and piano (1961); Concerto for Orchestra (1969); Symphony of Three Orchestras (1976–7); five string quartets.

ABOVE:

The American composer Elliott Carter (born 1908).

RIGHT: Carter rehearsing his Triple Duo at the Royal Academy of Music in London.

Witold Lutoslawski

Dissonances are only the more remote consonances.

ARNOLD SCHOENBERG (1874–1951)

Lutoslawski was the major Polish composer of the 20th century. He began to compose at the age of nine, and also studied piano and violin. In 1932 he entered the Warsaw Conservatory, and two years later his Piano Sonata was broadcast on Polish Radio. His Symphonic Variations were performed at the 1939 Krakow Festival.

The war disrupted Lutoslawski's promising career. He was taken prisoner, but escaped and eked out a precarious living playing the piano in Warsaw cafés. Many of his manuscripts disappeared during the wartime devastation: one exception was the *Variations on a Theme of Paganini* for two pianos, which Lutoslawski adapted in 1978 for piano and orchestra. In post-war communist Poland he wrote music for radio, film and television, and folk-based music for children. His First Symphony (1949) was denounced as formalist, and banned for a decade, but his Little Suite for orchestra (1950) and the Concerto for Orchestra (1950–4) – a worthy successor to Bartók's – found acceptance.

In the post-Stalinist thaw, Lutoslawski began to enlarge his harmonic language, exploring different ways of using the notes of the scale. *Funeral Music* (1958), dedicated to Bartók, established his international reputation, and his works of the 1960s, such as *Jeux vénitiens* (*Venetian Games*, 1961), *Trois poèmes d'Henri Michaux* (1963) and the 1964 String Quartet began to experiment with chance elements. His most important works of the late 1970s include *Paroles tissées* (*Woven Words*, 1965, written for Peter Pears), the Second Symphony (1967), *Livre pour orchestre* (1968), the Cello Concerto (1970, for Rostropovich), Preludes and Fugue for 13 solo strings, *Les espaces du sommeil* (*Sleep's Spaces*, 1975) for baritone and orchestra, and *Mi-parti* (1976).

Many works were commissioned by major artists and ensembles, including the Third Symphony by the Chicago Symphony Orchestra, *Chain I* by the London Sinfonietta, *Chain II* by the violinist Anne-Sophie Mutter (born 1963), and *Chain III* for the San Francisco Symphony Orchestra.

Lutoslawski's last major works included a Piano Concerto (1988), *Interludium* for chamber orchestra (1989) and *Chantefables et chantefleurs* (1990) for soprano and orchestra.

ABOVE: Witold Lutoslawski, the most important Polish composer of his generation.

LEFT: Lutoslawski rehearsing at the Royal Academy of Music in London in 1980.

Life and works

NATIONALITY: Polish

BORN: Warsaw, 1913; **DIED:** Warsaw, 1994

SPECIALIST GENRES: Orchestral works.

MAJOR WORKS: Concerto for Orchestra (1954); *Funeral Music* (1958); Cello Concerto (1970); four symphonies; Piano Concerto (1988).

György Ligeti

It is precisely a dread of deep significance and ideology that makes any kind of engaged art out of the question for me.

LIGETI

One of Hungary's most important composers, Ligeti was born in Transylvania of Hungarian Jewish parents, and studied privately during the war in Budapest. After the war he went to the Budapest Academy of Music, where from 1950–6 he was a professor. He left Hungary in 1956, the year of the Soviet invasion, and took up residence in Vienna. He was invited to work at the West German Radio electronic studios in Cologne, and caused a sensation at the 1960 International Society for Contemporary Music Festival with *Apparitions* (1958–9). From 1959 onwards he taught annually on the summer courses for new music at Darmstadt. Ten years later he moved to West Berlin, and from 1973–89 he was professor of composition at the Hamburg Musikhochschule.

ABOVE: The Hungarian composer György Ligeti (1923–2006), photographed in 1993.

Ligeti's early works were influenced by folk song and the music of Bartók. After a few experiments with electronic media in the late 1950s, he began to find an individual style in works such as *Apparitions* and *Atmosphères* for orchestra (1961), *Volumina* for organ (1961–2), and with the two works for solo voices and instruments called *Aventures* and *Nouvelles aventures* (1962–5). His works of the 1960s included a Requiem (1963–5), a Cello Concerto (1966), *Lux aeterna* for 16 solo voices (1966), the orchestral work *Lontano* (1967) and a chamber concerto for 13 instruments (1969–70). Some of his music was used – without

his permission – in the score of Stanley Kubrick's 1968 film *2001: A Space Odyssey*. Since the 1960s, Ligeti's most significant works have been *Clocks and Clouds* for 12-voice women's chorus and orchestra, *Melodien* (1971) and *San Francisco Polyphony* (1973–4), both for orchestra, a Double Concerto for flute and oboe (1972), a Piano Concerto (1985–8), a Violin Concerto (1992), a Horn Trio, subtitled "Homage to Brahms" (1982), a set of piano Etudes (1985), and the opera *Le grand macabre*. His individual style, which the composer described as "micropolyphony", is derived from Webern.

ABOVE: "The Horse of the Apocalypse" being prepared in rehearsal for a performance of Ligeti's opera Le grand macabre *at the 1997 Salzburg Festival.*

Life and works

NATIONALITY: Hungarian

BORN: Kolozsvár (now Cluj in Romania), 1923

DIED: Vienna, 2006

SPECIALIST GENRES: Orchestral and chamber music.

MAJOR WORKS: *Atmosphères* (1961); *Aventures* (1962); *Le grand macabre* (1976); *Clocks and Clouds* (1972).

Iannis Xenakis

Mathematics is music for the mind; music is mathematics for the soul.

ANONYMOUS

Iannis Xenakis was born in Romania, but his parents moved back to their native Greece when he was ten. He began studying music from the age of 12, but was trained as an engineer. During the war Xenakis fought in the Greek Resistance, losing an eye and narrowly escaping death. In 1947 he went to Paris, where he studied with Arthur Honegger and Darius Milhaud, and then with Messiaen in the early 1950s.

Between 1947 and 1960 he worked with the French avant-garde architect Le Corbusier (1887–1965), designing the much-admired Philips Pavilion for the 1958 Brussels Exhibition, in which Varèse's specially commissioned *Poème électronique* was played. Xenakis subsequently began to make his name as a composer, and thereafter concentrated on music. He has taught at Indiana University in the USA and also in Paris, where he was professor of music at the Sorbonne from 1972–89.

Xenakis's strong interest in mathematics led him to introduce mathematical concepts and theories into his compositions, some of which are scored for traditional instruments, others for electronic media. He applied the term "stochastic" to music, relating to the theory of probability, which assumes that a chance sequence of events can reach a predetermined conclusion. In his own works (many of which have Greek titles), the elements of chance are not left to the performer (as in works by Cage or Lutoslawski), but are controlled by the composer, normally by using a computer. Some of his earlier pieces, such as *Nomos gamma* (1967–8) place an orchestra among the audience. His later pieces vary in size from *Okho* (1989) for three players, to *Dox-Orkh* and *Troorkh* (both 1991), respectively for violin and trombone with 89 other players.

ABOVE: The works of Iannis Xenakis (1922–2001) are based on mathematical concepts and theories.

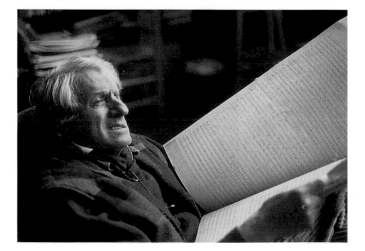

LEFT: Xenakis with one of his scores. He lost his sight in one eye while fighting in the Greek Resistance in 1947.

Life and works

NATIONALITY: Greek

BORN: Braïla, Romania, 1922;
DIED: Paris, 2001

SPECIALIST GENRES: Compositions based on mathematical concepts.

MAJOR WORKS: *Metastasis* (1953–4); *Oresteia* (1965–6); *Terretektorh* (1965–6); *Persephassa* (1969).

Luciano Berio

Abstract it may be, the human voice...

THOMAS MANN (1875–1955), "DR FAUSTUS"

Together with Bruno Maderna (1920–73), with whom he founded the Studio di Fonologia Musicale at Radiotelevisione Italiana in Milan in 1955, Luciano Berio was one of the most important Italian composers of his generation. He studied at the Milan Conservatory, and has been equally active as both teacher and composer. He has taught composition at Tanglewood; Mills College, California; Harvard University; and the Juilliard School, all in the USA; at Dartington in Britain; and at Darmstadt and Cologne in Germany. In the late 1970s he also worked with Boulez at IRCAM in Paris.

Berio's compositions reflect his fascination with the human voice, intensified by his marriage (1950–66)

ABOVE: Luciano Berio (1925–2003), the major Italian composer of his generation.

collage technique, in particular *Recital I (for Cathy)*, for mezzo-soprano and 17 instruments (1972).

Among Berio's best-known works are the *Quattro canzoni popolari* for voice and piano (1946–7); *Circles*, based on poems by e. e. cummings, for female voice, harp and percussion; *O King* (a homage to Martin Luther King), for mezzo and five players (1967); the series of solo works called *Sequenze I–XI* (*No. III*, for voice, was written for Berberian); and a related series called *Chemins* (*Paths*) for solo instrument(s) and ensemble or orchestra. He has written several theatre works, some in collaboration with distinguished writers such as Italo Calvino and Umberto Eco.

Life and works

NATIONALITY: Italian

BORN: Oneglia, 1925

DIED: Rome, 2003

SPECIALIST GENRES: Works for both conventional and electronic media.

MAJOR WORKS: *Epifanie* (1959–61); *Circles* (1960); *Sinfonia* (1968–9); *Coro* (1975–6); *Un re in ascolto* (*King in Waiting*, 1979–83); 11 *Sequenze* (1958–75); four *Chemins* (*Paths*, 1965–75).

to the American singer/actress Cathy Berberian (1925–83). He draws inspiration from the juxtaposition of different musical processes, from Baroque vocal styles to modern techniques of serialism, indeterminacy and the use of electronics and computer technology. His idiomatic use of collage technique is demonstrated in his most popular work, *Sinfonia* for eight voices and orchestra, which quotes from a wide range of sources, including works by Mahler, Wagner, Ravel and Richard Strauss. He has also reworked music by Brahms and Schubert, most recently in *Rendering* (1989), attributed to "Schubert/Berio". Several of his pieces written for Cathy Berberian also use

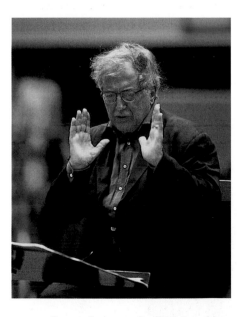

ABOVE: Berio rehearsing the BBC Symphony Orchestra in their Maida Vale recording studio in London, February 2000.

Hans Werner Henze

My profession…consists of bringing truths nearer to the point where they explode.

HENZE, "MUSIC AND POLITICS" (1982)

Henze was the eldest of six children of a schoolmaster, who discouraged him from taking up music. He began composing at 12, but received no formal musical training until after the war (during which he had been attached to a unit making Nazi propaganda films). In 1946 he began to study harmony and counterpoint with Wolfgang Fortner (born 1907), and serial techniques with René Leibowitz. In 1953, after finishing his first opera, *Boulevard Solitude*, he settled in Italy.

During the 1960s Henze's music became associated with radical, left-wing politics. He shot to international fame in 1966 when his opera *The Bassarids*, with a libretto by W. H. Auden and Chester Kallman, was produced at the

ABOVE: *Hans Werner Henze (born 1926), considered the major German opera composer of his generation.*

Salzburg Festival, and his 1968 oratorio *Das Floss der "Medusa"* (*The Raft of the "Medusa"*) – one of his best-known works – was written as a requiem for the guerrilla leader Che Guevara.

Henze also began to work with young musicians, and in 1976 founded the Montepulciano Cantiere in Umbria for communal international music-making. Since 1980 he has taught composition at the Cologne Academy and at the Royal Academy of Music in London, and in 1988 he founded the Munich International Festival of New Music Theatre. He combines composing with conducting, and has been a guest conductor of the Berlin Philharmonic Orchestra.

During the 1970s and '80s Henze collaborated with the British playwright Edward Bond on works such as the "action for music" *We Come to the River*, the ballet *Orpheus* (1979) and the opera *The English Cat* (1980–2). His highly coloured, richly orchestrated works include several operas, of which the early works *Der Prinz vom Homburg* (1958), *Elegy for Young Lovers* (1959–61) and *Der junge Lord* (*The Young Lord*, 1964) are perhaps the best known: the latest is *Venus and Adonis* (1993–5) for singers and dancers. A prolific composer for both instruments and voices, he has also written nine symphonies, two violin concertos, two piano concertos and other concertante works, five string quartets, several ballets, and a great deal of vocal music.

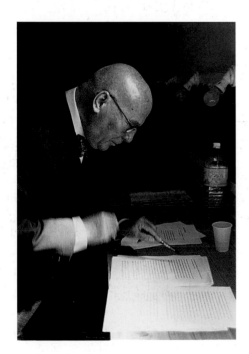

ABOVE: *Hans Werner Henze at work in 1996.*

Life and works

NATIONALITY: German

BORN: Gütersloh, Westphalia, 1926

SPECIALIST GENRES: Opera and theatre music.

MAJOR WORKS: *Boulevard Solitude* (1951); *König Hirsch* (*King Stag*, 1956); *The Bassarids* (1966); *Das Floss der "Medusa"* (1968); *We Come to the River* (1976).

Other Composers of the Era

It is fortunate that to assert itself in music, a new generation does not need to destroy the works of its ancestors.

ERNST KŘENEK (1900–91), "HORIZONS CIRCLED" (1974)

Although the demand for contemporary music is relatively limited compared with that of earlier periods, many talented composers have achieved widespread popularity over the last 50 years.

America

In the USA, a group of so-called "minimalists" came to attention in the 1970s and '80s. Among them is Steve Reich (born 1936), who founded his own ensemble in 1966. He was much influenced by African and Asian drumming techniques, and all his works, which range from vocal and orchestral pieces such as *The Desert Music* (1982–4) for 27 amplified voices and orchestra,

ABOVE: The American composer Steve Reich (born 1936) introduced the "phasing" technique, whereby instruments play the same patterns at slightly different speeds.

to the famous *Clapping Music* for two performers (1972), and *Different Trains* for string quartet and tape (1988), deal with *ostinato* patterns subtly altered by variations in time. Similar repetitive techniques govern the work of Terry Riley (born 1935), whose most famous piece is *In C* (1964).

Two other minimalists, Philip Glass (born 1937) and John Adams (born 1946) have developed the technique on a larger scale, including opera. Glass worked with Ravi Shankar (born 1920), and his style was influenced by Indian music. Of his many stage works, *Einstein on the Beach* (1974–5), *Akhnaten* (1980–3)

and *The Making of the Representative for Planet 8* (1988) are the best known; while his orchestral works include *Glassworks* (1981) for chamber orchestra, and a Third Symphony (1994). Adams's style is more eclectic, and he has a substantial international following. The subject-matter of both his operas, *Nixon in China* (1984–7) and *The Death of Klinghoffer* (1990–1), had contemporary resonance; while his *Grand Pianola Music* (1981–2) for two sopranos, two pianos and small orchestra, *The Wound Dresser* (1988–9) for baritone and orchestra, and his 1993 Violin Concerto have become widely known.

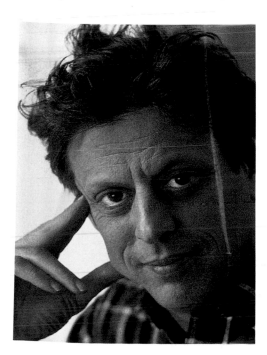

ABOVE: Philip Glass (born 1937), another American minimalist, has been influenced by Indian music.

ABOVE: John Adams (born 1947) successfully applied minimalist techniques to opera, including Nixon in China (1984–7).

Music since World War II **497**

double bass 55, **112–13**
double horn 161
double-strung spinet 225
double virginal 223
Dowland, John 271, **284**
drum kit **197**
drums 6, 7, 14, 17, 20–1, 24,
 38–9, 66, 73, 96, 127,
 138, 188–9, **190–7**, 229

duda 181
dudy 107, 181
Dufay, Guillaume 271, **275**,
 285
Dukas, Paul 87, 194, 429
dulcian 159
dulcimer 31, 137
Dvořák, Antonín 58, 261,
 375, **386–7**, 397, 433,
 446

E
eastern European pipes 181
Edward VII of England 417
Eichendorff, Joseph von 365,
 428
electric instruments 107,
 117, 119

electronic instruments 52,
 87, 96, **240–1**
electronic music 262, 478–9
Elgar, Edward 53, 58, 65,
 111, 159, 205, 261, 401,
 416–17, 418, 424, 473
Elizabeth I of England 281,
 282, 284

Elizabeth II of England 483
Esterházy, Prince Nikolaus
 324–5, 343, 366
euphonium 37, 167
experimental harmoniums
 236–7

F
fairground organ 233
Falla, Manuel de 117, 121,
 474
 fantasias 299, 302,
 303
 Fauré, Gabriel 59,
 401, **421**, 437,
 442
female composers 270, 272,
 479
fiddles 61, 70, 102, **122–3**
Field, John 342, 361, 371,
 376
fife 66, 147
flageolet 149
Flaubert, Gustave 378
flugelhorn 166, 177
flute 6, 7, 21, 23, 24, 25, **44**,
 46, 50, 52, 55, 56, 80,
 97, 117, 127, 142, **144–7**
folk music 60–1, 107, 182
Franck, César 155, 233, 429
French harmonium 236
fretted clavichord 218–19
Freud, Sigmund 414
fugue 303, 307, 337
Furtwängler, Wilhelm 450,
 472

G
Gabrieli, Domenico 110
Gabrieli, Giovanni 159, 175,
 246, 258, 285, 292
gadulka 101
gambang 207
gamelan 21, 207, 435–6,
 438
gardon 111

Gay, John 310, 459
George I of England 309–10
Gershwin, George 74, 131,
 155, 433, 459, **464**
Gershwin, Ira 459, 464
Gesualdo, Carlo **283**, 284
Giazotto, Remo 314
Gibbons, Orlando 282
Gide, André 468–9
Gilbert, William Schwenk
 247, 261, 350, 375, 392
gittern 118
Glass, Philip 478, 497
Glazunov, Alexander 426,
 428, 480
Glinka, Mikhail 59, 202,
 261, 375, **376**, 377, 379
glockenspiel 66, **212–13**
Gluck, Christoph Willibald
 117, 175, 198, 258,
 319, **320–1**
Goethe, Johann
 Wolfgang von 306,
 338, 346, 357,
 358–9, 365, 367,
 368, 396, 415, 428,
 429
gong chimes 21, 201
gong drum 195
gongs 15, 21, 24, 188, **201**
Górecki, Henryk 498
Gounod, Charles **368**
Grainger, Percy 235, 389, **452**
Granados, Enrique **391**
Grieg, Edvard 57, **59**, 261,
 375, **388–9**, 392, 445,
 451, 452
 Grillparzer, Franz 337, 341
 Gubaidulina, Sofia 263,
 479, 498
Guido d'Arezzo **29**, 255
guiro 189
guitar 55, 76, 77, 78, 79,
 96, 106–7, **118–21**, 202
guitarillo 121

H
Halévy, Jacques **369**, 370–1
Hammond organ 240
hand bells **210**

Handel, George Frideric 49,
 85, 108, 117, 130, 146,
 149, 151, 178, 212, 232,
 247, 258, 259, 288, 289,
 297, **308–11**, 312, 320,
 322, 359, 392
Hardanger fiddle (*Hardingfele*)
 106, 107
harmonica 35, 182
harmonium 21, 35, **236–7**
harp 16, 51, 55, 79, 100,
 114–17, 136
harpsichord 40, 44, 55, 56,
 63, 82, 88, **220–1**, 224,
 225, 226, 228
Hasse, Johann 288, 315
Hawaiian guitar 120
Haydn, Joseph 46, 47, 52,
 56, 57, 81, 84, 134, 194,
 204–5, 247, 259, 319,
 322–5, 332–3, 342, 343,
 370

Haydn, Michael 194
heckelphone 153
Heine, Heinrich 341, 361, 365
helicon 69, 167
Henze, Hans Werner 54, 80,
 263, **496**
hi-hats 200
Hildegard of Bingen 270, **272**
Hindemith, Paul 57, 78, 80,
 108–9, 113, 161, 167,
 433, **472**
Hoffman, Ernst Theodore
 Amadeus 371, 393, **396**,
 442
Holst, Gustav 65, 146, 151,
 167, 433, 443, **444**, 452
Honegger, Arthur 87, **461**,
 494
horn 15, 37, 52, 53, 66, 81,
 142, 143, 145, 159,
 160–1, 166, 168